Delivering Health Care in America

A SYSTEMS APPROACH SEVENTH EDITION

Leiyu Shi, DrPH, MBA, MPA

Professor, Bloomberg School of Public Health
Director, Johns Hopkins Primary Care Policy Center
Johns Hopkins University
Baltimore, Maryland

Douglas A. Singh, PhD, MBA

Associate Professor Emeritus of Management
School of Business and Economics
Indiana University, South Bend
South Bend, Indiana

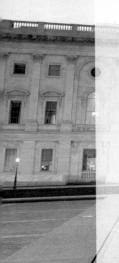

JONES & BARTLETT
LEARNING

World Headquarters
Jones & Bartlett Learning
5 Wall Street
Burlington, MA 01803
978-443-5000
info@jblearning.com
www.jblearning.com

Jones & Bartlett Learning books and products are available through most bookstores and online booksellers. To contact Jones & Bartlett Learning directly, call 800-832-0034, fax 978-443-8000, or visit our website, www.jblearning.com.

Substantial discounts on bulk quantities of Jones & Bartlett Learning publications are available to corporations, professional associations, and other qualified organizations. For details and specific discount information, contact the special sales department at Jones & Bartlett Learning via the above contact information or send an email to specialsales@jblearning.com.

21285-3

Production Credits

VP, Executive Publisher: David D. Cella
Publisher: Michael Brown
Associate Editor: Danielle Bessette
Production Editor: Vanessa Richards
Senior Marketing Manager: Sophie Fleck Teague
Manufacturing and Inventory Control Supervisor: Amy Bacus
Composition: codeMantra U.S. LLC
Cover Design: Scott Moden
Rights & Media Specialist: Merideth Tumasz
Media Development Editor: Shannon Sheehan
Cover Image (Title Page, Part Opener, Chapter Opener): © f11photo/ShutterStock
Printing and Binding: LSC Communications
Cover Printing: LSC Communications

Library of Congress Cataloging-in-Publication Data

Names: Shi, Leiyu, author. | Singh, Douglas A., 1946- author.
Title: Delivering health care in America : a systems approach / Leiyu Shi,
  Douglas A. Singh.
Description: Seventh edition. | Burlington, Massachusetts : Jones & Bartlett
  Learning, [2019] | Includes bibliographical references and index.
Identifiers: LCCN 2017015329 | ISBN 9781284124491 (pbk.)
Subjects: | MESH: Delivery of Health Care | Health Policy | Health Services |
United States
Classification: LCC RA395.A3 | NLM W 84 AA1 | DDC 362.10973—dc23
LC record available at https://lccn.loc.gov/2017015329

6048

Printed in the United States of America
23 22 21 20   10 9 8 7 6 5

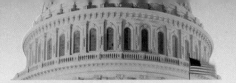

Contents

PART II System Resources   135

Chapter 4   Health Services Professionals.......................137

Chapter 5   Medical Technology.........175

Chapter 6   Health Services Financing ...217

PART III System Processes   267

Chapter 7   Outpatient and Primary Care Services 269

Chapter 8   Inpatient Facilities and Services. 315

Chapter 9   Managed Care and Integrated Organizations 359

Chapter 10   Long-Term Care 399

Chapter 11   Health Services for Special Populations 435

PART IV **System Outcomes**   485

Chapter 12 **Cost, Access, and Quality** . . . **487**

Chapter 13 **Health Policy** **537**

PART V **System Outlook**   563

Chapter 14 **The Future of Health Services Delivery**. **565**

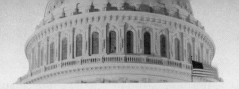

Preface

With this *Seventh Edition*, we celebrate 20 years of serving instructors, students, policymakers, and others, both at home and overseas, with up-to-date information on the dynamic U.S. health care delivery system. Much has changed, and much will continue to change in the future, as the nation grapples with critical issues of access, cost, and quality. Indeed, much of the developing and developed world will also be contending with similar issues.

People in the United States, in particular, have just gotten a taste of a far-reaching health care reform through President Barack Obama's signature Affordable Care Act (ACA), nicknamed "Obamacare." To date, this law has produced mixed results that are documented in this new edition.

At the time this edition went to press, we were left with promises of another reform under the slogan "Repeal and replace Obamacare," a move championed by President Donald Trump, who had made it one of the centerpieces of his presidential campaign. Much remains to be seen as to how this promise will play out.

On May 4, 2017, the U.S. House of Representatives passed the American Health Care Act (AHCA) by a vote of 217 to 213, with Republican support. The bill is likely to undergo significant changes in the U.S. Senate. Hence, what the new law may eventually look like was unknown at the time this manuscript went to press. As was the case with the ACA, for which the Democratic Party played an exclusive role in its passage, contentious debates, partisanship, and deal making among both Republicans and Democrats have marked the progress in moving the new law through Congress.

Although we have chosen to sidestep any premature speculation about the fate of the ACA and the shape of its replacement, wherever possible, we have presented trends and facts that support certain conclusions. Mainly, experiences and outcomes under the ACA have been highlighted in this edition.

On his first day in office in January 2017, President Trump signed an executive order to "waive, defer, grant exemptions from, or delay the implementation of any provision or requirement of the [Affordable Care] Act that would impose a fiscal burden on any State or a cost, fee, tax, penalty, or regulatory burden on individuals, families, health care providers, health insurers, patients, recipients of health care services, purchasers of health insurance, or makers of medical devices, products, or medications." This executive order effectively repealed small portions of the ACA that deal with taxation and fees.

Going forward, the issues of universal coverage and affordability of insurance and health care will be critical. Under the ACA, approximately 27 million people remained uninsured, even though the uninsurance rate in the United States dropped from 13.3% to 10.9% between 2013 and 2016. The majority of the newly insured individuals were covered under Medicaid, the nation's safety net health insurance program for the poor.

Another thorny issue will be how to provide health care for the millions of illegal immigrants who obtain services mainly through hospital emergency departments, and through charitable sources to some extent. Is there a better, more cost-effective way to address their needs?

The affordability of health insurance in the non-employment-based private market was severely eroded under the ACA, mainly for those who did not qualify for federal subsidies to buy insurance. The reason for the rate hikes in this segment was that few young and healthy people enrolled in health care plans under the ACA. Consequently, for many people, premium costs rose to unaffordable levels in 2016. People who really needed to use health care enrolled in much larger numbers than healthier individuals. Such an adverse selection prompted the chief executive of Aetna Insurance, Mark Bertolini, to remark that the marketplace for individual health insurance coverage was in a "death spiral." Some large insurance companies either pulled out of the government-sponsored health care exchanges or were planning to do so because of financial losses sustained under the ACA.

▶ New to This Edition

This edition continues to reference some of the main features of the ACA wherever it was important to provide contextual discussions from historical and policy perspectives. Several chapters cover the main provisions of the 21st Century Cures Act, which, after a long delay, was finally passed by Congress and signed by President Obama in December 2016.

As in the past, this text has been updated throughout with the latest pertinent data, trends, and research findings available at the time the manuscript was prepared. Copious illustrations in the form of examples, facts, figures, tables, and exhibits continue to make the text come alive. Following is a list of the main additions and revisions:

Chapter 1

- Updates the impact of the Affordable Care Act (ACA)

- Critical global health issues and health care reforms in other countries

Chapter 2

- Health insurance under the ACA
- Evaluation of progress made toward the *Healthy People 2020* goals
- Information on global pandemics and infectious diseases

Chapter 3

- Expanded section: Reform of mental health care
- Complete revision of the section: Era of health care reform

Chapter 4

- Major issues related to the health care workforce
- Updated information on nonphysician providers

Chapter 5

- New section: Electronic health records and quality of care
- Global trends in biomedical research and a new table on R&D expenditures
- New section: Drugs from overseas
- New section: Health care reform and medical technology

Chapter 6

- New section: Private coverage and cost under the Affordable Care Act
- New section: Medicaid experiences under the ACA

- New section: Issues with Medicaid
- New section: Long-term care hospital payment systems
- New section: Value-based reimbursement (discusses the MACRA and Medicare Shared Savings Program)
- Updated current directions and issues in financing

Chapter 7

- Research findings using the Primary Care Assessment Tool
- Measurement and achievement of the patient-centered medical home
- The impact of community health centers

Chapter 8

- New section: Comparative data from the Organization for Economic Cooperation and Development on hospital access and utilization
- Comparative hospital prices in selected countries
- New section: Factors that affect hospital employment
- New section: Rise in bad debts
- New section: State mental health institutions
- Update on physician-owned specialty hospitals
- Medicare designations of sole community hospitals and Medicare-dependent hospitals
- Patient outcomes at Magnet hospitals
- New section: Hospital costs

Chapter 9

- "Any willing provider" and "freedom of choice" laws under managed care regulations
- The latest on accountable care organizations

Chapter 10

- New section: Recent policies for community-based services

Chapter 11

- Updated information on vulnerable subpopulations
- Expanded coverage on chronically ill patients

Chapter 12

- Current issues in health care costs, access, and quality
- Pay-for-performance in health care
- Quality initiatives in both the public and private sectors

Chapter 13

- Current critical policy challenges
- Future health policy issues in both the United States and abroad

Chapter 14

- Almost all sections have been completely updated
- New section: No single payer
- New section: Reforming the reform
- New section: Universal coverage and access
- New section: Toward population health

As in the previous editions, our aim is to continue to meet the needs of both graduate and undergraduate students. We have attempted to make each chapter complete, without making it overwhelming for beginners. Instructors, of course, will choose the sections they decide are most appropriate for their courses.

As in the past, we invite comments from our readers. Communications can be directed to either or both authors:

Leiyu Shi
Department of Health Policy and Management
Bloomberg School of Public Health
Johns Hopkins University
624 North Broadway, Room 409
Baltimore, MD 21205-1996
lshi2@jhu.edu

Douglas A. Singh
dsingh@iusb.edu

We appreciate the work of Hailun Liang and Megha Parikh in providing assistance in the preparation of selected chapters of this text.

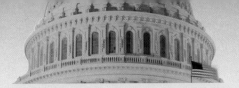
© f11photo/Shutterstock

List of Exhibits

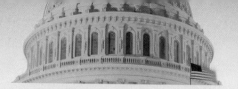

List of Figures

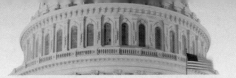
© f11photo/Shutterstock

List of Tables

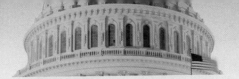

List of Abbreviations/Acronyms

A

AALL—American Association of Labor Legislation
AAMC—Association of American Medical Colleges
AA/PIs—Asian Americans and Pacific Islanders
AAs—Asian Americans
ACA—Affordable Care Act
ACNM—American College of Nurse-Midwives
ACO—accountable care organization
ACS—American College of Surgeons
ADA—American Dental Association
ADC—adult day care
ADLs—activities of daily living
ADN—associate's degree nurse
AFC—adult foster care
AHA—American Hospital Association
AHRQ—Agency for Healthcare Research and Quality
AIANs—American Indians and Alaska Natives
AIDS—acquired immunodeficiency syndrome
ALF—assisted living facility
ALOS—average length of stay
AMA—American Medical Association
AMDA—American Medical Directors Association
ANA—American Nurses Association
APCs—ambulatory payment classifications
APN—advanced practice nurse
ARRA—American Recovery and Reinvestment Act

ASPR—Assistant Secretary for Preparedness and Response

B

BBA—Balanced Budget Act
BPCI—bundled payments for care improvement
BSN—baccalaureate degree in nursing
BWC—Biological and Toxin Weapons Convention

C

CAH—critical access hospital
CAM—complementary and alternative medicine
CBO—Congressional Budget Office
CCAH—continuing care at home
CCRC—continuing care retirement center/community
CDC—Centers for Disease Control and Prevention
CDSS—clinical decision support system
CEO—chief executive officer
CEPH—Council on Education for Public Health
CER—comparative effectiveness research
CF—conversion factor
CHAMPVA—Civilian Health and Medical Program of the Department of Veterans Affairs
CHC—community health center
CHIP—Children's Health Insurance Program

CMGs—case-mix groups

C/MHCs—community and migrant health centers

CMS—Centers for Medicare and Medicaid Services

CNA—certified nursing assistant

CNM—certified nurse-midwife

CNS—clinical nurse specialist

COBRA—Consolidated Omnibus Budget Reconciliation Act

CON—certificate of need

COPC—community-oriented primary care

COTA—certified occupational therapy assistant

COTH—Council of Teaching Hospitals and Health Systems

CPI—consumer price index

CPOE—computerized provider order entry

CPT—Current Procedural Terminology

CQI—continuous quality improvement

CRNA—certified registered nurse anesthetist

CT—computed tomography

D

DC—Doctor of Chiropractic

DD—developmental disability

DDS—Doctor of Dental Surgery

DGME—Direct Graduate Medical Education

DHHS—U.S. Department of Health and Human Services

DHS—Department of Homeland Security

DMD—Doctor of Dental Medicine

DME—durable medical equipment

DO—Doctor of Osteopathic Medicine

DoD—Department of Defense

DPM—Doctor of Podiatric Medicine

DRA—Deficit Reduction Act

DRGs—diagnosis-related groups

DSM-5—*Diagnostic and Statistical Manual of Mental Disorders, Fifth Edition*

DTP—diphtheria/tetanus/pertussis (vaccine)

E

EBM—evidence-based medicine

EBRI—Employee Benefit Research Institute

ECG—electrocardiogram

ECU—extended care unit

ED—emergency department

EHRs—electronic health records

EMT—emergency medical technician

EMTALA—Emergency Medical Treatment and Active Labor Act

ENP—Elderly Nutrition Program

ERISA—Employee Retirement Income Security Act

ESRD—end-stage renal disease

F

FD&C Act—Federal Food, Drug, and Cosmetic Act

FDA—Food and Drug Administration

FMAP—Federal Medical Assistance Percentage

FPL—federal poverty level

FTE—full-time equivalent

FY—fiscal year

G

GAO—General Accounting Office

GDP—gross domestic product

GP—general practitioner

H

HAART—highly active antiretroviral therapy

HCBS—home- and community-based services

HCBW—home- and community-based waiver

HCH—Health Care for the Homeless

HCPCS—Healthcare Common Procedures Coding System

HDHP—high-deductible health plan

HDHP/SO—high-deductible health plan with a savings option

HEDIS—Healthcare Effectiveness Data and Information Set

HHRG—home health resource group

HI—hospital insurance

HIAA—Health Insurance Association of America

Hib—*Haemophilus influenzae* serotype b

HIO—health information organization

HIPAA—Health Insurance Portability and Accountability Act

HIT—health information technology

HITECH— Health Information Technology for Economic and Clinical Health Act

HIV—human immunodeficiency virus

HMO—health maintenance organization

HMO Act—Health Maintenance Organization Act

HPSAs—health professional shortage areas

HPV—human papillomavirus

HRA—health reimbursement arrangement

HRQL—health-related quality of life

HRSA—Health Resources and Services Administration

HSA—health savings account

HTA—health technology assessment

HUD—U.S. Department of Housing and Urban Development

I

IADLs—instrumental activities of daily living

ICF—intermediate care facility

ICF/IID—intermediate care facilities for individuals with intellectual disabilities

ICF/MR—intermediate care facilities for the mentally retarded

ID—intellectual disability

IDD—intellectual/developmental disability

IDEA—Individuals with Disabilities Education Act

IDS—integrated delivery systems

IDU—injection drug use

IHR—International Health Regulations

IHS—Indian Health Service

IME—Indirect Medical Education

IMGs—international medical graduates

IOM—Institute of Medicine

IPA—independent practice association

IRB—institutional review board

IRF—inpatient rehabilitation facility

IRMAA—Income-Related Monthly Adjustment Amount

IRS—Internal Revenue Service

IS—information systems

IT—information technology

IV—intravenous

L

LPN—licensed practical nurse

LTC—long-term care

LTCH—long-term care hospital

LVN—licensed vocational nurse

M

MA—Medicare Advantage

MA-PD—Medicare Advantage Prescription Drug Plan

MA-SNP—Medicare Advantage Special Needs Plan

MACPAC—Medicaid and CHIP Payment and Access Commission

MACRA—Medicare Access and CHIP Reauthorization Act

MBA—Master of Business Administration

MCOs—managed care organizations

MD—Doctor of Medicine

MDS—Minimum Data Set

MedPAC—Medicare Payment Advisory Commission

MEPS—Medical Expenditure Panel Survey

MERS—Middle East respiratory syndrome

MFP—Money Follows the Person

MHA—Master of Health Administration

MHS—multihospital system

MHSA—Master of Health Services Administration

MIPS—Merit-based Incentive Payment System

MLP—midlevel provider

MLR—medical loss ratio

MMA—Medicare Prescription Drug, Improvement, and Modernization Act

MMR—measles/mumps/rubella vaccine

MPA—Master of Public Administration/Affairs

MPFS—Medicare Physician Fee Schedule

MPH—Master of Public Health

MRHFP—Medicare Rural Hospital Flexibility Program

MRI—magnetic resonance imaging

MSA—metropolitan statistical area

MS-DRGs—Medicare severity diagnosis-related groups

MSO—management services organization

MSSP—Medicare Shared Savings Program

MUAs—medically underserved areas

N

NAB—National Association of Boards of Examiners of Long-Term Care Administrators

NAPBC—National Action Plan on Breast Cancer

NCCAM—National Center for Complementary and Alternative Medicine

NCCIH—National Center for Complementary and Integrative Health

NCHS—National Center for Health Statistics

NCQA—National Committee for Quality Assurance

NF—nursing facility

NGC—National Guideline Clearinghouse

NHC—neighborhood health center

NHE—national health expenditures

NHI—national health insurance

NHS—national health system

NHS—U.K. National Health Service

NHSC—National Health Service Corps

NICE—National Institute for Health and Clinical Excellence

NIH—National Institutes of Health

NIMH—National Institute of Mental Health

NP—nurse practitioner

NPP—nonphysician practitioner

NRP—National Response Plan

O

OAM—Office of Alternative Medicine

OBRA—Omnibus Budget Reconciliation Act

OD—Doctor of Optometry

OI—opportunistic infection

OPPS—Outpatient Prospective Payment System

OT—occupational therapist

OWH—Office on Women's Health

P

P4P—pay-for-performance
PA—physician assistant
PACE—Program of All-Inclusive Care for the Elderly
PAHPA—Pandemic and All-Hazards Preparedness Act
PASRR—Preadmission Screening and Resident Review
PBMs—pharmacy benefits managers
PCCM—primary care case management
PCGs—primary care groups
PCMH—patient-centered medical home
PCP--primary care physician
PDP—stand-alone prescription drug plan
PERS—personal emergency response system
PET—positron emission tomography
PFFS—private fee-for-service
PharmD—Doctor of Pharmacy
PhD—Doctor of Philosophy
PHI—personal health information
PHO—physician–hospital organization
PhRMA—Pharmaceutical Research and Manufacturers of America
PMPM—per member per month
POS—point-of-service (plan)
PPD—per-patient day (rate)
PPM—physician practice management
PPO—preferred provider organization
PPS—prospective payment system
PRO—peer review organization
PSO—provider-sponsored organization
PSRO—professional standards review organization
PsyD—Doctor of Psychology
PTA—physical therapy assistant
PTCA—percutaneous transluminal coronary angioplasty
PT—physical therapist

Q

QALY—quality-adjusted life year
QI—quality indicator
QIO—quality improvement organization

R

R&D—research and development
RBRVS—resource-based relative value scales
RN—registered nurse
RUGs—resource utilization groups
RVUs—relative value units
RWJF—Robert Wood Johnson Foundation

S

SAMHSA—Substance Abuse and Mental Health Services Administration
SARS—severe acute respiratory syndrome
SAV—small area variations
SES—socioeconomic status
SGR—sustainable growth rate
SHI—socialized health insurance
SMI—supplementary medical insurance
SNF—skilled nursing facility
SPECT—single-photon emission computed tomography
SSI—Supplemental Security Income
STD—sexually transmitted disease

T

TAH—total artificial heart
TANF—Temporary Assistance for Needy Families
TCU—transitional care unit

TEFRA—Tax Equity and Fiscal Responsibility Act
TPA—third-party administrator
TQM—total quality management

U

UCR—usual, customary, and reasonable
UR—utilization review

V

VA—Department of Veterans Affairs
VBP—Value-Based Purchasing

VHA—Veterans Health Administration
VISN—Veterans Integrated Service Network

W

WHO—World Health Organization
WIC—Special Supplemental Nutrition Program for Women, Infants, and Children

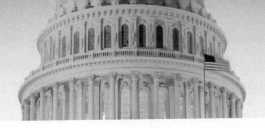

CHAPTER 1

An Overview of U.S. Health Care Delivery

LEARNING OBJECTIVES

- Understand the basic nature of the U.S. health care system.
- Outline the key functional components of a health care delivery system.
- Get a basic overview of the Affordable Care Act.
- Discuss the primary characteristics of the U.S. health care system.
- Emphasize why it is important for health care practitioners and managers to understand the intricacies of the health care delivery system.
- Get an overview of health care systems in selected countries.
- Point out global health challenges and reform efforts.
- Introduce the systems model as a framework for studying the health care system in the United States.

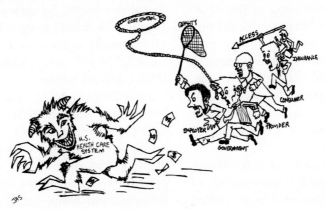

The U.S. health care delivery system is a behemoth that is almost impossible for any single entity to manage and control.

▶ Introduction

The United States has a unique system of health care delivery that is unlike any other health care system in the world. Almost all other developed countries have national health insurance programs run by the government and financed through general taxes. Nearly all citizens in such countries are entitled to receive health care services. Such is not yet the case in the United States, where Americans are not automatically covered by health insurance.

Though U.S. health care is often called a system because is has various features, components, and services, it may be misleading to talk about the American health care delivery "system," because a true, cohesive system does not exist (Wolinsky, 1988). Indeed, a major feature of the U.S. health care system is its fragmented nature, as different people obtain health care through different means. The system has continued to undergo periodic changes, mainly in response to concerns regarding costs, access, and quality.

Describing health care delivery in the United States can be a daunting task. To facilitate an understanding of the structural and conceptual basis for the delivery of health care services, this text is organized according to the systems framework presented at the end of this chapter. Also, for the sake of simplicity, the mechanisms of health care delivery in the United States are collectively referred to as a system throughout this text.

The main objective of this chapter is to provide a broad understanding of how health care is delivered in the United States. Examples of how health care is delivered in other countries are also presented for the sake of comparison. The overview presented here introduces the reader to several concepts discussed more extensively in later chapters.

▶ An Overview of the Scope and Size of the System

TABLE 1-1 demonstrates the complexity of health care delivery in the United States. Many organizations and individuals are involved in health care. To name just a few: educational and research institutions, medical suppliers, insurers, payers, and claims processors to health care providers. A multitude of providers are involved in the delivery of preventive, primary, subacute, acute, auxiliary, rehabilitative, and continuing care. A large number of managed care organizations (MCOs) and integrated networks now provide a continuum of care, covering many of the service components.

The U.S. health care delivery system is massive, with total employment that exceeded 16.4 million people in 2010 in various health delivery settings. This number included more than 838,000 professionally active doctors of medicine (MDs), 70,480 osteopathic physicians (DOs), and 2.6 million active nurses (U.S. Census Bureau, 2012). The majority of health care and health services professionals (5.98 million) work in ambulatory health service settings, such as the offices of physicians, dentists, and other health practitioners, medical and diagnostic laboratories, and home health care service locations. Smaller proportions of these professionals are employed by hospitals (4.7 million) and nursing and residential

TABLE 1-1 The Complexity of Health Care Delivery

Education/Research	Suppliers	Insurers	Providers	Payers	Government
Medical schools	Pharmaceutical companies	Managed care plans	***Preventive Care***	Blue Cross/ Blue Shield plans	Public insurance financing
Dental schools	Multipurpose suppliers	Blue Cross/ Blue Shield plans	Health departments	Commercial insurers	Health regulations
Nursing programs	Biotechnology companies	Commercial insurers	***Primary Care***	Employers	Health policy
Physician assistant programs		Self-insured employers	Physician offices	Third-party admin- istrators	Research funding
Nurse practitioner programs		Medicare	Community health centers	State agencies	Public health
Physical therapy, occupational therapy, speech therapy programs		Medicaid	Dentists		
Research organizations		Veterans Affairs	Nonphysician providers		
Private foundations		Tricare	***Subacute Care***		
U.S. Public Health Service (Agency for Healthcare Research and Quality, Agency for Toxic Substances and Disease Registry, Centers for Disease Control and Prevention, Food and Drug Administration, Health Resources and Services Administration, Indian Health Service, National Institutes of Health, Substance Abuse and Mental Health Services Administration)			Subacute care facilities		
Professional associations			Ambulatory surgery centers		
Trade associations			***Acute Care***		
			Hospitals		
			Auxiliary Services		
			Pharmacists		
			Diagnostic clinics		
			X-ray units		
			Suppliers of medical equipment		
			Rehabilitative Services		
			Home health agencies		
			Rehabilitation centers		
			Skilled nursing facilities		
			Continuing Care		
			Nursing homes		
			End-of-Life Care		
			Hospices		
			Integrated		
			Managed care organizations		
			Integrated networks		

care facilities (3.13 million). The vast array of health care institutions in the United States includes approximately 5,795 hospitals, 15,700 nursing homes, and 13,337 substance abuse treatment facilities (U.S. Census Bureau, 2012).

In 2015, 1,375 federally qualified health center grantees, with 188,851 full-time employees, provided preventive and primary care services to approximately 24.3 million people living in medically underserved rural and urban areas (Health Resources and Services Administration [HRSA], 2015). Various types of health care professionals are trained in 180 medical and osteopathic schools (Association of American Medical Colleges, 2017), 66 dental schools (American Dental Association, 2017), 136 schools of pharmacy (American Association of Colleges of Pharmacy, 2017), and more than 1,500 nursing programs located throughout the country. Multitudes of government agencies are involved with the financing of health care, medical research, and regulatory oversight of the various aspects of the health care delivery system.

▶ A Broad Description of the System

U.S. health care delivery does not function as a rational and integrated network of components designed to work together coherently. To the contrary, it is a kaleidoscope of financing, insurance, delivery, and payment mechanisms that remain loosely coordinated. Each of these basic functional components represents an amalgam of public (government) and private sources. Government-run programs finance and insure health care for select

groups of people who meet each program's prescribed criteria for eligibility. To a lesser degree, government programs also deliver certain health care services directly to certain recipients, such as veterans, military personnel, American Indians/Alaska Natives, and some uninsured people. Nevertheless, the financing, insurance, payment, and delivery functions largely remain in private hands.

The market-oriented economy in the United States attracts a variety of private entrepreneurs that pursue profits by facilitating the key functions of health care delivery. Employers purchase health insurance for their employees through private sources, and employees receive health care services delivered by the private sector. The government finances public insurance through Medicare, Medicaid, and the Children's Health Insurance Program (CHIP) for a significant portion of the country's low-income, elderly, disabled, and pediatric populations. However, insurance arrangements for many publicly insured people are made through private entities, such as health maintenance organizations (HMOs), and health care services are rendered by private physicians and hospitals. This blend of public and private involvement in the delivery of health care has resulted in the following characteristics of the U.S. system:

- A multiplicity of financial arrangements for health care services
- Numerous insurance agencies or MCOs that employ various mechanisms for insuring against risk
- Multiple payers that make their own determinations regarding how much to pay for each type of service
- A diverse array of settings where medical services are delivered

- Numerous consulting firms offering expertise in planning, cost containment, electronic systems, quality, and restructuring of resources

There is little standardization in a system that is functionally fragmented, and in which the various system components fit together only loosely. Because a central agency such as the government does not oversee the overall coordination of such a system, problems of duplication, overlap, inadequacy, inconsistency, and waste occur. Lack of system-wide planning, direction, and coordination leads to a complex and inefficient system. Moreover, the system as a whole does not lend itself to standard budgetary methods of cost control. Individual and corporate entities within a predominantly private entrepreneurial system seek to manipulate financial incentives to their own advantage, without regard to their impact on the system as a whole. Hence, cost containment remains an elusive goal.

In short, the U.S. health care delivery system is like a behemoth that is almost impossible for any single entity to manage or control. The United States consumes more health care services as a proportion of its total economic output than any other country in the world. The U.S. economy is the largest in the world and, compared to other nations, consumption of health care services in the United States represents a greater proportion of the country's total economic output. Although the system can be credited for delivering some of the best clinical care in the world, it falls short of delivering equitable services to every American. It certainly fails in terms of providing cost-efficient services.

An acceptable health care delivery system should have two primary objectives: (1) enable all citizens to obtain needed health care services; and (2) ensure that services are cost-effective and meet certain established standards of quality. While the U.S. health care delivery system falls short of both these basic ideals, the United States leads the world in providing the latest and the best in medical technology, training, and research. It offers some of the most sophisticated institutions, products, and processes of health care delivery.

▶ Basic Components of a Health Care Delivery System

FIGURE 1-1 illustrates that a health care delivery system incorporates four functional components—financing, insurance, delivery, and payment; hence, it is termed a **quad-function model**. Health care delivery systems differ depending on the arrangement of these components. The four functions generally overlap, but the degree of overlap varies between private and government-run systems, and between traditional health insurance and managed care–based systems. In a government-run system, the functions are more closely integrated and may be indistinguishable. Managed care arrangements also integrate the four functions to varying degrees.

Financing

Financing is necessary to obtain health insurance or to pay for health care services. For most privately insured Americans, health insurance is employment based; that is, the employers finance health care as a fringe benefit for their employees. A

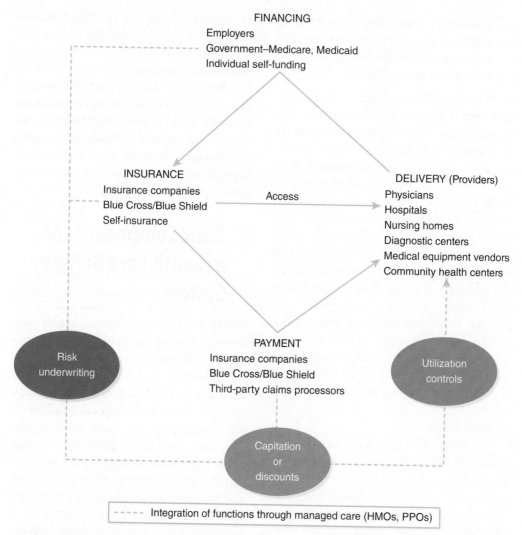

FIGURE 1-1 Basic health care delivery functions.

dependent spouse or children may also be covered by the working spouse's or working parent's employer. Most employers purchase health insurance for their employees through an MCO or an insurance company selected by the employer. Small employers may or may not be in a position to afford health insurance coverage for their employees. In public programs, the government functions as the financier; the insurance function may be carved out to an HMO.

Insurance

Insurance protects the insured against financial catastrophe by providing expensive health care services when needed. The insurance function determines the package of health services that the insured individual is entitled to receive. It specifies how and where health care services may be received. The MCO or insurance company also functions as a claims processor and manages the disbursement of funds to the health care providers.

Delivery

The term "delivery" refers to the provision of health care services by various providers. The term **provider** refers to any entity that delivers health care services and either independently bills for those services or is supported through tax revenues. Common examples of providers include physicians, dentists, optometrists, and therapists in private practices, hospitals, and diagnostic and imaging clinics, and suppliers of medical equipment (e.g., wheelchairs, walkers, ostomy supplies, oxygen). With few exceptions, most providers render services to people who have health insurance and even those covered under public insurance programs receive health care services from private providers.

Payment

The payment function deals with **reimbursement** to providers for services delivered. The insurer determines how much is paid for a certain service. Funds for actual disbursement come from the premiums paid to the MCO or insurance company. At the time of service, the patient is usually required to pay an out-of-pocket amount, such as $25 or $30, to see a physician. The remainder is covered by the MCO or insurance company. In government insurance plans, such as Medicare and Medicaid, tax revenues are used to pay providers.

▶ Insurance and Health Care Reform

The U.S. government finances health benefits for certain special populations, including government employees, the elderly (people ages 65 years and older), people with disabilities, some people with very low incomes, and children from low-income families. The program for the elderly and certain disabled individuals, which is administered by the federal government, is called **Medicare**. The program for the indigent, which is jointly administered by the federal government and state governments, is named **Medicaid**. The program for children from low-income families, another federal/state partnership, is called the Children's Health Insurance Program (CHIP).

However, the predominant employment-based financing system in the United States has left some employed individuals uninsured for two main reasons. First, some small businesses simply cannot get group insurance at affordable rates and, therefore, are not able to offer health insurance as a benefit to their employees. Second, in some work settings, participation in health insurance programs is voluntary, so employees are not required to join. Some employees choose not to sign up, mainly because they cannot afford the cost of health insurance premiums. Employers rarely pay 100% of the insurance premium; instead, most require their employees to pay a portion of the cost. This is called **premium cost sharing**. Self-employed people and other individuals who are not covered by employer-based plans have to obtain health insurance on their own. Individual rates are typically higher than group rates available to employers. In the United States, working people earning low wages have been the most likely to be uninsured because most cannot afford premium cost sharing and are not eligible for public benefits.

In the U.S. context, **health care reform** refers to the expansion of health insurance to cover the **uninsured**—those without private or public health insurance coverage. The Patient Protection and Affordable Care Act of 2010, more commonly known as the Affordable Care Act (ACA), was the most sweeping health care reform in recent U.S. history. One of the main objectives of the ACA was to reduce the number of uninsured.

The ACA was rolled out gradually starting in 2010, when insurance companies were mandated to start covering children and young adults younger than age 26 under their parents' health insurance plans. Most other insurance provisions went into effect on January 1, 2014, except for a mandate for employers to provide health insurance, which was postponed until 2015. The ACA required that all U.S. citizens and legal residents must be covered by either public or private insurance. The law also relaxed standards to qualify additional numbers of people for Medicaid, although many states chose not to implement the Medicaid expansion based on a 2012 ruling by the U.S. Supreme Court. Individuals without private or public insurance had to obtain health insurance from participating insurance companies through Web-based, government-run exchanges; if they failed to do so, they had to pay a tax. The exchanges—also referred to as health insurance marketplaces—would determine whether an applicant qualified for Medicaid or CHIP programs. If an applicant did not qualify for a public program, the exchange would enable the individual to purchase a government-approved health plan offered by private insurers through the exchange. Federal subsidies enabled low-income people to partially offset the cost of health insurance.

A predictive model developed by Parente and Feldman (2013) estimated that, at best, full implementation of the ACA would reduce the number of uninsured by more than 20 million. Nevertheless, by its own design, the ACA failed to achieve **universal coverage** that would enable all citizens and legal residents to have health insurance. Possible future scenarios for health care reform are discussed later in this text.

By March 2015, approximately 16.5 million uninsured Americans had gained health insurance coverage due to the Affordable Care Act ("Impact of Obamacare on Coverage," 2016). By 2016, an estimated 20 million had gained coverage (Uberoi et al., 2016), and by 2017, 31 states and the District of Columbia had expanded Medicaid through the ACA's provisions (Kaiser Family Foundation, 2017). By March 2016, states that had expanded Medicaid experienced an 8.1% decline in their uninsured rate (from 18.2% to 10.1%). States that had not expanded Medicaid experienced a comparably smaller decline of 7.3%—from 23.4% to 16.1% ("Impact of Obamacare on Coverage," 2016). The uninsured rate declined among all race/ethnicity categories, with the greatest decreases seen among African Americans and Hispanics, compared to whites (Uberoi et al., 2016). The uninsured rate declined from 22.4% to 10.6% among African Americans, from 41.8% to 30.5% among Hispanics, and from 14.3% to 7.0% among whites (Uberoi et al., 2016). Additionally, females experienced a greater decline in their uninsured rate (49.7% decline) compared to males (37.6% decline). Specifically, the uninsured rate among females decreased from 18.9% to 9.5%, whereas the uninsured rate among males decreased from 21.8% to 13.6% (Uberoi et al., 2016). Despite these gains, however, the ACA left more than 27.3 million Americans uninsured in 2016 (Cohen et al., 2016).

During his first week in office in January 2017, President Donald Trump signed an Executive Order to repeal and replace the ACA (commonly referred to as Obamacare) in an effort to minimize the ACA's economic and regulatory burdens and to waive any requirement imposing a fiscal burden on states or families, individuals, health care providers, insurers, or other parties.

▶ Role of Managed Care

Under traditional insurance, the four basic health delivery functions have been fragmented; with few exceptions, the financiers, insurers, providers, and payers have been different entities. However, during the 1990s, health care delivery in the United States underwent a fundamental change involving a tighter integration of the basic functions through managed care.

Previously, fragmentation of the four functions meant a lack of control over utilization and payments. The quantity of health care consumed refers to **utilization** of health services. Traditionally, determination of the utilization of health services and the price charged for each service had been left up to the insured individuals and the providers of health care. However, due to rising health care costs, current delivery mechanisms have instituted some controls over both utilization and price.

Managed care is a system of health care delivery that (1) seeks to achieve efficiency by integrating the four functions of health care delivery discussed earlier; (2) employs mechanisms to control (manage) utilization of medical services; and (3) determines the price of services and, consequently, how much the providers are paid. The primary financier is still the employer or the government. Instead of purchasing health insurance through a traditional insurance company, the employer contracts with an MCO, such as an HMO or a preferred provider organization (PPO), to offer a selected health plan to its employees. In this case, the MCO functions like an insurance company and promises to provide health care services contracted under the health plan to the enrollees of the plan. The term **enrollee** (member) refers to the individual covered under the plan. The contractual arrangement between the MCO and the enrollee—including the collective array of covered health services that the enrollee is entitled to—is referred to as the **health plan** (or "plan," for short). The health plan uses selected providers from whom the enrollees can choose to receive services.

Compared with health services delivery under fee-for-service plans, managed care was successful in accomplishing cost control and greater integration of health care delivery. By ensuring access to needed health services, emphasizing preventive care, and maintaining a broad provider network, managed care can implement effective cost-saving measures without compromising access and quality, thereby achieving a health care budget predictability unattainable by other kinds of health care delivery.

▶ Major Characteristics of the U.S. Health Care System

In any country, certain external influences shape the basic character of the health services delivery system. These forces consist of a national political climate, economic development, technological progress, social and cultural values, physical environment, population characteristics (i.e., demographic and health trends), and global influences (**FIGURE 1-2**). The combined interaction of these environmental forces influence the course of health care delivery.

Ten basic characteristics differentiate the U.S. health care delivery system from most other countries:

1. No central agency governs the system.
2. Access to health care services is selectively based on insurance coverage.
3. Health care is delivered under imperfect market conditions.

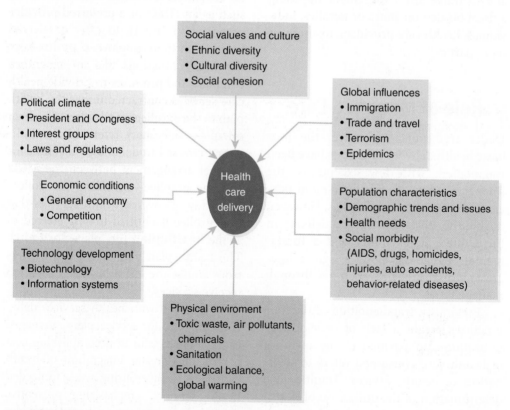

FIGURE 1-2 External forces affecting health care delivery.

4. Insurers from a **third party** act as intermediaries between the financing and delivery functions.
5. The existence of multiple payers makes the system cumbersome.
6. The balance of power among various players prevents any single entity from dominating the system.
7. Legal risks influence the practice behavior of physicians.
8. Development of new technology creates an automatic demand for its use.
9. New service settings have evolved along a continuum.
10. Quality is no longer accepted as an unachievable goal.

No Central Agency

Unlike health care systems in most developed nations, the U.S. health care system is not administratively controlled by a department or agency. Most other developed nations have a national health care program in which citizens are entitled to receive a defined set of health care services. To control costs, these systems use **global budgets** that determine total health care expenditures on a national scale and allocate resources within budgetary limits. As a consequence, both availability of services and payments to providers are subject to such budgetary constraints. The governments of these nations also control the proliferation of health care services, especially costly medical technology. System-wide controls over the allocation of resources determine the extent to which government-sponsored health care services are available to citizens. For instance, the availability of specialized services is restricted.

By contrast, the United States has a mainly private system of financing and delivery. Private financing, predominantly through employers, accounts for approximately 52% of total health care expenditures; the government finances the remaining 48% (Centers for Medicare and Medicaid, 2015). Private delivery of health care means that the majority of hospitals and physician clinics are private businesses, which are independent of the government. No central agency monitors total expenditures through global budgets or controls the availability and utilization of services. Nevertheless, federal and state governments play important roles in health care delivery. They determine public-sector expenditures and reimbursement rates for services provided to Medicare, Medicaid, and CHIP beneficiaries. The federal government also formulates **standards of participation** through health policy and regulation, meaning providers must comply with the standards established by the government to be certified to provide services to Medicare, Medicaid, and CHIP beneficiaries. Certification standards are regarded as minimum standards of quality in most sectors of the health care industry.

Partial Access

Access means the ability of an individual to obtain health care services when needed, which is not the same as having health insurance. Americans can access health care services if they (1) have health insurance through their employers; (2) are covered under a government health care program; (3) can afford to buy insurance with their own private funds; (4) are able to pay for services privately; or (5) can obtain charity or subsidized care. Health insurance is the primary means for ensuring access. Although the uninsured can access certain types of services, they often encounter barriers to obtaining needed health care. For example, while federally supported health centers provide physician services to anyone regardless of ability to pay, such centers and free clinics are located only in certain geographic areas and provide limited specialized services. However, under U.S. law, hospital emergency departments (EDs) are required to evaluate a patient's condition and render medically needed services for which the hospital does not receive any direct payments unless the patient is able to pay. Therefore, even uninsured are able to obtain medical care for acute illness. While one can say that the United States does have a form of universal catastrophic health insurance, it does not guarantee the uninsured access to continual basic and routine care, commonly referred to as **primary care** (Altman and Reinhardt, 1996).

Countries with national health care programs provide universal coverage. However, even in these countries, access to services may be restricted because no health care system has the capacity to deliver every type of service on demand. Hence, **universal access**—the ability of all citizens to obtain health care when needed—remains mostly a theoretical concept.

As previously mentioned, having coverage does not necessarily equate to having access. The cost of insurance and care and availability of services have continued to present barriers to receiving health care services in a timely manner.

Imperfect Market

Though the U.S. health care delivery system is largely in private hands, this system is only partially governed by free-market forces. The delivery and consumption of health care in the United States does not quite pass the basic test of a **free market**, so the system is best described as a quasi-market or an imperfect market.

In a free market, patients (buyers) and providers (sellers) act independently, with patients able to choose services from any provider. Providers do not collude to fix prices, and prices are not fixed by an external agency. Rather, prices are governed by the free and unencumbered interaction of the forces of supply and demand (**FIGURE 1-3**). **Demand**—the quantity of health care purchased—is driven by the prices prevailing in the free market. Under free-market conditions, the quantity demanded will increase as the price is lowered for a given product or

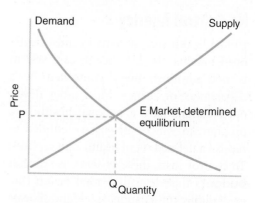

FIGURE 1-3 Relationship between price, supply, and demand under free-market conditions.

Note: Under free-market conditions, there is an inverse relationship between the quantity of medical services demanded and the price of medical services. That is, quantity demanded goes up when the prices go down, and vice versa. In contrast, there is a direct relationship between price and the quantity supplied by the providers of care. In other words, providers are willing to supply higher quantities at higher prices, and vice versa. In a free market, the quantity of medical care that patients are willing to purchase, the quantity of medical care that providers are willing to supply, and the price reach a state of equilibrium. This equilibrium is achieved without the interference of any nonmarket forces. It is important to keep in mind that these conditions exist only under free-market conditions, which are not characteristic of the U.S. health care market.

service. Conversely, the quantity demanded will decrease as the price increases.

At first glance, it might appear that multiple patients and providers do exist. Most patients, however, are now enrolled in either a private health plan or one or more government-sponsored programs. These plans act as intermediaries for the patients, and the enrollment of patients into health plans has the effect of shifting the power from the patients to the administrators of the plans. The result is that the health plans—not the patients—are the real buyers in the health care services market. Private health plans, in many instances, offer their enrollees a limited choice of providers rather than an open choice.

Theoretically, prices are negotiated between the payers and providers. In practice, prices are determined by payers, such as MCOs, Medicare, and Medicaid. Because prices are set by agencies external to the market, they are not governed by the unencumbered forces of supply and demand.

For the health care market to be free, unrestrained competition must occur among providers based on price and quality. However, the consolidation of buying power in the hands of private health plans has been forcing providers to form alliances and integrated delivery systems on the supply side. In certain geographic sectors of the country, a single giant medical system has taken over as the sole provider of major health care services, restricting competition. As the overall health care system continues to move in this direction, it appears that only in large metropolitan areas will there be more than one large integrated system competing to get the business of the health plans.

A free market requires that patients have information about the appropriateness of various services to their needs. Such information is difficult to obtain because technology-driven medical care has become highly sophisticated. Knowledge about new diagnostic methods, intervention techniques, and more effective drugs fall in the domain of the professional physician, not the patient. Moreover, because medical interventions are commonly required in a state of urgency, patients have neither the skills nor the time and resources to obtain accurate information when needed. Channeling all health care needs through a primary care provider can reduce this information gap when the primary care provider acts as the patient's advocate or agent. In recent years, consumers have been seizing some measure of control over the flow of information: The Internet is becoming a prominent source of medical information for patients, and medical advertising is influencing consumer expectations.

In a free market, patients must directly bear the cost of services received. The purpose of insurance is to protect against the risk of unforeseen catastrophic events. Since the fundamental purpose of insurance is to reimburse major expenses when unlikely events occur, having insurance for basic and routine health care undermines the principle of insurance. When you buy home insurance to protect your property against the unlikely event of a fire, you do not anticipate the occurrence of a loss. The probability that you will suffer a loss by fire is very small. If a fire does occur and cause major damage, insurance will cover the loss, but insurance does not cover routine wear and tear on the house, such as chipped paint or a leaky faucet. However, unlike other types of insurance, health insurance generally covers basic and routine services that are predictable. Coverage for minor services, such as colds and coughs, earaches, and so forth, amounts to prepayment for such services. In this sense, health insurance has the effect of insulating patients from the full cost of health care. This situation may also create a **moral hazard** in that, once enrollees have purchased health insurance, they may use more health care services than if they were to pay for these services on an out-of-pocket basis.

At least two additional factors limit the ability of patients to make decisions in the health care system. First, decisions about the utilization of health care are often determined by need rather than by price-based demand. **Need** has been defined as the amount of medical care that medical experts believe a person should have to remain or become healthy (Feldstein, 1993). Second, the delivery of health care can result in demand creation. This follows from self-assessed need, which, coupled with moral hazard, leads to greater utilization, creating an artificial demand because prices are not taken into consideration. Practitioners who have a financial interest in additional treatments also create artificial demand (Hemenway and Fallon, 1985). This is referred to as **provider-induced demand**, or supplier-induced demand. Functioning as patients' agents, physicians exert enormous influence on the demand for health care services (Altman and Wallack, 1996). Demand creation occurs when physicians prescribe medical care beyond what is clinically necessary. This can include practices such as making more frequent follow-up appointments than necessary, prescribing

excessive medical tests, or performing unnecessary surgery (Santerre and Neun, 1996).

In a free market, patients have information on the price and quality of each provider. The current system, however, has drawbacks that obstruct information-seeking efforts. Item-based pricing is one such hurdle. Surgery is a good example to illustrate item-based (also known as fee-for-service) pricing. Patients can generally obtain the fees the surgeon would charge for a particular operation. But the final bill, after the surgery has been performed, is likely to include charges for supplies, use of the hospital's facilities, and services performed by other providers, such as anesthesiologists, nurse anesthetists, and pathologists. These providers, sometimes referred to as **phantom providers**, function in an adjunct capacity and bill for their services separately. Item billing for such additional services, which sometimes cannot be anticipated, makes it extremely difficult to ascertain the total price before services have actually been received. Package pricing can help overcome these drawbacks, but it has made relatively little headway for pricing medical procedures. **Package pricing** refers to a bundled fee for a package of related services. In the surgery example, this would mean one all-inclusive price for the surgeon's fees, hospital facilities, supplies, diagnostics, pathology, anesthesia, and postsurgical follow-up.

Third-Party Insurers and Payers

Insurance often functions as the intermediary among those who finance, deliver, and receive health care. The insurance intermediary does not have an incentive to be the patient's advocate on either price or quality. At best, employees can air their dissatisfactions with the plan to their employer, who has the power to discontinue the current plan and choose another company. In reality, however, employers may be reluctant to change plans if the current plan offers lower premiums than a different plan.

Multiple Payers

A national health care system is sometimes also referred to as a **single-payer system** because there is one primary payer, the government. When delivering services, providers send the bill to a government agency that subsequently sends payments to each provider. By contrast, the United States has a multiplicity of health plans. Multiple payers often represent a billing and collection nightmare for the providers of services. Multiple payers make the system more cumbersome in several ways:

- It is extremely difficult for providers to keep tabs on numerous health plans. It is challenging for providers to keep up with which services are covered under each plan and how much each plan will pay for those services.
- Providers must hire claims processors to bill for services and monitor receipt of payments. Billing practices are not standardized, and each payer establishes its own format.
- Payments can be denied for not precisely following the requirements set by each payer.
- Denied claims necessitate rebilling.
- When only partial payment is received, some health plans may allow the provider to **balance bill** the patient for the amount the health plan did not pay, the

difference between provider charges and insurance payment. Other plans prohibit balance billing. Even when the balance billing option is available to the provider, it triggers a new cycle of billings and collection efforts.

- Providers must sometimes engage in lengthy collection efforts, including writing collection letters, turning delinquent accounts over to collection agencies, and finally writing off as bad debt amounts that cannot be collected.
- Government programs have complex regulations for determining whether payment is made for services actually delivered. Medicare, for example, requires that each provider maintain lengthy documentation on services provided. Medicaid is known for lengthy delays in paying providers.

It is generally believed that the United States spends far more on **administrative costs**—costs associated with billing, collections, bad debts, and maintaining medical records—than do the national health care systems in other countries.

Power Balancing

The U.S. health care system involves multiple players, not just multiple payers. The key players in the system have traditionally been physicians, administrators of health service institutions, insurance companies, large employers, and the government. Big business, labor, insurance companies, physicians, and hospitals make up the powerful and politically active special-interest groups represented before lawmakers by high-priced lobbyists. Each set of players has its own economic interests to protect. Physicians, for instance, want to maintain their incomes and have minimum interference with the way they practice medicine; institutional administrators seek to maximize reimbursement from private and public insurers; insurance companies and MCOs are interested in maintaining their share of the health insurance market; large employers want to contain the costs they incur providing health insurance to their employees; the government tries to maintain or enhance existing benefits for those covered under public insurance programs and simultaneously contain the cost of providing these benefits. The problem is that the self-interests of different players are often at odds. For example, providers seek to increase government reimbursement for services delivered to Medicare, Medicaid, and CHIP beneficiaries, but the government wants to contain cost increases. Employers dislike rising health insurance premiums. Health plans, under pressure from the employers, may limit fees for the providers, who then resent these cuts.

The fragmented self-interests of the various players produce competing forces within the system. In an environment that is rife with motivations to protect conflicting self-interests, achieving comprehensive system-wide reform has been next to impossible, and cost containment has remained a major challenge. Consequently, the approach to health care reform in the United States has been characterized as incremental or piecemeal, and the focus of reform initiatives has been confined to health insurance coverage and payment cuts to providers rather than focusing on the better provision of health care.

Litigation Risks

The United States is a litigious society. Motivated by the prospects of enormous jury awards, many Americans are quick to drag an alleged offender into a courtroom at the slightest perception of incurred harm. Private health care providers, too, have become increasingly susceptible to litigation and the risk of malpractice lawsuits is a real consideration in the practice of medicine. To protect themselves against the possibility of litigation, practitioners may engage in what is referred to as **defensive medicine** by prescribing additional diagnostic tests, scheduling return checkup visits, and maintaining copious documentation. Many of these additional efforts may be unnecessary, costly, and inefficient.

High Technology

The United States has been the hotbed of research and innovation in new medical technology. Growth in science and technology often creates demand for new services despite shrinking resources to finance sophisticated care. People generally equate high-tech care with high-quality care. They want "the latest and the best," especially when health insurance will pay for new treatments. Physicians and technicians want to try the latest gadgets. Hospitals compete on the basis of having the most modern equipment and facilities. Once capital investments in these new services are made, those costs must be recouped through utilization. Legal risks for providers and health plans may also play a role in discouraging denial of new technology. Thus, several factors promote the use of costly new technology once it is developed.

Continuum of Services

Medical care services are classified into three broad categories: curative (i.e., drugs, treatments, and surgeries), restorative (e.g., physical, occupational, and speech therapies), and preventive (i.e., prenatal care, mammograms, and immunizations). Health care settings are no longer confined to the hospital and the physician's office. Additional settings, such as home health, subacute care units, and outpatient surgery centers, have emerged in response to the changing configuration of economic incentives. **TABLE 1-2** describes the continuum of health care services. The

TABLE 1-2 The Continuum of Health Care Services	
Types of Health Services	**Delivery Settings**
Preventive care	Public health programs Community programs Personal lifestyles Primary care settings
Primary care	Physician's office or clinic Community health centers Self-care Alternative medicine
Specialized care	Specialist provider clinics
Chronic care	Primary care settings Specialist provider clinics Home health Long-term care facilities Self-care Alternative medicine
Long-term care	Long-term care facilities Home health
Subacute care	Special subacute units (hospitals, long-term care facilities) Home health Outpatient surgical centers
Acute care	Hospitals
Rehabilitative care	Rehabilitation departments (hospitals, long-term care facilities) Home health Outpatient rehabilitation centers
End-of-life care	Hospice services provided in a variety of settings

health care continuum in the United States remains lopsided, with a heavier emphasis on specialized services than on preventive services, primary care, and management of chronic conditions.

Quest for Quality

Even though the definition and measurement of quality in health care are not as clear-cut as they are in other industries, the delivery sector of health care has come under increased pressure to develop quality standards and demonstrate compliance with those standards. There are higher expectations for improved health outcomes at the individual and community levels. The concept of continual quality improvement has also received much emphasis in managing health care institutions.

▶ Trends and Directions

Since the 1980s, the U.S. health care delivery system has continued to undergo fundamental shifts in emphasis, summarized in **FIGURE 1-4**. Later chapters discuss these

◊ Illness ⟶ Wellness

◊ Acute care ⟶ Primary care

◊ Inpatient ⟶ Outpatient

◊ Individual health ⟶ Community well-being

◊ Fragmented care ⟶ Managed care

◊ Independent institutions ⟶ Integrated systems

◊ Service duplication ⟶ Continuum of services

FIGURE 1-4 Trends and directions in health care delivery.

transformations in greater detail and focus on the factors driving them.

These trends have been primarily driven by the desire to promote health while reducing costs. An example of a fundamental shift is the concept of health itself. Health is now increasingly seen as the presence of wellness rather than solely the absence of illness. Such a change requires new methods for wellness promotion, although the treatment of illness remains the primary goal of the health care delivery system. The ACA had partially shifted the focus from disease treatment to disease prevention, better health outcomes for individuals and communities, and lower health care costs.

At present, the greatest challenge to the U.S. health care system is the quest to control costs while still meeting the increasing health care demands of an aging population, a population with more chronic diseases and comorbidities. This is challenging because patients are more informed about high-tech discoveries while economic conditions are also more uncertain. In response, players in the health care system have been moving toward providing more effective and efficient quality care. Recent trends have focused more on delivery of services by mid-level health professionals and health coaches as well as use of health information technology (HIT). However, the health care system continues to face challenges related to managing costs, focusing on care delivery, adopting new technologies, delivering new operating models, and meeting various federal and state regulations (Deloitte, 2017).

Patients with multiple chronic conditions use the most health services and each chronic condition increases costs by a factor of three (DeVore, 2014). Managing chronic diseases has been a major focus of efforts to control health care costs. Chronic care models, patient-centered care, and continuous care are being implemented as means to improve health care delivery performance, quality, and patient health outcomes. In particular, patient-centered medical homes (PCMHs) and ambulatory intensive care units (A-ICUs) are being incorporated into accountable care organizations (ACOs). The main objective in establishing these programs is to better manage chronic conditions exclusively within a "clinically integrated, financially accountable primary care practice" (DeVore, 2014). Ultimately, providers hope these measures can address behavioral health needs, lower hospital utilization rates, decrease inpatient bed-days, shorten lengths of stay, limit admissions and readmissions, and minimize ED visits.

Mid-level health care professionals and health coaches are important for managing chronic conditions and reducing costs. Health coaches, for examples, complement medical professionals by getting to know patients through one-on-one contact and can keep the clinical staff apprised of financial struggles, issues with housing, family concerns, or other obstacles that may stand in the way of the patient following a prescribed care plan (DeVore, 2014). Health coaches do not need a medical degree, can be recruited from various professional backgrounds, and help improve the effectiveness and efficiency of care.

Similarly, HIT has helped improve access to information and, consequently, health. The market for telemedicine and remote monitoring applications was estimated to double from $11.6 billion in 2011 to $27.3 billion in 2016 (DeVore, 2014).

This growth is in part driven by the increased demands for care owing to expansion of insurance coverage through the ACA; the health system may not have the capacity to treat each individual in person. For example, the Johns Hopkins Hospital at Home program delivers acute care services at the homes of patients with chronic illnesses who might otherwise need inpatient care. In this way, HIT also increases access to care, particularly for patients living in rural areas where distance to the closest hospital is a major barrier.

Electronic health records (EHRs) have helped provide clinical measures and decision support tools, enabled providers to automate processes to reduce redundancy, and captured more clinical data (DeVore, 2014). Trends toward greater interoperability of health information systems, along with open source interfaces, will allow for greater transparency, increased availability of data, and more creative use of data.

▶ Significance for Health Care Practitioners

An understanding of the intricacies within the health services system would be beneficial to all those who come in contact with the system. In their respective training programs, health professionals, such as physicians, nurses, technicians, therapists, dietitians, and pharmacists may understand their own individual clinical roles but remain ignorant of the forces outside their profession that could significantly impact both current and future clinical practices. An understanding of the health care delivery system can attune health professionals to their relationship with the rest of the health care environment. It can help them understand changes and the impact of those changes on their own practice. Adaptation and relearning are strategies that can prepare health professionals to cope with an environment that will see ongoing change long into the future, particularly as the U.S. health care system is expected to further evolve under subsequent efforts to reform the system.

▶ Significance for Health Care Managers

An understanding of the health care system has specific implications for both private and public health services managers, who must understand the macro environment in which they make critical planning and management decisions. Such decisions will ultimately affect the efficiency and quality of services delivered. The interactions between the system's key components and the implications of these interactions must be well understood because the operations of health care institutions are strongly influenced, either directly or indirectly, by the financing of health services, reimbursement rates, insurance mechanisms, delivery modes, new statutes and legal opinions, and government regulations.

For the foreseeable future, the environment of health care delivery will remain fluid and dynamic. The viability of delivery and the success of health care managers often depends on how the managers react to the system dynamics. Timeliness of action is often a critical factor that can make the difference between

failure and success. Following are some more specific reasons why understanding the health care delivery system is indispensable for health care managers.

Positioning the Organization

Managers need to understand their own organizational position within the macro environment of the health care system. Senior managers, such as chief executive officers, must constantly gauge the nature and impact of the fundamental shifts illustrated in Figure 1-4. Managers need to consider which changes in the current configuration of financing, insurance, payment, and delivery might affect their organization's long-term stability. Middle and first-line managers also need to understand their roles in the current configuration and how these roles might change in the future.

How should resources be realigned to effectively respond to those changes? As an example, managers need to evaluate whether certain functions in their departments must be eliminated, modified, or added. Would the changes involve further training? Which processes are likely to change, and how? Which steps do the managers need to take to maintain the integrity of their institution's mission, the goodwill of the patients they serve, and the quality of care? Well-thought-out and appropriately planned changes are likely to cause less turbulence for both the providers and the recipients of care.

Handling Threats and Opportunities

Changes in any of the functions of financing, insurance, payment, and delivery can present new threats or opportunities in the health care market. Health care managers will be more effective if they proactively deal with any threats to their institution's profitability and viability. Managers need to find ways to transform certain threats into new opportunities.

Evaluating Implications

Managers are better able to evaluate the implications of health policy and new reform proposals when they understand the relevant issues and appreciate how such issues link to the delivery of health services in the establishments they manage. Health care reform has brought more individuals into the U.S. health care system, creating greater demand for health services. Planning and staffing to ensure the right mix of health care workers are available to meet this anticipated surge in demand are critical.

Planning

Senior managers are often responsible for strategic planning regarding which services should be added or discontinued, which resources should be committed to facility expansion, and what should be done with excess capacity. Any long-range planning must take into consideration the current makeup of health services delivery, the evolving trends, and the potential impact of these trends.

Capturing New Markets

Health care managers will be in a better position to capture new health services markets if they understand emerging trends in the financing, insurance, payment, and delivery functions. New

opportunities must be explored before any newly evolving segments of the market become crowded with competition. An understanding of the dynamics within the system is essential to forging new marketing strategies that will let the institution stay ahead of the competition and, in some cases, find a service niche.

Complying with Regulations

Delivery of health care services is heavily regulated. Health care managers must comply with government regulations, such as standards of participation in government programs, licensing rules, and security and privacy laws regarding patient information, and they must operate within the constraints of reimbursement rates. On a periodic basis, the Medicare and Medicaid programs have made drastic changes to their reimbursement methodologies that have triggered the need for operational changes in the way services are organized and delivered. Private agencies, such as the Joint Commission, also play an indirect regulatory role, mainly in the monitoring of quality of services. Health care managers have no choice but to play by the rules set by the various public and private agencies that regulate the health care marketplace. Hence, it is paramount that health care managers acquaint themselves with the rules and regulations governing their areas of operation.

Following the Organizational Mission

Knowledge of the health care system and its development is essential for effective management of health care organizations. By keeping up-to-date on community needs, technological progress, consumer demand, and economic prospects, managers can be in a better position to fulfill their organizational missions to enhance access, improve service quality, and achieve efficiency in the delivery of services.

▶ Health Care Systems of Other Countries

Except for the United States, the 25 wealthiest nations in the world all have some form of universal health care coverage (Rodin and de Ferranti, 2012). Canada and Western European nations have used three basic models for structuring their national health care systems:

- In a system based on **national health insurance (NHI)**, such as that found in Canada, the government finances health care through general taxes, but the actual care is delivered by private providers. In the context of the quad-function model, NHI requires a tighter consolidation of the financing, insurance, and payment functions coordinated by the government. Delivery is characterized by detached private arrangements.

- In a **national health system (NHS)**, such as that found in the United Kingdom, in addition to financing a tax-supported NHI program, the government manages the infrastructure for the delivery of medical care. Thus, the government operates most of the country's medical institutions. Most health care providers, such as physicians, either are government employees or are tightly organized in

a publicly managed infrastructure. In the context of the quad-function model, NHS requires a tighter consolidation of all four functions.

- In a **socialized health insurance (SHI)** system, such as that found in Germany, government-mandated contributions from employers and employees finance health care. Private providers deliver health care services. Private, not-for-profit insurance companies, called sickness funds, are responsible for collecting the contributions and paying physicians and hospitals (Santerre and Neun, 1996). The insurance and payment functions are closely integrated in a SHI system, and the financing function is better coordinated with the insurance and payment functions than in the United States. Delivery is characterized by independent private arrangements, but the government exercises overall control of the system.

In the remainder of this text, the terms "national health care program" and "national health insurance" are used generically and interchangeably to refer to any type of government-supported universal health insurance program. Following is a brief discussion of health care delivery in selected countries from various parts of the world to illustrate the application of the three models discussed and to provide a sample of the variety of health care systems in the world.

Australia

In the past, Australia had switched from a universal national health care program to a privately financed system. In 1984, it returned to a national program—called Medicare—financed by income taxes and an income-based Medicare levy. This system is built on the philosophy that everyone should contribute to the cost of health care according to his or her capacity to pay. In addition to carrying Medicare, approximately 49% of Australians carry private health insurance (Australian Government, Department of Health, 2016) to cover gaps in public coverage, such as dental services and care received in private hospitals (Willcox, 2001). Although private health insurance is voluntary, it is strongly encouraged by the Australian government through tax subsidies for purchasers and tax penalties for nonpurchasers (Healy, 2002). Public hospital spending is funded by the government, but private hospitals offer better choices. Costs incurred by patients receiving private medical services, whether in or out of the hospital, are reimbursed in whole or in part by Medicare. Private patients are free to choose and change their doctors. The medical profession in Australia is composed mainly of private practitioners, who provide care predominantly on a fee-for-service basis (Hall, 1999; Podger, 1999).

In 2011, the Council of Australian Governments (COAG) signed the National Health Reform Agreement, which established the architecture for national health insurance reform. In particular, the Agreement provides for more sustainable funding arrangements for Australia's health system. At the same time, the National Health Reform Act 2011 establishes a new Independent Hospital Pricing Authority and a National Health Performance Authority. The Pricing Authority determines and publishes the national price for services provided by public hospitals. The Commonwealth Government determines its contribution to funding public hospitals on the basis of these prices. The Performance Authority is charged with monitoring and reporting on the performance of local hospital networks, public and private hospitals, primary health care organizations, and other bodies or organizations that provide health care services. The 2011 act also provides a new statutory framework for the Australian Commission on Safety and Quality in Health Care (Australian Government, 2011).

Australia is focused on developing various health service delivery models to contain costs and provide quality and accessible care (Brownie et al., 2014). Notably, Australia has encouraged interprofessional practice as a means to enhance socioeconomic development and improve health outcomes (Brownie et al., 2014). COAG defined new Australian Health Care Agreements (AHCAs), under which each state and territory funds a portion of the public hospital operation costs, commits to providing equitable access to free public hospital services based on clinical need, and agrees to match the rate of growth in the Australian government's hospital funding (Australian Institute of Health and Welfare, 2017).

Additionally, Australia has developed a National Primary Health Care Strategy and established a Preventative Health Taskforce to lead its National Preventative Health Strategy (Policy Review, 2010). The National Primary Health Care Strategy aims to better incentivize prevention, promote evidence-based management of chronic disease, support the role of general practitioners in health care teams, encourage a focus on interprofessional team-based care, and address the increased need for access to various health professionals such as practice nurses and allied health professionals, such as physiotherapists and dieticians (Policy Review, 2010). The Preventative Health Taskforce aims to stop the obesity epidemic, reduce the prevalence of daily smoking to less than 9%, reduce the prevalence of binge consumption and other harmful alcohol consumption habits by 30%, and reduce the 17-year life expectancy gap between indigenous and non-indigenous people by the year 2020 (Policy Review, 2010). Other health reforms seek to achieve continuity of care, provide high-quality education and training for existing and incoming health care workers, and embed a culture of interprofessional practice (Brownie et al., 2014).

Canada

Canada implemented its national health insurance system—referred to as Medicare—under the Medical Care Act of 1966. Medicare consists of 13 provincial and territorial health insurance plans, sharing basic standards of coverage, as defined by the Canada Health Act (Health Canada, 2013). The bulk of financing for Medicare comes from general provincial tax revenues; the federal government provides a fixed amount that is independent of actual expenditures. Public-sector health expenditures account for 70% of the total Canadian health care expenditures. The remaining 30% consists of private-sector expenditures, which include household out-of-pocket expenditures, commercial and not-for-profit insurance expenditures,

and nonconsumption expenditures (Canadian Institute for Health Information, 2012). Many employers also offer private insurance that gives their employees supplemental coverage.

Provincial and territorial departments of health have the responsibility to administer medical insurance plans, determine reimbursement for providers, and deliver certain public health services. Provinces are required by law to provide reasonable access to all medically necessary services and to provide portability of benefits from province to province. Patients are free to select their providers (Akaho et al., 1998). According to Canada's Fraser Institute, specialist physicians surveyed across 12 specialties and 10 Canadian provinces reported a total waiting time of 20.0 weeks between referral from a general practitioner and delivery of treatment in 2016—an increase from 18.3 weeks in 2015. Patients had to wait the longest to undergo neurosurgery surgery (46.9 weeks) (Barua et al., 2016).

Nearly all the Canadian provinces—Ontario is one of the exceptions—have resorted to regionalization of health care services, through the creation of administrative districts within each province. The objective of regionalization is to decentralize authority and responsibility in order to more efficiently address local needs and to promote citizen participation in health care decision making (Church and Barker, 1998). The majority of Canadian hospitals are operated as private nonprofit entities run by community boards of trustees, voluntary organizations, or municipalities, and most physicians are in private practice (Health Canada, 2013). Most provinces use global budgets and allocate set reimbursement amounts for each hospital. Physicians are paid fee-for-service rates, which are negotiated between each provincial government and medical association (MacPhee, 1996; Naylor, 1999).

In 2004, Canada created the 10-Year Plan to Strengthen Health Care, which focuses on problems with wait times, health human resources, pharmaceutical management, EHRs, health innovation, accountability and reporting, public health, and Aboriginal health. Overall, progress has been made in these areas, but the goals have not yet been fully achieved (Health Council of Canada, 2013).

Although most Canadians are quite satisfied with their health care system, sustaining the current health care delivery and financing remains a challenge. Spending on health care has increased dramatically in recent decades, from approximately 7% of program spending at the provincial level in the 1970s to almost 41% in 2015. It is expected to surpass 50% in every province and territory within the next few years (Barua et al., 2016).

With global pressure on health reforms, Canada is also transitioning to patient-centered care (Dickson, 2016), but has not implemented major country-wide health reform since 2005 (Health Systems and Policy Monitor [HSPM], 2012). In addition to leadership challenges, two reasons that Canada has been reluctant to reform its health system are (1) resistance from long-standing professional associations; and (2) a lack of follow-through from provincial governments (Dickson, 2016).

The 2014 version of the Canada Health Act expanded services such as nursing home intermediate care, adult residential care, home care services, and ambulatory care services (Canada Minister and Attorney General, 2016). Other initiatives include collaboration between provincial and territorial governments to purchase drugs in bulk and cut costs in order to make drugs more affordable to patients and also a program to improve access to high-quality mental health services, particularly for veterans and first-responders (Granovsky, 2016).

China

Since the economic reforms initiated in the late 1970s, health care in the People's Republic of China has undergone significant changes. In urban China, health insurance has evolved from a predominantly public insurance (either government or public enterprise) system to a multipayer system. Government employees are covered under government insurance as a part of their benefits. Employees for public enterprises are largely covered through public enterprise insurance, but the actual benefits and payments vary according to the financial well-being of the enterprises. Employees of foreign businesses or joint ventures are typically well insured through private insurance arrangements. Almost all of these plans contain costs through a variety of means, such as experience-based premiums, deductibles, copayments, and health benefit dollars (i.e., pre-allocated benefit dollars for health care that can be converted into income if not fully used). The unemployed, self-employed, and employees working for small enterprises (public or private) are largely uninsured. They can purchase individual or family plans in the private market or pay for services out of pocket. In rural China, the New Cooperative Medical Scheme (NCMS), discussed later, has become widespread; it relies on funds pooled from national and local governments, as well as private citizens. Although the insurance coverage rate is high (more than 90%) in China, the actual benefits are still very limited.

Similarly to the United States, China has been facing the growing problems of a large uninsured population and health care cost inflation. Although health care funding was increased by 87% in 2006 and 2007, the country has yet to reform its health care system into an efficient and effective scheme. Employment-based insurance in China does not cover dependents, nor does it cover migrant workers, leading to high out-of-pocket cost sharing as part of total health spending. Rural areas in China are most vulnerable to poor access to health care because of a lack of true insurance plans and accompanying comprehensive coverage. Health care cost inflation is also growing 7% faster than the growth rate for China's gross domestic product (GDP), which is 16% per year (Yip and Hsiao, 2008).

In recent years, health care delivery in China has undergone significant changes. The former three-tier referral system (primary, second, tertiary) has been largely abolished. Patients can now go to any hospital of their choice as long as they are insured or can pay out of pocket. As a result, large (tertiary) hospitals are typically overutilized, whereas smaller (primary and secondary) hospitals are underutilized. Use of large hospitals contributes to both escalation of medical costs and greater medical specialization.

Major changes in health insurance and delivery have made access to medical care more difficult for the poor, uninsured, and underinsured. Consequently, wide and growing disparities in access, quality, and outcomes are becoming apparent between rural and urban areas, and between the rich and the poor. After the severe acute respiratory syndrome (SARS) epidemic in 2003, the Chinese government created an electronic disease-reporting system at the district level. Each district in China now has a hospital dedicated to infectious diseases. However, these are still flaws in this system, particularly in monitoring infectious diseases in the remote localities that comprise some districts (Blumenthal and Hsiao, 2005).

To fix some of its problems, the Chinese government has pushed through health reform initiatives in five major areas: health insurance, pharmaceuticals, primary care, public health, and public/community hospitals. For example, it created the New Cooperative Medical Scheme to provide rural areas with a government-run voluntary insurance program. This program is intended to prevent individuals living in these areas from becoming impoverished due to illness or catastrophic health expenses (Yip and Hsiao, 2008). In 2008, a similar program was established in urban areas, called the Urban Resident Basic Medical Insurance scheme. It targets uninsured children, elderly persons, and other nonworking urban residents and enrolls them into the program at the household level rather than at the individual level (Wagstaff et al., 2009).

To improve access to primary care, China has reestablished community health centers (CHCs) that provide preventive and primary care services so patients no longer need to seek expensive outpatient services at hospitals. The goal is to reduce hospital utilization and increase CHCs that can provide prevention, home care, and rehabilitative services (Yip and Hsiao, 2008; Yip and Mahal, 2008). The CHCs have not been very popular among the public because of their perceived lack of quality and because of their poor reputation from perceived lack of quality. It remains uncertain whether China will restore its previously integrated health care delivery system, aimed at achieving universal access, or continue on its current course toward greater medical specialization and privatization.

Another major component of Chinese health reform has been the establishment of an essential drug system that aims to enhance access to and reduce out-of-pocket spending for essential medicines. The reform policies specified a comprehensive system including selection, procurement, pricing, prescription, and quality and safety standards (Barber et al., 2013).

In terms of public hospital reform, quality, efficiency, and development of a hospital governance structure have been emphasized. Several pilot reforms have been launched in various cities in China, but no national implementation plan has been formulated (Yip et al., 2012).

China's National Health and Family Planning Commission (previously the Ministry of Health) and State Council have detailed several health reform objectives, such as constraining drug prices, enhancing the affordability of medical services at public hospitals, and improving staff performance (Hsu, 2015). Eliminating markups on drug sales in hospitals has led to financial losses in country-level pilot programs, although

government subsidies to these programs have increased.

In 2012, China lifted restrictions on foreign investments in private hospitals in an effort to increase the number of hospitals and improve access to care (Hsu, 2015). By 2015, the State Council aimed to increase use of private health services by 20%. Health insurance reform is also being developed. The Chinese government plans to give tax breaks to private health insurance policyholders in an attempt to increase insurance coverage. Some of these tax breaks include allowing those privately insured to deduct 2,400 Renminbi per year from their assessable income for health insurance premiums (Hsu, 2015).

In 2015, China announced a 5-year plan for the health system, which outlined key areas for development by 2020 (Zhu, 2015). Despite broad reforms, the Chinese health care system continues to be plagued by resource shortages and underdevelopment in rural areas. Thus, the latest reforms target three main areas: infrastructure development, reduction of costs expansion of insurance coverage, and investment in novel technologies. Importantly, these reforms will open up new opportunities for foreign investments.

Germany

Health insurance has been mandatory for all citizens and permanent residents in Germany since 2009 (Blumel and Busse, 2016). As mentioned earlier, the German health care system is based on the SHI model, and voluntary substitutive private health insurance is available. "About 86 percent of the population receive their primary coverage through SHI and 11 percent through substitutive PHI" and there are also special programs to cover the rest of the population (Blumel and Busse, 2016). Sickness funds act as purchasing entities by negotiating contracts with hospitals. However, paying for the increasing costs of medical care has proved challenging in Germany because of an aging population, fewer people in the workforce, and stagnant wage growth during recessions.

During the 1990s, Germany adopted legislation to promote competition among sickness funds (Brown and Amelung, 1999). To further control costs, its national system employs global budgets for the hospital sector and places annual limits on spending for physician services. Inpatient care is paid per admission based on diagnosis-related groups (DRGs)—a system that was made obligatory in 2004 (Blumel and Busse, 2016).

Health reforms in Germany have focused on improving the efficiency and appropriateness of care. In 2011, the Pharmaceutical Market Reform Act introduced an assessment scheme for all new pharmaceuticals, under which only those drugs that offer additional benefits relative to existing alternatives can be reimbursed at a higher rate (World Health Organization [WHO], 2014). The Hospital Financing Reform Act of 2009 requires performance-based flat-rate grants for investments in hospitals, rather than non-performance-based flat-rate grants on a case-by-case basis as of 2012 (WHO, 2014).

One of Germany's biggest challenges is the division between SHI and private health insurance. The differences in risk pools, financing structures, access, and provisions in these alternative insurance plans contribute to inequalities in care (WHO, 2014). Additionally, more work is needed to improve quality of medical services, patient satisfaction, and accessibility of health services in rural communities (WHO, 2014).

The most recent reforms in Germany have focused on improving services for SHI-covered patients and enhancing hospital quality. In June 2015, the Act to Strengthen SHI Health Care Provision gave municipalities the right to establish medical treatment centers, gave patients the right to see a specialist within 4 weeks, and promoted innovative forms of care in an effort to strengthen services for SHI-covered patients (HSPM, 2016). This act improves prevention services and health promotion through investments in schools, the workplace, and long-term care facilities. In addition, the 2016 Hospital Care Structure Reform Act introduced quality aspects in the regulation of hospital volume and payments (Blumel and Busse, 2016). Substantial funds will be invested to improve the hospital care structure in Germany.

United Kingdom

The United Kingdom follows the national health system model. Its health delivery system is called the National Health Service (NHS). The NHS is founded on the principles of primary care and has a strong focus on community health services. The system owns its hospitals and employs its hospital-based specialists and other staff on a salaried basis. The primary care physicians, referred to as general practitioners (GPs), are mostly private practitioners. All NHS-insured patients are required to register with a local GP. In 2014, there were on average 7,171 patients per practice and 1,530 patients per GP (Thorlby and Arora, 2016).

The NHS emphasizes free point of access and equal access to all (HSPM, 2015). In England, the Health and Social Care Act abolished the Primary Care Trust and Strategic Health Authority in 2012, replacing them with the Clinical Commissioning Group. In 2013, the Better Care Fund was enacted to improve integration of health and social care. In 2014, the Care Act was introduced to cap out-of-pocket expenditures (HSPM, 2015).

Delivery of primary care occurs through primary care trusts (PCTs) in England, local health groups in Wales, health boards in Scotland, and primary care partnerships in Northern Ireland. PCTs have geographically assigned responsibility for community health services; each person living in a given geographic area is assigned to a particular PCT. A typical PCT is responsible for approximately 50,000 to 250,000 patients (Dixon and Robinson, 2002). PCTs function independently of the local health authorities and are governed by a consumer-dominated board. A fully developed PCT has its own budget allocations, used for both primary care and hospital-based services. In this respect, PCTs function like MCOs in the United States.

Approximately 83% of U.K. health expenditures in 2013 went to the public sector (Office of National Statistics, 2015). Private expenditures involve mainly drugs and other medical products as well as private hospital care. Despite having a national health care system, 10.9% of the British population maintains private health insurance (Arora et al., 2013).

England, Scotland, Wales, and Northern Ireland are taking their own approaches to health care. England is moving toward decentralization, reinforcement of an internal market, and more localized decision making (HSPM, 2015). Scotland and Wales are dissolving the internal market and centralizing authority. While Scotland is embracing a publicly funded universal health system, England is emphasizing private partnerships and internal competition. Costs are increasing in the United Kingdom owing to infrastructure improvements, technology innovations, an aging and growing population, more patients with chronic diseases, heightened focus on quality of care, informed and empowered consumers, and innovative treatments (Deloitte, 2017).

In 2014, NHS England introduced the Five Year Forward View plan, which lays out strategies for addressing the most pressing challenges in the health care system (National Health Services England, 2015). This plan places a greater emphasis on prevention, integration of services, and patient-centered care. It sets out strategies and new care models whose goals include integrating primary and acute care systems, creating multispecialty community providers, and fostering collaborations in acute care. These models will redesign services and change the way health services are administered, financed and regulated in coming years.

Israel

Until 1995, Israel had a system of universal coverage based on the German SHI model, financed through an employer tax and income-based contributions from individuals. When the National Health

Insurance (NHI) Law went into effect in 1995, it made insurance coverage mandatory for all Israeli citizens. Adults are required to pay a health tax. General tax revenues supplement the health tax revenues, which the government distributes to the various health plans based on a capitation formula. Each year, the government determines how much from the general tax revenue should be contributed toward the NHI. In 2013, public funds accounted for 60% of NHI revenues. The remaining share came from individuals' copayments, supplemental health insurance, and sales of health products (Rosen, 2016).

Health plans (or sickness funds) offer a predefined basic package of health care services and are prohibited from discriminating against those who have preexisting medical conditions. Recent reforms have added mental health and dental care for children to the benefits package (WHO, 2015). The capitation formula has built-in incentives for the funds to accept a larger number of elderly and chronically ill members. Rather than relying on a single-payer system, the health care reform supported the development of multiple health plans (today there are four competing, nonprofit sickness funds) to foster competition among funds, under the assumption that competition would lead to better quality of care and an increased responsiveness to patient needs. The plans also sell private health insurance to supplement the basic package. The system is believed to provide a high standard of care (Rosen et al., 2016).

Israel has a highly efficient health care system due to the regulated competition between the health plans, the country's strict regulatory controls on the supply of hospital beds, its accessible and high-quality primary care, and its reliance on EHRs (WHO, 2015). In 2014, the Ministry of Health created a national health information exchange for sharing clinical patient data across all general hospitals, health plans, and other providers in the country. Emerging challenges include an increasing reliance on private financing, which affects equity and efficiency, the need to expand public financing and improve the efficiency of the public system, reduction of health inequalities, and goals related to measuring and improving quality of hospital care, reducing surgical waiting times, and enhancing dissemination of comparative data on performance (WHO, 2015).

Japan

Since 1961, Japan has been providing universal coverage to its citizens through two main health insurance schemes: (1) an employer-based system, modeled after Germany's SHI program; and (2) a national health insurance program. Generally, large employers (with more than 300 employees) have their own health programs. Nearly 2,000 private, nonprofit health insurance societies manage insurance for large firms. Smaller companies either band together to provide private health insurance or belong to a government-run plan. Day laborers, seamen, agricultural workers, the self-employed, and retirees are all covered under the national health care program. Individual employees pay roughly 8% of their salaries as premiums and receive coverage for approximately 90% of the cost of medical services, with some limitations. Dependents receive slightly less than 90% coverage. Employers and the national government subsidize the cost of private premiums. Coverage is comprehensive, including most dental care and approved prescription drugs, and patients are free to select their providers (Matsuda, 2016). Providers are paid on a national fee-for-service basis set by the government, and have little control over reimbursement (Ikegami and Anderson, 2012).

Several health policy issues have emerged in Japan in the past few years. First, since 2002, some business leaders and economists have urged the Japanese government to lift its ban on mixed public/private payments for medical services, arguing that private payments should be allowed for services not covered by medical insurance (i.e., services involving new technologies or drugs). The Japan Medical Association and the Ministry of Health, Labor, and Welfare have argued against these recommendations, stating such a policy would favor the wealthy and create disparities in access to care. Although the ban on mixed payments has not been lifted, Prime Minister Koizumi expanded the existing "exceptional approvals system" for new medical technologies in 2004 to allow private payments for selected technologies not covered by medical insurance (Nomura and Nakayama, 2005).

Another policy development in Japan is hospitals' increased use of a system of reimbursement for inpatient care services, called diagnosis–procedure combinations (DPCs). With the DPCs, hospitals receive daily fees for each condition and treatment, proportionate to patients' length of stay regardless of actual provision of tests and interventions. In theory, the DPC system will incentivize hospitals to become more efficient (Nomura and Nakayama, 2005).

Japan's economic stagnation in the last several years has led to an increased pressure to contain the country's health care costs (Ikegami and Campbell, 2004). In 2005, Japan implemented reform initiatives in long-term care (LTC) delivery in an effort to contain the rapidly rising costs in this growing health care sector. The policy required residents in LTC facilities to pay for room and board. It also established new preventive benefits for seniors with low needs. Charging nursing home residents a fee for room and board was a departure from past policies, which had promoted institutionalization of elderly individuals (Tsutsui and Muramatsu, 2007).

Despite their overall success, Japan's health and long-term care systems face sustainability issues similar to those found in the United States, including rising costs and increasing demands for services. The Japanese government is considering and pursuing several options: preventive services, promotion of community-based services, and increases in taxes, premiums, and fees. In 2011, reform centered on the comprehensive community care model was implemented. This model ensures access to long-term care, medical or hospital care, preventive services, residential care facilities, and "life support" (or legal services) within a community where an elder lives. The focus on prevention and service consolidation is expected to result in health populations and, therefore, decreased use of more expensive services.

More recently, health reforms in Japan have introduced the general practitioner (GP) and family physician (FP) system. Starting in 2017, the Japan Primary Care Society will run a training program to qualify doctors as GP/FP specialists (Takamura, 2015). By permitting the Japan Primary Care Society to run this program, the Japanese government aims not only to increase the number of systematically trained GPs/FPs, but also to maintain good community care, improve health outcomes through prevention and primary care, and lower medical expenses. Challenges arising from the GP/FP reform include questions about where to place GPs and FPs (clinics or hospitals), how organ-specialists currently providing primary care will be affected, and whether the GP/FP culture will be accepted by Japanese patients and citizens at large.

Singapore

Prior to 1984, Singapore had a British-style NHS program, in which medical services were provided mainly by the public sector and financed through general taxes. Since then, the nation has designed a system based on market competition and self-reliance. Singapore has achieved universal coverage through a policy that requires mandatory private contributions but little government financing. The program, known as Medisave, mandates every working person, including the self-employed, to deposit a portion of earnings into an individual Medisave account. Employers are required to match employee contributions. These savings can be withdrawn only for two purposes: (1) to pay for hospital services and some selected, expensive physician services; or (2) to purchase a government-sponsored insurance plan, called MediShield, for catastrophic (expensive and major) illness. For basic and routine services, people are expected to pay out of pocket. Out-of-pocket expenditures can be quite high, as only 38% of health spending is publicly funded (Salkeld, 2014). Those who cannot afford to pay for health care services receive government assistance (Hsiao, 1995). In 2002, the government introduced ElderShield, which defrays out-of-pocket medical expenses for elderly persons and severely disabled individuals who require long-term care (Singapore Ministry of Health, 2007). The fee-for-service system of payment is widely used throughout Singapore (McClellan and Kessler, 1999).

In 2006, the Ministry of Health launched the Chronic Disease Management Program. By November 2011, this program covered 10 chronic diseases, including mental health illnesses. More than 700 GP clinics and GP groups are supported by the Ministry to provide comprehensive chronic disease management to patients. Patients can use their own Medisave accounts or their family members' accounts to pay for outpatient services under the program (Singapore Ministry of Health, 2012).

Future challenges in Singapore include adjusting copayments to avoid discouraging patients from seeking necessary primary care and preventive services that might lower their risk of developing chronic diseases. Overall, Singapore faces the challenge of ensuring positive health outcomes and containing costs given an aging population that is facing an increased prevalence of chronic disease (Tan et al., 2014).

Developing Countries

Developing countries, which are home to almost 85% of the world's population, are responsible for only 11% of the world's total health spending—even though they account for 93% of the worldwide burden of disease. The six developing regions of the world are East Asia and the Pacific, Europe (mainly Eastern Europe) and Central Asia, Latin America and the Caribbean, the Middle East and North Africa, South Asia, and sub-Saharan Africa. Of these regions, the latter two have the least resources and the greatest health burden. On a per-capita basis, industrialized countries have six times as many hospital beds and three times as many physicians than do developing countries. People with private financial means can find reasonably good health care in many parts of the developing world. Unfortunately, the majority of the populations have to depend on limited government services that are often of questionable quality, when evaluated by Western standards. As a general observation, government financing for health services increases in countries with higher per-capita incomes (Schieber and Maeda, 1999).

Developing countries are moving toward adopting universal health coverage to decrease the financial impoverishment due to health spending, improve health, and increase access to care (Lagomarsino et al., 2012). Trends in health reforms in developing countries include increasing enrollment in government-sponsored health insurance, expanded benefits packages, decreasing out-of-pocket expenditures, and increasing the government's share of health spending. Countries that have successfully met the Millennium

Development Goals—the world's time-bound and quantified targets for addressing extreme poverty in its many dimensions (income poverty, hunger, disease, lack of adequate shelter, and exclusion) while promoting gender equality, education, and environmental sustainability—have used a comprehensive set of strategies to reduce maternal and child mortality, improve health financing, address workforce challenges, and improve quality of care (Ahmed et al., 2016).

▶ Global Health Challenges and Reform

There is a huge gap in health care and health status between developing and developed countries. For example, in 2014, the global life expectancy at birth was 71.4 years of age, but life expectancy in the African region was only 60 years (WHO, 2016). In that same year, infant mortality rates varied between 2 deaths per 1,000 live births and 110 deaths per 1,000 live births. There were also wide variations in health care for pregnant women, availability of skilled health personnel for childbirth, and access to medicine.

The poor quality and low efficiency of health care services in many countries—especially services provided by the public sector, which is often the main source of care for poor people—have become a serious issue for decision makers in these countries (Sachs, 2012). This issue, combined with the rising out-of-pocket costs and high numbers of uninsured, has forced many governments to launch health care reform efforts. Many low and middle-income countries are moving toward universal health coverage (Lagomarsino et al., 2012). Even so, international health assistance continues to play a significant role in health care in many developing countries. Global aid for health care increased from $10 billion in 2000 to $27 billion in 2010 (Sachs, 2012), but then began to decrease in 2011 because of a global recession (Organization for Economic Cooperation and Development [OECD], 2012).

Since 1999, the Bill and Melinda Gates Foundation (2017) has invested $7 billion in international health delivery programs. This foundation's focus is on coordination of delivery efforts, strengthening of country health systems, and building of integrated delivery systems. Funded initiatives include community health worker programs, information and communications technology, and investment into data systems. From 2010 to 2015, USAID dedicated $50 billion to strengthening international health systems. This U.S. agency set forth a plan for continuing its progress, from 2015 to 2019, by strengthening six interrelated health system functions: (1) human resources for health; (2) health finance; (3) health governance; (4) health information; (5) medical products, vaccines, and technologies; and (6) service delivery (USAID, 2015). The ultimate goal of that initiative is to strengthen these systems so they will contribute to positive health outcomes and create an environment for universal health coverage.

▶ The Systems Framework

A **system** consists of a set of interrelated and interdependent, logically coordinated components designed to achieve common goals. Even though the various functional components of the health services delivery structure in the United States are, at best, only loosely coordinated, the main components can be identified using a systems model. The systems framework used here helps one understand that the structure of health care services in the United States is based on some foundations, provides a logical arrangement of the various components, and demonstrates a progression from inputs to outputs. The main elements of this arrangement are system inputs (resources), system structure, system processes, and system outputs (outcomes). In addition, system outlook (future directions) is a necessary feature of a dynamic system. This systems framework is used as the conceptual base for organizing later chapters in this text (**FIGURE 1-5**).

System Foundations

The current health care system is not an accident. Historical, cultural, social, and economic factors explain its current structure. These factors also affect forces that shape new trends and developments, as well as those that impede change. The chapters titled *Beliefs, Values, and Health* and *The Evolution of Health Services in the United States* provide a discussion of the system foundations.

System Resources

No mechanism for health services delivery can fulfill its primary objective without deploying the necessary human and nonhuman resources. Human resources consist of the various types and categories of workers directly engaged in the

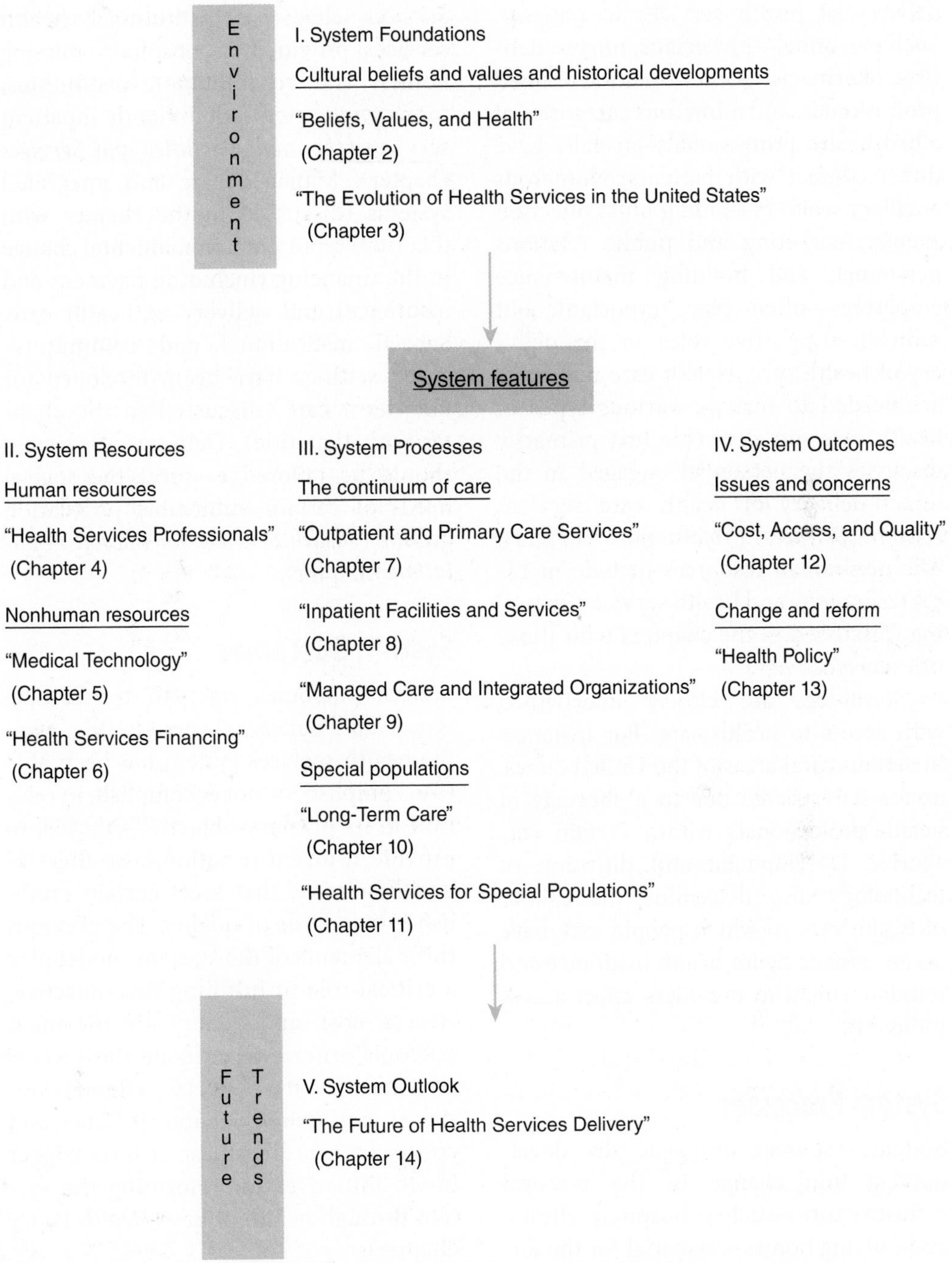

Environment

I. System Foundations

Cultural beliefs and values and historical developments

"Beliefs, Values, and Health"
(Chapter 2)

"The Evolution of Health Services in the United States"
(Chapter 3)

System features

II. System Resources

Human resources

"Health Services Professionals"
(Chapter 4)

Nonhuman resources

"Medical Technology"
(Chapter 5)

"Health Services Financing"
(Chapter 6)

III. System Processes

The continuum of care

"Outpatient and Primary Care Services"
(Chapter 7)

"Inpatient Facilities and Services"
(Chapter 8)

"Managed Care and Integrated Organizations"
(Chapter 9)

Special populations

"Long-Term Care"
(Chapter 10)

"Health Services for Special Populations"
(Chapter 11)

IV. System Outcomes

Issues and concerns

"Cost, Access, and Quality"
(Chapter 12)

Change and reform

"Health Policy"
(Chapter 13)

Future Trends

V. System Outlook

"The Future of Health Services Delivery"
(Chapter 14)

FIGURE 1-5 The systems model and related chapters.

delivery of health services to patients. Such personnel—physicians, nurses, dentists, pharmacists, other doctoral-trained professionals, and numerous categories of allied health professionals—usually have direct contact with patients. Numerous ancillary workers—billing and collection agents, marketing and public relations personnel, and building maintenance employees—often play important, but indirect, supportive roles in the delivery of health care. Health care managers are needed to manage various types of health care services. This text primarily discusses the personnel engaged in the direct delivery of health care services (*Health Services Professionals* chapter). The nonhuman resources include medical technology and health services financing (discussed in the chapters with those titles, respectively).

Resources are closely intertwined with access to health care. For instance, in certain rural areas of the United States, access is restricted due to a shortage of health professionals within certain categories. Development and diffusion of technology also determine the caliber of health care to which people may have access. Financing for health insurance and reimbursement to providers affect access indirectly.

System Processes

System resources influence the development and change in the physical infrastructure—such as hospitals, clinics, and nursing homes—essential for the different processes of health care delivery. Most health care services are delivered in noninstitutional settings, mainly associated with processes referred to as outpatient care (*Outpatient and Primary Care*

Services chapter). Institutional health services provided in hospitals, nursing homes, and rehabilitation institutions, for example, are predominantly inpatient services (*Inpatient Facilities and Services* chapter). Managed care and integrated systems (discussed in the chapter with that title) represent a fundamental change in the financing (including payment and insurance) and delivery of health care. Special institutional and community-based settings have been developed for long-term care (discussed in the chapter with that title). Delivery of services should be tailored to meet the special needs of certain vulnerable population groups (*Health Services for Special Populations* chapter).

System Outcomes

System outcomes refer to the critical issues and concerns surrounding what the health services system has been able to accomplish, or not accomplish, in relation to its primary objective—that is, to provide, to an entire nation, cost-effective health services that meet certain established standards of quality. The previous three elements of the systems model play a critical role in fulfilling this objective. Access, cost, and quality are the main outcome criteria to evaluate the success of a health care delivery system (*Cost, Access, and Quality* chapter). Issues and concerns regarding these criteria trigger broad initiatives for reforming the system through health policy (*Health Policy* chapter).

System Outlook

A dynamic health care system must be forward looking. In essence, it must project into the future the accomplishment of desired system outcomes in view of anticipated social, economic, political, technological, informational, ecological, anthro-cultural, and global forces of change (*The Future of Health Services Delivery* chapter).

▶ Summary

The United States has a unique system of health care delivery. Its basic features characterize it as a patchwork of subsystems. Health care is delivered through an amalgam of private and public financing, through private health insurance and public insurance programs; the latter programs are reserved for special groups. Contrary to popular opinion, health care delivery in the United States is not governed by free-market principles; at best, it is an imperfect market. Yet, the system is not dominated or controlled by a single entity as would be the case in national health care systems.

No country in the world has a perfect health care insurance system, and most nations with a national health care program also have a private sector that varies in size. Because of resource limitations, universal access remains a theoretical concept even in countries that offer universal health insurance coverage. The developing countries of the world also face serious challenges due to the scarcity of resources and strong underlying needs for services in those nations.

Health care managers must understand how the health care delivery system works and evolves. Such an understanding can help them maintain a strategic position within the macro environment of the health care system. The systems framework provides an organized approach to an understanding of the various components of the U.S. health care delivery system.

▶ Test Your Understanding

Terminology

access
administrative costs
balance bill
defensive medicine
demand
enrollee
free market
global budgets
health care reform
health plan
managed care
Medicaid
Medicare

moral hazard
national health
    insurance (NHI)
national health
    system (NHS)
need
package pricing
phantom providers
premium cost sharing
primary care
provider
provider-induced
    demand

quad-function model
reimbursement
single-payer system
socialized health
    insurance (SHI)
standards of
    participation
system
third party
uninsured
universal access
universal coverage
utilization

Review Questions

1. Why does cost containment remain an elusive goal in U.S. health services delivery?
2. What are the two main objectives of a health care delivery system?
3. Name the four basic functional components of the U.S. health care delivery system. Which role does each play in the delivery of health care?
4. What is the primary reason for employers to purchase insurance plans to provide health benefits to their employees?
5. Why is it that, despite public and private health insurance programs, some U.S. citizens are without health care coverage?
6. What is managed care?
7. Why is the U.S. health care market referred to as "imperfect"?
8. Discuss the intermediary role of insurance in the delivery of health care.
9. Who are the major players in the U.S. health services system? What are the positive and negative effects of the often conflicting self-interests of these players?
10. Which main roles does the government play in the U.S. health services system?
11. Why is it important for health care managers and policymakers to understand the intricacies of the health care delivery system?
12. What is the difference between national health insurance (NHI) and a national health system (NHS)?
13. What is socialized health insurance (SHI)?
14. Provide a general overview of the Affordable Care Act. What is its main goal?

▶ References

Ahmed, S. M., et al. 2016. Cross-country analysis of strategies for achieving progress towards global goals for women's and children's health. *Bulletin of the World Health Organization* 94, no. 5: 351–361.

Akaho, E., et al. 1998. A proposed optimal health care system based on a comparative study conducted between Canada and Japan. *Canadian Journal of Public Health* 89, no. 5: 301–307.

Altman, S. H., and U. E. Reinhardt. 1996. Introduction: Where does health care reform go from here? An uncharted odyssey. In: *Strategic choices for a changing health care system*. S. H. Altman and U. E. Reinhardt, eds. Chicago, IL: Health Administration Press. pp. xxi–xxxii.

Altman, S. H., and S. S. Wallack. 1996. Health care spending: Can the United States control it? In: *Strategic choices for a changing health care system*. S. H. Altman and U. E. Reinhardt, eds. Chicago, IL: Health Administration Press. pp. 1–32.

American Association of Colleges of Pharmacy. 2017. *Academic pharmacy's vital statistics*. Available at: http://www.aacp.org/about/Pages /Vitalstats.aspx. Accessed April 2017.

American Dental Association. 2017. *Education*. Available at: http://www.ada.org/en/science -research/health-policy-institute/dental -statistics/education. Accessed April 2017.

Arora, S., et al. 2013. *Public payment and private provision: The changing landscape of health care in the 2000s.* Nuffield Trust. Available at: https://www.nuffieldtrust.org.uk/research/public-payment-and-private-provision-the-changing-landscape-of-health-care-in-the-2000s. Accessed February 2017.

Association of American Medical Colleges. 2017. *2016 data book.* Available at: https://www.aamc.org/data/databook/tables/. Accessed April 2017.

Australian Government. 2011. *Improving primary health care for all Australians.* Canberra, Australian: Commonwealth of Australia. Available at: http://www.g21.com.au/sites/default/files/dmdocuments/ImprovingPHCforallAustralians.pdf. Accessed April 2017.

Australian Government, Department of Health. 2016. *Department of Health annual report 2015–16.* Canberra, Australia: Commonwealth of Australia. Available at: http://www.health.gov.au/internet/main/publishing.nsf/Content/annual-report2015-16. Accessed February 2017.

Australian Institute of Health and Welfare. 2017. *Australia's health system.* Available at: http://www.aihw.gov.au/australias-health/2016/health-system/. Accessed April 2017.

Barber, S. L., et al. 2013. The reform of the essential medicines system in China: A comprehensive approach to universal coverage. *Journal of Global Health* 3, no. 1: 10303.

Barua, B., et al. 2016. *The sustainability of health care spending in Canada.* Vancouver, Canada: Fraser Institute.

Bill and Melinda Gates Foundation. 2017. *Integrated delivery strategy system.* Available at: http://www.gatesfoundation.org/What-We-Do/Global-Development/Integrated-Delivery. Accessed February 2017.

Blumel, M., and R. Busse. 2016. *The German health care system.* The Commonwealth Fund. Available at: http://international.commonwealthfund.org/countries/germany/. Accessed February 2017.

Blumenthal, D., and W. Hsiao. 2005. Privatization and its discontents: The evolving Chinese health care system. *New England Journal of Medicine* 353, no. 11: 1165–1170.

Brown, L. D., and V. E. Amelung. 1999. "Manacled competition": Market reforms in German health care. *Health Affairs* 18, no. 3: 76–91.

Brownie, S., et al. 2014. Australian health reforms: Enhancing interprofessional practice and competency within the health workforce. *The Journal of Interprofessional Care* 28, no. 3: 252–253.

Canada Minister and Attorney General. 2016. *Canada Health Act.* Available at: http://laws-lois.justice.gc.ca/eng/acts/c-6/. Accessed April 2017.

Canadian Institute for Health Information. 2012. *National health expenditure trends, 1975 to 2012.* Ottawa, ON: The Institute. Available at: https://secure.cihi.ca/free_products/NHEXTrendsReport2012EN.pdf. Accessed December 2013.

Centers for Medicare and Medicaid. 2015. *National health expenditures 2015 highlights.* Available at: https://www.cms.gov/research-statistics-data-and-systems/statistics-trends-and-reports/nationalhealthexpenddata/downloads/highlights.pdf. Accessed February 2017.

Church, J., and P. Barker. 1998. Regionalization of health services in Canada: A critical perspective. *International Journal of Health Services* 28, no. 3: 467–486.

Cohen, R. A., et al. 2016. *Health insurance coverage: Early release of estimates from the National Health Interview Survey, January–March 2016.* National Center for Health Statistics. Available at: http://www.cdc.gov/nchs/nhis/releases.htm. Accessed February 2017.

Deloitte. 2017. *2017 global health care sector outlook: Making progress against persistent challenges.* Available at: https://www2.deloitte.com/global/en/pages/life-sciences-and-healthcare/articles/global-health-care-sector-outlook.html. Accessed February 2017.

DeVore, S. 2014. *The changing health care world: Trends to watch in 2014.* Available at: http://healthaffairs.org/blog/2014/02/10/the-changing-health-care-world-trends-to-watch-in-2014/. Accessed May 2016.

Dickson, G. 2016. Health reform in Canada: Enabling perspectives for health leadership. *Healthcare Manage Forum* 29, no. 2: 53–58.

Dixon, A., and R. Robinson. 2002. The United Kingdom. In: *Health care systems in eight* countries: Trends and challenges. A. Dixon and E. Mossialos, eds. London, UK: European Observatory on Health Care Systems, London School of Economics & Political Science. pp. 103–114.

Feldstein, P. J. 1993. Health care economics. 4th ed. New York, NY: Delmar.

Granovsky, D. 2016. A new government: A new open and collaborative era? Canadian Nurse 112, no. 1: 15–18.

Hall, J. 1999. Incremental change in the Australian health care system. Health Affairs 18, no. 3: 95–110.

Health Canada. 2013. Available at: http://laws-lois .justice.gc.ca/eng/acts/C-6/index.html. Accessed July 2013.

Health Council of Canada. 2013. Progress report 2013. Available at: http://www.healthcouncilcanada .ca/rpt_det.php?id=481. Accessed July 2013.

Health Resources and Services Administration (HRSA). 2015. 2015 health center data: Health center program grantee data. Available at: https://bphc.hrsa.gov/uds/datacenter.aspx. Accessed February 2017.

Health Systems and Policy Monitor (HSPM). 2012. Health systems in transition (HiT) profile of Canada. Available at: http://www.hspm .org/countries/canada22042013/livinghit .aspx?Section=6.1%20Analysis%20of% 20recent%20reforms&Type=Section. Accessed April 2017.

Health Systems and Policy Monitor (HSPM). 2015. United Kingdom. Available at: http://www.hspm .org/countries/england11032013/countrypage .aspx. Accessed May 2016.

Health Systems and Policy Monitor (HSPM). 2016. Country page: Germany. Available at: http:// www.hspm.org/countries/germany28082014 /countrypage.aspx. Accessed February 2017.

Healy, J. 2002. Australia. In: Health care systems in eight countries: Trends and challenges. A. Dixon and E. Mossialos, eds. London, UK: European Observatory on Health Care Systems, London School of Economics & Political Science. pp. 3–16.

Hemenway, D., and D. Fallon. 1985. Testing for physician-induced demand with hypothetical cases. Medical Care 23, no. 4: 344–349.

Hsiao, W. C. 1995. Medical savings accounts: Lessons from Singapore. Health Affairs 14, no. 2: 260–266.

Hsu, S. 2015. China's health care reforms. Available at: http://thediplomat.com/2015/05/chinas-health -care-reforms/. Accessed May 2016.

Ikegami, N., and G. F. Anderson. 2012. In Japan, all-payer rate setting under tight government control has proved to be an effective approach to containing costs. Health Affairs 31, no. 5: 1049–1056.

Ikegami, N., and J. C. Campbell. 2004. Japan's health care system: Containing costs and attempting reform. Health Affairs 23: 26–36.

Impact of Obamacare on coverage. 2016. Congressional Digest 95, no. 3: 7–32.

Kaiser Family Foundation. 2017. Current status of state Medicaid expansion decisions. Available at: http://kff.org/health-reform/slide/current-status -of-the-medicaid-expansion-decision/. Accessed February 2017.

Lagomarsino, G., et al. 2012. Moving towards universal health coverage: Health insurance reforms in nine developing countries in Africa and Asia. Lancet 380, no. 9845, 933–943.

MacPhee, S. 1996. Reform the watchword as OECD countries struggle to contain health care costs. Canadian Medical Association Journal 154, no. 5: 699–701.

Matsuda, R. 2016. The Japanese health care system, 2015. In: International profiles of health care systems, 2015. E. Mossialos, M. Wenzl, R. Osborn, and D. Sarnak, eds. New York, NY: The Commonwealth Fund. pp. 107–114. Available at: http://www.commonwealthfund.org/~/media /files/publications/fund-report/2016/jan/1857 _mossialos_intl_profiles_2015_v7.pdf. Accessed February 2017.

McClellan, M., and D. Kessler. 1999. A global analysis of technological change in health care: The case of heart attacks. Health Affairs 18, no. 3: 250–257.

National Health Services England. (2015). Five Year Forward View: Time to deliver. Available at: https://www.england.nhs.uk/wp-content/uploads /2015/06/5yfv-time-to-deliver-25-06.pdf. Accessed February 2017.

Naylor, C. D. 1999. Health care in Canada: Incrementalism under fiscal duress. Health Affairs 18, no. 3: 9–26.

Nomura, H., and T. Nakayama. 2005. The Japanese healthcare system. BMJ 331: 648–649.

Office of National Statistics. 2015. Expenditure on healthcare in the UK, 2013. Available at: https://

socialwelfare.bl.uk/subject-areas/services -activity/health-services/ons/176574dcp171766 _399822.pdf. Accessed April 2017.

Organization for Economic Cooperation and Development (OECD). 2012. *Development: Aid to developing countries falls because of global recession.* Available at: http://www.oecd .org/newsroom/developmentaidtodeveloping countriesfallsbecauseofglobalrecession.htm. Accessed April 2017.

Parente, S. T., and R. Feldman. 2013. Micro-simulation of private health insurance and Medicaid take-up following the U.S. Supreme Court decision upholding the Affordable Care Act. *Health Services Research* 48, no. 2 Pt 2: 826–849.

Podger, A. 1999. Reforming the Australian health care system: A government perspective. *Health Affairs* 18, no. 3: 111–113.

Rodin, J., and D. de Ferranti. 2012. Universal health coverage: The third global health transition? *Lancet* 380, no. 9845: 861–862.

Rosen, B. 2016. The Israeli health care system, 2015. In: *International profiles of health care systems, 2015.* E. Mossialos, M. Wenzl, R. Osborn, and D. Sarnak, eds. New York, NY: The Commonwealth Fund. pp. 87-95. Available at: http://www.commonwealthfund.org/~/media /files/publications/fund-report/2016/jan/1857 _mossialos_intl_profiles_2015_v7.pdf. Accessed February 2017.

Rosen, B., et al. 2016. Israel: Health system review. *Health Systems in Transition* 17, no. 6: 1–243.

Sachs, J. D. 2012. Achieving universal health coverage in low-income settings. *Lancet* 380, no. 9845: 944–947.

Salkeld, G. 2014. *Creating a better health system: lessons from Singapore.* The Conversation. Available at: http://theconversation.com/creating -a-better-health-system-lessons-from -singapore-30607. Accessed May 2016.

Santerre, R. E., and S. P. Neun. 1996. *Health economics: Theories, insights, and industry studies.* Chicago, IL: Irwin.

Schieber, G., and A. Maeda. 1999. Health care financing and delivery in developing countries. *Health Affairs* 18, no. 3: 193–205.

Singapore Ministry of Health. 2007. *Eldershield experience 2002-2007.* Available at: https://www.moh.gov.sg/content/dam/moh_web /Publications/Information%20Papers/2007 /ESH_Experience_2002-2007.pdf. Accessed April 2017.

Singapore Ministry of Health. 2012. *Medisave for Chronic Disease Management Programme (CDMP) and vaccinations.* Available at: http://www.moh.gov.sg/content/moh_web/home /policies-and-issues/elderly_healthcare.html. Accessed December 2013.

Takamura, A. 2015. The present circumstance of primary care in Japan. *Quality in Primary Care* 23, no. 5: 262.

Tan, K. B., et al. 2014. Monitoring and evaluating progress towards universal health coverage in Singapore. *PLoS Medicine* 11, no. 9: e1001695.

Thorlby, R., and S. Arora. 2016. The English health care system, 2015. In: *International profiles of health care systems, 2015.* E. Mossialos, M. Wenzl, R. Osborn, and D. Sarnak, eds. New York, NY: The Commonwealth Fund. pp. 49–58. Available at: http://www.commonwealthfund.org/~/media /files/publications/fund-report/2016/jan/1857 _mossialos_intl_profiles_2015_v7.pdf. Accessed February 2017.

Tsutsui, T., and N. Muramatsu. 2007. Japan's universal long-term care system reform of 2005: Containing costs and realizing a vision. *Journal of the American Geriatrics Society* 55: 1458–1463.

Uberoi, N., et al. 2016. *Health insurance coverage and the Affordable Care Act, 2010–2016. ASPE Issue Brief.* Washington, DC: Office of the Assistant Secretary for Planning and Evaluation.

USAID. 2015. *USAID's vision for health systems strengthening: 2015–2019.* Available at: https://www.usaid.gov/what-we-do/global-health /health-systems/usaids-vision-health-systems -strengthening. Accessed February 2017.

U.S. Census Bureau. 2012. *The 2012 statistical abstract.* Available at: https://www2.census .gov/library/publications/2011/compendia /statab/131ed/2012-statab.pdf. Accessed April 2017.

Wagstaff, A., et al. 2009. China's health system and its reform: A review of recent studies. *Health Economics* 18: S7–S23.

Willcox, S. 2001. Promoting private health insurance in Australia. *Health Affairs* 20, no. 3: 152–161.

Wolinsky, F. D. 1988. *The sociology of health: Principles, practitioners, and issues.* 2nd ed. Belmont, CA: Wadsworth.

World Health Organization (WHO). 2014. Germany: Health system review. *Health Systems in Transition* 16, no. 2. Available at: http://www.euro.who.int/__data/assets/pdf _file/0008/255932/HiT-Germany.pdf?ua=1. Accessed May 2016.

World Health Organization (WHO). 2015. Israel: Health system review. *Health Systems in Transition* 17, no. 6. Available at: http://www.euro .who.int/__data/assets/pdf_file/0009/302967 /Israel-HiT.pdf. Accessed May 2016.

World Health Organization (WHO). 2016. *World health statistics 2016*. Available at: http://www

.who.int/gho/publications/world_health _statistics/2016/en/. Accessed February 2017.

Yip, W., and W. C. Hsiao. 2008. The Chinese health system at a crossroads. *Health Affairs* 27: 460–468.

Yip, W., and A. Mahal. 2008. The health care systems of China and India: Performance and future challenges. *Health Affairs* 27: 921–932.

Yip, W. C., et al. 2012. Early appraisal of China's huge and complex health-care reforms. *Lancet* 379, no. 9818: 833–842.

Zhu, C. 2015. *Healthy China 2020*. Singapore: People's Medical Publishing House.

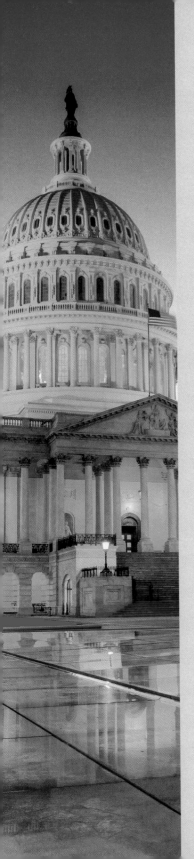

PART I

System Foundations

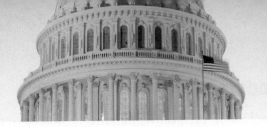

CHAPTER 2

Beliefs, Values, and Health

LEARNING OBJECTIVES

- Study the concepts of health and disease, risk factors, and the role of health promotion and disease prevention.
- Summarize the disease prevention requisites under the Affordable Care Act.
- Get an overview of public health and appreciate its expanding role in health protection both in the United States and globally.
- Explore the determinants of health and measures related to health.
- Understand the American anthro-cultural values and their implications for health care delivery.
- Evaluate justice and equity in health care according to contrasting theories.
- Explore the integration of individual and population health.

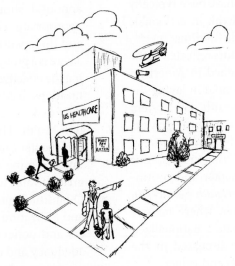

"This is the market justice system. Social justice is over there."

▶ Introduction

From an economic perspective, curative medicine appears to produce decreasing returns in health improvement while increasing health care expenditures (Saward and Sorensen, 1980). There has also been a growing recognition of the benefits afforded to society by the promotion of health and the prevention of disease, disability, and premature death. Even so, progress in this direction has been slow because of the prevailing social values and beliefs, which continue to focus on curing diseases rather than promoting health. The common definitions of health, as well as measures for evaluating health status, reflect similar inclinations. This chapter proposes a balanced approach to health, although fully achieving such an ideal is not without difficult challenges. The 10-year *Healthy People* initiatives, undertaken by the U.S. Department of Health and Human Services (DHHS) since 1980, illustrate steps taken in this direction, even though these initiatives have been typically strong in rhetoric but weak in actionable strategies and sustainable funding.

Anthro-cultural factors reflected in the beliefs and values ingrained in American culture have been influential in laying the foundations of a U.S. health care system that has remained predominantly private, as opposed to a tax-financed national health care program. Discussion of this theme begins in this chapter and continues in the *Evolution of Health Services in the United States* chapter, where failures of past proposals to create a nationalized health care system are discussed in the context of cultural beliefs and values.

This chapter further explores the issue of equity in the distribution of health services, using contrasting theories of market justice and social justice. U.S. health care delivery incorporates both principles, which are complementary in some ways and create conflicts in other areas.

▶ Significance for Managers and Policymakers

Materials covered in this chapter have several implications for health services managers and policymakers alike:

- The health status of a population has tremendous bearing on the utilization of health services, assuming the services are readily available. Planning of health services must be governed by demographic and health trends and initiatives toward reducing disease and disability.
- The basic meanings of health, determinants of health, and health risk appraisal should be used to design appropriate educational, preventive, and therapeutic initiatives.
- There is a growing emphasis on evaluating the effectiveness of health care organizations based on the contributions they make to community and population health. The concepts discussed in this chapter can guide administrators in implementing programs that have the greatest value to their communities.
- Quantified measures of health status and utilization can be used by managers and policymakers to evaluate the adequacy and effectiveness of existing programs, plan new strategies, measure progress, and discontinue ineffective services.

▶ Basic Concepts of Health

Health

In the United States, the concepts of health and health care have largely been governed by the medical model, more specifically referred to as the biomedical model. The **medical model** defines health as the absence of illness or disease. This definition implies that optimal health exists when a person is free of symptoms and does not require medical treatment. However, it is not a definition of health in the true sense. This prevailing view of health emphasizes clinical diagnoses and medical interventions to treat disease or symptoms of disease, but fails to account for prevention of disease and health promotion. Therefore, when the term "health care delivery" is used, in reality it refers to *medical* care delivery.

Medical sociologists have gone a step further in defining health as the state of optimal capacity of an individual to perform his or her expected social roles and tasks, such as work, school, and household chores (Parsons, 1972). A person who is unable (as opposed to unwilling) to perform his or her social roles in society is considered sick. However, this concept also seems inadequate because many people continue to engage in their social obligations despite suffering from pain, cough, colds, and other types of temporary disabilities, including mental distress. Their efforts are counterbalanced by individuals who shirk their social responsibilities even when they may be in good health. In other words, optimal health is not necessarily reflected in a person's engagement in social roles and responsibilities.

An emphasis on both the physical and mental dimensions of health is found in the definition of health proposed by the Society for Academic Emergency Medicine. According to this organization, health is "a state of physical and mental well-being that facilitates the achievement of individual and societal goals" (Ethics Committee, Society for Academic Emergency Medicine, 1992). This view of health recognizes the importance of achieving harmony between the physiological and emotional dimensions.

The definition of health developed by the World Health Organization (WHO) is most often cited as the ideal for health care delivery systems; it recognizes that optimal health is more than the absence of disease or infirmity. WHO (1948) defines health as "a state of complete physical, mental and social well-being and not merely the absence of disease or infirmity." As a biopsychosocial model, WHO's definition specifically identifies social well-being as a third dimension of health. For example, having a social support network is positively associated with resilience to life stresses, self-esteem, and social relations. Conversely, many studies show that social isolation is associated with a higher risk of poor health and mortality (Pantell et al., 2013).

WHO has also defined a health care system as all the activities whose primary purpose is to promote, restore, or maintain health (McKee, 2001). As this chapter points out, health care should include much more than medical care. Thus, **health care** can be defined as a variety of services believed to improve a person's health and well-being.

In recent decades, increased interest has been directed toward **holistic health**, which emphasizes the well-being of every aspect of what makes a person whole and complete. Thus, **holistic medicine** seeks to treat the individual as a whole person (Ward, 1995). For example, within this approach, diagnosis and treatment would take into account the mental, emotional, spiritual, nutritional, environmental, and other factors surrounding the origin of disease (Cohen, 2003).

In addition to the physical, mental, and social aspects necessary for optimal health, the spiritual dimension is incorporated as a fourth element in holistic health (**FIGURE 2-1**). A growing volume of medical literature, both in the United States and abroad, points to the healing effects of a person's religion and spirituality on morbidity and mortality. The importance of spirituality as an aspect of health care is also reflected in a number of policy documents produced by the WHO (2003) and other bodies.

Based on their extensive review of the literature, Chida et al. (2009) concluded that religious practice/spirituality is associated with reductions in deaths from all causes as well as deaths from cardiovascular diseases. Patients with heart disease who attend regular religious services have been found to have a significant survival advantage (Oman et al., 2002). Religious and spiritual beliefs and practices have been shown to have a positive impact on a person's physical, mental, and social well-being. In addition, many studies have identified a positive relationship between religious practice and protective health behaviors (Chida et al., 2009). Several religious communities promote healthy lifestyles in terms of (lack of) tobacco use, (lack of) alcohol consumption, and diet. An examination of the literature found a reduced risk for cancer in these communities (Hoff et al., 2008). Spiritual well-being has also been recognized as an important internal resource for helping people cope with illness. For instance, in a study conducted at the University of Michigan, 93% of the women undergoing cancer treatment indicated that their religious lives helped them sustain their hope (Roberts et al., 1997). Studies have also found that a large percentage of patients want their physicians to consider their spiritual needs, and almost half express a desire for the physicians to pray with them if they can (Post et al., 2000).

The spiritual dimension is frequently tied to one's religious beliefs, values, morals, and practices. Broadly, this dimension is described as meaning, purpose, and fulfillment in life; hope and will to live; faith; and a person's relationship with God (Marwick, 1995; Ross, 1995; Swanson, 1995). A clinically tested scale to measure spiritual well-being included categories such as belief in a power greater than oneself, purpose in life, faith, trust in providence, prayer, meditation, group worship, ability to forgive, and gratitude for life (Hatch et al., 1998). In addition, several formal assessments have been developed

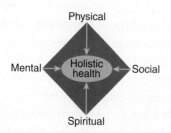

FIGURE 2-1 The four dimensions of holistic health.

to help physicians address the spiritual needs of their patients. One such tool is the HOPE Questions, which enable physicians to speak about spirituality with their patients so as to obtain important information about patients' view of health care and faith (Anandarajoh and Hight, 2001).

Respect for patient values and beliefs is increasingly recognized as an important aspect of culturally appropriate care by the medical community. An increasing number of medical schools and continuing education courses now offer formal courses in spirituality in medicine (Fortin and Barnett, 2004). Furthermore, the Joint Commission (2003) recommends that health care institutions accommodate and assess patients' spiritual beliefs and practices as a routine part of care.

The Committee on Religion and Psychiatry of the American Psychiatric Association has issued a position statement to emphasize the importance of maintaining respect for a patient's religious/spiritual beliefs. In fact, in 2013, "religious or spiritual problem" was included as a diagnostic category for the first time in the most recent edition of the *Diagnostic and Statistical Manual of Mental Disorders, Fifth Edition* (DSM-5). The holistic approach to health also alludes to the need to incorporate alternative therapies into the predominant medical model.

▶ Quality of Life

The term **quality of life** is used to capture the essence of overall satisfaction with life during and following a person's encounter with the health care delivery system. This term is employed in two ways. First, it is an indicator of how satisfied a person is with his or her experiences while receiving health care. Specific life domains—such as comfort factors, respect, privacy, security, degree of independence, decision-making autonomy, and attention to personal preferences—are significant to most people. These factors, in turn, are now regarded as rights that patients can demand during any type of health care encounter. Second, quality of life can refer to a person's overall satisfaction with life and with self-perceptions of health, particularly after some medical intervention. The implication is that desirable processes during medical treatment and successful outcomes should subsequently have a positive effect on an individual's ability to function, carry out social roles and obligations, and have a sense of fulfillment and self-worth.

▶ Risk Factors and Disease

The occurrence of disease involves more than just a single factor. For example, the mere presence of the tubercle bacillus does not automatically mean the infected person will develop tuberculosis. Other factors, such as poverty, overcrowding, and malnutrition, may be essential for development of the disease (Friedman, 1980). Hence, tracing **risk factors**—attributes that increase the likelihood of developing a particular disease or negative health condition in the future—requires a broad approach.

One useful explanation of disease occurrence (for communicable diseases, in particular) is provided by the tripartite model, sometimes referred to as the Epidemiology Triangle (**FIGURE 2-2**). In this model, the **host** is the organism—generally, a human—that becomes sick. Factors associated with the host include

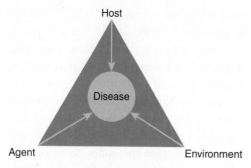

FIGURE 2-2 The Epidemiology Triangle.

genetic makeup, level of immunity, fitness, and personal habits and behaviors. For the host to become sick, an **agent** must be present, although presence of an agent does not ensure that disease will occur. In the previous example, tubercle bacillus is the agent for tuberculosis. Other examples of agents include chemicals, radiation, tobacco smoke, dietary indiscretions, and nutritional deficiencies. The third entity, **environment**, is external to the host and includes the physical, social, cultural, and economic aspects of the environment. Examples include sanitation, air pollution, anthro-cultural beliefs, social equity, social norms, and economic status. The environmental factors play a moderating role that can either enhance or reduce susceptibility to disease. Because the three entities of host, agent, and environment often interact to produce disease, disease prevention efforts should focus on a broad approach to mitigate or eliminate risk factors associated with all three entities.

Behavioral Risk Factors

Certain individual behaviors and personal lifestyle choices represent important risk factors for illness and disease. For example, smoking has been identified as the leading cause of preventable disease and death in the United States because it significantly increases the risk of heart disease, stroke, lung cancer, and chronic lung disease (DHHS, 2004). Substance abuse, inadequate physical exercise, a high-fat diet, irresponsible use of motor vehicles, and unsafe sex are additional examples of behavioral risk factors. **TABLE 2-1** presents the percentages of the U.S. population with selected behavioral risks.

Acute, Subacute, and Chronic Conditions

Disease can be classified as acute, subacute, or chronic. An **acute condition** is relatively severe, episodic (of short duration), and often treatable and subject to recovery. Treatments are generally provided in a hospital. Examples of acute conditions include a sudden interruption of kidney function and a myocardial infarction (heart attack). A **subacute condition** is a less severe phase of an acute illness. It can be a postacute condition, requiring continuity of treatment after discharge from a hospital. Examples include ventilator and head trauma care. A **chronic condition** is one that persists over time, is not severe, but is generally irreversible. A chronic condition may be kept under control through appropriate medical treatment, but if left untreated, it may lead to severe and life-threatening health problems. Examples of chronic conditions are hypertension, asthma, arthritis, heart disease, and diabetes. Contributors to chronic disease include ethnic, cultural, and behavioral factors and the social and physical environment, as discussed later in this chapter.

TABLE 2-1 Percentage of U.S. Population with Behavioral Risks

Behavioral Risks	Percentage of Population	Year
Alcohol (12 years and older)	52.7	2014
Marijuana (12 years and older)	8.4	2014
Cocaine use (12th graders)	1.0	2014
Cocaine use (10th graders)	0.6	2014
Cocaine use (8th graders)	0.5	2014
Cigarette smoking (18 years and older)	16.8	2014
Hypertension (20 years and older)	30.4	2011–2014
Overweight and obese (20 years and older)	69.5	2011–2014
Serum cholesterol (20 years and older)	12.1	2011–2014

Note: Data are based on household interviews of a sample of the civilian noninstitutionalized population 12 years of age and older in the coterminous United States.

Data from National Center for Health Statistics (NCHS). 2016. *Health, United States, 2015.* Hyattsville, MD: Department of Health and Human Services. pp. 2, 192, 194, 202, 216.

In the United States, chronic diseases have become the leading cause of death and disability. Almost 50% of Americans have at least one chronic illness (Robert Wood Johnson Foundation [RWJF], 2010), and 8.7 out of every 10 deaths are attributable to chronic disease, with heart disease and cancer accounting for nearly 50% of all deaths (WHO, 2011). Cardiovascular diseases are responsible for one-fourth of all deaths annually. While heart disease is largely preventable, the burden associated with this disease continues to grow.

Approximately half of Americans have at least one of the major clinical risk factors: high low-density lipoprotein (LDL) cholesterol, high blood pressure, or smoking (Centers for Disease Control and Prevention [CDC], 2011). Other major risk factors include physical inactivity, diabetes, and obesity (Kannel and Abbott, 1984).

Cancer is the second leading cause of death in the United States, with more than 1.5 million people being diagnosed with cancer annually (Xu et al., 2016). The most commonly diagnosed types of cancer are breast cancer, prostate cancer, lung cancer, and colon cancer (CDC, 2016a). Although the specific risk factors vary by type of cancer, general risk factors include family history, age, exposure to cancerous substances, diet, obesity and tobacco use.

As of 2016, more than 29 million Americans were living with diabetes and another 86 million were living with pre-diabetes, a health condition that increases the risk of type 2 diabetes (CDC, 2016b). The major risk factor for diabetes is obesity.

Chronic diseases have a major impact on the economy, in terms of both medical costs and lost productivity. Approximately 71% of all health care spending is attributable to people with at least one chronic condition (Gerteis et al., 2014). For example, the estimated cost of diagnosed diabetes in 2012 was $245 billion, which includes $69 billion in reduced productivity. The high costs of prescription medications, hospital inpatient care, and diabetes supplies contribute to the $176 billion in medical costs associated with this disease (American Diabetes Association, 2013). The economic burden of heart disease and stroke is also high, with these conditions costing the U.S. economy approximately $207 billion each year for health care services, medications, and lost productivity (Mozaffarian et al., 2016). In total, cardiovascular disease is responsible for an estimated $317 billion annually in direct and indirect costs. The direct medical costs for cancer are approximately $88 billion per year in the United States, and the economic burden of this disease is expected to increase significantly in the future due to the growth and aging of the population, improvements in survival, and increased costs of care (Yabroff et al., 2011).

Three main reasons underlie the rise of chronic conditions in the U.S. population:

- New diagnostic methods, medical procedures, and pharmaceuticals have significantly improved the treatment of acute illnesses, survival rates, and longevity, but these achievements have had the consequence of creating a larger population living with chronic conditions. The prevalence of chronic disease is expected to continue to rise with an aging population and longer life expectancy.
- Screening and diagnosis have expanded in scope, frequency, and accuracy (RWJF, 2010).
- Lifestyle choices, such as consumption of high-salt and high-fat diets and sedentary lifestyles, are risk factors that contribute to the development of chronic conditions.

Some risk factors that contribute to the most common chronic diseases can be modified through prevention. For example, smoking, obesity, physical inactivity, and poor nutrition are risk factors for most chronic diseases. Proven prevention methods include lifestyle change programs, though such programs are notoriously difficult to sustain. Increasing prevention efforts and awareness of the need to reduce cholesterol levels and hypertension so as to prevent heart disease and stroke remains a challenge (Franco et al., 2011). In the United States, obesity and diabetes rates have increased over the last several decades, at least in part due to changes in food consumption and technological advances, which have reduced energy expenditure in labor-intensive occupations (Caballero, 2007; Finkelstein et al., 2005; Franco et al., 2009). State and local health departments face challenges in enacting health-promotion programs such as budget restrictions. Moreover, many state and local programs directed at people with chronic diseases have been reduced or eliminated (Johnson et al., 2011). Chronic disease programs are not standardized or comprehensive in most health care settings (Bauer et al., 2014; Maylahn et al., 2013).

The CDC supports strengthened collaboration between public health agencies and private health care providers to prevent chronic diseases and improve population health. One comprehensive initiative geared toward meeting this aim was launched by the DHHS with funding of $650 million allocated to the American Recovery and Reinvestment Act of 2009. The goal of this initiative, called Communities Putting Prevention to Work (CPPW), is to "reduce risk factors, prevent/delay chronic disease, promote wellness in children and adults, and provide positive, sustainable health change in communities" (DHHS, 2010a). By June 2013, CPPW had met 73% of its objectives (CDC, 2013a). CPPW was successful in increasing access to environments with healthy food and beverage options in communities nationwide. It also created bike lanes in cities, supported the development of walking trails, and provided guidelines for daily physical activity in schools to increase access to physical activity activities. The program decreased exposure to second-hand smoke through expansion of smoke-free areas and expanded smoking cessation services. In addition, CPPW increased local capacity to improve public health interventions, developed products to support public health departments, and guided the development of programs to better support long-term community

health. It is estimated that if these health improvements are sustained in CPPW communities beyond the intervention period, there will be 14,000 fewer deaths and $2.4 billion in health care costs will be averted through 2020 (Khavjou et al., 2014).

▶ Health Promotion and Disease Prevention

A program of health promotion and disease prevention is built on three main principles:

- Risk factors associated with host, agent, environment, and their health consequences are evaluated through a process called **health risk appraisal**. Only when the risk factors and their health consequences are known can interventions be developed to help individuals adopt healthier lifestyles.
- Interventions for counteracting the key risk factors include two main approaches: (1) behavior modification geared toward the goal of adopting healthier lifestyles; and (2) therapeutic interventions.
- Adequate public health and social services, as discussed later in this chapter, include all health-related services designed to minimize risk factors and their negative effects so as to prevent disease, control disease outbreaks, and contain the spread of infectious agents.

Various avenues can be used in motivating individuals to alter behaviors that may contribute to disease, disability, or death. Behavior can be modified through educational programs and incentives directed at specific high-risk populations.

For example, in the case of cigarette smoking, health promotion efforts aim to build people's knowledge, attitudes, and skills to avoid or quit smoking. These efforts also seek to reduce the number of advertisements and environmental enticements that promote nicotine addiction. Likewise, financial incentives and disincentives, such as higher cigarette taxes, have been used to discourage purchase of cigarettes.

Therapeutic interventions fall into three areas of preventive effort: primary prevention, secondary prevention, and tertiary prevention. **Primary prevention** refers to activities undertaken to reduce the probability that a disease will develop in the future (Kane, 1988). The objective of primary prevention is to restrain the development of a disease or negative health condition before it occurs. For example, therapeutic interventions can include community health efforts to assist patients in smoking cessation and exercise programs to prevent conditions such as lung cancer and heart disease. Safety training and practices at the workplace can reduce serious work-related injuries. Prenatal care is known to lower infant mortality rates. Immunization has had a greater impact on prevention against childhood diseases and mortality reduction than has any other public health intervention besides providing clean water (Plotkin and Plotkin, 2012). Hand washing, refrigeration of foods, garbage collection, sewage treatment, and protection of the water supply are other examples of primary prevention (Timmreck, 1994). There have been numerous incidents where training on food safety and proper cooking could have prevented outbreaks of potentially deadly episodes, such as those caused by *Escherichia coli*.

Secondary prevention refers to early detection and treatment of disease. Health screenings and periodic health examinations are just two examples. Screening for hypertension, cancers, and diabetes, for example, has been instrumental in prescribing early treatment for these conditions. The main objective of secondary prevention is to block the progression of a disease or an injury—that is, to keep it from developing into an impairment or disability (Timmreck, 1994).

Tertiary prevention refers to interventions that could prevent complications from chronic conditions and prevent further illness, injury, or disability. For example, regular turning of bed-bound patients prevents pressure sores, rehabilitation therapies can prevent permanent disability, and infection control practices in hospitals and nursing homes are designed to prevent **iatrogenic illnesses** (i.e., illnesses or injuries caused by the process of health care).

As shown in **TABLE 2-2**, prevention, early detection, and treatment efforts helped reduce cancer mortality quite significantly between 1991 and 2013. This decrease was the first sustained decline since record keeping was instituted in the 1930s.

▶ Disease Prevention Under the Affordable Care Act

Prevention and wellness received significant emphasis under the Affordable Care Act (ACA). At least partially as a result of the ACA, an estimated 137 million Americans, including 28.5 million children, received no cost coverage for preventive services (Office of

TABLE 2-2 Annual Percentage Decline in U.S. Cancer Mortality, 1991–2013

Type of Cancer	1991–1995	1994–2003	1998–2007	2001–2010	2009–2013
All cancers	3.0	1.1	1.4	1.5	1.5
Breast cancer	6.3	2.5	2.2	2.2	1.9
Cervical cancer	9.7	3.6	2.6	1.5	0.8
Ovarian cancer	4.8	0.5	0.8	2.0	2.1
Prostate cancer	6.3	3.5	3.1	2.7	3.6

Data from National Center for Health Statistics, Centers for Disease Control and Prevention, National Cancer Institute, SEER Cancer Statistics Review, 1975–2010; National Cancer Institute. 2016. *State cancer profiles*. Available at: https://statecancerprofiles.cancer.gov/recenttrend/index.php.

the Assistant Secretary for Planning and Evaluation, 2015).

Other ACA initiatives included the Prevention and Public Health Fund (PPHF) for national preventive efforts and programs geared toward improving health outcomes and enhancing quality of health care (American Public Health Association, 2013). The Office of the Surgeon General developed a National Prevention Strategy to encourage partnerships among federal, state, tribal, local, and territorial governments; business, industry, and other private-sector entities; philanthropic organizations; community and faith-based organizations; and everyday Americans to improve health through prevention (National Prevention Council, 2011).

As one example of a federally driven effort directed toward reducing chronic disease, the CDC established a National Diabetes Prevention Program (NDPP). In 2012, six organizations received $6.75 million to develop partnerships with the aim of reaching people with prediabetes

(CDC, 2013b, 2013c). Through the NDPP, organizations nationwide offer diabetes prevention lifestyle programs in health care clinics, pharmacies, wellness centers, worksites, and other community centers. These organizations also work to increase awareness of lifestyle changes. Organizations encourage health professionals to refer patients with prediabetes to a lifestyle change program. The program has also increased awareness across employers, some of which now provide coverage for lifestyle change programs as health benefits for their employees. The NDPP is working to ensure quality and standardized reporting and to monitor and evaluate program effectiveness (CDC, 2016c).

In 2011, $10 million in federal funding was made available to establish and evaluate comprehensive workplace wellness programs (DHHS, 2011b). Beginning in 2014, $200 million in wellness grants was made available to small businesses to encourage the establishment of wellness programs and employee health-promotion incentives (Anderko et al., 2012). In 2015, 46.8 million employees worked in firms that offered wellness programs. Although workplace wellness programs are diverse and vary in the services and activities offered, they are all required to promote health and/or prevent disease to qualify for federal funding support. Of the companies that provided health benefits in 2015, 50% offered wellness programs for tobacco cessation, weight control, nutrition, and other lifestyle or behavioral coaching (Mattke et al., 2013). Health-promotion activities, such as on-site vaccination services, biometric screenings, fitness benefits, and health food options at the workplace, are also common. The majority of workplaces that offer wellness programs offer a combination of screening and intervention services. These programs have been shown to generate savings in medical costs of approximately $3 for every $1 spent on the program and to reduce absenteeism (Baicker et al., 2010).

▶ Public Health

Public health remains poorly understood by its prime beneficiaries, the public. For some people, public health evokes images of a massive social enterprise or welfare system. To others, the term means health care services for everyone. Still another image of public health is of a body of knowledge and techniques that can be applied to health-related problems (Turnock, 1997). However, none of these ideas adequately reflects what public health is.

The Institute of Medicine (1988) has proposed that the mission of public health should be understood as fulfilling "society's interest in assuring conditions in which people can be healthy." **Public health** deals with broad societal concerns about ensuring conditions that promote optimal health for the society as a whole. It involves the application of scientific knowledge to counteract any threats that may jeopardize the health and safety of the general population. Because of its extensive scope, the vast majority of public health efforts are carried out by government agencies, such as the CDC in the United States.

Three main distinctions can be seen between the practices of medicine and public health:

- Medicine focuses on the individual patient—diagnosing symptoms, treating and preventing disease, relieving pain and suffering, and maintaining or restoring normal function. Public health, in contrast, focuses on populations (Shi and Johnson, 2014).
- The emphases in modern medicine are the biological causes of disease and the development of treatments and therapies. In contrast, public health focuses on (1) identifying environmental, social, and behavioral risk factors as well as emerging or potential risks that may threaten people's health and safety; and (2) implementing population-wide interventions to minimize these risk factors (Peters et al., 2001).
- Medicine focuses on the treatment of disease and recovery of health, whereas public health deals with various efforts to prevent disease and counteract threats that may negatively affect people's health.

Public health activities range from providing education on nutrition to passing laws that enhance automobile safety. For example, public health includes dissemination, both to the public and to health professionals, of timely information about important health issues, particularly when communicable diseases pose potential threats to large segments of a population.

Compared to medicine, public health involves a broader range of professionals. The medical sector encompasses physicians, nurses, dentists, therapists, social workers, psychologists, nutritionists, health educators, pharmacists, laboratory technicians, health services administrators, and so forth. In addition to these professionals, the public health forum includes professionals such as sanitarians, epidemiologists, statisticians, industrial hygienists, environmental health specialists, food and drug inspectors, toxicologists, and economists (Lasker, 1997).

Health Protection and Environmental Health

Health protection is one of the main public health functions. In the 1850s, John Snow successfully traced cholera outbreaks in London to contamination of the Broad Street water pump (Rosen, 1993). Since then, **environmental health** has specifically dealt with preventing the spread of disease through water, air, and food (Schneider, 2000). Environmental health science, along with other public health measures, was instrumental in reducing the risk of infectious diseases during the 1900s. For example, in 1900, pneumonia, tuberculosis, and diarrhea, along with enteritis, were the top three killers in the United States (CDC, 1999); that is no longer the case today (**TABLE 2-3**). With the rapid industrialization that occurred

during the 20th century, environmental health faced new challenges due to serious health hazards from chemicals, industrial waste, infectious waste, radiation, asbestos, and other toxic substances. In the 21st century, the possession of chemical, biological, and nuclear agents by terrorists and rogue nations have emerged as a new environmental threat.

Health Protection During Global Pandemics

Over time, public health has become a complex global undertaking. Its main goal of protecting the health and safety of populations from a variety of old and new threats cannot be achieved without global cooperation. Influenza is the most common infectious disease on a global scale, affecting nearly 3 to 5 million people annually and resulting in 250,000 to 500,000 deaths (Thompson et al., 2009). It spreads around the world in a yearly outbreak.

The global threat of avian influenza has also elicited a public health response. The CDC launched a website dedicated to educating the public about avian influenza, the means by which it is spread, and past and current outbreaks. This website contains specific information for health professionals, travelers, the poultry industry, state departments of health, and people with possible exposures to avian influenza (CDC, 2007).

Although several strains of influenza exist, the subtypes currently circulating among humans are H1N1 and H3N2 (WHO, 2016a). After a novel H1N1 influenza virus emerged from Mexico in April 2009, U.S. health officials anticipated

TABLE 2-3 Leading Causes of Death, 2014

Cause of Death	Deaths	Percentage of All Deaths
All causes	2,626,418	100.0
Diseases of the heart	614,348	23.4
Malignant neoplasms	591,699	22.5
Chronic lower respiratory diseases	147,101	5.6
Unintentional injuries	136,053	5.2
Cerebrovascular diseases	133,103	5.1
Alzheimer's disease	93,541	3.6
Diabetes mellitus	76,488	2.9
Influenza and pneumonia	55,227	2.1
Nephritis, nephrotic syndrome, and nephrosis	48,146	1.8
Suicide	42,773	1.6

Data from National Center for Health Statistics (NCHS). 2016. *Health, United States, 2015*. Hyattsville, MD: Department of Health and Human Services. p. 107.

and prepared for an influenza pandemic, and these efforts stretched the response capabilities of the public health system. The virus affected every U.S. state, and Americans were left unprotected because of the unavailability of antiviral medications. Since then, a global effort has been undertaken to establish collaborative networks to exchange information and contain global pandemics (WHO, 2013).

Coronaviruses are believed to cause a large percentage of all common colds in adults (Committee on Infectious Diseases et al., 2015). However, two strains of coronavirus have particularly serious health effects. Severe acute respiratory syndrome (SARS) and Middle East respiratory syndrome (MERS) coronavirus outbreaks occurred in 2003 and 2012, respectively. In 2003, SARS—a contagious disease that is accompanied by fever and symptoms of pneumonia or other respiratory illness—spread from China to Canada. Worldwide, more than 8,000 people were affected by this infection (CDC, 2012). MERS still occurs in parts of the Middle East. Since 2012, 27 countries have reported cases of MERS, for a total of

1,888 cases and 670 deaths from this disease (WHO, 2016b).

WHO's (2016c) *2016 World Malaria Report* provides estimates of the global prevalence and mortality due to malaria. In 2015, there were an estimated 212 million malaria cases and 429,000 malaria deaths worldwide. The majority of cases were in Africa (90%), followed by southeast Asia (7%). The global incidence of malaria decreased by 21% between 2010 and 2015, and the number of deaths decreased by 29% in the same time period.

The *Global Tuberculosis (TB) Report*, also published by WHO (2016d), provides current estimates of the worldwide TB epidemic. In 2015, there were an estimated 10.4 million incident TB cases worldwide. Sixty percent of cases were concentrated in six countries: India, Indonesia, China, Nigeria, Pakistan, and South Africa. Multidrug-resistant TB cases are especially problematic, with 480,000 new cases in 2015 and an additional 100,000 new cases of rifampicin-resistant TB. An estimated 1.4 million deaths due to TB occurred in 2015. Nevertheless, the number of TB deaths fell 22% between 2000 and 2015, and TB treatment averted 49 million deaths globally. Even so, TB remains among the top 10 causes of death worldwide.

Prevent HIV, Test and Treat All: Progress Report 2016, a WHO (2016e) report, provides estimates of the global human immunodeficiency virus (HIV)/acquired immunodeficiency syndrome (AIDS) epidemic. As of 2015, 36.7 million people were living with HIV/AIDS worldwide; in that same year, 1.1 million people died of AIDS-related illnesses. This mortality was the lowest number of deaths from HIV/AIDS in 2 decades. The burden of the pandemic is greatest in sub-Saharan Africa, where an estimated 25.5 million people are living with the disease (70% of all people living with HIV worldwide) as of 2017. In 2015, 800,000 people in this region died from HIV/AIDS. Approximately 66% of all new HIV infections occur in this region as well. As of June 2016, 18.2 million people living with HIV globally were receiving life-prolonging antiretroviral therapy (ART), compared to 7.5 million people in 2010 and fewer than 1 million people in 2000. Additionally, access to ART to prevent transmission of HIV from mother to baby is increasing, with new HIV infections among newborns declining by 50% since 2010.

While some types of hepatitis are more problematic (i.e., hepatitis B and C) than others, all variants of this infection are viral in nature and present in the global population. An estimated 400 million people are affected by at least one type of viral hepatitis, and 6 to 10 million are newly infected annually. In total, approximately 1.4 million people die from hepatitis each year globally (GBD 2013 Mortality and Causes of Death Collaborators, 2015; Jacobsen and Wiersma, 2010). Hepatitis B accounts for approximately 686,000 deaths each year, and an estimated 240 million chronic infections. In sub-Saharan Africa and East Asia, 5% to 10% of the population is chronically infected with hepatitis B; in the Middle East and India, an estimated 2% to 5% of the population is chronically infected. Approximately 130 to 150 million people have chronic hepatitis C, and 700,000 die annually from related liver diseases. Africa, Central Asia, and East Asia are the regions most affected by the hepatitis C pandemic.

The most current outbreak of the Ebola virus, which started in December 2013 and ended in April 2016, led to more than 28,000 cases and 11,000 deaths in Africa (WHO, 2016f). The countries most severely affected by the recent major Ebola outbreak—Guinea, Sierra Leone, and Liberia—are all in West Africa. Now that the outbreak has ended, the current focus is on preparedness and prevention of future epidemics (WHO Ebola Response Team et al., 2016). In December 2016, scientists reported highly promising results for an experimental Ebola vaccine (Henao-Restrepo et al., 2017). The first vaccine to prevent infections from this virus, it is estimated to be 70% to 100% effective.

▶ Health Protection and Preparedness in the United States

Since the horrific events of what is commonly referred to as 9/11 (the terrorism attacks on September 11, 2001), the United States has begun a new chapter in health protection. These efforts to protect the health and safety of Americans began in June 2002 when President George W. Bush signed into law the Public Health Security and Bioterrorism Preparedness Response Act of 2002. Subsequently, the Homeland Security Act of 2002 created the Department of Homeland Security (DHS) and called for a major restructuring of the nation's resources, with the primary mission of helping prevent, protect against, and respond to any acts of terrorism in the United States. It also provided better tools to contain attacks on food and water supplies, protect the nation's vital infrastructures (i.e., nuclear facilities), and track biological materials anywhere in the United States. The term **bioterrorism** encompasses the use of chemical, biological, and nuclear agents to cause harm to relatively large civilian populations.

Today, health protection and preparedness comprises a massive operation to deal with any natural or human-made threats. Dealing with such threats requires large-scale preparations, which include appropriate tools and training for workers in medical care, public health, emergency care, and civil defense agencies at the federal, state, and local levels. It requires national initiatives to develop countermeasures, such as new vaccines, a robust public health infrastructure, and coordination among numerous agencies. It also requires development of an infrastructure that can handle large numbers of casualties and isolation facilities for contagious patients. Hospitals, public health agencies, and civil defense must be linked together through information systems. Containment of infectious agents, such as smallpox, necessitates quick detection, treatment, isolation, and organized efforts to protect the unaffected population. Rapid cleanup, evacuation of the affected population, and transfer of victims to medical care facilities require detailed plans and logistics.

The United States has confronted several major natural disasters in the 21st century, such as Hurricane Katrina in 2005, Hurricane Sandy in 2012, and tornadoes in Oklahoma in 2013, as well as human-made mass casualties such as the Boston Marathon bombing on April 15, 2013. Health protection and preparedness have become ongoing efforts through revitalized initiatives such as the Pandemic and All-Hazards Preparedness

Act (PAHPA) of 2006, which also authorized a new Assistant Secretary for Preparedness and Response (ASPR) within the DHHS and called for the establishment of a quadrennial National Health Security Strategy (NHSS). The CDC has developed the National Biosurveillance Strategy for Human Health, which covers six priority areas: electronic health information exchange, electronic laboratory information exchange, unstructured data, integrated biosurveillance information, global disease detection and collaboration, and biosurveillance workforce. Based on the National Health Security Strategy developed by the DHHS in 2009, *Healthy People 2020* focused on four areas for reinforcement under an overarching goal to "improve the Nation's ability to prevent, prepare for, respond to, and recover from a major health incident": time to release official information about a public health emergency, time for designated personnel to respond to an emergency, Laboratory Response Network (LRN) laboratories, and time to develop after-action reports and improvement plans in states (DHHS, 2010b). A progress report shows that most states and localities have strong biological laboratory capabilities and capacities, with nearly 90% of laboratories in the LRN reachable around the clock (CDC, 2010b).

In 2011, the Health Alert Network (HAN) was established; this nationwide program is designed to facilitate communication, information, and distance learning related to health threats, including bioterrorism (DHHS, 2011a). When fully established, the network will link together local health departments and other components of bioterrorism preparedness and response, such as laboratories and state health departments.

One of the key concepts of preparedness is **surge capacity**, defined as "the ability of a health care facility or system to expand its operations to safely treat an abnormally large influx of patients" (Bonnett and Peery, 2007). The initial response is conducted at a local health care facility, such as a hospital. Strategies for expanding the surge capacity of a hospital include early discharge of stable patients, cancellation of elective procedures and admissions, conversion of private rooms to double rooms, reopening of closed areas, revision of staff work hours to a 12-hour disaster shift, callback of off-duty personnel, and establishment of temporary external shelters for patient holding (Hick et al., 2004).

If the local level response becomes overloaded or incapacitated, a second tier of disaster response can be activated: community-level surge capacity. Cooperative regional planning necessitates sharing of staff and supplies across a network of regional health care facilities (Hick et al., 2004). An important aspect of disaster planning at the community level entails the transportation logistics for the region. The number of ambulances in the area and the means of accessing such resources during an event is crucial to delivering proper care to critical patients (Kearns et al., 2013).

The final tier of disaster response involves federal aid under the National Disaster Medical System (NDMS), which dates back to the 1980s and was designed to accommodate large numbers of military casualties. Disaster Medical Assistance Teams (DMATs) are a vital component of the NDMS that directly respond to the needs of an overwhelmed community. DMATs deploy with trained personnel (in both medical and ancillary services), equipped with tents, water filtration, generators, and medical supplies (Stopford, 2005).

Developments in technology have made major contributions to advances in disaster preparedness. For example, the United States is using new information and communication technologies to streamline emergency responses among various organizations. Social media is increasingly being used as a tool by governments, communities, and organizations for a range of purposes in disaster preparedness (i.e., detecting an event; connecting individuals following a disaster; and preparing and receiving disaster preparedness information, warnings, and signals) (Houston et al., 2015).

Despite the progress that has been made, disaster preparedness efforts in the United States remain fragmented and underfunded. For example, review, rotation, replacement, and upgrading of equipment and supplies in the system on a regular basis remain challenging (Cohen and Mulvaney, 2005). Given the differences in institutional and local structures, it is difficult to develop clear and objective standards and methods while still respecting local authorities (Nelson et al., 2007). Other challenges include retention of high-quality staff in emergency departments and having insufficient funding and resources to provide education and training opportunities (Walsh et al., 2015).

▶ Determinants of Health

Health determinants are major factors that affect the health and well-being of individuals and populations. An understanding of health determinants is necessary to plan and implement any positive interventions that improve health and longevity.

Blum's Model of Health Determinants

In 1974, Blum (1981) proposed an "Environment of Health" model, later called the "Force Field and Well-Being Paradigms of Health." Blum proposed that four major inputs contribute to health and well-being ("force fields"): environment, lifestyle, heredity, and medical care. All of these factors must be considered simultaneously when addressing the health status of an individual or a population. In other words, there is no single pathway to better health because health determinants interact in complex ways. Consequently, improvement in health requires a multipronged approach.

The four wedges in Blum's model represent the four major force fields. The size of each wedge signifies its relative importance. Thus, the most important force field is environment, followed by lifestyle and heredity. Medical care has the least impact on health and well-being.

Blum's model also explains that the four main forces operate within a much broader context, and are affected by broad national and international factors, such as a nation's population characteristics, natural resources, ecological balance, human satisfactions, and cultural systems. One of these factors is the type of health care delivery system. In the United States, the majority of health care expenditures is devoted to the treatment of medical conditions, rather than to the prevention of factors that produce those medical conditions in the first place.

Environment

Environmental factors encompass the physical, socioeconomic, sociopolitical, and sociocultural dimensions. Among physical environmental factors are air pollution, food and water contaminants, radiation, toxic chemicals, wastes, disease vectors, safety hazards, and habitat alterations.

The positive relationship between socioeconomic status (SES) and health may be explained by the general likelihood that people who have better education also have higher incomes. The greater the economic gap between the rich and the poor is in a given geographic area, the worse the health status of the overall population in that area is likely to be. It has been suggested that wide income gaps produce less social cohesion, greater psychosocial stress, and consequently, poorer health (Wilkinson, 1997). For example, social cohesion—characterized by a hospitable social environment in which people trust each other and participate in communal activities—is linked to lower overall mortality and better self-rated health (Kawachi et al., 1997, 1999). Even countries with national health insurance programs, such as the United Kingdom, Australia, Denmark, and Sweden, experience persistent and widening disparities in health according to socioeconomic status (Pincus et al., 1998). The joint relationship of income inequality and availability of primary care has also been found to be significantly associated with individuals' self-rated health status (Shi et al., 2002).

Lifestyle

Lifestyle factors, also known as behavioral risk factors, were discussed earlier in this chapter. This section provides some illustrations of how lifestyle factors are related to health. Studies have shown that diet plays a major role in most of today's significant health problems. Heart disease, diabetes, stroke, and cancer are some of the diseases with direct links to dietary

choices. Throughout the world, incidence and mortality rates for many forms of cancer are rising, though research has clearly indicated that a significant portion of cancer is preventable. Researchers estimate that 30% to 50% of all cancers and as many as 30% to 35% of cancer deaths are linked to diet (World Cancer Research Fund and American Institute for Cancer Research, 2007). Research also shows that a diet rich in fruits, vegetables, and low-fat dairy foods, and a diet low in saturated and total fat, can substantially lower blood pressure (see, for example, the DASH Eating Plan recommended by DHHS [2006]).

Increasing exercise and physical activity is a potentially useful, effective, and acceptable method for reducing the risk of colon cancer (Macfarlane and Lowenfels, 1994) and many other health problems. Smoking and alcohol consumption are also important lifestyle factors that impact health. In addition to increasing the risk of lung cancer, smoking increases the risk of coronary heart disease and stroke by 2 to 4 times (DHHS, 2014). Half of all cancer deaths and nearly half of all cancer diagnoses could potentially be prevented through a healthy lifestyle that includes not smoking, drinking in moderation, maintaining a healthy weight, and exercising regularly (Song and Giovannucci, 2016).

Heredity

Genetic factors may predispose individuals to certain diseases. While cancer is not entirely genetic, cancer can occur when the body's healthy genes lose their ability to suppress malignant growth or when other genetic processes stop working properly (Davis and Webster, 2002). While people can do little about the genetic makeup they have inherited, their lifestyle and behavior can significantly impact their progeny. Finally, advances in gene therapy hold the promise of treating a variety of inherited or acquired diseases.

Medical Care

Although the factors of lifestyle, environment, and heredity are more important in the determination of health, medical care is, nevertheless, a key factor affecting health. Though, according to Blum, medical care is the least important factor in determining health and well-being, the United States focuses more on medical research and development of new medical technologies than it does on the other three factors. It can be noted that significant declines in mortality rates were achieved well before the modernization of Western medicine and the escalation in medical care expenditures.

The availability of primary care may be one way in which income inequality influences population-level health outcomes. Research by Shi and colleagues (Shi and Starfield, 2001; Shi et al., 1999) suggests that access to primary care significantly correlates with reduced mortality, increased life expectancy, and improved birth outcomes. Access to primary care includes access to and use of preventive services, which can prevent illness or detect disease at an earlier, often more treatable stage. In the United States, individuals living in states with a higher primary care physician-to-population ratio are more likely to report good health than those living in states with a lower ratio (Shi et al., 2002).

Contemporary Models of Health Determinants

More recent models have built upon and extended Blum's framework of health determinants. For example, the model proposed by Dahlgren and Whitehead (2006) identifies age, sex, and genetic makeup as fixed factors, but state that other factors can be modified to positively influence population health. While individual lifestyle factors can benefit or damage health, broader social, economic, cultural, and environmental conditions often have greater influence on both individual and population health.

Another model by Ansari and colleagues (2003) have proposed a public health model of the social determinants of health in which the determinants are categorized into four major groups: social determinants, health care system attributes, disease-inducing behaviors, and health outcomes.

The WHO Commission on Social Determinants of Health (2008) concluded that "the social conditions in which people are born, live, and work are the single most important determinant of one's health status" (Satcher, 2010). The WHO model provides a conceptual framework for understanding the socioeconomic and political contexts, structural determinants, intermediary determinants (including material circumstances, social–environmental circumstances, behavioral and biological factors, social cohesion, and the health care system), and the impact on health equity and well-being measured as health outcomes (**FIGURE 2-3**).

U.S. government agencies, such as the CDC and DHHS, have recognized the need to address health inequities. The CDC's National Center for HIV/AIDS, Viral Hepatitis, STD, and TB Prevention adopted the WHO framework on social determinants of health as a guide for its activities.

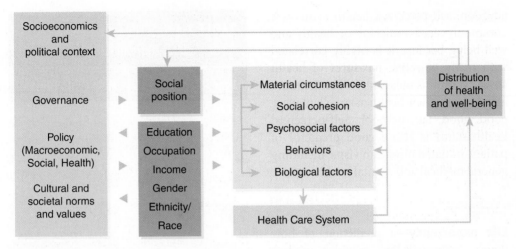

FIGURE 2-3 WHO Commission on Social Determinants of Health conceptual framework.

Reproduced from Centers for Disease Control and Prevention (CDC). 2010a. *Establishing a holistic framework to reduce inequities in HIV, viral hepatitis, STDs, and tuberculosis in the United States.* Available at: https://www.cdc.gov/socialdeterminants/docs/SDH-White-Paper-2010.pdf. Accessed April 2017. Modified from Solar, O., and A. Irwin; World Health Organization (WHO). 2010. *A conceptual framework for action on the social determinants of health. Social Determinants of Health Discussion Paper 2 (Policy and Practice).* Geneva, Switzerland: WHO.

▶ Measures Related to Health

Certain quantitative measures are commonly applied to health, health status, and the utilization of health care. The conceptual approaches for defining health and its distribution help form a vision for the future, and objective measures play a critical role in evaluating the success of programs and directing future planning activities. Practical approaches for measuring health are, however, quite limited, and mental health is more difficult to quantify and measure than physical health. An objective evaluation of social and spiritual health is even more obscure.

The concept of population, as it applies to population health, has been borrowed from the disciplines of statistics and epidemiology. The term "population" is not restricted to describing the total population. Although commonly used in this way, the term population may also apply to a defined subpopulation—for example, age groups, marital categories, income levels, occupation categories, racial/ethnic groups, people having a common disease, people in a certain risk category, or people in a certain community or geographic region of a country. The main advantage of studying subpopulations is that it helps trace the existence of health problems to a defined group. Doing so avoids the likelihood that serious problems in a minority group will be hidden within the favorable statistics of the majority. By pinpointing health problems in certain well-defined groups, targeted interventions and new policy initiatives can be deployed in the most effective manner.

Measures of Physical Health

Physical health status is often interpreted through **morbidity** (disease and disability) and **mortality** (death) rates. In addition, self-perceived health status is a commonly used indicator of health and well-being because it is highly correlated with many objective measures of health status. With this measure, respondents are asked to rate their health as excellent, very good, good, fair, or poor. Self-perceived health status is also a good predictor of patient-initiated physician visits, including general medical and mental health visits.

Longevity

Life expectancy—a prediction of how long a person will live—is widely used as a basic measure of health status. The two common measures are life expectancy at birth (**TABLE 2-4**)—or how long a newborn can expect to live—and life expectancy at age 65—expected remaining years of life for someone at age 65. These measures are actuarially determined and published by government agencies such as the National Center for Health Statistics (NCHS). The U.S. Census Bureau (2016) has projected that life expectancy in the United States will increase from 78.8 years in 2014 to 84.1 years in 2050.

Morbidity

The measurement of morbidity or disease, such as cancer or heart disease, is expressed as a ratio or proportion of those who have the problem and the **population at risk**. The population at risk includes all the people in the same community or population group who could acquire a disease or condition (Smith, 1979).

Incidence and prevalence are two widely used indicators for the number of **cases**, people who end up acquiring a negative health condition. Both incidence and prevalence rates can apply to disease, disability, or death.

TABLE 2-4 U.S. Life Expectancy at Birth—2002, 2007, and 2014

Year	Total	Male	Female
2002	77.0	74.4	79.6
White	77.5	74.9	80.1
Black	72.2	68.7	75.4
2007	78.1	75.5	80.6
White	78.5	76.0	80.9
Black	73.8	70.3	77.0
2014	78.8	76.4	81.2
White	79.0	76.7	81.4
Black	75.6	72.5	78.4

Data from National Center for Health Statistics (NCHS). 2016. *Health, United States, 2015*. Hyattsville, MD: Department of Health and Human Services. p. 95.

Incidence counts the number of new cases occurring in the population at risk within a certain period of time, such as a month or a year (Smith, 1979; **FORMULA 2-1**). It describes the extent to which people in a given population acquire a given disease during a specified time period. Incidence is particularly useful in estimating the significance or

FORMULA 2-1

Incidence = Number of new cases during a specified period/Population at risk magnitude of conditions of relatively short duration. Declining levels of incidence indicate successful health promotion and disease prevention efforts because they prevent new cases (Ibrahim, 1985). High levels of incidence may suggest an impending **epidemic**, a large number of people who get a specific disease from a common source.

Prevalence determines the total number of cases at a specific point in time, in a defined population (**FORMULA 2-2**). Prevalence is useful in quantifying the magnitude of illnesses of a relatively long duration. Decreased prevalence indicates success of treatment programs by shortening the duration of illness (Ibrahim, 1985).

FORMULA 2-2

Prevalence = Total number of cases at a specific point in time/Specified population

---

The calculation of rates often requires dividing a small number by a large number representing a defined population. The result is a fraction. To make the fractions meaningful and interpretable, they are multiplied by 100 (to get a percentage), by 1,000 (to get a rate per 1,000 people), by 10,000 (to get a rate per 10,000 people), or by a higher multiple of 10.

Disability

Disease and injury can lead to temporary or permanent, as well as partial or total, disability. Although the idea of morbidity includes disabilities, as well as disease, specific measures of disability have been developed. Some commonly used

measures are the number of days of bed confinement, days missed from work or school, and days of restricted activity. All measures are in reference to a specific time period, such as a year.

One of the most widely used measures of physical disability among the elderly, in particular, is the **activities of daily living (ADLs)** scale. The ADLs identify personal care functions with which a disabled person may need assistance. Depending on the extent of disability, personal care needs can be met through adaptive devices; care rendered by another individual, such as a family member; or care in a nursing facility. Consequently, the ADL scale is appropriate for evaluating disability in both community-dwelling and institutionalized adults. The classic ADL scale, developed by Katz and Akpom (1979), includes six basic activities: eating, bathing, dressing, using the toilet, maintaining continence, and transferring from bed to chair. To evaluate disability in community-dwelling adults, a modified Katz scale, which consists of seven items, is used (Ostir et al., 1999). Five of these items—feeding, bathing, dressing, using the toilet, and transferring from bed to chair—have been retained from the original Katz scale. The additional two items are grooming and walking a distance of 8 feet. Thus, the modified scale includes items measuring self-care and mobility.

Another commonly used measure of physical function is the **instrumental activities of daily living (IADLs)** scale. This scale measures activities that are necessary for living independently in the community, such as using the telephone, driving a car or traveling alone on a bus or by taxi, shopping, preparing meals, doing light housework, taking medicines, handling money, doing heavy housework, walking up and down stairs, and walking a half-mile without help. IADLs typically require higher cognitive functioning than ADLs and, as such, are not purely physical tests of functional disability. The IADL scale measures the level of functioning in activities that are important for self-sufficiency, such as the ability to live independently.

Mortality

Death rates are computed in different forms as indicators of population health. **Crude rates** refer to the total population; they are not specific to any age group or disease category (**FORMULA 2-3**).

FORMULA 2-3

Crude death rate = Total deaths (usually in 1 year)/Total population

---

Specific rates are useful because death rates vary greatly by race, sex, age, and type of disease or condition. Specific rates allow health care professionals to target programs at the appropriate population subgroups (Dever, 1984). Examples of specific rates are the age-specific mortality rate (**FORMULA 2-4**) and the cause-specific mortality rate (**FORMULA 2-5**). The age-specific mortality rate provides a measure of the risk (or probability) of dying when a person is in a certain age group. The cause-specific mortality rate provides

---

FORMULA 2-4

Age-specific mortality rate = Number of deaths within a certain age group/Total number of persons in that age group

---

FORMULA 2-5

Cause-specific mortality rate = Number of deaths from a specific disease/Total population

---

a measure of the risk (or probability) of dying from a specific cause.

The infant mortality rate (actually a ratio; **FORMULA 2-6**) is an indicator that reflects the health status of the mother and the child throughout pregnancy and the birth process. It also reflects the level of prenatal and postnatal care (Timmreck, 1994).

FORMULA 2-6

Infant mortality rate = Number of deaths from birth to 1 year of age (in 1 year)/Number of live births during the same year

---

Demographic Change

In addition to measures of disease and mortality, changes in the composition of a population over time are important in planning health services. Population change involves three components: births, deaths, and migration (Dever, 1984). For example, the migration of elderly individuals to the southern and southwestern states requires planning of adequate retirement and long-term care services in those states. Longevity is also an important factor that determines demographic change. For example, lower death rates, lower birth rates, and greater longevity, taken collectively, indicate an aging population. This section presents measures of births and migration.

Births

Natality and fertility are two measures associated with births. **Natality**, or the birth rate, is useful in assessing the influence of births on demographic change and is measured by the crude birth rate (**FORMULA 2-7**).

FORMULA 2-7

Crude birth rate = Number of live births (usually in 1 year)/Total population

Fertility refers to the capacity of a population to reproduce (**FORMULA 2-8**). Fertility is a more precise measure than natality because fertility relates actual births to the sector of the population capable of giving birth.

FORMULA 2-8

Fertility rate = Number of live births (usually in 1 year)/Number of females aged 15–44

Migration

Migration refers to the geographic movement of populations between defined geographic units and involves a permanent change of residence. The net migration rate (**FORMULA 2-9**) defines the change in the population as a result of **immigration** (in-migration) and **emigration**

FORMULA 2-9

Net migration rate = (Number of immigrants – Number of emigrants)/Total population (during a specific period of time)

(out-migration) (Dever, 1984). This rate is calculated for a specified period, such as 1 year, 2 years, 5 years, and so on.

Measures of Mental Health

Measurement of mental health is less objective than measurement of mortality and morbidity because mental health often encompasses feelings that cannot be observed. In contrast, physical functioning, as reflected in behaviors and performances, can be more readily observed. Hence, measurement of mental health more appropriately refers to assessment rather than measurement. Mental health can be assessed by the presence of certain symptoms, including both psychophysiologic and psychological symptoms. Examples of psychophysiologic symptoms are low energy, headache, and upset stomach. Examples of psychological symptoms are nervousness, depression, and anxiety.

Self-assessment of one's psychological state may also be used for mental health assessment. Self-assessment can be obtained through self-reports of frequency and intensity of psychological distress, anxiety, depression, and psychological well-being.

Measures of Social Health

Measures of social health extend beyond the individual to encompass the extent of social contacts across various facets of life, such as family life, work life, and community life. Breslow (1972) attempted to measure social health along four dimensions: (1) employability based on educational achievement, occupational status, and job experience; (2) marital satisfaction; (3) sociability, determined by the number of close friends and relatives; and

(4) community involvement, encompassing attendance at religious services, political activity, and organizational membership.

Social health status is sometimes evaluated in terms of social contacts and social resources. **Social contacts** are the number of social contacts or social activities a person engages in within a specified period. Examples are visits with friends and relatives, as well as attendance at social events, such as conferences, picnics, or other outings. **Social resources** refer to social contacts that can be relied on for support, such as relatives, friends, neighbors, and members of a religious congregation. Social contacts can be observed, and they are the more objective of the two categories; however, one criticism of social contact measures is their focus on events and activities, with little consideration of how the events are personally experienced. Unlike social contacts, social resources cannot be directly observed and are best measured by asking the individuals direct questions. Evaluative questions include whether these individuals can rely on their social contacts to provide tangible support and needed companionship and whether they feel cared for, loved, and wanted.

Measures of Spiritual Health

Depending on the person's individual, social, and cultural context, spiritual well-being can have a large variety of connotations. Such variations make it extremely difficult to propose standardized approaches for measuring the spiritual dimension. Attempts to measure this dimension are illustrated in the General Social Survey, which includes people's self-perceptions about happiness, religious experiences, and their degree of involvement in activities, such as prayer and attending religious services.

A wide range of tools for spiritual assessment are now available. Generic methods of spiritual assessment are not associated with any particular religion or practice, so they do not require a detailed understanding of any particular religious tradition (Draper, 2012). An example of a generic scale is the tool developed by Vella-Brodrick and Allen (1995), which evaluates items such as reaching out for spiritual intervention; engaging in meditation, yoga, or prayer; duration of meditation or prayer for inner peace; frequency of meditation or prayer; reading about one's religious beliefs; and discussions or readings about ethical and moral issues. Quantitative measurement scales are also available to assess dimensions such as general spirituality, spiritual well-being, spiritual needs, and spiritual coping (Monod et al., 2011), but their use has been confined mainly to clinical research.

Measures of Health Services Utilization

Utilization refers to the consumption of health care services and the extent to which health care services are used. Measures of utilization can be used to determine which individuals in a population group do or do not receive certain types of medical services. With this type of measure, a health care provider, such as a hospital, can find out the extent to which its services are used. Managers can use these measures to decide whether certain services should be added or eliminated, and health planners can determine whether programs have been effective in reaching their targeted populations. For example, managers can use these measures to ascertain how many hospital beds are required to meet the acute care needs of a given population (Pasley et al.,1995). Therefore, measures of utilization play a critical role in the planning of health care delivery capacity. Measures of utilization are too numerous to be covered here, but some common measures are provided (**FORMULAS 2-10** to **2-16**).

Crude Measures of Utilization

FORMULA 2-10

Access to primary care services = Number of persons in a given population who visited a primary care provider in a given year/Size of the population

(This measure is generally expressed as a percentage; that is, the fraction is multiplied by 100.)

FORMULA 2-11

Utilization of primary care services = Number of primary care visits by people in a given population in a given year/Size of the population

(This measure is generally expressed as number of visits per person per year.)

Specific Measures of Utilization

FORMULA 2-12

Utilization of targeted services = Number of people in a specific targeted population using special services (or visits)/Size of the targeted population group

(The fraction obtained is multiplied by 100, 1,000, or a higher multiple of 10 to facilitate interpretation of the result.)

FORMULA 2-13

Utilization of specific inpatient services = Number of inpatient days/Size of the population

(The fraction obtained is multiplied by 100, 1,000, or a higher multiple of 10 to facilitate interpretation of the result.)

Measures of Institution-Specific Utilization

FORMULA 2-14

Average daily census = Total number of inpatient days in a given time period/Number of days in the same time period

FORMULA 2-15

Occupancy rate = Total number of inpatient days in a given time period/Total number of available beds during the same time period
or
Average daily census/Total number of beds in the facility

(This measure is expressed as a percentage; that is, the fraction is multiplied by 100.)

FORMULA 2-16

Average length of stay = Total number of inpatient days during a given time period/Total number of patients served during the same time period

Measures of Global Health

Global monitoring of changes in the health of various populations requires the use of "tried and true" global health indicators. Global health indicators can be divided into those that directly measure health phenomena (e.g., diseases, deaths, use of services) and indirect measures (e.g., social development, education and poverty indicators); these are also referred to as proximal and distal indicators, respectively. As one example, when using population statistics to describe levels of educational attainment and access to safe water and sanitation, it is possible to accurately categorize a country as having a population with high, medium, or low burden of disease (Larson and Mercer, 2004).

WHO (2015) compiles more than 100 indicators of a broad range of key public health issues. Commonly used indicators of life expectancy and mortality include life expectancy at age 60, healthy life expectancy at birth, infant and under-5 mortality rates, and the adult mortality rate. Cause-specific mortality rates are collected for selected communicable and noncommunicable diseases. Health services indicators reflect the extent to which people receive important health interventions. These services include unmet needs for family planning, prenatal care coverage, births attended by skilled health personnel, vaccination coverage, and other prevention and treatment coverage for common diseases among children. It is also important to report indicators of risk factors that are associated with increased mortality and morbidity. In order to assess the risk of transmission of diarrheal disease, it is important to know the percentage of the population that do not have safe water supplies and sanitation. Use of solid fuels in households is a

proxy indicator for household pollution. Indicators of the prevalence of diabetes, hypertension, and obesity all signal the risk of cardiovascular disease and several types of cancer.

Indirect indicators of global health include health system indicators related to the workforce, infrastructure, medical technologies and devices, and government expenditures on health. Demographic and socioeconomic factors that are major determinants of health include primary school enrollment, population living in poverty, population size, crude birth and death rates, total fertility rates, and per-capita gross national income.

▶ Anthro-Cultural Beliefs and Values

A value system orients the members of a society toward defining what is desirable for that society. It has been observed that even a society as complex and highly diverse as that found in the United States can be said to have a relatively well-integrated system of institutionalized common values at the societal level (Parsons, 1972). Although such a view still prevails, American society now includes distinct subcultures whose membership has increased significantly due to a steady influx of immigrants from different parts of the world.

The current system of health services delivery has roots in the traditional beliefs and values espoused by the American people. This belief and value system governs the training and general orientation of health care providers, the type of health delivery settings, the financing and allocation of resources, and access to health care in the United States.

Among the main beliefs and values prevalent in the American culture are those outlined here.

1. The United States has a strong belief in the advancement of science and the application of scientific methods to medicine. This belief was instrumental in the creation of the medical model that primarily governs U.S. health care delivery. As a result, the United States has long led the world in medical breakthroughs. These developments have had numerous implications for health services delivery:

    a. They increase the demand for the latest treatments and raise patients' expectations for finding cures.

    b. Because medical professionals focus on clinical interventions, they do not provide adequate emphasis on the holistic aspects of health and use of alternative therapies.

    c. Health care professionals have been trained to focus on physical symptoms rather than the underlying causes of disease.

    d. Integrating diagnosis and treatment with disease prevention has lagged behind other concerns.

    e. Most research efforts have focused on the development of medical technology. Fewer resources have been committed to the preservation and enhancement of health and well-being.

    f. Medical specialists, using the latest technologies, are held in higher esteem and earn higher incomes than do general practitioners.

    g. The desirability of health care delivery institutions such as hospitals is often evaluated based on their acquisition of advanced technology.

    h. Whereas biomedicine has taken central stage in the biomedical model, mental health diagnosis and treatment have been relegated to a lesser status.

    i. The biomedical model has neglected the social and spiritual elements of health.

2. The United States has been a champion of capitalism. Due to the public's strong belief in capitalism, health care has largely been viewed as an economic good (or service), not as a public resource.

3. A culture of capitalism promotes entrepreneurial spirit and self-determination. Hence, individual capabilities to obtain health services have largely determined the production and consumption of health care (i.e.,

which services will be produced, where and in which quantities, and who will have access to those services). Some key implications are as follows:

a. Upper-tier access to health care services is available mainly through private health insurance. Those with public insurance fall in a second tier. The uninsured make up a third tier.

b. A clear distinction exists between the types of services for poor and affluent communities, and between the types of services available in rural and inner-city locations.

c. The culture of individualism emphasizes individual health rather than population health. Consequently, medical practice has been directed at keeping the individual healthy, rather than the entire community.

d. A concern for the most underprivileged classes in society—the poor, elderly, disabled, and children—led to the creation of the public programs Medicaid, Medicare, and the Children's Health Insurance Program (CHIP).

4. U.S. health care delivery is guided by principles of free enterprise and a general distrust of big government. Hence, health care delivery is largely in private hands, and a separation exists between public health functions and the private practice of medicine.

Equitable Distribution of Health Care

Scarcity of economic resources is a central economic concept. From this perspective, health care can be viewed as an economic good. Two fundamental questions arise with regard to how scarce health care resources ought to be used:

- How much health care should be produced?
- How should health care be distributed?

The first question concerns the appropriate combination of health services that should be produced in relation to all other goods and services in the overall economy. If more health care is produced, a society may concomitantly devote fewer resources to producing some other goods, such as food, clothing, and transportation. The second question affects individuals at a more personal level—namely, it deals with who can receive which type of medical service, and how access to services will be restricted.

The production, distribution, and subsequent consumption of health care must be perceived as equitable by a society. No society has found a perfectly equitable method to distribute limited economic resources. In fact, any method of resource distribution inevitably leaves some inequalities in its wake. Therefore, societies try to allocate resources according to some guiding principles that are deemed acceptable by the particular society. Such principles are ingrained in a society's value and belief system. It is recognized, for example, that not everyone can receive everything medical science has to offer.

A just and fair allocation of health care poses conceptual and practical difficulties. Hence, a theory of justice is necessary to resolve the problem of health care allocation (Jonsen, 1986). Even though various ethical principles can be used to guide decisions pertaining to just and fair allocation of health care in individual circumstances, the concern about providing equitable access to health services on a population level is addressed by two contrasting theories referred to as market justice and social justice.

Market Justice

The principle of **market justice** leaves the fair distribution of health care up to the market forces in a free economy. Medical care and its benefits are distributed based on people's willingness and ability to pay (Santerre and Neun, 2010). In other words, people are entitled to purchase a share of the available goods and services that they value; they purchase these valued goods and services by means of wealth acquired through their own efforts. This is how most goods and services are distributed in a free market. The free market implies that giving people something they have not earned would be morally and economically wrong.

The *Overview of U.S. Health Care Delivery* chapter discussed several characteristics that describe a free market. These market characteristics are a precondition to the distribution of health care services according to market justice principles. As previously mentioned, health care in the United States is not delivered in a free

market; it is delivered in a quasi-market. Hence, market justice principles are only partially applicable to the U.S. health care delivery system. Distribution of health care according to market justice is based on the following key assumptions:

- Health care is like any other economic good or service, the distribution and consumption of which are determined by the free market forces of supply and demand.
- Individuals are responsible for their own achievements. With the rewards of their achievements, people are free to obtain various economic goods and services, including health care. When individuals pursue their own best interests, the interests of society as a whole are best served (Ferguson and Maurice, 1970).
- People make rational choices in their decisions to purchase health care products and services. Grossman (1972) proposed that health is also an investment commodity—in other words, people consider the purchase of health services an investment. For example, the investment has a monetary payoff when it reduces the number of sick days, making extra time available for productive activities, such as earning a living. Alternatively, it can have a utility payoff—a payoff in terms of satisfaction—when it makes life more enjoyable and fulfilling.
- People, in consultation with their physicians, know what is best for them. This assumption implies that people place a certain degree of trust in their physicians and that the physician–patient relationship is ongoing.
- The marketplace works best with minimum interference from the government. In other words, the market,

rather than the government, can allocate health care resources in the most efficient and equitable manner.

Under market justice, the production of health care is determined by how much consumers are willing and able to purchase health care at the prevailing market prices. Thus, prices and ability to pay ration the quantity and type of health care services that people consume. The uninsured and individuals who lack sufficient income to pay for private health care services face barriers to obtaining health care. Such limitations to obtaining health care are referred to as **demand-side rationing**, or "rationing by ability to pay" (Feldstein, 1994). To some extent, the uninsured may be able to overcome some barriers through charitable services.

The key characteristics of the market justice system and their implications are summarized in **TABLE 2-5**. Market justice emphasizes individual—rather than collective—responsibilityforhealth.Itproposes private—rather than government—solutions to social problems of health.

Social Justice

The idea of social justice is at odds with the principles of capitalism and market justice. The term "social justice" was invented in the 19th century by the critics of capitalism to describe the "good society" (Kristol, 1978). According to the principle of **social justice**, the equitable distribution of health care is a societal responsibility, which is best achieved by letting the government take over the production and distribution of health care. Social justice regards health care as a social good rather than an economic good that should be collectively financed and available to all

citizens regardless of the individual recipient's ability to pay. The main characteristics and implications of social justice are summarized in Table 2-5.

Canadians and Europeans long ago reached a broad consensus that health care is a social good (Reinhardt, 1994). Public health also has a social justice orientation (Turnock, 1997). Under the social justice system, inability to obtain medical services because of a lack of financial resources is considered inequitable. Accordingly, a just distribution of health care must be based on need, not simply on the individual's ability to purchase such care in the marketplace (demand). Need for health care is determined either by the patient or by a health professional.

The principle of social justice is also based on certain assumptions:

- Health care is different from most other goods and services. Health-seeking behavior is governed primarily by need rather than by ability to pay.
- Responsibility for health is shared. Individuals are not held completely responsible for their condition because factors outside their control may have brought on the condition. Society is held responsible because individuals cannot control certain environmental factors, such as economic inequalities, unemployment, or unsanitary conditions.
- Society has an obligation to the collective good. The well-being of the community is superior to that of the individual. An unhealthy individual is a burden on society. A person carrying a deadly infection, for example, is a threat to society. Society, therefore, is obligated to cure the problem by providing health care to the individual. By doing so, the whole society will benefit.

TABLE 2-5 Comparison of Market Justice and Social Justice	
Market Justice	**Social Justice**
Characteristics	
▪ Views health care as an economic good	▪ Views health care as a social resource
▪ Assumes free-market conditions for health services delivery	▪ Requires active government involvement in health services delivery
▪ Assumes that markets are more efficient in allocating health resources equitably	▪ Assumes that the government is more efficient in allocating health resources equitably
▪ Production and distribution of health care determined by market-based demand	▪ Medical resource allocation determined by central planning
▪ Medical care distribution based on people's ability to pay	▪ Ability to pay is inconsequential for receiving medical care
▪ Access to medical care viewed as an economic reward of personal effort and achievement	▪ Equal access to medical services viewed as a basic right
Implications	
▪ Individual responsibility for health	▪ Collective responsibility for health
▪ Benefits based on individual purchasing power	▪ Everyone is entitled to a basic package of benefits
▪ Limited obligation to the collective good	▪ Strong obligation to the collective good
▪ Emphasis on individual well-being	▪ Community well-being supersedes that of the individual
▪ Private solutions to social problems	▪ Public solutions to social problems
▪ Rationing based on ability to pay	▪ Planned rationing of health care

▪ The government, not the market, can better decide through central planning how much health care to produce and how to distribute it to all citizens.

Just as true market justice does not exist in health care, so true social justice also does not exist. In the real world, no society can afford to provide unlimited amounts of health care to all its citizens (Feldstein, 1994). The government may offer insurance coverage to all, but must also find ways to limit the availability of certain health care services. For example, under the social justice principle, the government decides how technology will be dispersed and who will be allowed access to certain types of costly high-tech services, even though basic services may be available to all. The government engages in **supply-side rationing**, which is also referred to as **planned rationing**, or nonprice rationing. In social justice systems, the government uses "health planning" to limit the supply of health care services, although the limited resources are often more equally dispersed throughout the country than is generally the case under a market justice system. The necessity of rationing health care explains why citizens of a country can be given universal coverage but not universal access. Even when a covered individual has a medical need, depending on the nature of health services required, he or she may have to wait until services become available.

Justice in the U.S. Health Delivery System

In a quasi-perfect or imperfect market, such as the market for health care delivery in the United States, elements of both the market and social justice principles exist. In some areas, the principles of market and social justice complement each other. In other areas, the two present conflicts.

The two contrasting principles complement each other in the employer-based health insurance available to most middle-class working Americans (market justice) and the publicly financed Medicare, Medicaid, and CHIP coverage for certain disadvantaged groups (social justice). Insured populations access health care services delivered mainly by private practitioners and private institutions (market justice). Tax-supported county and city hospitals, public health clinics, and community health centers can be accessed by the uninsured in areas where such services are available (social justice).

Market and social justice principles create conflicts when health care resources are not uniformly distributed throughout the United States, and when there is a general shortage of primary care physicians (an issue discussed in the *Health Services Professionals* chapter). Consequently, in spite of having public insurance, many Medicaid-covered patients have difficulty obtaining timely access, particularly in rural and inner-city areas. This conflict is partly created by artificially low reimbursement from public programs; in comparison, reimbursement from private payers is more generous.

Limitations of Market Justice

The principles of market justice work well for allocating economic goods when their unequal distribution does not affect the larger society. For example, based on individual success, people live in different sizes and styles of homes, drive different types of automobiles, and spend their money on a variety of things. In other cases, the allocation of resources has wider repercussions for society. In these areas, market justice has severe limitations:

■ Market justice principles fail to rectify critical human concerns. Pervasive social problems, such as crime, illiteracy, and homelessness, can significantly weaken the cohesion of a society. Indeed, the United States has recognized such issues and instituted programs based on the social justice principle to combat such problems. These programs have added police protection, publicly supported education, and subsidized housing for many poor and elderly populations. Health care is an important social issue because it not only affects human productivity and achievement but also provides basic human dignity.

■ Market justice does not always protect a society. Individual health issues can have negative consequences for society because ill health is not always confined to the individual. The AIDS epidemic is an example of how a society can be put at serious risk by illness originally affecting just a few subpopulations. The initial spread of the SARS epidemic in Beijing, China, was largely due to patients with SARS symptoms being turned away by hospitals because they were not able to pay in advance for the cost of the treatment. Similar to clean air and water, health care is a social concern that, in the long run, protects against the burden of preventable disease and disability—a burden that is ultimately borne by society at large.

■ Market justice does not work well in health care delivery. On the one hand, a growing national economy and prosperity in the past did not materially reduce the number of uninsured Americans. On the other hand, the number of uninsured increases during economic downturns. For example, during the 2007–2009 recession, 5 million Americans lost employment-based health insurance (Holahan, 2011).

▶ ## Integration of Individual and Population Health

It has been recognized that the typical emphasis on the treatment of acute illness in hospitals, biomedical research, and high technology has not significantly improved the population's health. Instead, the medical model should be integrated with a disease-prevention, health-promotion, primary care–based model to produce significant gains in health. Society will always need the benefits of modern science and technology for the treatment of disease, but health promotion and primary care can prevent and delay the onset of many diseases, disability, and premature death. An integrated approach will improve the overall health of the population, enhance people's quality of life, and conserve health care resources.

The real challenge for the health care delivery system is incorporating the medical and wellness models within the holistic context of health. For instance, the Ottawa Charter for Health Promotion mentions caring, holism, and ecology as essential issues in developing strategies for health promotion (de Leeuw, 1989). "Holism" and "ecology" refer to the complex relationships that exist among (1) the individual; (2) the health care delivery system;

and (3) the physical, social, cultural, and economic environmental factors. In addition, as noted by an increasing body of research, the spiritual dimension must be incorporated into the integrated model.

Another equally important challenge for the health care delivery system is focusing on both individual and population health outcomes. The nature of health is complex, and the interrelationships among the physical, mental, social, and spiritual dimensions are not well understood. Translating this multidimensional framework of health into specific actions that are efficiently configured to achieve better individual and community health is one of the greatest challenges that today's health care systems face.

For an integrated approach to become reality, the best American ingenuity must be applied in addressing health-spending reductions and coordination of services among public health agencies, hospitals, and other health care providers. Community hospitals, in particular, are increasingly held accountable for the health status of the communities in which they are located. To fulfill this mission, hospitals must first conduct a health assessment of their communities. Such assessments provide broad perspectives of the local population's health and point to specific needs that health care providers can address. These assessments can help pinpoint interventions that should be given priority to improve the population's health status or address critical issues pertaining to certain subgroups within the population.

Healthy People Initiatives

Since 1980, the United States has undertaken 10-year plans outlining certain key national health objectives to be accomplished during each of the 10-year periods. The objectives are developed by a consortium of national and state organizations under the leadership of the U.S. Surgeon General. The first of these programs, with objectives for 1990, provided national goals for reducing premature deaths among all age groups and for reducing the average number of days of illness among persons older than age 65. A final review of this program concluded that positive changes in premature deaths had been achieved for all age categories except adolescents, but that illness among the elderly had not been reduced. However, the review set the stage to develop and modify the goals and objectives for the subsequent 10-year program (Chrvala and Bulger, 1999).

Healthy People 2000: National Health Promotion and Disease Prevention Objectives identified three main goals to be reached by the year 2000: (1) increase the span of healthy life for Americans; (2) reduce health disparities and wasteful care; and (3) promote individual responsibility and accountability for one's health as well as improved access to basic services. In a broad sense, these services include medical care, preventive services, health promotion, and social policy to improve education, lifestyle, employment, and housing (**FIGURE 2-4**). According to the final review, the major accomplishments of *Healthy People 2000* included surpassing the targets for reducing deaths from coronary heart disease and cancer; meeting the targets for mammography exams, violent deaths, tobacco-related deaths, and incidence rates of AIDS and syphilis; nearly meeting the targets for infant mortality and number of children

INDIVIDUAL HEALTH

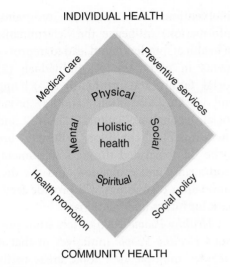

FIGURE 2-4 Integrated model for holistic health.

COMMUNITY HEALTH

with elevated levels of lead in their blood; and making some progress toward reducing health disparities among special populations.

The Ottawa Charter has proposed achieving health objectives through social public policy and community action. An integrated approach also necessitates creation of a new model for training health care professionals that forms partnerships with the community (Henry, 1993). The following paragraphs describe examples of community partnerships reflected in community health assessments and *Healthy People* initiatives. **Community health assessment** is a method used to conduct broad assessments of populations at a local or state level. To integrate individual and community health, the assessment is best conducted through collaboration with community members and local authorities (DHHS, 1992).

Healthy People 2010: Healthy People in Healthy Communities continued the earlier tradition as an instrument to improve the health of the American people in the first decade of the 21st century. It focused on two broad goals: (1) to increase quality and years of healthy life; and (2) to eliminate health disparities. It went a step beyond the previous initiatives by emphasizing the role of community partners (businesses, local governments, and civic, professional, and religious organizations) as effective agents for improving health in their local communities (DHHS, 1998). The final report revealed that 23% of the targets were met or exceeded and that the nation had made progress toward 48% of the targets. Specifically, life expectancy at birth, expected years in good or better health, and expected years free of activity limitations all improved, though expected years free of selected chronic diseases decreased. While many of the targets have been met or are in progress, the goal of reducing health disparities has not been achieved. Health disparities identified in approximately 80% of the objectives have not changed, and they even increased in another 13% of the objectives (NCHS, 2012). Hence, challenges remain in the reduction of chronic conditions and health disparities among population groups.

Healthy People 2020

Launched in 2010, *Healthy People 2020* (DHHS, 2010b) has a fivefold mission: (1) identify nationwide health improvement priorities; (2) increase public awareness and understanding of the determinants of health, disease, and disability and the opportunities for progress; (3) provide measurable objectives and goals that can be used at the national, state, and local levels; (4) engage multiple sectors to take actions that are driven by the best available evidence and knowledge; and (5) identify critical research and data collection needs. This initiative also has four overarching goals:

- Attain high-quality and longer lives free of preventable disease, disability, injury, and premature death.
- Achieve health equity, eliminate disparities, and improve the health of all groups.
- Create social and physical environments that promote good health for all.
- Promote quality of life, healthy development, and healthy behaviors across all life stages.

These overarching goals are in line with the tradition of earlier *Healthy People* initiatives but place particular emphasis on the determinants of health.

FIGURE 2-5 illustrates the action model to achieve the *Healthy People 2020* overarching goals. This model illustrates that interventions (i.e., policies, programs, information) influence the determinants of health at four levels and lead to improvements in outcomes: (1) individual; (2) social, family, and community; (3) living and working conditions; and (4) broad social, economic, cultural, health, and environmental conditions. Results are to be demonstrated through assessment, monitoring, and evaluation, and the dissemination of findings will provide feedback for future interventions.

Healthy People 2020 differs from previous *Healthy People* initiatives in that it includes multiple new topic areas to its objectives list, such as adolescent health, genomics, global health, health communication and health information technology, and social determinants of health. *Healthy People 2020* has 42 topic areas, with 13 new areas (**TABLE 2-6**).

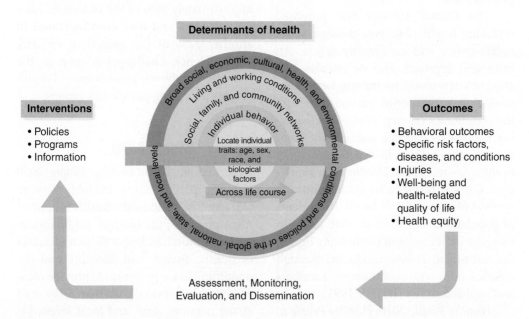

FIGURE 2-5 Action model to achieve U.S. *Healthy People 2020* overarching goals.

TABLE 2-6 *Healthy People 2020* Topic Areas

1. Access to health services	22. HIV
2. Adolescent health[1]	23. Immunization and infectious diseases
3. Arthritis, osteoporosis, and chronic back conditions	24. Injury and violence prevention
4. Blood disorders and blood safety[1]	25. Lesbian, gay, bisexual, and transgender health[1]
5. Cancer	26. Maternal, infant, and child health
6. Chronic kidney disease	27. Medical product safety
7. Dementias, including Alzheimer's disease[1]	28. Mental health and mental disorders
8. Diabetes	29. Nutrition and weight status
9. Disability and health	30. Occupational safety and health
10. Early and middle childhood[1]	31. Older adults[1]
11. Educational and community-based programs	32. Oral health
12. Environmental health	33. Physical activity
13. Family planning	34. Preparedness[1]
14. Food safety	35. Public health infrastructure
15. Genomics[1]	36. Respiratory diseases
16. Global health[1]	37. Sexually transmitted diseases
17. Health communication and health information technology	38. Sleep health[1]
18. Health care-associated infections[1]	39. Social determinants of health[1]
19. Health-related quality of life and well-being[1]	40. Substance abuse
20. Hearing and other sensory or communication disorders	41. Tobacco use
21. Heart disease and stroke	42. Vision

[1] New topic area.

Measurement of *Healthy People 2020*

Healthy People 2020 establishes four foundational health measures to monitor progress toward achieving its goals. The foundational health measures include general health status, health-related quality of life and well-being, determinants of health, and disparities. Measures of general health status include life expectancy, healthy life expectancy, years of potential life lost, physically and mentally unhealthy days, self-assessed health status, limitations of activity, and chronic disease prevalence. Measures of health-related quality of life and well-being include physical, mental, and social health-related quality of life, well-being/satisfaction, and participation in common activities. *Healthy People 2020* defines determinants of health as "a range of personal, social, economic, and environmental factors that influence health status. Determinants of health include such things as biology, genetics, individual behavior, access to health services, and the environment in which people are born, live, learn, play, work, and age." Measures of disparities and inequity include differences in health status based on race/ethnicity, gender, physical and mental ability, and geography (DHHS, 2010b).

Global health is also an important topic area in *Healthy People 2020*. The measurement of global health focuses on two aspects: (1) measuring the reduction of global diseases in the United States, including malaria and tuberculosis (TB); and (2) measuring "global capacity in support of the International Health Regulations to detect and contain emerging health threats" (DHHS, 2010b). The indicators include the number of global disease detection (GDD) regional centers worldwide, the number of public health professionals trained by GDD programs worldwide, the number of public health professionals trained by GDD programs worldwide, and the number of diagnostic tests established or improved by GDD programs (DHHS, 2010b).

Achievement of *Healthy People 2020*

Ongoing review has focused on how well the health care system is working toward achieving its delineated goals (*Healthy People 2020*, 2014). The findings of these ongoing studies are compared to the baseline data from the beginning of the 10-year period to determine whether adequate progress has occurred.

In total, *Healthy People 2020* contains 42 topic areas with more than 1,200 objectives. A subset of 26 of the objectives, known as the leading health indicators (LHI), is used to track the progress of the initiative and communicate high-priority health issues. Of the 26 LHIs, 4 indicators have met or exceeded their *Healthy People 2020* targets, 10 show improvement, 8 show little or undetectable change, and 3 are getting worse. One indicator has only baseline data available.

To date, indicators for access to health services show little change in this area. Although the proportion of people with medical insurance increased under the ACA, the target of 100% has not been reached. Similarly, access to a usual-care provider has increased but has not met *Healthy People 2020*'s target.

Many of the LHIs for clinical preventive services show improvement. The percentage of adults receiving colorectal cancer screenings, adults with hypertension whose blood pressure is controlled, and children receiving recommended vaccines have all increased significantly, moving toward the *Healthy People 2020* target (Egan et al., 2014). In contrast, the rate of adults with diabetes who also have poor glycemic control has not shown any significant improvement.

Some environmental quality indicators have not only met their *Healthy People 2020* goals, but actually exceeded them. The Air Quality Index, which assesses changes in air quality by number and severity of unhealthy days, met its goal. Likewise, the goal for reducing the percentage of children exposed to secondhand smoke has been achieved.

So far, the LHIs for injury and violence show positive progress. Injury deaths have decreased by 43% and the homicide rate has declined by 13%, both of which meet the *Healthy People 2020* targets.

Maternal and child health LHIs are significantly improving, with infant deaths and total preterm live births almost achieving their *Healthy People 2020* targets. Conversely, the LHIs for mental health appear to be significantly worse than those measures at baseline. The suicide rate has increased by 7%, and the percentage of adolescents with major depressive episodes has increased by almost 10%.

The LHIs for nutrition, physical activity, and obesity mostly show little or no detectable change. Rates of obesity among adults, children, and adolescents have all increased between 4% and 5%, although these changes are not statistically significant. Intake of vegetables remains stagnant. In a promising development, the percentage of adults meeting the federal physical activity guidelines has increased by 13%, exceeding the *Healthy People 2020* target.

In the area of oral health, the LHI is moving away from the target, showing a 6% decrease in the percentage of children, adolescents, and adults who had a dental visit in the past year. In contrast, the LHIs for reproductive and sexual health and social determinants show some progress toward the *Healthy People 2020* goals. Substance abuse indicators are mixed. While the number of adolescents using alcohol or illicit drugs has decreased, the prevalence of binge drinking among adults shows no change. The prevalence of adolescent cigarette smoking has slightly decreased, with the overall cigarette smoking rate showing an even larger decrease of approximately 12%.

▶ Summary

The delivery of health care is primarily driven by the medical model, which emphasizes illness rather than wellness. Holistic concepts of health, along with the integration of medical care with preventive and health promotional efforts, need to be adopted to significantly improve the health of Americans. Such an approach would require individuals to take responsibility for their own health-oriented behaviors, as well as the establishment of community partnerships to improve both personal and community health. Understanding the determinants of health, providing health education, utilizing community health assessment, and promoting national initiatives, such as *Healthy People*, are essential to accomplish these goals. *Healthy People 2020*, launched in 2010, continues its goals of improving health and eliminating health disparities in the United States. Public health has drawn increased attention in recent times because of the growing recognition of its role in health protection, environmental health, and preparedness for natural disasters and bioterrorism. Moreover, public health has now become global in its scope.

Programs to address the various facets of health and its determinants, and ongoing initiatives in the areas of prevention, health promotion, health protection, and equality, are complex undertakings and require substantial financial resources. Objective measures play a critical role both in evaluating the success of various programs and in directing future planning activities.

The broad concern of achieving equitable access to health services can be addressed by considering the contrasting theories of market justice and social justice. Countries offering universal coverage have adopted the principles of social justice, under which the government finances health care services and decides on the distribution of those services. However, because no country can afford to provide unlimited amounts of health care to all citizens, supply-side rationing becomes inevitable in such a system. Many of the characteristics of the U.S. health care system trace back to the beliefs and values underlying the American culture. Under market justice, not all citizens have health insurance coverage, a phenomenon called demand-side rationing.

▶ Test Your Understanding

Terminology

activities of daily living (ADLs)	health determinants	planned rationing
acute condition	health risk appraisal	population at risk
agent	holistic health	prevalence
bioterrorism	holistic medicine	primary prevention
cases	host	public health
chronic condition	iatrogenic illnesses	quality of life
community health assessment	immigration	risk factors
crude rates	incidence	secondary prevention
demand-side rationing	instrumental activities of daily living (IADLs)	social contacts
emigration	life expectancy	social justice
environment	market justice	social resources
environmental health	medical model	subacute condition
epidemic	migration	supply-side rationing
fertility	morbidity	surge capacity
health care	mortality	tertiary prevention
	natality	utilization

health determinants
health risk appraisal
holistic health
holistic medicine
host

Review Questions

1. What is the role of health risk appraisal in health promotion and disease prevention?
2. Health promotion and disease prevention may require both behavioral modification and therapeutic intervention. Discuss.
3. Discuss the definitions of health presented in this chapter in terms of their implications for the health care delivery system.
4. What are the main objectives of public health?
5. Discuss the significance of an individual's quality of life from the health care delivery perspective.
6. Which "preparedness"-related measures have been taken to cope with potential natural and human-made disasters since the tragic events of 9/11? Assess their effectiveness.
7. The Blum model points to four key determinants of health. Discuss their implications for health care delivery.
8. What has been the main cause of the dichotomy between the way physical and mental health issues have traditionally been addressed by the health care delivery system?
9. Discuss the main cultural beliefs and values in American society that have influenced health care delivery, including how they have shaped the health care delivery system.
10. Briefly describe the concepts of market justice and social justice. In which ways do the two principles complement each other, and in which ways are they in conflict in the U.S. system of health care delivery?
11. Describe how health care is rationed in the market justice and social justice systems.
12. To what extent do you think the objectives set forth in *Healthy People* initiatives can achieve the vision of an integrated approach to health care delivery in the United States?
13. What are the major differences between *Healthy People 2020* and the previous *Healthy People* initiatives?
14. How can health care administrators and policymakers use the various measures of health status and service utilization? Please use examples to illustrate your answer.
15. Using the data given in the table:
    a. Compute crude birth rates for 2005 and 2010.
    b. Compute crude death rates for 2005 and 2010.
    c. Compute cancer mortality rates for 2005 and 2010.
    d. Answer the following questions:
        i. Did the infant death rates improve between 2005 and 2010?
        ii. Which conclusions can you draw about the demographic change in this population?
        iii. Have efforts to prevent death from heart disease been successful in this population?

Population	2005	2010
Total	248,710	262,755
Male	121,239	128,314
Female	127,471	134,441
Whites	208,704	218,086
Blacks	30,483	33,141
Number of live births	4,250	3,840
Number of infant deaths (birth to 1 year)	39	35
Number of total deaths	1,294	1,324
Deaths from heart disease	378	363
Deaths from cancer	336	342

▶ References

American Diabetes Association. 2013. Economic costs of diabetes in the U.S. in 2012. *Diabetes Care* 36: 1033–1046.

American Public Health Association. 2013. *Prevention and Public Health Fund allocations*. Available at: https://www.hhs.gov/open/prevention/fy2013-allocation-pphf-funds.html. Accessed April 2017.

Anandarajah, G., and E. Hight. 2001. Spirituality and medical practice: Using the HOPE questions as a practical tool for spiritual assessment. *American Family Physician* 63, no. 1: 81–89.

Anderko, L., et al. 2012. Promoting prevention through the Affordable Care Act: Workplace wellness. *Preventing Chronic Disease* 9: E175.

Ansari, Z., et al. 2003. A public health model of the social determinants of health. *Sozial und Präventivmedizin (Social and Preventive Medicine)* 48, no. 4: 242–251.

Baicker, K., et al. 2010. Workplace wellness programs can generate savings. *Health Affairs (Millwood)* 29, no. 2: 304–311.

Bauer, U. E., et al. 2014. Prevention of chronic disease in the 21st century: Elimination of the leading preventable causes of premature death and disability in the USA. *Lancet* 384: 45–52.

Blum, H. L. 1981. *Planning for health*. 2nd ed. New York, NY: Human Sciences Press.

Bonnett, C., and B. C. Peery. 2007. Surge capacity: A proposed conceptual framework. *American Journal of Emergency Medicine* 25: 297–306.

Breslow, L. 1972. A quantitative approach to the World Health Organization definition of health: Physical, mental, and social well-being. *International Journal of Epidemiology* 4: 347–355.

Caballero, B. 2007. The global epidemic of obesity: An overview. *Epidemiology Review* 29: 1–5.

Centers for Disease Control and Prevention (CDC). 1999. Achievements in public health, 1900–1999: Control of infectious diseases. *Morbidity and Mortality Weekly Report* 48, no. 29: 621–629.

Centers for Disease Control and Prevention (CDC). 2007. *Avian influenza (bird flu)*. Available at: http://www.cdc.gov/flu/avian/. Accessed January 2007.

Centers for Disease Control and Prevention (CDC). 2010a. *Establishing a holistic framework to reduce inequities in HIV, viral hepatitis, STDs, and tuberculosis in the United States*. Available at: https://www.cdc.gov/socialdeterminants/docs/SDH-White-Paper-2010.pdf. Accessed April 2017.

Centers for Disease Control and Prevention (CDC). 2010b. Office of Public Health Preparedness and Response. *Public health preparedness: Strengthening the nation's emergency response state by state*. Available at: https://www.cdc.gov/phpr/publications/2010/phprep_report_2010.pdf. Accessed April 2017.

Centers for Disease Control and Prevention (CDC). 2011. *Million Hearts: Strategies to reduce the prevalence of leading cardiovascular disease risk factors—United States, 2011*. Available at: https://www.cdc.gov/mmwr/preview/mmwrhtml/mm6036a4.htm. Accessed April 2017.

Centers for Disease Control and Prevention (CDC). 2012. *SARS basics fact sheet*. Available at: http://www.cdc.gov/sars/about/fs-SARS.html. Accessed October 2013.

Centers for Disease Control and Prevention (CDC). 2013a. *Community based interventions: Brief executive summary*. Available at: https://www.cdc.gov/nccdphp/dch/programs/communitiesputtingpreventiontowork/pdf/community-based-interventions-executive-brief-update.pdf. Accessed April 2017.

Centers for Disease Control and Prevention (CDC). 2013b. *National Diabetes Prevention Program*. Available at: https://www.cdc.gov/diabetes/prevention/index.html. Accessed April 2017.

Centers for Disease Control and Prevention (CDC). 2013c. *National Diabetes Prevention Program: Find a program near you*. Available at: https://nccd.cdc.gov/DDT_DPRP/Programs.aspx. Accessed April 2017.

Centers for Disease Control and Prevention (CDC). 2016a. U.S. Cancer Statistics Working Group. *United States cancer statistics: 1999–2013 incidence and mortality web-based report*. Available at: https://nccd.cdc.gov/uscs/. Accessed April 2017.

Centers for Disease Control and Prevention (CDC). 2016b. *Diabetes: Working to reverse the US epidemic*. Available at: https://www.cdc.gov/chronicdisease/resources/publications/aag/pdf/2016/diabetes-aag.pdf. Accessed April 2017.

Centers for Disease Control and Prevention (CDC). 2016c. Facts about the National DPP. Available at: https://www.cdc.gov/diabetes/prevention/facts-figures/facts.html. Accessed April 2017.

Chida, Y., et al. 2009. Religiosity/spirituality and mortality. *Psychotherapy and Psychosomatics* 78: 81–90.

Chrvala, C. A., and R. J. Bulger, eds. 1999. *Leading health indicators for Healthy People 2010: Final report*. Washington, DC: National Academy of Sciences.

Cohen, M. H. 2003. *Future medicine*. Ann Arbor, MI: University of Michigan Press.

Cohen, S., and K. Mulvaney. 2005. Field observations: Disaster medical assistance team response for Hurricane Charley, Punta Gorda, Florida, 2004. *Disaster Management and Response*, 22–27.

Committee on Infectious Diseases, American Academy of Pediatrics; Kimberlin, D., et al. 2015. *Red book: 2015 report of the Committee of Infectious Diseases*. 30th ed. Elk Grove Village, Illinois: American Academy of Pediatrics.

Dahlgren, G., and M. Whitehead. 2006. *European strategies for tackling social inequities in health: Levelling up (part 2). Studies on Social and Economic Determinants of Population Health, No. 3*. Copenhagen, Denmark: World Health Organization. Available at: http://www.euro.who.int/__data/assets/pdf_file/0018/103824/E89384.pdf. Accessed December 2010.

Davis, D. L., and P. S. Webster. 2002. The social context of science: Cancer and the environment. *Annals of the American Academy of Political and Social Science* 584, 13–34.

De Leeuw, E. 1989. Concepts in health promotion: The notion of relativism. *Social Science and Medicine* 29, no. 11: 1281–1288.

Department of Health and Human Services (DHHS). 1992. *Healthy People 2000: National health promotion and disease prevention objectives*. Boston, MA: Jones and Bartlett.

Department of Health and Human Services (DHHS). 1998. *Healthy People 2010 objectives: Draft for public comment*. Washington, DC: U.S. Government Printing Office.

Department of Health and Human Services (DHHS). 2004. *The health consequences of smoking: A report of the Surgeon General.* Available at: http://www.surgeongeneral.gov/library/smoking consequences/. Accessed December 2010.

Department of Health and Human Services (DHHS). 2006. *Your guide to lowering blood pressure.* Available at: http://www.nhlbi.nih.gov/health/public/heart/hbp/dash/new_dash.pdf. Accessed December 2013.

Department of Health and Human Services (DHHS). 2008. *The Secretary's Advisory Committee on National Health Promotion and Disease Prevention Objectives for 2020. 2008. Phase I report: Recommendations for the framework and format of Healthy People 2020. Section IV. Advisory Committee findings and recommendations.* Available at: http://www.healthypeople.gov/2010/hp2020/advisory/phasei/sec4.htm. Accessed April 2017.

Department of Health and Human Services (DHHS). 2010a. *Summary of the prevention and wellness initiative.* Available at: http://www.cdc.gov/chronicdisease/recovery/docs/PW_Community_fact_sheet_final.pdf. Accessed November 2010.

Department of Health and Human Services (DHHS). 2010b. *Healthy People 2020.* Available at: http://healthypeople.gov/2020. Accessed December 2010.

Department of Health and Human Services (DHHS). 2011a. *National Health Security Strategy 2009.* Available at: http://www.phe.gov/Preparedness/planning/authority/nhss/Pages/default.aspx. Accessed August 2013.

Department of Health and Human Services (DHHS). 2011b. *$10 million in Affordable Care Act funds to help create workplace health programs* [News release]. Available at: http://www.businesswire.com/news/home/20110623005954/en/10-Million-Affordable-Care-Act-funds-create. Accessed April 2017.

Department of Health and Human Services (DHHS). 2014. *The health consequences of smoking—50 years of progress: A report of the Surgeon General.* Atlanta, GA: DHHS, Centers for Disease Control and Prevention, National Center for Chronic Disease Prevention and Health Promotion, Office on Smoking and Health.

Department of Health and Human Services (DHHS). 2017. *2020 Topics and Objectives—Objectives A–Z.* Available at: https://www.healthypeople.gov/2020/topics-objectives. Accessed April 2017.

Dever, G. E. 1984. *Epidemiology in health service management.* Gaithersburg, MD: Aspen.

Draper, P. 2012. An integrative review of spiritual assessment: Implications for nursing management. *Journal of Nursing Management* 20, no. 8: 970–980.

Egan, B. M., et al. 2014. Hypertension in the United States, 1999 to 2012: Progress toward *Healthy People 2020* goals. *Circulation* 130: 1692–1699.

Ethics Committee, Society for Academic Emergency Medicine. 1992. An ethical foundation for health care: An emergency medicine perspective. *Annals of Emergency Medicine* 21, no. 11: 1381–1387.

Feldstein, P. J. 1994. *Health policy issues: An economic perspective on health reform.* Ann Arbor, MI: AUPHA/HAP.

Ferguson, C. E., and S. C. Maurice. 1970. *Economic analysis.* Homewood, IL: Richard D. Irwin.

Finkelstein, E. A., et al. 2005. Economic causes and consequences of obesity. *Annual Review of Public Health* 26: 239–257.

Fortin, A. H., and K. G. Barnett. 2004. Medical school curricula in spirituality and medicine. *Journal of the American Medical Association* 291, no. 23: 2883.

Franco, M., et al. 2011. Challenges and opportunities for cardiovascular disease prevention. *American Journal of Medicine* 124: 95–102.

Franco, M., et al. 2009. Availability of healthy foods and dietary patterns: The Multi-Ethnic Study of Atherosclerosis. *American Journal of Clinical Nutrition* 89: 897–904.

Friedman, G. D. 1980. *Primer of epidemiology.* New York, NY: McGraw-Hill.

GBD 2013 Mortality and Causes of Death Collaborators. 2015. Global, regional, and national age–sex specific all-cause and cause-specific mortality for 240 causes of death, 1990–2013: A systematic analysis for the Global Burden of Disease Study 2013. *Lancet* 385: 117–171.

Gerteis, J., et al. 2014. *Multiple chronic conditions chartbook: 2010 medical expenditure panel survey data.* Rockville, MD: Agency for Healthcare Research and Quality.

Grossman, M. 1972. On the concept of health capital and the demand for health. *Journal of Political Economy* 80, no. 2: 223–255.

Hatch, R. L., et al. 1998. The Spiritual Involvement and Beliefs Scale: Development and testing of a new instrument. *Journal of Family Practice* 46: 476–486.

Healthy People 2020. 2014. Leading health indicators: Progress update. Available at: https://www.healthypeople.gov/2020/leading-health-indicators/Healthy-People-2020-Leading-Health-Indicators%3A-Progress-Update. Accessed April 2017.

Henao-Restrepo, A. M., et al. 2017. Efficacy and effectiveness of an rVSV-vectored vaccine in preventing Ebola virus disease: Final results from the Guinea ring vaccination, open-label, cluster-randomised trial (Ebola Ça Suffit!). *Lancet* 389: 505–518.

Henry, R. C. 1993. Community partnership model for health professions education. *Journal of the American Podiatric Medical Association* 83, no. 6: 328–331.

Hick, J., et al. 2004. Health care facility and community strategies for patient care surge capacity. *Annals of Emergency Medicine, 44,* 253–261.

Hoff, A., et al. 2008. Religion and reduced cancer risk—what is the explanation? A review. *European Journal of Cancer* 44, no. 17: 2573–2579.

Holahan, J. 2011. The 2007–09 recession and health insurance coverage. *Health Affairs* 30, no. 1: 145–152.

Houston, J. B., et al. 2015. Social media and disasters: A functional framework for social media use in disaster planning, response, and research. *Disasters* 39, no. 1: 1–22.

Ibrahim, M. A. 1985. *Epidemiology and health policy.* Gaithersburg, MD: Aspen.

Institute of Medicine, National Academy of Sciences. 1988. *The future of public health.* Washington, DC: National Academies Press.

Jacobsen, K. H., and S. T. Wiersma. 2010. Hepatitis A virus seroprevalence by age and world region, 1990 and 2005. *Vaccine* 28: 6653–6657.

Johnson, N., et al. 2011. *An update on state budget cuts: At least 46 states have imposed cuts that hurt vulnerable residents and the economy.* Washington DC: Center on Budget and Policy Priorities.

Joint Commission on the Accreditation of Healthcare Organizations. 2003. *2003 comprehensive accreditation manual for healthcare organizations: The official handbook.* Chicago, IL: Joint Commission.

Jonsen, A. R. 1986. Bentham in a box: Technology assessment and health care allocation. *Law,* *Medicine, and Health Care* 14, no. 3–4: 172–174.

Kane, R. L. 1988. Empiric approaches to prevention in the elderly: Are we promoting too much? In: *Health promotion and disease prevention in the elderly.* R. Chernoff and D. A. Lipschitz, eds. New York, NY: Raven Press. pp. 127–141.

Kannel, W. B., and R. D. Abbott. 1984. Incidence and prognosis of unrecognized myocardial infarction: An update on the Framingham Study. *New England Journal of Medicine* 311: 1144–1147.

Katz, S., and C. A. Akpom. 1979. A measure of primary sociobiological functions. In: *Sociomedical health indicators.* J. Elinson and A. E. Siegman, eds. Farmingdale, NY: Baywood. pp. 127–141.

Kawachi, I., et al. 1997. Social capital, income inequality, and mortality. *American Journal of Public Health* 87: 1491–1498.

Kawachi, I., et al. 1999. Social capital and self-rated health: A contextual analysis. *American Journal of Public Health* 89: 1187–1193.

Kearns, R., et al. 2013. Disaster planning: Transportation resources and considerations for managing a burn disaster. *Journal of Burn Care and Research* 35, e21–e32.

Khavjou, O. A., et al. 2014. Collecting costs of community prevention programs: Communities Putting Prevention to Work Initiative. *American Journal of Preventive Medicine* 47, no. 2: 160–165.

Kristol, I. 1978. A capitalist conception of justice. In: *Ethics, free enterprise, and public policy: Original essays on moral issues in business.* R. T. De George and J. A. Pichler, eds. New York, NY: Oxford University Press. pp. 57–69.

Larson, C., and A. Mercer. 2004. Global health indicators: An overview. *Canadian Medical Association Journal* 171, no. 10: 1199–1200.

Lasker, R. D. 1997. *Medicine and public health: The power of collaboration.* New York, NY: New York Academy of Medicine.

Macfarlane, G. J., and A. B. Lowenfels. 1994. Physical activity and colon cancer. *European Journal of Cancer Prevention* 3, no. 5: 393–398.

Marwick, C. 1995. Should physicians prescribe prayer for health? Spiritual aspects of well-being considered. *Journal of the American Medical Association* 273, no. 20: 1561–1562.

Mattke, S., et al. 2013. *Workplace wellness study: Final report*. Santa Monica, CA: RAND Health. Available at: https://www.dol.gov/sites/default /files/ebsa/researchers/analysis/health-and -welfare/workplacewellnessstudyfinal.pdf. Accessed April 2017.

Maylahn, C., et al. 2013. Health departments in a brave New World. *Preventing Chronic Disease* 10: E41.

McKee, M. 2001. Measuring the efficiency of health systems. *British Medical Journal* 323, no. 7308: 295–296.

Monod, S., et al. 2011. Instruments measuring spirituality in clinical research: A systematic review. *Journal of General Internal Medicine* 26, no. 11: 1345–1357.

Mozaffarian, D., et al. 2016. Executive summary: Heart disease and stroke statistics—2016 update: A report from the American Heart Association. *Circulation* 133: 447–454.

National Cancer Institute. 2016. *State cancer profiles*. Available at: https://statecancerprofiles.cancer .gov/recenttrend/index.php.

National Center for Health Statistics (NCHS). 2012. *Healthy People 2010 final review*. Hyattsville, MD. Available at: http://www.cdc.gov/nchs /healthy_people/hp2010/hp2010_final_review .htm. Accessed August 2013.

National Center for Health Statistics (NCHS). 2016. *Health, United States, 2015*. Hyattsville, MD: Department of Health and Human Services.

National Prevention Council. 2011. *Nation prevention strategy: America's plan for better health and wellness*. Washington, DC: U.S. Department of Health and Human Services.

Nelson, C., et al. 2007. Assessing public health emergency preparedness: Concepts, tools, and challenges. *Annual Review of Public Health* 28: 1–18.

Office of the Assistant Secretary for Planning and Evaluation. 2015. *The Affordable Care Act is improving access to preventive services for millions of Americans*. Available at: https:// aspe.hhs.gov/pdf-report/affordable-care-act -improving-access-preventive-services-millions -americans. Accessed April 2017.

Oman, D., et al. 2002. Religious attendance and cause of death over 31 years. *International Journal of Psychiatry and Medicine* 32: 69–89.

Ostir, G. V., et al. 1999. Disability in older adults 1: Prevalence, causes, and consequences. *Behavioral Medicine* 24, no. 4: 147–156.

Pantell, M., et al. 2013. Social isolation: A predictor of mortality comparable to traditional clinical risk factors. *American Journal of Public Health* 103, no. 11: 2056–2062.

Parsons, T. 1972. Definitions of health and illness in the light of American values and social structure. In: *Patients, physicians and illness: A sourcebook in behavioral science and health*. 2nd ed. E. G. Jaco, ed. New York, NY: Free Press. pp. 97–117.

Pasley, B. H., et al. 1995. Excess acute care bed capacity and its causes: The experience of New York State. *Health Services Research* 30, no. 1: 115–131.

Peters, K. E., et al. 2001. *Cooperative actions for health programs: Lessons learned in medicine and public health collaboration*. Chicago, IL: American Medical Association.

Pincus, T., et al. 1998. Social conditions and self-management are more powerful determinants of health than access to care. *Annals of Internal Medicine* 129, no. 5: 406–411.

Plotkin, S. L., and S. A. Plotkin. 2012. A short history of vaccination. In: *Vaccines*. 6th ed. S. A. Plotkin, W. A. Orenstein, and P. Offit, eds. Philadelphia, PA: W. B. Saunders. pp. 1–13.

Post, S. G., et al. 2000. Physicians and patient spirituality: Professional boundaries, competency, and ethics. *Annals of Internal Medicine* 132, no. 7: 578–583.

Reinhardt, U. E. 1994. Providing access to health care and controlling costs: The universal dilemma. In: *The nation's health*. 4th ed. P. R. Lee and C. L. Estes, eds. Boston, MA: Jones and Bartlett. pp. 263–278.

Robert Wood Johnson Foundation (RWJF). 2010. *Chronic care: Making the case for ongoing care*. Available at: http://www.rwjf.org/pr/product.jsp ?id=50968. Accessed April 2017.

Roberts, J. A., et al. 1997. Factors influencing the views of patients with gynecologic cancer about end-of-life decisions. *American Journal of Obstetrics and Gynecology* 176: 166–172.

Rosen, G. 1993. *A history of public health*. Baltimore, MD: Johns Hopkins University Press.

Ross, L. 1995. The spiritual dimension: Its importance to patients' health, well-being and quality of life and its implications for nursing practice. *International Journal of Nursing Studies* 32, no. 5: 457–468.

Santerre, R. E., and S. P. Neun. 2010. *Health economics: Theory, insights, and industry studies*. Mason, OH: South-Western Cengage Learning.

Satcher, D. 2010. Include a social determinants of health approach to reduce health inequities. *Public Health Reports* 4, no. 25: 6–7.

Saward, E., and A. Sorensen. 1980. The current emphasis on preventive medicine. In: *Issues in health services.* S. J. Williams, ed. New York: John Wiley & Sons. pp. 17–29.

Schneider, M. J. 2000. *Introduction to public health.* Gaithersburg, MD: Aspen.

Shi, L., and J. Johnson, eds. 2014. *Public health administration: Principles for population-based management.* 3rd ed. Burlington, MA: Jones & Bartlett Learning.

Shi, L., and B. Starfield. 2001. Primary care physician supply, income inequality, and racial mortality in U.S. metropolitan areas. *American Journal of Public Health* 91, no. 8: 1246–1250.

Shi, L., et al. 1999. Income inequality, primary care, and health indicators. *Journal of Family Practice* 48, no. 4: 275–284.

Shi, L., et al. 2002. Primary care, self-rated health, and reduction in social disparities in health. *Health Services Research* 37, no. 3: 529–550.

Smith, B. C. 1979. *Community health: An epidemiological approach.* New York, NY: Macmillan. pp. 197–213.

Solar, O., and A. Irwin; World Health Organization (WHO). 2010. *A conceptual framework for action on the social determinants of health. Social Determinants of Health Discussion Paper 2 (Policy and Practice).* Geneva, Switzerland: WHO.

Song, M., and E. Giovannucci. 2016. Preventable incidence and mortality of carcinoma associated with lifestyle factors among white adults in the United States. *JAMA Oncology* 9: 1154–1161.

Stopford, B. 2005. The National Disaster Medical System: America's medical readiness force. *Disaster Management and Response,* 53–56.

Swanson, C. S. 1995. A spirit-focused conceptual model of nursing for the advanced practice nurse. *Issues in Comprehensive Pediatric Nursing* 18, no. 4: 267–275.

Thompson, W. W., et al. 2009. Estimates of US influenza-associated deaths made using four different methods. *Influenza and Other Respiratory Viruses* 3: 37–49.

Timmreck, T. C. 1994. *An introduction to epidemiology.* Boston, MA: Jones and Bartlett.

Turnock, B. J. 1997. *Public health: What it is and how it works.* Gaithersburg, MD: Aspen.

U.S. Census Bureau. 2016. *An aging world: 2015 international population reports.* Available at: https://www.census.gov/content/dam/Census/library/publications/2016/demo/p95-16-1.pdf. Accessed February 2017.

Vella-Brodrick, D. A., and F. C. Allen. 1995. Development and psychometric validation of the mental, physical, and spiritual well-being scale. *Psychological Reports* 77, no. 2: 659–674.

Walsh, L., et al. 2015. Building health care system capacity to respond to disasters: Successes and challenges of disaster preparedness health care coalitions. *Prehospital Disaster Medicine* 30, no. 2: 112–122.

Ward, B. 1995. Holistic medicine. *Australian Family Physician* 24, no. 5: 761–762, 765.

WHO Ebola Response Team et al. 2016. After Ebola in West Africa: Unpredictable risks, preventable epidemics. *New England Journal of Medicine* 375, no. 6: 587–596.

Wilkinson, R. G. 1997. Comment: Income, inequality, and social cohesion. *American Journal of Public Health* 87: 1504–1506.

World Cancer Research Fund, and American Institute for Cancer Research (AICR). 2007. *Food, nutrition, physical activity, and the prevention of cancer: A global perspective.* Washington DC: AICR. Available at: http://www.aicr.org/assets/docs/pdf/reports/Second_Expert_Report.pdf. Accessed April 2017.

World Health Organization (WHO). 1948. *Preamble to the constitution.* Geneva, Switzerland: WHO. Available at: http://www.who.int/governance/eb/who_constitution_en.pdf. Accessed April 2017.

World Health Organization (WHO). 2003. *WHO definition of palliative care.* Geneva, Switzerland: WHO.

World Health Organization (WHO). 2008. *Closing the gap in a generation: health equity through action on the social determinants of health. Report from the Commission on Social Determinants of Health.* Geneva, Switzerland. WHO. Available at: http://www.who.int/social_determinants/thecommission/finalreport/en/index.html. Accessed April 2017.

World Health Organization (WHO). 2011. *Noncommunicable diseases country profiles.* Available at: http://www.who.int/nmh/countries/usa_en.pdf. Accessed August 2013.

World Health Organization (WHO). 2013. *Pandemic influenza preparedness framework.* Available at:

http://www.who.int/influenza/resources/pip_framework/en/. Accessed August 2013.

World Health Organization (WHO). 2015. *World health statistics. Part II: Global health indicators.* Available at: http://www.who.int/gho/publications/world_health_statistics/EN_WHS2015_Part2.pdf. Accessed April 2017.

World Health Organization (WHO). 2016a. *Recommended composition of influenza virus vaccines for use in the 2017 southern hemisphere influenza season.* Available at: http://www.who.int/influenza/vaccines/virus/recommendations/2017_south/en/. Accessed January 2017.

World Health Organization (WHO). 2016b. *MERS-CoV global summary and risk assessment.* Geneva, Switzerland: WHO.

World Health Organization (WHO). 2016c. *World malaria report.* Geneva, Switzerland: WHO.

World Health Organization (WHO). 2016d. *Global Tuberculosis Programme: Global tuberculosis report 2016.* Geneva, Switzerland: WHO.

World Health Organization (WHO). 2016e. *Prevent HIV, test and treat all: WHO support for country impact: Progress report 2016.* Geneva, Switzerland: WHO.

World Health Organization (WHO). 2016f. *Fact sheet: Ebola virus disease.* Available at: http://www.who.int/mediacentre/factsheets/fs103/en/. Accessed January 2017.

Xu, J., et al. 2016. *Deaths: Final data for 2013. National Vital Statistics Reports.* Atlanta, GA: Centers for Disease Control and Prevention.

Yabroff, K. R., et al. 2011. Economic burden of cancer in the United States: Estimates, projections, and future research. *Cancer Epidemiology, Biomarkers, & Prevention* 20: 2006–2014.

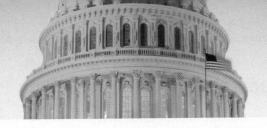

CHAPTER 3

The Evolution of Health Services in the United States

LEARNING OBJECTIVES

- Discover historical developments that have shaped the U.S. health care delivery system.
- Understand the history of mental health care in the United States.
- Evaluate why the system has been resistant to national health insurance reforms.
- Explore the corporatization of health care.
- Identify the globalization of health care.
- Obtain a historical perspective on the Affordable Care Act.
- Assess the prospects of new health care reform efforts.

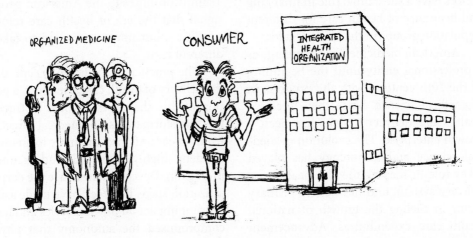

Where's the market?

▶ Introduction

Delivery of health care in the United States evolved quite differently from the systems in Europe. The U.S. health care system has been shaped by the country's anthro-cultural values and a series of social, political, and economic antecedents. Because social, political, and economic contexts are not static, their shifting influences lend a certain dynamism to the health care delivery system. Conversely, cultural beliefs and values remain relatively stable over time. As a consequence of the persistent resistance of American anthro-cultural values to a government-run national health care program, initiatives toward establishing such a system had long failed to make any significant progress. Instead, the interaction of forces just mentioned led to certain compromises that resulted in incremental changes over time. Incremental changes, both small and large, since 1935 have gradually shifted U.S. health care from a mainly private enterprise to one in which both the private and public sectors have a substantial role in financing and insurance of health care for different population groups in the United States.

American medicine did not emerge as a professional entity until the beginning of the 20th century, with the progress in biomedical science. Since then, the U.S. health care delivery system has been a growth enterprise. The evolution of medical science and technology has played a key role in shaping the U.S. health care delivery system, and has been a primary factor in fueling the growth of national health care expenditures. Advancement of technology has influenced other factors as well, such as medical education, growth of alternative settings for health services

delivery, and corporatization of medicine. In many respects, health care delivery has also become a global enterprise.

This chapter traces the evolution of health care delivery through historical phases, each demarcating a major change in the structure of the delivery system. The first evolutionary phase is the preindustrial era from the middle of the 18th century to the latter part of the 19th century. The second phase is the postindustrial era beginning in the late 19th century. The third phase— called the corporate era—became recognized in the latter part of the 20th century. Corporatization of medicine has played a major role in the globalization of health care.

Since the Obama presidency, health care reform has taken center stage in American politics. The Affordable Care Act (ACA) was passed in 2010 to bring about sweeping changes in U.S. health care delivery; however, many of its promises remained unfulfilled. These issues could very well have been one main reason behind the victory of Donald Trump in the 2016 presidential election. President Trump's promises to the American people signal that the era of health care reform continues, but now is expected to take a different turn.

The practice of medicine is central to the delivery of health care; therefore, a portion of this chapter is devoted to tracing the transformations in medical practice from a weak and insecure trade to an independent, highly respected, and lucrative profession. Developments since the corporatization stage, however, have made a significant impact on practice styles and have compromised the autonomy that physicians had historically enjoyed. **EXHIBIT 3-1** provides a snapshot of the historical developments in U.S. health care delivery.

EXHIBIT 3-1 Evolution of the U.S. Health Care Delivery System

Development of science and technology

Mid-18th to Late 19th Century	Late 19th to Late 20th Century	Late 20th to 21st Century
■ Open entry into medical practice ■ Intense competition ■ Weak and unorganized profession ■ Apprenticeship training ■ Undeveloped hospitals ■ Almshouses and pesthouses ■ Dispensaries ■ Mental asylums ■ Private payment for services ■ Low demand for services ■ Private medical schools providing only general education	■ Scientific basis of medicine ■ Urbanization ■ Emergence of the modern hospital ■ Emergence of organized medicine ■ Reform of medical training ■ Licensing ■ Specialization in medicine ■ Development of public health ■ Community mental health ■ Birth of workers' compensation ■ Emergence of private insurance ■ Failure of national health insurance ■ Medicaid and Medicare	■ Corporatization - Managed care - Organizational integration - Diluted physician autonomy ■ Globalization - Global telemedicine - Medical tourism - U.S. health care investment abroad - Migration of professionals - Global health ■ Era of health care reform - The Affordable Care Act - Prospects for new reforms
Consumer sovereignty	**Professional dominance**	**Government and corporate dominance**

Beliefs and values/Social, economic, and political constraints

▶ Medical Services in the Preindustrial Era

From colonial times to the beginning of the 20th century, American medicine lagged behind the advances in medical science, experimental research, and medical education that were taking place in Great Britain, France, and Germany. While London, Paris, and Berlin flourished as major research centers, Americans had a tendency to neglect research in basic sciences and to place more emphasis on applied science (Shryock, 1966). In addition, American attitudes about medical treatment placed strong emphasis on natural history and conservative common sense (Stevens, 1971). Consequently, the practice of medicine in the United States had a strong domestic—rather than professional—character. Medical services, when deemed appropriate by the consumer, were purchased out of one's private funds because there was no health insurance. The health care market was characterized by competition among providers, and the consumer decided who the provider would be. Thus, the consumer was sovereign in the health care market and health care was delivered under free-market conditions.

Five main factors explain why the medical profession remained largely an insignificant trade in preindustrial America:

1. Medical practice was in disarray.
2. Medical procedures were primitive.
3. An institutional core was missing.
4. Demand was unstable.
5. Medical education was substandard.

Medical Practice in Disarray

The early practice of medicine could be regarded more as a trade than a profession. It did not require the rigorous course of study, clinical practice, residency training, board exams, or licensing without which it is impossible to practice today. At the close of the Civil War (1861–1865), "anyone who had the inclination to set himself up as a physician could do so, the exigencies of the market alone determining who would prove successful in the field and who would not" (Hamowy, 1979). The clergy, for example, often combined medical services and religious duties.

The generally well-educated clergyman or government official was more learned in medicine than physicians were at the time (Shryock, 1966). Tradesmen, such as tailors, barbers, commodity merchants, and persons engaged in numerous other trades, also practiced the healing arts by selling herbal prescriptions, nostrums, elixirs, and cathartics. Likewise, midwives, homeopaths, and naturalists could practice medicine without being subject to any restrictions. The red-and-white striped poles (symbolizing blood and bandages) seen outside barbershops are reminders that barbers also functioned as surgeons at one time, using the same blade to cut hair, shave beards, and bleed the sick.

This era of medical pluralism has been referred to as a "war zone" by Kaptchuk and Eisenberg (2001) because it was marked by bitter antagonism among the various practicing sects. Eventually, in 1847, the American Medical Association (AMA) was founded with the main purpose of erecting a barrier between orthodox practitioners and the "irregulars" (Rothstein, 1972).

In the absence of minimum standards of medical training, entry into private practice was relatively easy for both trained and untrained practitioners, creating intense competition. Medicine as a profession was weak and unorganized. Hence, physicians did not enjoy the prestige, influence, and incomes that they later earned. Many physicians found it necessary to engage in a second occupation because income from medical practice alone was inadequate to support a family. It is estimated that most physicians' incomes in the mid-19th century placed them at the lower end of the middle class (Starr, 1982). In 1830, there were approximately 6,800 physicians in the United States, serving primarily the upper classes (Gabe et al., 1994). It was not until 1870 that medical education was reformed and licensing laws were passed in the United States.

Primitive Medical Procedures

Up until the mid-1800s, medical care was based more on primitive medical traditions than on science. In the absence of diagnostic tools, a theory of "intake and outgo" served as an explanation for all diseases (Rosenberg, 1979). It was believed that diseases needed to be expelled from the body. Hence, bleeding, use of emetics (to induce vomiting) and diuretics (to increase urination), and purging with enemas and purgatives (to clean the bowels) were popular forms of clinical therapy.

When George Washington became ill with an inflamed throat in 1799, he, too, was bled by physicians. One of the attending physicians argued, unsuccessfully, in favor of making an incision to open the trachea, which today would be considered a more enlightened procedure. The bleeding most likely weakened Washington's resistance, and historians have debated whether it played a role in his death (Clark, 1998).

Surgeries were limited because anesthesia had not yet been developed and antiseptic techniques were not known. Stethoscopes and x-rays had not been discovered, clinical thermometers were not in use, and microscopes were not available for a better understanding of pathology. Physicians relied mainly on their five senses and experience to diagnose and treat medical problems. Hence, in most cases, physicians did not possess any technical expertise greater than that of

the mothers and grandparents at home or experienced neighbors in the community.

Missing Institutional Core

In the United States, widespread development of hospitals did not occur before the 1880s. A few isolated hospitals were either built or developed in rented private houses in large cities, such as Philadelphia, New York, Boston, Cincinnati, New Orleans, and St. Louis. By contrast, general hospital expansion began much before the 1800s in France and Great Britain (Stevens, 1971).

In Europe, medical professionals were closely associated with hospitals. New advances in medical science were being pioneered, which European hospitals readily adopted. The medical profession came to be highly regarded because of its close association with an establishment that was scientifically advanced. In contrast, American hospitals played only a small part in medical practice because most hospitals served a social welfare function by taking care of the poor, those without families, or those who were away from home on travel.

The Almshouse and the Pesthouse

In the United States, the **almshouse**, also called a poorhouse, was the common ancestor of both hospitals and nursing homes. The poorhouse program was adopted from the Elizabethan system of public charity based on English Poor Laws. The first poorhouse in the United States is recorded to have opened in 1660 in Boston (Wagner, 2005). Almshouses served primarily general welfare functions by providing food and shelter to the destitute of society. Therefore, the main function of the almshouse was custodial. Caring for the sick was incidental because some of the residents would inevitably become ill and would be cared for in an adjoining infirmary. Almshouses were unspecialized institutions that admitted poor and needy persons of all kinds: the elderly, the orphaned, the insane, the ill, and the disabled. Hence, the early hospital-type institutions emerged mainly to take care of indigent people whose families could not care for them.

Another type of institution, the **pesthouse**, was operated by local governments (primarily in seaports) to quarantine people who had contracted a contagious disease, such as cholera, smallpox, typhoid, or yellow fever. The main function of a pesthouse was to isolate people with contagious diseases to prevent the spread of disease among the population. These institutions were the predecessors of contagious-disease and tuberculosis hospitals.

The Dispensary

Dispensaries were established as outpatient clinics, independent of hospitals, to provide free care to those who could not afford to pay. Urban workers and their families often depended on such charity (Rosen, 1983).

Starting with Philadelphia in 1786, dispensaries gradually spread to other cities. These private institutions were financed by bequests and voluntary subscriptions. Their main function was to provide basic medical care and to dispense drugs to ambulatory patients (Raffel, 1980). Generally, young physicians and medical students desiring clinical experience staffed the dispensaries,

as well as hospital wards, on a part-time basis for little or no income (Martensen, 1996). This model served a dual purpose: It provided needed services to the poor and enabled both physicians and medical students to gain experience diagnosing and treating a variety of cases. Later, as the practice of specialized medicine, as well as teaching and research, was transferred to hospital settings, many dispensaries were gradually absorbed into hospitals as outpatient departments. Indeed, outpatient or ambulatory care departments became an important locale for specialty consultation services within large hospitals (Raffel, 1980).

The Mental Asylum

Mental health care was seen as largely the responsibility of state and local governments. At this time, little was known about what caused mental illness or how to treat it. Although some mental health patients were confined to almshouses, asylums were built by states for patients with untreatable, chronic mental illness. The first such asylum was built around 1770 in Williamsburg, Virginia. When the Pennsylvania Hospital opened in Philadelphia in 1752, its basement was used as a mental asylum. Attendants in these asylums employed physical and psychological techniques in an effort to return patients to some level of rational thinking. Techniques such as bleeding, forced vomiting, and hot and ice-cold baths were also used.

Between 1894 and World War I, the State Care Acts were passed, centralizing financial responsibility for mentally ill patients in every state government. Local governments took advantage of this opportunity to send all those persons with a mental illness, including dependent older citizens, to the state asylums. The quality of care in public asylums deteriorated rapidly, as overcrowding and underfunding ran rampant (U.S. Surgeon General, 1999). Subsequent reforms are discussed in the section "Reform of Mental Health Care."

The Dreaded Hospital

Not until the 1850s were hospitals similar to those in Europe developed in the United States. These early hospitals had deplorable conditions due to a lack of resources. Poor sanitation and inadequate ventilation were hallmarks of these facilities. Unhygienic practices prevailed because nurses were unskilled and untrained. The early hospitals also had an undesirable image of being houses of death. The mortality rate among hospital patients, both in Europe and America, stood around 74% in the 1870s (Falk, 1999). People went into hospitals because of dire consequences, not by personal choice. It is not hard to imagine why members of the middle and upper classes, in particular, shunned such establishments.

Unstable Demand

Professional services suffered from low demand in the mainly rural, preindustrial society, and much of the medical care was provided by people who were not physicians. The most competent physicians were located in more populated communities (Bordley and Harvey, 1976). In the small communities of rural America, a strong spirit of self-reliance prevailed. Families and communities were accustomed to treating the sick, often using folk remedies passed from one generation to the next. It was also common to consult published books and pamphlets that gave advice on home remedies (Rosen, 1983).

The market for physicians' services was also limited by economic conditions. Many families could not afford to pay for medical services. Two factors contributed to the high costs associated with obtaining professional medical care:

- The indirect costs of transportation and the "opportunity cost" of travel (i.e., forgone value of time that could have been used for something more productive) could easily outweigh the direct costs of physicians' fees.
- The costs of travel often doubled because two people, the physician and an emissary, had to make the trip back and forth. For a farmer, a trip of 10 miles into town could mean an entire day's work lost. Farmers had to cover travel costs and the opportunity cost of time spent traveling. Mileage charges amounted to four or five times the basic fee for a visit if a physician had to travel 5 to 10 miles. Hence, most families obtained only occasional intervention from physicians, generally for nonroutine and severe conditions (Starr, 1982).

Personal health services had to be purchased without the help of government or private insurance. Private practice and **fee for service**—the practice of billing separately for each individual type of service performed—became firmly embedded in American medical care.

Similar to physicians, dentists were private entrepreneurs who made their living by private fee-for-service (PFFS) dental practice. Their services were not in great demand, however, because there was little public concern about dental health during this era (Anderson, 1990).

Substandard Medical Education

From about 1800 to 1850, medical training was largely received through individual apprenticeship with a practicing physician, referred to as a preceptor, rather than through university education. Many of the preceptors were themselves poorly trained, especially in basic medical sciences (Rothstein, 1972). By 1800, only four small medical schools were operating in the United States: College of Philadelphia (whose medical school was established in 1756, and which later became the University of Pennsylvania), King's College (whose medical school was established in 1768, and which later became Columbia University), Harvard Medical School (opened in 1782), and the Geisel School of Medicine at Dartmouth College (started in 1797).

American physicians later established medical schools in large numbers, partly to enhance their professional status and prestige and partly to enhance their income. Medical schools were inexpensive to operate and often quite profitable. All that was required was a faculty of four or more physicians, a classroom, a back room in which to conduct dissections, and legal authority to confer degrees. Operating expenses were met totally out of student fees that were paid directly to the physicians (Rothstein, 1972). Physicians would affiliate with a local college for the conferral of degrees and use of classroom facilities. Large numbers of men entered medical practice, as education in medicine

became readily available and unrestricted entry into the profession was still possible (Hamowy, 1979). Gradually, as physicians from medical schools began to outnumber those from the apprenticeship system, the Doctor of Medicine (MD) degree became the standard of competence. The number of medical schools tripled between 1800 and 1820, then tripled again between 1820 and 1850, with 42 being in operation by 1850 (Rothstein, 1972). Academic preparation gradually replaced apprenticeship training.

At this point, medical education in the United States was seriously deficient in science-based training, unlike European medical schools. Medical schools in the United States did not have laboratories, and clinical observation and practice were not part of the curriculum. In contrast, European medical schools, particularly those in Germany, emphasized laboratory-based medical research. At the University of Berlin, for example, professors were expected to conduct research as well as teach, and were paid by the state. In contrast, in American medical schools, students were taught by local practitioners, who were ill equipped in education and training. Unlike in Europe, where medical education was financed and regulated by the government, proprietary medical schools in the United States set their own standards (Numbers and Warner, 1985). A "year" of medical school in the United States generally lasted only 4 months and only 2 years of attendance was required for graduation. In addition, American medical students customarily repeated the same courses they had taken during their first year again during their second year (Numbers and Warner, 1985; Rosner, 2001). The physicians' desire to keep their schools profitable also contributed to low standards and a lack of rigor: They feared that higher standards in medical education would drive enrollments down, which could force the schools into bankruptcy (Starr, 1982).

▶ Medical Services in the Postindustrial Era

In the postindustrial period, American physicians, unlike other physicians in the world, were highly successful in retaining private practice of medicine and resisting national health care. Physicians delivered scientifically and technically advanced services to insured patients; became an organized medical profession; and gained power, prestige, and financial success. Notably, much of this transformation occurred in the aftermath of the Civil War. Social and scientific changes in the period following the war were accompanied by a transition from a rural, agricultural economy to a system of industrial capitalism. Mass production techniques used in the war were applied to peacetime industries. Railroads linked the east and west coasts of the United States, and small towns became cities (Stevens, 1971).

The American system for delivering health care took its current shape during this period. The well-defined role of employers in providing workers' compensation for work-related injuries and illnesses, together with other economic considerations, was instrumental in the growth of private health insurance. Even though attempts to pass national health care legislation failed, rising costs of health care prompted Congress to create the publicly financed programs, such as Medicare and Medicaid, for the most vulnerable members of society.

Growth of Professional Sovereignty

The 1920s represented a milestone in the consolidation of physicians' professional power. During and after World War I, physicians' incomes grew sharply, and their prominence as members of a true profession finally emerged. Of course, this prestige and power did not materialize overnight. Through the years, several factors interacted to gradually transform medicine from a weak, insecure, and isolated trade into a profession of power and authority. Seven key factors contributed to this transformation:

- Urbanization
- Science and technology
- Institutionalization
- Dependency
- Autonomy and organization
- Licensing
- Educational reform

Urbanization

Urbanization created increased reliance on the specialized skills of paid professionals in several ways. First, it distanced people from their families and the neighborhoods where family-based care was traditionally given. Women began working outside the home and could no longer care for sick members of the family.

Second, physicians became less expensive to consult as telephones, automobiles, and paved roads reduced the opportunity cost of time and travel and medical care became more affordable.

Urban development attracted more and more Americans to the growing towns and cities. In 1840, only 11% of the U.S. population lived in urban areas; by 1900, the proportion of the U.S. population living in urban areas grew to 40% (Stevens, 1971).

The trend away from home visits and toward office practice also began to develop around this time (Rosen, 1983). Physicians moved to cities and towns in large numbers to be closer to their growing markets. Better geographic proximity of patients enabled physicians to see more patients in a given amount of time. Whereas physicians in 1850 saw, on average, only 5 to 7 patients per day, by the early 1940s, the average patient load

of general practitioners had risen to 18 to 22 patients per day (Starr, 1982).

Science and Technology

EXHIBIT 3-2 summarizes some of the groundbreaking scientific discoveries in medicine. Advances in bacteriology, antiseptic surgery, anesthesia, immunology, and diagnostic techniques, along with an expanding repertoire of new drugs, gave medicine an aura of legitimacy and complexity, and the therapeutic effectiveness of scientific medicine became widely recognized.

When advanced technical knowledge becomes essential to practice a profession and the benefits of professional services

---

EXHIBIT 3-2 Groundbreaking Medical Discoveries

- The discovery of anesthesia was instrumental in advancing the practice of surgery. Nitrous oxide (laughing gas) was first employed as an anesthetic around 1846 for tooth extraction by Horace Wells, a dentist. Ether anesthesia for surgery was first successfully used in 1846 at Massachusetts General Hospital. Before anesthesia was discovered, strong doses of alcohol were used to dull the sensations. A surgeon who could do procedures, such as limb amputations, in the shortest length of time was held in high regard.
- Around 1847, Ignaz Semmelweis, a Hungarian physician practicing in a hospital in Vienna, implemented the policy of hand washing. Thus, aseptic technique was born. Semmelweis was concerned about the high death rate from puerperal fever among women after childbirth. Even though the germ theory of disease was unknown at this time, Semmelweis surmised that there might be a connection between puerperal fever and the common practice by medical students of not washing their hands before delivering babies and right after doing dissections. Semmelweis's hunch was right.
- Louis Pasteur, a French scientist, is generally credited with pioneering the germ theory of disease and microbiology around 1860. Pasteur demonstrated sterilization techniques, such as boiling to kill microorganisms and withholding exposure to air to prevent contamination.
- Joseph Lister, a British surgeon, is often referred to as the father of antiseptic surgery. Around 1865, Lister used carbolic acid to wash wounds and popularized the chemical inhibition of infection (antisepsis) during surgery.
- Advances in diagnostics and imaging can be traced to the discovery of x-rays in 1895 by Wilhelm Roentgen, a German professor of physics. Radiology became the first machine-based medical specialty. Some of the first training schools in x-ray therapy and radiography in the United States attracted photographers and electricians to become doctors in roentgenology (from the inventor's name).
- Alexander Fleming, a Scottish scientist, discovered the antibacterial properties of penicillin in 1929.

are widely recognized, a greater acceptance and a legitimate need for the services of that profession are simultaneously created. **Cultural authority** refers to the general acceptance of and reliance on the judgment of the members of a profession (Starr, 1982) because of their superior knowledge and expertise. Cultural authority legitimizes a profession in the eyes of common people. Advances in medical science and technology bestowed this legitimacy on the medical profession because medical practice could no longer remain within the domain of lay competence.

Scientific and technological change also required improved therapeutic competence of physicians in the diagnosis and treatment of disease. Developing these skills was no longer possible without specialized training. Science-based medicine created an increased demand for advanced services that were no longer available through family and neighbors.

Physicians' cultural authority was further bolstered when medical decisions became necessary in various aspects of health care delivery. For example, physicians decide whether a person should be admitted to a hospital or a nursing home and for how long, whether surgical or nonsurgical treatments should be used, and which medications should be prescribed. Physicians' decisions have a profound influence on other providers and nonproviders alike. The judgment and opinions of physicians even affect aspects of a person's life outside the delivery of health care. For example, physicians often evaluate the fitness of persons for jobs during the preemployment physical examinations many employers demand. Physicians assess the disability of the ill and the injured in workers' compensation cases. Granting of

medical leave for sickness and release back to work require authorizations from physicians. Payment of medical claims requires physicians' evaluations. Other health care professionals, such as nurses, therapists, and dietitians, are expected to follow physicians' orders for treatment. Thus, during disease and disability, and sometimes even in good health, people's lives have become increasingly governed by decisions made by physicians.

Institutionalization

The evolution of medical technology and the professionalization of medical and nursing staffs enabled advanced treatments that necessitated the pooling of resources in a common arena of care (Burns, 2004). As had already occurred in Europe, in the United States, hospitals became the core around which the delivery of medical services was organized. Thus, development of hospitals as the center for the practice of scientific medicine and the professionalization of medical practice became closely intertwined.

Indeed, physicians and hospitals developed a symbiotic relationship. For economic reasons, as hospitals expanded, their survival became increasingly dependent on physicians to keep the beds filled because the physicians decided where to hospitalize their patients. Therefore, hospitals had to make every effort to keep the physicians satisfied, which enhanced physicians' professional dominance, even though they were not employees of the hospitals. In turn, physicians exerted enormous influence over hospital policy. Also, for the first time, hospitals began conforming to both physician practice patterns and public expectations about medicine as a modern scientific enterprise. The expansion of surgery, in particular, had profound implications for hospitals, physicians, and the public. As hospitals added specialized facilities and staff, their regular use became indispensable to physicians and surgeons, who in earlier times had been able to manage their practices with little reference to hospitals (Martensen, 1996).

Hospitals in the United States did not expand and become more directly related to medical care until the late 1890s. However, as late as the 1930s, hospitals continued to experience frequent deaths among their patients due to infections that could not be prevented or cured. Despite these problems, hospital use increased due to the great influx of immigrants into large American cities (Falk, 1999). From only a few dozen facilities in 1875, the number of general hospitals in the United States exploded to 4,000 facilities by 1900 (Anderson, 1990) and to 5,000 facilities by 1913 (Wright, 1997).

Dependency

Patients depend on the medical profession's judgment and assistance. This dependency is created because society expects a sick person to seek medical help and try to get well. The patient is then expected to comply with medical instructions. In addition, dependency is created by the profession's cultural authority because its medical judgments must be relied on to (1) legitimize a person's sickness; (2) exempt the individual from social role obligations, such as work or school; and (3) provide competent medical care so the person can get well and resume his or her social role obligations. Moreover, in conjunction with the physician's cultural authority, the need for hospital services for critical illness and surgery creates dependency when patients are transferred from their homes to a hospital or surgery center.

Once physicians' cultural authority became legitimized, the sphere of their influence expanded into nearly all aspects of health care delivery. For example, laws were passed that prohibited individuals from obtaining certain classes of drugs without a physician's prescription. Health insurance paid for treatments only when they were rendered or prescribed by physicians. Thus, beneficiaries of health insurance became dependent on physicians to obtain covered services. The referral role (gatekeeping) of primary care physicians in some managed care plans has also increased patients' dependency on primary care physicians for referral to specialized services.

Autonomy and Organization

For a long time, physicians' ability to remain free of control from hospitals and insurance companies remained a prominent feature of American medicine. Hospitals and insurance companies could have hired physicians on salary to provide medical services, but individual physicians who took up practice in a corporate setting were castigated by the medical profession and pressured to abandon such practices. In some states, courts ruled that corporations could not employ licensed physicians without engaging in the unlicensed practice of medicine, a legal doctrine that became known as the "corporate practice doctrine" (Farmer and Douglas, 2001). Independence from corporate control enhanced private entrepreneurship and put American physicians in an enviable strategic position in relation to hospitals and insurance companies. Later, a formally organized medical profession was in a much better position to resist control from outside entities.

The AMA was formed in 1847, but it had little clout during its first half-century of existence. Its membership was small, with no permanent organization and scant resources. The AMA did not attain real strength until it was organized into county and state medical societies and until state societies were incorporated, delegating greater control at the local level. As part of the organizational reform, the AMA also began, in 1904, to concentrate attention on medical education (Bordley and Harvey, 1976). Since then, it has been the chief proponent for the practitioners of conventional medicine in the United States. Although the AMA often stressed the importance of raising the quality of care for patients and protecting the uninformed consumer from "quacks" and "charlatans," its principal goal—like that of other professional associations—was to advance the professionalization, prestige, and financial well-being of its members. The AMA vigorously pursued its objectives by promoting the establishment of state medical licensing laws and the legal requirement that, to be licensed to practice, a physician must be a graduate of an AMA-approved medical school. The concerted activities of physicians through the AMA are collectively referred to as **organized medicine**, to distinguish them from the uncoordinated actions of individual physicians competing in the marketplace (Goodman and Musgrave, 1992).

Licensing

Under the Medical Practice Acts established in the 1870s, medical licensure in the United States became a function of the states (Stevens, 1971). By 1896, 26 states had enacted medical licensure laws (Anderson, 1990). Licensing of physicians and upgrading of medical school standards developed hand in hand. At first, licensing required only a medical school diploma. Later, candidates could be rejected if the school they had attended was judged inadequate (Starr, 1982).

Through both licensure and upgrading of medical school standards, physicians obtained a clear monopoly on the practice of medicine (Anderson, 1990). The early licensing laws served to protect physicians from the competitive pressures posed by potential new entrants into the medical profession. Physicians led the campaign to restrict the practice of medicine. As biomedicine gained political and economic ground, the biomedical community expelled providers such as homeopaths, naturopaths, and chiropractors from medical societies; prohibited professional association with them; and encouraged prosecution of such providers for unlicensed medical practice (Rothstein, 1972). In 1888, in a landmark Supreme Court decision, *Dent v. West Virginia*, Justice Stephen J. Field wrote that no one had the right to practice "without having the necessary qualifications of learning and skill" (Haber, 1974). In the late 1880s and 1890s, many states revised laws to require all candidates for licensure, including those holding medical degrees, to pass an examination (Kaufman, 1980).

Educational Reform

Reform of medical education started around 1870, with the affiliation of medical schools with universities. In 1871, Harvard Medical School, under the leadership of a new university president, Charles Eliot, completely revolutionized the system of medical education. The academic year was extended from 4 to 9 months, and the length of medical education was increased from 2 to 3 years. Following the European model, laboratory instruction and clinical subjects, such as chemistry, physiology, anatomy, and pathology, were added to the curriculum.

Johns Hopkins University took the lead in further reforming medical education when it opened its medical school in 1893, under the leadership of William H. Welch, who trained in Germany. For the first time, medical education became a graduate training course, requiring a college degree—not a high school diploma—as an entrance requirement. Johns Hopkins had well-equipped laboratories, a full-time faculty for teaching the basic science courses, and its own teaching hospital (Rothstein, 1972). Standards at Johns Hopkins became the model of medical education in other leading institutions around the country. The heightened standards made it difficult for proprietary schools to survive, and, in time, those schools were closed.

The Association of American Medical Colleges (AAMC) was founded in 1876 by 22 medical schools (Coggeshall, 1965). Later, the AAMC set minimum standards for medical education, including a 4-year curriculum, but it was unable to enforce its recommendations.

In 1904, the AMA created the Council on Medical Education, which inspected the existing medical schools and found that fewer than half provided acceptable levels of training. The AMA did not publish its findings but did obtain the help of the Carnegie Foundation for the Advancement of Teaching to provide a rating of medical schools (Goodman and Musgrave, 1992). The Carnegie Foundation appointed Abraham Flexner to investigate medical schools located in both the United States and Canada. The Flexner Report, published in 1910, had a profound effect on medical education reform. Its recommendations were widely accepted by both the profession and the public. Schools that did not meet the proposed standards were forced to close. State laws were established, requiring graduation from a medical school accredited by the AMA as the basis for obtaining a license to practice medicine (Haglund and Dowling, 1993).

Once advanced graduate education became an integral part of medical training, it further legitimized the profession's authority and galvanized its sovereignty. Stevens (1971) noted that American medicine moved toward professional maturity between 1890 and 1914, mainly as a direct result of educational reform.

Specialization in Medicine

Specialization has been a hallmark of American medicine, albeit one that has resulted in an oversupply of specialists in relation to generalists. This distinctive aspect of medical practice in the United States explains why the structure of medicine did not develop around a nucleus of primary care.

Lack of a rational coordination of medical care in the United States has been one consequence of the preoccupation with specialization. In Great Britain, for example, the medical profession has divided itself into general practitioners (GPs), who practice in the community, and consultants, who hold specialist positions in hospitals. This kind of stratification did not develop in American medicine. Primary care physicians (PCPs) in America were not assigned the role that GPs had in Britain, where patients could consult a specialist only by referral from a GP. Unlike Great Britain, where GPs hold a key intermediary position in relation to the rest of the health care delivery system, the United States has lacked such a gatekeeping and coordinating role. Only since the early 1990s, under health maintenance organizations (HMOs), has the **gatekeeping** model, which requires initial contact with a generalist and the generalist's referral to a specialist, gained prominence in the United States.

Reform of Mental Health Care

At the turn of the 20th century, the scientific study and treatment of mental illnesses, called neuropathology, had just begun. Later, in 1946, federal funding was made available under the National Mental Health Act for psychiatric education and research. Signed by President Harry Truman, this law was enacted in response to the large number of World War II veterans who suffered from "battle fatigue" (National Association of State Mental Health Program Directors [NASMHPD], 2014). At about the same time, several reports and studies exposed poor and abusive conditions in state mental asylums.

In 1949, the National Institute of Mental Health (NIMH) was established with the goal of creating a better understanding of mental health issues through research. Six years later, the Mental Health Study Act of 1955 called for a thorough nationwide analysis of mental health and related problems. The task was assigned to a

Joint Commission on Mental Illness and Health, which produced a comprehensive report, *Action for Mental Health*, in 1960. In 1963, President John F. Kennedy called for a shift from institutional care to community-based services, and for integration of people with mental disorders into the mainstream of American life (Kennedy, 1963). Several factors contributed to the emerging belief that early treatment of mental disorders and early intervention in the community would be effective in preventing subsequent hospitalization (Grob, 2005). In addition, reformers of the mental health system argued that long-term institutional care was neglectful, ineffective, and even harmful (U.S. Surgeon General, 1999).

By the 1960s, the concept of community mental health was born, and deinstitutionalization became a major thrust of mental health reform. By this time, new drugs for treating psychosis and depression had become available. The NIMH played a leading role in championing the substitution of confinement to asylums with community-oriented care (Grob, 2005). Passage of the Community Mental Health Centers Act of 1963, signed by President Kennedy, lent support to the joint policies of "community care" and "deinstitutionalization." Under this act, federal funding became available to build community mental health centers. For the first time, federal money was granted to the states for mental health treatment (Ramsey, 2011). This policy change ushered in the era of community mental health services and the end of the state psychiatric hospital as the core of the mental health care system in the United States (NASMHPD, 2014).

From 1970 to 2002, state-run psychiatric hospital beds dropped from 207 to 20 beds per 100,000 population (Foley et al., 2006). The deinstitutionalization movement further intensified after the U.S. Supreme Court's 1999 decision in *Olmstead v. L.C.*, which directed U.S. states to provide community-based services, whenever appropriate, to people with mental illness. Today, state mental institutions still provide long-term treatment to people with severe and persistent mental illness (Patrick et al., 2006).

Around 1994, state-controlled money spent on community-based mental health services started to exceed the spending for institutionalized care. By 2012, fewer than 6% of people receiving mental health treatment used inpatient care (Substance Abuse and Mental Health Services Administration, 2013), and approximately 23% of all state funds for mental health were used for care in psychiatric hospitals (NASMHPD, 2014). By comparison, in the mid-1950s, inpatient services accounted for roughly 84% of the state and local funds devoted to mental health care (Fein, 1958). In achieving such remarkable results, income support programs for the disabled and low-income people—mainly Social Security Disability Insurance, Supplemental Security Income, and housing subsidies—played a critical role, along with the establishment of Medicare and Medicaid and the expansion of private insurance to cover mental health services on par with health care (Glied and Frank, 2016). As a result of these changes, mental health care in the United States is now an example of conjoint social and health policies.

Mental health parity acts were passed in 1996 and 2008 to address equality in insurance coverage for mental and physical health. The 1996 law did not mandate coverage for mental health, but mainly focused on parity for annual or lifetime dollar limits in coverage, and allowed waivers for certain cost increases. The 2008 law added to the previous law by prohibiting differences in cost sharing between treatments for mental and physical health; it also applied to substance abuse, which the previous law did not (Goodell, 2014). Both the laws, however, left loopholes in coverage for mental health treatments.

The 21st Century Cures Act, which had been held up in the U.S. Senate for nearly 1.5 years, was finally passed by Congress and signed by President Obama in December 2016. Among other initiatives, the law provided funds to strengthen parity laws, improve health care for people with serious mental illness, fight the opioid epidemic, and advance research into treating Alzheimer's disease ("Major provisions of the 21st Century Cures Act," 2017).

Development of Public Health

Historically, public health practices in the United States concentrated on sanitary regulation, the study of epidemics, and vital statistics. The growth of urban centers for the purpose of commerce and industry, unsanitary living conditions in densely populated areas, inadequate methods of sewage and garbage disposal, limited access to clean water, and long work hours in unsafe and exploitative industries led to periodic epidemics of cholera, smallpox, typhoid, tuberculosis, yellow fever, and other diseases. Such outbreaks led to arduous efforts to protect the public interest. For example, in 1793, the national capital had to be moved out of Philadelphia due to a devastating outbreak of yellow fever. This epidemic prompted the city to develop its first board of health that same year. Subsequently, in 1850, Lemuel Shattuck outlined the blueprint for the development of a public health system in Massachusetts. Shattuck also called for the establishment of state and local health departments.

A threatening outbreak of cholera in 1873 mobilized the New York City Health Department to alleviate the worst sanitary conditions within the city. Previously, cholera epidemics in 1832 and 1848–1849 had swept through American cities and towns, killing thousands within a few weeks (Duffy, 1971). Until about 1900, infectious diseases posed the greatest health threat to society. The development of public health played a major role in curtailing the spread of infection among populations. Simultaneously, widespread public health measures and better medical care were instrumental in reducing mortality and increasing life expectancy.

By 1900, most states had health departments that were responsible for a variety of public health efforts, such as sanitary inspections, communicable disease control, operation of state laboratories, vital statistics, health education, and regulation of food and water (Turnock, 1997; Williams, 1995). Public health functions were later extended to fill gaps in the medical care system. Such functions, however, were limited mainly to child immunizations, care of mothers and infants, health screening in public schools, and family planning. Federal grants were also made available to state and local governments for programs in substance abuse, mental health, and disease prevention services (Turnock, 1997).

Public health has remained separate from the private practice of medicine because of the skepticism of private physicians, who feared that the government could use the boards of health to regulate the private practice of medicine (Rothstein, 1972). Fear of government intervention, loss of autonomy, and erosion of personal incomes created a wall of separation between public health and private medical practice. Under this dichotomous relationship, medicine has concentrated on the physical health of the individual, whereas public health has focused on the health of whole populations and communities. The extent of collaboration between the two has been largely confined to the requirement by public health departments that private practitioners report cases of contagious diseases, such as sexually transmitted diseases, human immunodeficiency virus (HIV) infection, and acquired immune deficiency syndrome (AIDS), and any outbreaks of cases such as West Nile virus and other types of infections.

Health Services for Veterans

Shortly after World War I, the U.S. government started to provide hospital services to veterans with service-related disabilities and for non-service-related disabilities if the veteran declared an inability to pay for private care. At first, the federal government contracted for services with private hospitals. Over time, however, the Department of Veterans Affairs (formerly called Veterans Administration) built its own hospitals, outpatient clinics, and nursing homes.

Birth of Workers' Compensation

The first broad-coverage health insurance in the United States emerged in the form of workers' compensation programs, which were introduced in 1914 (Whitted, 1993). The theory underlying workers' compensation is that all accidents that occur during the course of employment and all illnesses directly attributable to the workplace must be regarded as risks of industry. In other words, the employer is financially liable for the full cost of such injuries and illnesses regardless of who is at fault.

Workers' compensation was originally concerned with cash payments to workers for wages lost due to job-related injuries and disease. Compensation for medical expenses and death benefits to the survivors were later added. Looking at the trend, some reformers believed that, since Americans had been persuaded to adopt compulsory insurance against industrial accidents, they could also be persuaded to adopt compulsory insurance against sickness. In essence, workers' compensation served as a trial balloon for the idea of government-sponsored universal health insurance in the United States. However, the growth of private health insurance, along with other key factors discussed later, has prevented any proposals for a national health care program from taking hold.

Rise of Private Health Insurance

Historically, private health insurance was commonly referred to as **voluntary health insurance**, in contrast to proposals for a government-sponsored compulsory health insurance system. At least some private insurance coverage—albeit limited to bodily injuries—has been available since approximately 1850. By 1900, health insurance policies became available, but their initial role was to protect against loss of income during sickness and temporary disability (Whitted, 1993). Later, coverage was added for surgical fees, but the emphasis remained on replacing lost income. Thus, the coverage was, in reality, disability insurance rather than health insurance (Mayer and Mayer, 1984).

As detailed in subsequent sections, technological, social, and economic factors created a general need for health insurance. However, economic conditions that prompted private initiatives, the self-interests of the well-organized medical profession, and the momentum of a successful health insurance enterprise gave private health insurance a firm footing in the United States. Later, economic conditions during the World War II period laid the foundations for health insurance to become an employment-based benefit.

Technological, Social, and Economic Factors

The health insurance movement of the early 20th century was the product of three converging developments—technological, social, and economic. From a technological perspective, medicine offered new and better treatments. Because of its well-established healing values, medical care had become individually and socially desirable, which created a growing demand for medical services. From an economic perspective, people could predict neither their future needs for medical care nor the costs, both of which had been gradually increasing. In short, scientific and technological advances made health care more desirable but less affordable. These developments pointed to the need for some kind of insurance that could spread the financial risks over a large number of people.

Early Blanket Insurance Policies

In 1911, insurance companies began to offer blanket policies for large industrial populations, usually covering life insurance, accidents, sickness, and nursing services. A few industrial and railroad companies set up their own medical plans, covering specified medical benefits, as did several unions and fraternal orders. Nevertheless, the total amount of voluntary health insurance remained minute (Stevens, 1971).

Economic Necessity and the Baylor Plan

The Great Depression, which started at the end of 1929, forced hospitals to turn from philanthropic donations to patient fees for support. Patients now faced not only loss of income from illness, but also increased debt from medical care costs when they became sick. People needed protection from the economic consequences of sickness and hospitalization, while hospitals needed protection from economic instability (Mayer and Mayer, 1984). During the Depression, occupancy rates in hospitals fell, income from endowments and contributions dropped sharply, and the charity patient load almost quadrupled (Richardson, 1945).

In 1929, the blueprint for modern health insurance was established when Justin F. Kimball began a hospital insurance plan for public school teachers at the Baylor University Hospital in Dallas,

Texas. Kimball was able to enroll more than 1,200 teachers, who paid 50 cents per month for a maximum of 21 days of hospital care. Within a few years, the Baylor plan became the model for Blue Cross plans around the country (Raffel, 1980). At first, other independent hospitals copied Baylor and started offering single-hospital plans. It was not long before community-wide plans, offered jointly by more than one hospital, became popular because they provided consumers a choice of hospitals. The hospitals agreed to provide services in exchange for a fixed monthly payment by the plans. In essence, these were prepaid plans for hospital services. A **prepaid plan** is a contractual arrangement under which a provider must provide all needed services to a group of members (or enrollees) in exchange for a fixed monthly fee paid in advance. This concept was later adopted by managed care.

Successful Private Enterprise: The Blue Cross Plans

A hospital plan in Minnesota was the first to use the name Blue Cross in 1933 (Davis, 1996). The American Hospital Association (AHA) lent support to the hospital plans and became the coordinating agency to unite these plans into the Blue Cross network (Koch, 1993; Raffel, 1980). The Blue Cross plans were nonprofit—that is, they had no shareholders who would receive profit distributions—and covered only hospital charges, as not to infringe on the domain of private physicians (Starr, 1982).

Later, control of the plans was transferred to a completely independent body, the Blue Cross Commission, which subsequently became the Blue Cross Association (Raffel, 1980). In 1946, Blue Cross plans in 43 states served 20 million members. Between 1940 and 1950, driven by the widespread adoption of these plans, the proportion of the U.S. population covered by hospital insurance increased from 9% to 57% (Anderson, 1990).

Self-Interests of Physicians: Birth of Blue Shield

Voluntary health insurance had received the AMA's endorsement, but the AMA had also made it clear that private health insurance plans should include only hospital care. Given the AMA's position, it is not surprising that the first Blue Shield plan designed to pay for physicians' bills was started by the California Medical Association, which established the California Physicians' Service in 1939 (Raffel, 1980). By endorsing hospital insurance and by actively developing medical service plans, the medical profession committed itself to private health insurance as the means to spread the financial risk of sickness and to ensure that its own interests would not be threatened.

From the medical profession's point of view, voluntary health insurance, in conjunction with PFFS practice by physicians, was regarded as a desirable feature of the evolving U.S. health care system (Stevens, 1971). Throughout the Blue Shield movement, physicians dominated the boards of directors not only because they underwrote the plans, but also because the plans were, in a very real sense, their response to the challenge of national health insurance. In addition, the plans met the AMA's stipulation of keeping medical matters in the hands of physicians (Raffel and Raffel, 1994).

Combined Hospital and Physician Coverage

Even though Blue Cross and Blue Shield developed independently and were financially and organizationally distinct, they often worked together to provide hospital and physician coverage (Law, 1974). In 1974, the New York Superintendent of Insurance approved a merger of the Blue Cross and Blue Shield plans of Greater New York (Somers and Somers, 1977). Similar mergers occurred in other states. Today, Blue Cross and Blue Shield plans operate throughout the United States and other countries under the umbrella of the Blue Cross–Blue Shield Association.

The for-profit insurance companies were initially skeptical of the Blue Cross plans and adopted a wait-and-see attitude toward entering the health care insurance market. Their apprehension was justified because no actuarial information was available to predict losses. Nevertheless, within a few years, lured by the success of the Blue Cross plans, commercial insurance companies also started offering health insurance.

Employment-Based Health Insurance

Between 1916 and 1918, 16 state legislatures, including New York and California, attempted to enact legislation mandating employers to provide health insurance, but these efforts were unsuccessful (Davis, 1996). Subsequently, three main developments pushed private health insurance to become employment based in the United States:

- To control high inflation in the economy during the World War II period, Congress imposed wage freezes. In response, many employers started offering health insurance to their workers in lieu of wage increases.

- In 1948, the U.S. Supreme Court ruled that employee benefits, including health insurance, were a legitimate part of union–management negotiations. Health insurance then became a permanent part of employee benefits in the postwar era (Health Insurance Association of America [HIAA], 1991).
- In 1954, Congress amended the Internal Revenue Code to make employer-paid health coverage nontaxable. In terms of its economic value, employer-paid health insurance was equivalent to getting additional salary without having to pay taxes on it, which provided an incentive to obtain health insurance as an employer-furnished benefit.

Employment-based health insurance expanded rapidly. The economy was strong during the postwar years of the 1950s, and employers started offering more extensive benefits. This expansion led to the birth of "major medical" expense coverage to protect against prolonged or catastrophic illness or injury (Mayer and Mayer, 1984). Thus, private health insurance became the primary vehicle for the financing of health care services in the United States.

Failure of National Health Care Initiatives During the 1990s

Starting in Germany in 1883, compulsory sickness insurance had spread throughout Europe by 1912. Sickness insurance was seen as a natural outgrowth of insurance against workplace accidents. In the United States, the American Association of Labor Legislation (AALL) had been primarily responsible for leading the successful drive for workers' compensation. Some social academics and labor leaders were the prominent members of the AALL, whose stated agenda was to initiate social reform through government action. Emboldened by its success in bringing about workers' compensation, the AALL spearheaded the drive to establish a government-run health insurance system for the general population (Anderson, 1990). It also supported the Progressive (i.e., liberal) movement headed by former President Theodore Roosevelt, who was again running for the presidency in 1912 on a platform of social reform. Roosevelt, who might have been a national political sponsor for compulsory health insurance, was defeated by Woodrow Wilson, but the Progressive movement for national health insurance did not die.

The AALL continued its efforts to win support for a model for national health insurance by appealing to both social and economic concerns. The reformers argued that national health insurance would relieve poverty because sickness usually brought wage loss and high medical costs to individual families. Reformers also argued that national health insurance would contribute to economic efficiency by reducing illness, lengthening life, and diminishing the causes of industrial discontent (Starr, 1982). At the time, the leadership of the AMA outwardly supported a national plan, and the AALL and the AMA formed a united front to secure legislation meeting this goal. A standard health insurance bill was introduced in 15 states in 1917 (Stevens, 1971).

As long as compulsory health insurance was only under study and discussion, potential opponents paid no heed to it.

Once bills were introduced into state legislatures, however, opponents expressed vehement disapproval of them. Eventually, the AMA's support proved only superficial.

Historically, the repeated attempts to pass national health insurance legislation in the United States have failed for several reasons, which can be classified into four broad categories: political inexpediency, institutional dissimilarities, ideological differences, and tax aversion.

Political Inexpediency

At the time when they embarked on their national health programs, countries in Western Europe—notably Germany and England—were experiencing labor unrest that threatened their political stability. Social insurance was seen as a means to obtain workers' loyalty and ward off political threats. Conditions in the United States, by comparison, were quite different. There was no real threat to the country's political stability. Unlike the governments in Europe, the U.S. government was highly decentralized and engaged in little direct regulation of the economy or social welfare. Although Congress had set up a system of compulsory hospital insurance for merchant seamen as early as 1798, it was an exceptional measure.[1] Matters related to health and welfare were typically left to state and local governments, and as a general rule, these levels of government left as much as possible to private and voluntary action.

---

[1] Important seaports, such as Boston, were often con-fronted with the challenge of dealing with sickness or injuries of seamen. Congress enacted a law requiring that 20 cents per month be withheld from the wages of each seaman on American ships to support merchant marine hospitals (Raffel and Raffel, 1994).

The entry of the United States into World War I in 1917 dealt a final political blow to the health insurance movement, as anti-German feelings were aroused among the U.S. populace. The U.S. government denounced German social insurance, and opponents of health insurance called it a Prussian menace, inconsistent with American values (Starr, 1982).

After attempts to pass compulsory health insurance laws failed at the state levels in California and New York, the AALL itself lost interest in an obviously lost cause. In 1920, the AMA's House of Delegates approved a resolution condemning compulsory health insurance that would be regulated by the government (Numbers, 1985). The main aim of this resolution was to solidify the medical profession against government interference with the practice of medicine.

Institutional Dissimilarities

Germany and England established mutual benefit funds to provide insurance against the cost of sickness for a sector of the working population. Voluntary sickness funds were less developed in the United States than in Europe, reflecting less interest in health insurance and less familiarity with this concept. More important, American hospitals were mainly private, whereas in Europe they were largely government-operated facilities (Starr, 1982).

In the United States, national financing and payment mechanisms were viewed as inconsistent with health care delivered predominantly by private institutions. For instance, the compulsory health insurance proposals put forth by the AALL were regarded by individual members of the medical profession as a threat to their private practice because such proposals would shift the primary source of income of medical professionals from individual patients to the government (Anderson, 1990). Any efforts that would potentially erode the fee-for-service payment system and let private practice of medicine be controlled by a powerful third party—particularly the government—were opposed.

The insurance industry feared losing the income it derived from disability insurance, some insurance against medical services, and funeral benefits[2] (Anderson, 1990). The pharmaceutical industry feared the government would curtail its profits by acting as a monopoly buyer, and retail pharmacists feared that hospitals would establish their own pharmacies under a government-run national health care program (Anderson, 1990). Employers also saw the proposals as contrary to their interests. Spokespersons for U.S. business rejected the argument that national health insurance would add to productivity and efficiency. It may seem ironic, but the labor unions—the American Federation of Labor, in particular—also denounced compulsory health insurance at the time. Union leaders were afraid the government would usurp their own legitimate role of providing social benefits, thereby weakening the unions' influence in the workplace. Organized labor was the largest and most powerful interest group at that time, and its lack of support is considered instrumental in the defeat of national health insurance (Anderson, 1990).

---

[2] Patients admitted to a hospital were required to pay a burial deposit so the hospital would not have to incur a funeral expense if they died (Raffel and Raffel, 1994). Therefore, many people bought funeral policies from insurance companies.

Ideological Differences

In the American experience, individualism and self-determination, distrust of government, and reliance on the private sector to address social concerns—collectively seen as typical American values—have stood as a bulwark against anything perceived as an attack on individual liberties. These beliefs and values have typically represented the sentiments of the American middle class, whose support was necessary for any broad-based health care reform. Conversely, during times of national distress, such as the Great Depression, pure necessity may have legitimized the advancement of social programs, such as the New Deal programs of the Franklin Roosevelt era (for example, Social Security legislation providing old-age pensions and unemployment compensation).

In the early 1940s, during Roosevelt's presidency, several bills on national health insurance were introduced in Congress, but they all failed to pass. Perhaps the most notable bill was the Wagner-Murray-Dingell bill, drafted in 1943 and named after the bill's congressional sponsors. World War II diverted the nation's attention to other issues, however, and without the president's active support the bill died quietly (Numbers, 1985).

In 1946, Harry Truman became the first president to make an appeal for a national health care program (Anderson, 1990). Unlike the Progressives, who had proposed a plan for the working class, Truman proposed a single health insurance plan that would include all classes of society. At the president's behest, the Wagner-Murray-Dingell bill was redrafted and reintroduced. The AMA was vehement in opposing the plan. Other interest groups, such as the AHA, also opposed it.

By this time, private health insurance had expanded. Initial public reaction to the Wagner-Murray-Dingell bill was positive; however, when a government-controlled medical plan was compared to private insurance, polls showed that only 12% of the public favored extending Social Security to include health insurance (Numbers, 1985).

During this era of the Cold War,[3] any attempts to introduce national health insurance were met with the stigmatizing label of **socialized medicine**—a label that has since become synonymous with any large-scale government-sponsored expansion of health insurance or intrusion in the private practice of medicine. The Republicans took control of Congress in 1946, and any interest in enacting national health insurance was put to rest. However, to the surprise of many, Truman was reelected in 1948, and he promised to establish a national health insurance system if the Democrats were returned to power (Starr, 1982). Fearing the inevitable, the AMA levied a $25 fee on each of its members to build a war chest of $3.5 million (Anderson, 1990), which was a substantial sum of money at the time. The AMA hired the public relations firm of Whitaker and Baxter and spent $1.5 million, in 1949 alone, to launch one of the most expensive lobbying efforts in American history. The campaign directly linked national health insurance with Communism so that the idea of "socialized medicine" was firmly implanted in the public's minds. In 1952, the election of a Republican president, Dwight Eisenhower, effectively ended any further debate over national health insurance.

---

[3] Rivalry and hostility after World War II between the United States and the former Soviet Union.

Tax Aversion

Americans have generally supported the idea that the government ought to help people who are in financial need to pay for their medical care. However, most Americans have not favored an increase in their own taxes to pay for such care. This reluctance is perhaps why health care reform failed in 1993.

While seeking the presidency in 1991, then Governor Bill Clinton made health system reform a major campaign issue. Not since Harry Truman's initiatives in the 1940s had such a bold attempt to overhaul the U.S. health care system been made by a presidential candidate. In the Pennsylvania U.S. Senate election in November 1991, the victory of Democrat Harris Wofford over Republican Richard Thornburgh sent a clear signal that the time for a national health care program might be ripe. Wofford's call for national health insurance was widely supported by middle-class Pennsylvanians. Election results in other states were not quite as decisive on the issue of health care reform, but various public polls seemed to suggest that the rising cost of health care was a concern for many people. Against this backdrop, both Bill Clinton and the running incumbent, President George H. W. Bush, advanced health care reform proposals.

After taking office in 1992, President Clinton made health system reform a top priority. His wife, Hillary Clinton, was given the leadership role for the Task Force on National Health Reform. A complex piece of legislation, the Health Security Act, was introduced in November 1993, but within the first year it died in Congress. Policy experts and public opinion leaders have debated over what went wrong. Some of the fundamental causes for the failure of the Clinton plan were no doubt historical in nature, as discussed previously in this chapter. According to one seasoned political observer, James J. Mongan, the reform debate in Congress was not about the expansion of health care services, but rather about the financing of the proposed services. Avoiding tax increases, it appeared, took priority over expanding health insurance coverage and caused the demise of Clinton's health care reform initiatives (Mongan, 1995).

Creation of Medicare and Medicaid

The year 1965 marked a major turning point in U.S. health policy. Up to this point, private health insurance was the only widely available source of payment for health care, and it was available primarily to middle-class working Americans and their families. Many of the elderly, the unemployed, and the poor had to rely on their own resources, on limited public programs, or on charity from hospitals and individual physicians. Often, when charity care was provided, private payers were charged more to make up the difference, a practice referred to as **cost shifting** or **cross-subsidization**. In 1965, Congress passed the amendments to the Social Security Act and created the Medicare and Medicaid programs. Thus, for the first time in U.S. history, the government assumed direct responsibility for paying for health care on behalf of two vulnerable population groups—the elderly and the poor (Potter and Longest, 1994).

Through both the debates over how to protect the public from the rising costs of health care and the opposition to national health insurance, one thing had become clear: Government intervention was not

desired insofar as it pertained to how most Americans received health care, with one exception. That exception came into play when reform initiatives were proposed for the underprivileged and vulnerable classes. In principle, the poor were considered a special class who could be served through a government-sponsored program. The elderly—those 65 years of age and older—were another group who had started to receive increased attention in the 1950s. On their own, most of the poor and the elderly could not afford the increasing costs of health care. Also, because the health status of these subpopulations was significantly worse than that of the general population, they required a higher level of health care services. The elderly, in particular, had higher incidence and prevalence of disease compared to younger groups. It was also estimated that less than half of the elderly population was covered by private health insurance. By this time, the growing elderly middle class was also becoming a politically active force.

In 1957, a bill introduced in Congress by Aime Forand provided momentum for including necessary hospital and nursing home care as an extension of Social Security benefits for the elderly (Stevens, 1971). In response, the AMA undertook a massive public relations campaign that portrayed the proposed government insurance plan as a threat to the physician–patient relationship. The bill stalled, but public hearings around the country, which were packed with elderly attendees, produced intense grassroots support that pushed the issue onto the national agenda (Starr, 1982). A compromise bill, the Medical Assistance Act (Public Law 86–778), also known as the Kerr-Mills Act, was passed and went into effect in 1960. Under this act, federal grants were given to the states to extend health services provided by the state welfare programs to those low-income elderly who previously did not qualify for such services (Anderson, 1990). Since the program was based on a **means test** that limited eligibility to people below a pre-determined income level, it was opposed by liberal congressional representatives, who labeled it as a source of humiliation to the elderly (Starr, 1982). Within 3 years, the program was declared ineffective because many states did not even implement it (Stevens, 1971). In 1964, however, health insurance for the aged and the poor became top priorities of President Lyndon Johnson's Great Society programs.

During the debate over Medicare, the AMA developed its own "Eldercare" proposal, which called for a federal–state program to subsidize private insurance policies for hospital and physician services. Representative John W. Byrnes introduced yet another proposal, dubbed "Bettercare." It proposed a federal program based on partial premium contributions by the elderly, with the remainder subsidized by the government. Other proposals included tax credits and tax deductions for health insurance premiums.

In the end, a three-layered program emerged from the debate. The first two layers constituted Part A and Part B of **Medicare**, or **Title XVIII** of the Social Security Amendment of 1965, which sought to provide health insurance to the elderly. Based on Forand's initial bill, the administration's proposal to finance hospital insurance and partial nursing home coverage for the elderly through Social Security became **Part A** of Medicare. The Byrnes proposal to cover physicians' bills through government-subsidized insurance became

Part B of Medicare. An extension of the Kerr-Mills program of federal matching funds to the states, based on each state's financial needs, became **Medicaid**, or **Title XIX** of the Social Security Amendment of 1965. The Medicaid program was intended for indigent persons, based on means tests established by each state, but was expanded to include all age groups, not just the poor elderly (Stevens, 1971).

Although adopted together, Medicare and Medicaid reflected sharply different traditions. Medicare enjoyed broad grassroots support and, because it was attached to the Social Security program, had no class distinction. Medicaid, however, was burdened by the stigma of public welfare. Medicare had uniform national standards for eligibility and benefits; Medicaid varied from state to state in terms of eligibility and benefits. Medicare allowed physicians to **balance bill**—that is, charge the patient the amount above the program's set fees and recoup the difference. In contrast, Medicaid prohibited balance billing and, consequently, had limited participation from physicians (Starr, 1982). Medicaid, in essence, created a two-tier system of medical care delivery because, even today, many physicians refuse to accept Medicaid-covered patients due to the low fees paid by the government for their care.

Not surprisingly, shortly after Medicare and Medicaid became operational, national spending for health services began to rise, as did public outlays of funds in relation to private spending for health services (Anderson, 1990). For example, national health expenditures (NHE), which had increased by 50% from 1960 to 1965, jumped by 78% from 1965 to 1970, and by 71% from 1970 to 1975. Similarly, public expenditures for health care, which were stable at 25% of NHE for 1955, 1960, and 1965, increased to 36.5% of NHE in 1970, and to 42.1% of NHE in 1975 (based on data from Bureau of the Census, 1976).

Regulatory Role of Public Health Agencies

With the expansion of the publicly financed Medicare and Medicaid programs, the regulatory powers of government have increasingly encroached upon the private sector. This incursion is possible because the government provides financing for the two programs, but services are delivered by the private sector. After the federal government developed the standards for participation in the Medicare program, states developed their own regulations in conjunction with the Medicaid program. The regulations often overlapped, and the federal government delegated authority to the states to carry out the monitoring of regulatory compliance. As a result, the regulatory powers assigned to state public health agencies increased dramatically. Thus, most institutions of health care delivery are subject to annual scrutiny by public health agencies under the authority delegated to them by the federal and state governments.

▶ Medical Care in the Corporate Era

Early Developments

As pointed out previously, corporate practice of medicine—that is, delivery of medical care by for-profit corporations—was historically prohibited by law, being labeled as "commercialism" in medicine. The AMA, however, recognized the need for certain industries located in remote areas—such as railroads, mining, and lumber companies—to employ or contract with practicing physicians. As early as 1882, companies such as Northern Pacific Railroad started to provide direct medical care to their employees.

In the early- to mid-1900s, the health care delivery landscape began to change. Physicians in specialty practices were brought together into group practices. The Mayo Clinic, started in Rochester, Minnesota, in 1887, became the model for consolidating specialists into group practice—an arrangement that presented certain economic advantages, such as sharing of expenses and incomes. Family practitioners joined in, and many group practices started to offer multi-specialty services. These innovations led to the formation of prepaid group plans.

Prepaid group plans began enrolling employee groups under capitated fee arrangements, through which these groups received comprehensive services for a fixed monthly fee paid in advance. Prepaid group practice plans first became popular in some large urban markets in the United States. The AMA opposed the first such plan, the Group Health Association of Washington (started in 1937 in Washington, D.C.), but was found guilty of restraint of trade, in violation of the Sherman Antitrust Act. This verdict may have been crucial in paving the way for the growth of other prepaid group practice plans. For example, the HIP Health Plan of New York, started in 1947, stands as one of the most successful programs, providing comprehensive medical services through organized medical groups of family physicians and specialists (Raffel, 1980). Similarly, Kaiser-Permanente, started in 1942, has grown on the West Coast.

The corporate era began in earnest in the latter part of the 20th century, as employment of physicians by certain industries, group practices, and capitation plans sowed the seeds of managed care, which first appeared in the form of HMOs.

The HMO Act of 1973

The Health Maintenance Organization Act (HMO Act) of 1973 was passed during the Richard Nixon administration, with the objective of stimulating growth of HMOs by providing federal funds for the establishment and expansion of new HMOs (Wilson and Neuhauser, 1985). The underlying reason for supporting the growth of HMOs was the belief that prepaid medical care, as an alternative to traditional fee-for-service practice, would stimulate competition among health plans, enhance efficiency, and control the rising health care expenditures. The HMO Act required employers with 25 or more employees to offer an HMO alternative if one was available in their geographic area. The objective was to create 1,700 HMOs to enroll 40 million members by 1976 (Iglehart, 1994). Ultimately, the HMO Act failed to achieve this objective. By 1976, only 174 HMOs had formed, with an enrollment of 6 million (Public Health Service, 1995). Employers did not take the HMO option seriously and continued to offer traditional fee-for-service insurance until their own health insurance expenses started to grow rapidly during the 1980s.

Corporatization of Health Care Delivery

By the dawn of the 21st century, business environment in the United States—and indeed around the world—had become the domain of large corporations. At the same time, tremendous advances were occurring in global communications, transportation, medical and information technology, and international trade. Health care delivery has not remained immune to these transformations.

Managed care organizations (MCOs) are, in many regards, indistinguishable from large insurance corporations. The rising tide of managed care consolidated immense purchasing power on the demand side. To counteract this imbalance, providers began to consolidate their practices, and larger, integrated health care organizations began forming. As a result, many large hospitals and group practices have become part of larger health systems that deliver hospital services in addition to outpatient care, long-term care, and specialized rehabilitation.

In a health care landscape that is increasingly dominated by corporations, individual physicians have struggled to preserve their autonomy. As a matter of survival, many physicians have consolidated their services within large clinics, formed strategic partnerships with hospitals, or started their own specialty hospitals. There is also a growing trend of physicians choosing to become employees of hospitals and other medical corporations.

Corporatization has shifted marketplace power from individuals to corporations. The days of consumer dominance in health care are long gone.

▶ Globalization of Health Care

Globalization, from social and economic perspectives, has been another hallmark of the 21st century. **Globalization** refers to various forms of cross-border economic activities, characterized by transnational movement and exchange of goods, services, people, and capital. Corporatization, transportation, and telecommunications have been key enabling factors in globalization.

From the standpoint of cross-border trade in health services, Mutchnick and colleagues (2005) identified four different modes of economic interrelationships:

- Telemedicine enables cross-border information exchange and delivery of certain services. For example, teleradiology (the electronic transmission of radiologic images over a distance) enables physicians in the United States to transmit radiologic images to Australia, where they are interpreted and reported back the next day (McDonnell, 2006). Telemedicine consulting services in pathology and radiology are being delivered to other parts of the world by cutting-edge U.S. medical institutions, such as Johns Hopkins Hospital.

- Consumers travel abroad to receive elective, nonemergency medical care, referred to as **medical tourism**. The Centers for Disease Control and Prevention (CDC, 2102) has estimated that as many as 750,000 U.S. residents travel abroad each year to receive medical and dental care. Specialty hospitals, such as the Apollo chain in India and Bumrungrad International Hospital in Thailand, offer state-of-the-art medical facilities to foreigners at a fraction of the cost for the same procedures done in the United States or Europe. Physicians and hospitals outside the United States have clear competitive advantages: reasonable malpractice costs, minimum regulation, and lower costs of labor. As

a result of these efficiencies, Indian specialty hospitals can do quality liver transplants for one-tenth of the cost in U.S. hospitals (Mutchnick et al., 2005). Some health insurance companies have also started to explore cheaper options for their covered members to receive certain costly services overseas. Conversely, dignitaries and other wealthy foreigners come to multispecialty centers in the United States, such as the Mayo Clinic, to receive highly specialized services.

- Foreign direct investment in health services enterprises benefits foreign citizens. For example, Chindex International, a U.S. corporation, provides medical equipment, supplies, and medical services in China. Chindex's United Family Healthcare serves Beijing, Shanghai, and Guangzhou.

- Health professionals move to other countries that have high demand for their services and offer better economic opportunities than their native countries. For example, nurses from other countries are moving to the United States and the United Kingdom to relieve the existing personnel shortages in those nations. Health care workers from Indonesia are migrating to Japan for similar reasons (Shinohara, 2016).

To this list, we can add three more aspects of globalization of health care:

- Corporations based in the United States have increasingly expanded their operations overseas. As a result, an increasing number of Americans are now working overseas as expatriates. Health insurance companies based in the United States are, in turn, having to develop benefit plans for these expatriates. According to a survey of 87 insurance companies, health care is also becoming one of the most sought-after employee benefits worldwide, even in countries that have national health insurance programs. Moreover, the cost of medical care overseas is rising at a faster rate than the rate of inflation in the general economy (Cavanaugh, 2008). Hence, the cost-effective delivery of health care is becoming a major challenge worldwide.

- Medical care delivery by U.S. providers is in demand overseas. American provider organizations—such as Johns Hopkins Hospital, Cleveland Clinic, Mayo Clinic, Duke University Medical Center, and several others— are now delivering medical services in various developing countries.
- The realities of globalization have resulted in a discipline called **global health**—that is, efforts to protect the entire global community against threats to people's health and to deliver cost-effective public health and clinical services to the world's population. It is now widely recognized that no country can ensure the health of its own population in isolation from the rest of the world (DeCock et al., 2013).

Cross-border collaborations in health care are also on the rise, mainly triggered by worldwide health care budgetary constraints. For example, the United States and Japan are collaboratively developing and testing medical devices (Uchida et al., 2013). India's Apollo Group is exporting telemedicine services from its Apollo Gleneagles Hospital in Kolkata (India) to patients in Bangladesh, Nepal, Bhutan, and Myanmar. It provides telediagnostic and teleconsultation from its center in

Karaganda Oblast in Kazakhstan to the region, and partners with Health Services America and Medstaff International in the United States for billing, documentation of clinical and administrative records, coding of medical processes, and insurance claims processing (Smith et al., 2009).

Globalization has also produced some negative effects. The developing world pays a steep price when emigration leaves these countries with shortages of trained professionals. The burden of disease in these countries is often greater than it is in the developed world, and emigration merely exacerbates these countries' inability to provide adequate health care to their own populations (Norcini and Mazmanian, 2005). As developing countries become more prosperous, their citizens tend to acquire Western tastes and lifestyles. In some instances, negative health consequences follow. For example, increased use of motorized vehicles results in a lack of physical exercise, which, along with changes in diet, greatly increases the prevalence of chronic diseases, such as heart disease and diabetes, in the developing world.

Globalization has also brought some new threats to health. For instance, the threat of infectious diseases has increased, as diseases appearing in one country can spread rapidly to other countries. HIV/AIDS, hepatitis B, and hepatitis C infections have spread worldwide.

▶ The Era of Health Care Reform

Efforts to reform the health care system in a comprehensive way have had a checkered past in the United States, as discussed previously. Passage of the ACA in

2010 was a bold undertaking that sought to bring about major reforms. Under the Trump presidency, however, there is every indication that the ACA, as crafted, may be short-lived.

Passage of the Affordable Care Act

On March 21, 2010, the U.S. House of Representatives passed, by a narrow vote of 219–212, the Patient Protection and Affordable Care Act, which was signed into law 2 days later by President Barack Obama. A week later, on March 30, the president signed the Health Care and Education Reconciliation Act of 2010, which amended certain provisions of the first law, mainly to raise additional revenues through taxation to pay for expanded health care services. Together the two laws comprise the principal features of what came to be known as the Affordable Care Act, commonly known as Obamacare. Not a single Republican in Congress voted in favor of these bills.

At least six factors can be cited that led to the ACA's successful passage. First, the Democratic Party held not only the presidency, but also majorities in the two houses of Congress. That made it easier for Obama to push forward his agenda. In fact, in the early days of his presidency, Obama confidently stated that this was "the best chance of reform we have ever had" (White House, 2009).

Second, there is some question as to whether the Democrats had intended to make health care reform a bipartisan effort—but their control of the executive and legislative branches gave them great power to set the agenda for health care reform, despite any Republican demurrals.

A public option[4] was initially included in the bill, but was later dropped because of opposition from both Republican and Democratic lawmakers.

Third, deliberations in Congress over the reform bill took place behind closed doors so that the American public had little to no participation and scant understanding of the bill. Without any knowledge of the content in these proceedings, opponents were unable to mount a challenge to specific aspects of the ACA.

Fourth, the benefits of the proposed health care reform were overstated, making them more attractive to the public. For example, in a televised address to the nation on August 8, 2009, Obama claimed that his reform would "protect people against unfair insurance practices; provide quality, affordable insurance to every American; and bring down rising costs that are swamping families, businesses, and our budgets" (White House, 2009). In that same address, the president said, "Under the reforms we seek, if you like your doctor, you can keep your doctor. If you like your health care plan, you can keep your health care plan." This refrain was repeated numerous times to "sell" the plan to the American public. Obama may also have created the illusion of universal coverage by stating that "while reform is obviously essential for the 46 million Americans who don't have health insurance, it will also provide more stability and security to the hundreds of millions who do" (White House, 2009). Unfortunately, the final version of the ACA did not fully meet those lofty goals.

Fifth, the ACA won the backing of major health care industry representatives.

---

[4] A government-sponsored insurance plan as an alternative to private insurance.

Even the AMA reluctantly pledged its support for the legislation, in a complete reversal of its traditional stance toward major health care reform proposals.

Sixth, subsequent to the Clinton presidency, the White House was held by a Republican, George W. Bush. For half of his 8-year tenure, both houses of Congress were under Republican control. Yet, Bush's focus remained on incremental reform, even though a large segment of the U.S. population did not have health insurance. While the United States was still mired in a deep economic recession, Obama made health care reform a top priority and tied his reform proposals to future economic growth and prosperity—a winning strategy, as it turned out (White House, 2009).

The Patchy Legacy of the ACA

The ACA was partially successful in reducing the number of Americans without health insurance, which stood at 43 million in 2013, before the ACA's main provisions went into effect. Under the ACA, approximately 17 million of the uninsured gained health insurance coverage (Carman et al., 2015). Frean and colleagues (2016) analyzed the insurance coverage gains in 2014 when the main insurance provisions of the law went into effect. They reported that the biggest gains were attributed to Medicaid enrollment, although, at the time, only approximately half of the states had chosen to expand their Medicaid[5]

programs to enroll people who became newly eligible under the ACA. While Medicaid accounted for roughly 60% of ACA coverage gains, the other 40% was attributed to the law's income-based federal subsidies,[6] which enabled low-income individuals to purchase coverage on the new government-established health insurance exchanges.[7]

Another key feature of the law was the individual mandate, which required all legal residents of the United States to either have what the law had designated as "minimum essential coverage" or pay a penalty tax. Frean and colleagues (2016) found that overall coverage rates did not respond to the mandate. Indeed, many people chose to pay the penalty instead of buying health insurance because of the high cost of insurance relative to the size of penalty. Moreover, the ACA's effects on employer-sponsored insurance were found to be essentially nil.

In short, the primary gains under Obamacare were made by the newly qualified Medicaid beneficiaries and those who received adequate federal subsidies to purchase insurance through the exchanges. Thus, Obamacare did help low-income people to obtain health insurance, but significant numbers of Americans were still left without coverage. For example, despite the ACA's promise to achieve near-universal health coverage, approximately 24 million working-age adults remained

---

[5] The ACA's mandate for all states to expand Medicaid was struck down by the U.S. Supreme Court in a decision rendered on June 28, 2012. Expanding or not expanding Medicaid became an option for each state. Eventually, 31 states and the District of Columbia expanded Medicaid under the ACA.

[6] Subsidies in the form of tax credits were made available to people with incomes between 100% and 400% of the federal poverty level (FPL). In 2014, 100% of the FPL was an annual income of $23,850 for a family of four.

[7] The exchanges (also called marketplaces) were established by either the state or the federal government. Health insurance was sold on these exchanges by private insurance companies.

uninsured in 2016. These uninsured adults were disproportionately poor, young (ages 19–34), and employed by small businesses. Lack of affordability proved to be a major reason for not purchasing health insurance through the exchanges (Collins et al., 2016). Thus, the label "affordable" in the law's title turned out to be a misnomer for many Americans.

While insurance coverage is often the focus of attention in most published reports, the ability to obtain health care services—that is, access—is much more valuable for assessing a program's success. A recent report concluded that a significant number of people who obtained insurance thanks to the ACA were also able to obtain a regular source of care and medical checkups. The authors cautioned, however, that the large increase in Medicaid enrollment under the ACA might stretch the capacity of a system that already had problems with provider participation in Medicaid (Kirby and Vistnes, 2016). Indeed, expanded access to services came mainly from obtaining care from hospital emergency departments (EDs) and community health centers (CHCs) (Goozner, 2015). Hence, the ACA did not respond to the problem of overcrowded EDs. Additionally, not all low-income Americans have access to CHCs because the centers are unevenly distributed in the United States. The ACA, however, enabled people with preexisting medical conditions to obtain health insurance, and young adults (up to age 26) were able to enroll under their parents' plans.

Unfortunately, many Americans did not benefit from the ACA, and some actually lost ground. For a large segment of the American middle class, the ACA's legacy was marred by unmet expectations. Many Americans found that their existing health insurance did not comply with the new rules established under the ACA, and many consequently received cancellation notices from their insurance companies. These people were generally left with no choice but to purchase insurance through the government-run exchanges.

In 2013, the Congressional Budget Office (CBO) had projected that in 2016, 24 million people would gain private coverage by purchasing health insurance through the exchanges. When 2016 came, that estimate was cut by 50% to 12 million people (CBO, 2016). It is not entirely clear why health insurance sold through the exchanges did not prove more popular. Notably, ACA-compliant plans sold outside the exchanges carried higher premiums (McCue and Hall, 2015), making them less attractive to consumers.

Late 2016 may well have been a turning point for the ACA's survival. The presidential election coincided with significant hikes in premiums as well as fewer choices for those consumers purchasing health insurance through the exchanges. The average premium increase for benchmark plans was 25%; it was more than 50% in some states. Also, three of the largest U.S. insurance companies—Aetna, United Health, and Humana—announced their decision to discontinue selling health insurance on most exchanges. In turn, a handful of states found themselves with only one insurer in the exchange (Muchmore, 2016a). Concerned about the unraveling of the exchanges, Obama called for more government intervention by proposing

the "public option" that had been eliminated from the originally planned ACA,
advocating for increased subsidies, and
encouraging the 19 states that had chosen not to expand Medicaid to now do so
(Muchmore, 2016b). These developments
came even as some pundits announced
that the ACA's health insurance market
reforms were working as intended, both
inside and outside the exchanges (McCue
and Hall, 2015).

Prospects for New Reforms

The victory of Donald Trump in the
November 2016 presidential election
stunned the pundits and the pollsters
alike, but his message resonated with
middle-class Americans despite fierce
opposition to his candidacy from many
quarters. Along with promises to grow
the economy and secure the nation's borders, Trump also promised to "repeal and
replace Obamacare." In contrast, his opponent, Hillary Clinton, proposed to morph
Obamacare into a single-payer national
health system in which the government
would become the primary insurer and
payer for people's health care. Since the
law's inception, those who had favorable
opinions of the ACA and those who had
unfavorable opinions were about evenly
split in polls conducted by the Henry
J. Kaiser Family Foundation. As late as
October 2016, polls showed an even split.
The same polls also showed that small
employers were worse off under the ACA.
For most families, the ACA had made no
difference, but 29% said they were worse
off, whereas only 19% indicated that they
were better off (Kirzinger et al., 2016).
With a majority of Republicans in both
houses of Congress, the Trump presidency had opened a new chapter in health
care reform.

The Secretary of the Department of
Health and Human Services in the Trump
administration is Tom Price, an orthopedic surgeon, who was chairman of the
House Budget Committee before assuming his new position. Price was a fierce
critic of the ACA, and was assigned the
responsibility to dismantle the ACA and
replace it with a program featuring less
government involvement in health care.
Although the political environment may
appear favorable, the task will not be easy.
Reform will likely emerge after meander-
ing through many efforts to tweak and
derail this process—though that is nothing new in American policymaking.

Although there is little clarity at the
time of this writing, we can speculate on
five main fronts about the prospects for
a full replacement of the ACA, based on
observations in several areas since the
2016 election. First, the ACA is highly
complex and many of its features are
firmly entrenched in the U.S. health care
system. Hence, full replacement of the
ACA will be a daunting task. Second, any
major changes to the ACA will be fiercely
opposed by the Democrats in Congress.
Third, the American media is not likely
to present unbiased reporting of the proposed changes and their likely effects on
insurance coverage and access to health
care. Fourth, public protests by supporters
of the ACA will add to a distorted message.
Fifth, court challenges to repeal the legislation will be mounted, perhaps in greater
numbers than was the case with enactment
of the ACA. The U.S. Supreme Court may
again become the final arbiter of a new law.

While both opponents to and proponents of the ACA will have many hurdles to cross, change appears inevitable. Hours after taking the oath of office on January 20, 2017, President Trump signed his first executive order to "waive, defer, grant exemptions from, or delay the implementation of any provision or requirement of the Act that would impose a fiscal burden on any State or a cost, fee, tax, penalty, or regulatory burden on individuals, families, healthcare providers, health insurers, patients, recipients of healthcare services, purchasers of health insurance, or makers of medical devices, products, or medications" (Bernstein, 2017). In effect, this executive order suspended the collection of individual penalties under the ACA for not having health insurance.

Whereas Trump's executive order is a small step, Congress is responsible for the formulation and passage of a reform bill. During deliberations over the ACA, Republican lawmakers were in general agreement with the Democrats on four areas (Talev et al., 2009), which are likely to be incorporated in some form in a new reform bill: (1) All Americans should have access to coverage regardless of pre-existing conditions; (2) small businesses should be able to receive insurance at prices comparable to large companies and labor unions; (3) government should provide some form of assistance to those who cannot afford insurance; and (4) insurers should offer incentives for preventive health behavior.

▶ Summary

The evolution of health care services in the United States, which has spanned approximately 150 years, has come a long way—from the delivery of primitive care, to technologically advanced services delivered by small and large medical corporations that have increasingly crossed national boundaries. The need for health insurance was first recognized and addressed during the Great Depression. Unlike in Europe, where government-sponsored health insurance took root, health insurance in the United States began mainly as a private endeavor because of circumstances that did not parallel those in Europe. Even so, social, political, and economic exigencies and opportunities led to the creation of two major government health insurance programs, Medicare and Medicaid, in 1965. Since then, small-scale incremental reforms have been undertaken because they were politically and socially more acceptable than large-scale changes in how most middle-class Americans obtained health care services.

Historically, traditional American beliefs and values have acted as strong forces against attempts to initiate fundamental changes in the financing and delivery of health care. The ACA was passed without seeking consensus among Americans on how it fit with the basic values and ethics of the populace. Its provisions helped mainly low-income Americans obtain health insurance, but put greater financial burdens on the middle class. Repealing and replacing the ACA was one of President Trump's campaign promises. The task of actually undoing the ACA, however, is challenging and faces many hurdles.

▶ Test Your Understanding

Terminology

almshouse	globalization	pesthouse
balance bill	means test	prepaid plan
cost shifting	Medicaid	socialized medicine
cross-subsidization	medical tourism	Title XVIII
cultural authority	Medicare	Title XIX
fee for service	organized medicine	voluntary health
gatekeeping	Part A	insurance
global health	Part B	

Review Questions

1. Why did the professionalization of medicine start later in the United States than in some Western European nations?

2. Why did medicine have a domestic—rather than professional—character in the preindustrial era? How did urbanization change that?

3. Which factors explain why the demand for the services of a professional physician was inadequate in the preindustrial era? How did scientific medicine and technology change that?

4. How did the emergence of general hospitals strengthen the professional sovereignty of physicians?

5. Discuss the relationship of dependency within the context of the medical profession's cultural and legitimized authority. What role did medical education reform play in galvanizing professional authority?

6. How did the organized medical profession manage to remain free of control by business firms, insurance companies, and hospitals until the latter part of the 20th century?

7. In general, discuss how technological, social, and economic factors created the need for health insurance.

8. Which conditions during the World War II period lent support to employer-based health insurance in the United States?

9. Discuss, with particular reference to the roles of (a) organized medicine, (b) the middle class, and (c) American beliefs and values, why reform efforts to bring in national health insurance have historically been unsuccessful in the United States.

10. Which particular factors that earlier may have been somewhat weak in bringing about national health insurance later led to the passage of Medicare and Medicaid?

11. On what basis were the elderly and the poor regarded as vulnerable groups for whom special government-sponsored programs needed to be created?

12. Discuss the government's role in the delivery and financing of health care, with specific reference to the

dichotomy between public health and private medicine.

13. Explain how contract practice and prepaid group practice were the prototypes of today's managed care plans.

14. Discuss the main ways in which current delivery of health care has become corporatized.

15. In the context of globalization in health services, which main economic activities are discussed in this chapter?

16. From the standpoint of health insurance, what were the main accomplishments of the Affordable Care Act?

▶ References

Anderson, O. W. 1990. *Health services as a growth enterprise in the United States since 1875.* Ann Arbor, MI: Health Administration Press.

Bernstein, L. 2017. *Trump's executive order to repeal Obamacare could go further than critics suggest.* KEPR tv.com. Available at: http://keprtv.com/news/nation-world/trumps-executive-order-to-repeal-obamacare-goes-further-than-critics-suggest. Accessed February 2017.

Bordley, J., and A. M. Harvey. 1976. *Two centuries of American medicine 1776–1976.* Philadelphia, PA: W. B. Saunders.

Bureau of the Census. 1976. *Statistical abstract of the United States, 1976.* Washington, DC: U.S. Department of Commerce.

Burns, J. 2004. Are nonprofit hospitals really charitable? Taking the question to the state and local level. *Journal of Corporate Law* 29, no. 3: 665–683.

Carman, K. G., et al. 2015. Trends in health insurance enrollment, 2013–2015. *Health Affairs* 34, no. 6: 1044–1048.

Cavanaugh, B. B. 2008. Building the worldwide health network. *Best's Review* 108, no. 12: 32–37.

Centers for Disease Control and Prevention (CDC). 2012. *Medical tourism: Getting medical care in another country.* Available at: http://www.cdc.gov/Features/MedicalTourism. Accessed July 2013.

Clark, C. 1998, October 20. A bloody evolution: Human error in medicine is as old as the practice itself. *The Washington Post,* Z10.

Coggeshall, L. T. 1965. *Planning for medical progress through education.* Evanston, IL: Association of American Medical Colleges.

Collins, S. R., et al. 2016. *Who are the remaining uninsured and why haven't they signed up for coverage?* Washington, DC: Commonwealth Fund.

Congressional Budget Office (CBO). 2013. *CBO's February 2013 estimate of the effects of the Affordable Care Act on health insurance coverage.* Available at: https://www.cbo.gov/sites/default/files/51298-2013-02-ACA.pdf. Accessed November 2016.

Congressional Budget Office (CBO). 2016. *Federal subsidies for health insurance coverage for people under age 65: Tables from CBO's March 2016 baseline.* Available at: https://www.cbo.gov/sites/default/files/51298-2016-03-HealthInsurance.pdf. Accessed November 2016.

Davis, P. 1996. The fate of Blue Shield and the new blues. *South Dakota Journal of Medicine* 49, no. 9: 323–330.

DeCock, K. M., et al. 2013. The new global health. *Emerging Infectious Diseases* 19, no. 8: 1192–1197.

Duffy, J. 1971. Social impact of disease in the late 19th century. *Bulletin of the New York Academy of Medicine* 47, no. 7: 797–811.

Falk, G. 1999. *Hippocrates assailed: The American health delivery system.* Lanham, MD: University Press of America.

Farmer, G. O., and J. H. Douglas. 2001. Physician "unionization": A primer and prescription. *Florida Bar Journal* 75, no. 7: 37–42.

Fein, R. 1958. *Economics of mental illness.* New York, NY: Basic Books.

Foley, D. J., et al. 2006. Highlights of organized mental health services in 2002 and major national and state trends. In: *Mental health, United States, 2004.* R. W. Manderscheid and J. T. Berry, eds. Washington, DC: U.S. Government Printing Office. pp. 200–236.

Frean, M., et al. 2016. Disentangling the ACA's coverage effects: Lessons for policymakers. *New England Journal of Medicine* 375, no. 17: 1605–1608.

Gabe, J., et al. 1994. *Challenging medicine.* New York, NY: Routledge.

Glied, S, and R. G. Frank. 2016. Economics and the transformation of the mental health system. *Journal of Health Politics, Policy and Law* 41, no. 4: 541–558.

Goodell, S. 2014. Health policy brief: Mental health parity. *Health Affairs.* Available at: http://healthaffairs.org/healthpolicybriefs/brief_pdfs/healthpolicybrief_112.pdf. Accessed February 2017.

Goodman, J. C., and G. L. Musgrave. 1992. *Patient power: Solving America's health care crisis.* Washington, DC: Cato Institute.

Goozner, M. 2015. Medicaid's enduring pay problem. *Modern Healthcare* 45, no. 22: 24.

Grob, G. N. 2005. Public policy and mental illnesses: Jimmy Carter's Presidential Commission on Mental Health. *Milbank Quarterly* 83, no. 3: 425–456.

Haber, S. 1974. The professions and higher education in America: A historical view. In: *Higher education and labor markets.* M. S. Gordon, ed. New York, NY: McGraw-Hill.

Haglund, C. L., and W. L. Dowling. 1993. The hospital. In: *Introduction to health services.* 4th ed. S. J. Williams and P. R. Torrens, eds. New York, NY: Delmar. pp. 135–176.

Hamowy, R. 1979. The early development of medical licensing laws in the United States, 1875–1900. *Journal of Libertarian Studies* 3, no. 1: 73–119.

Health Insurance Association of America (HIAA). 1991. *Source book of health insurance data.* Washington, DC: Health Insurance Association of America.

Iglehart, J. K. 1994. The American health care system: Managed care. In: *The nation's health.* 4th ed. P. R. Lee and C. L. Estes, eds. Boston, MA: Jones and Bartlett. pp. 231–237.

Kaptchuk, T. J., and D. M. Eisenberg. 2001. Varieties of healing 1: Medical pluralism in the United States. *Annals of Internal Medicine* 135, no. 3: 189–195.

Kaufman, M. 1980. American medical education. In: *The education of American physicians: Historical essays.* R. L. Numbers, ed. Los Angeles, CA: University of California Press. pp. 7–28.

Kennedy, J. F. 1963. Message from the President of the United States relative to mental illness and mental retardation. *American Journal of Psychiatry* 120, no. 8: 729–737.

Kirby, J. B., and J. P. Vistnes. 2016. Access to care improved for people who gained Medicaid or marketplace coverage in 2014. *Health Affairs* 35, no. 10: 1830–1834.

Kirzinger, A., et al. 2016. *Data note: Americans' opinions of the Affordable Care Act.* Available at: http://kff.org/health-reform/poll-finding/data-note-americans-opinions-of-the-affordable-care-act. Accessed November 2016.

Koch, A. L. 1993. Financing health services. In: *Introduction to health services.* 4th ed. S. J. Williams and P. R. Torrens, eds. New York, NY: Delmar. pp. 299–331.

Law, S. A. 1974. *Blue Cross: What went wrong?* New Haven, CT: Yale University Press.

Major provisions of the 21st Century Cures Act. 2017. *Congressional Digest* 96, no. 2: 2, 32.

Martensen, R. L. 1996. Hospital hotels and the care of the "worthy rich." *Journal of the American Medical Association* 275, no. 4: 325.

Mayer, T. R., and G. G. Mayer. 1984. *The health insurance alternative: A complete guide to health maintenance organizations.* New York, NY: Putnam.

McCue, M. J., and M. A. Hall. 2015. *Comparing individual health coverage on and off the Affordable Care Act's insurance exchanges.* Washington, DC: Commonwealth Fund.

McDonnell, J. 2006. Is the medical world flattening? *Ophthalmology Times* 31, no. 19: 4.

Mongan, J. J. 1995. Anatomy and physiology of health reform's failure. *Health Affairs* 14, no. 1: 99–101.

Muchmore, S. 2016a. ACA exchanges to reopen amid political, pricing pressures. *Modern Healthcare* 46, no. 44: 4.

Muchmore, S. 2016b. Obama calls for public option, more subsidies to improve ACA. *Modern Healthcare* 46, no. 43: 2.

Mutchnick, I. S., et al. 2005. Trading health services across borders: GATS, markets, and caveats. *Health Affairs* 24, web suppl. 1: W5-42–W5-51.

National Association of State Mental Health Program Directors (NASMHPD). 2014. *The vital role of state psychiatric hospitals.* J. Parks and A. Q. Radke, eds. Alexandria, VA: NASMHPD.

Norcini, J. J., and P. E. Mazmanian. 2005. Physician migration, education, and health care. *Journal of Continuing Education in the Health Professions* 25, no. 1: 4–7.

Numbers, R. L. 1985. The third party: Health insurance in America. In: *Sickness and health in America: Readings in the history of medicine and public health.* J. W. Leavitt and R. L. Numbers, eds. Madison, WI: University of Wisconsin Press.

Numbers, R. L., and J. H. Warner. 1985. The maturation of American medical science. In: *Sickness and health in America: Readings in the history of medicine and public health.* J. W. Leavitt and R. L. Numbers, eds. Madison, WI: University of Wisconsin Press.

Patrick, V., et al. 2006. Facilitating discharge in state psychiatric institutions: A group intervention strategy. *Psychiatric Rehabilitation Journal* 29, no. 3: 183–188.

Potter, M. A., and B. B. Longest. 1994. The divergence of federal and state policies on the charitable tax exemption of nonprofit hospitals. *Journal of Health Politics, Policy and Law* 19, no. 2: 393–419.

Public Health Service. 1995. *Health United States, 1994.* Washington, DC: Government Printing Office.

Raffel, M. W. 1980. *The U.S. health system: Origins and functions.* New York, NY: John Wiley & Sons.

Raffel, M. W., and N. K. Raffel. 1994. *The U.S. health system: Origins and functions.* 4th ed. Albany, NY: Delmar.

Ramsey, D. D. 2011. Evolution of mental health organizations in the United States. *Journal of Global Health Care Systems* 1, no. 3: 1–11.

Richardson, J. T. 1945. The origin and development of group hospitalization in the United States, 1890–1940. *University of Missouri Studies XX*, no. 3.

Rosen, G. 1983. *The structure of American medical practice 1875–1941.* Philadelphia, PA: University of Pennsylvania Press.

Rosenberg, C. E. 1979. The therapeutic revolution: Medicine, meaning, and social change in nineteenth-century America. In: *The therapeutic revolution.* M. J. Vogel, ed. Philadelphia, PA: University of Pennsylvania Press. pp. 3–25.

Rosner, L. 2001. The Philadelphia medical marketplace. In: *Major problems in the history of American medicine and public health.* J. H. Warner and J. A. Tighe, eds. Boston, MA: Houghton Mifflin. pp. 80–89.

Rothstein, W. G. 1972. *American physicians in the nineteenth century: From sect to science.* Baltimore, MD: Johns Hopkins University Press.

Shinohara, C. 2016. Health-care work in globalization: News reports on care worker migration to Japan. *International Journal of Japanese Sociology* 25, no. 1: 7–26.

Shryock, R. H. 1966. *Medicine in America: Historical essays.* Baltimore, MD: Johns Hopkins Press.

Smith, R. D., et al. 2009. Trade in health-related services. *Lancet* 373, no. 9663: 593–601.

Somers, A. R., and H. M. Somers. 1977. *Health and health care: Policies in perspective.* Germantown, MD: Aspen Systems.

Starr, P. 1982. *The social transformation of American medicine.* Cambridge, MA: Basic Books.

Stevens, R. 1971. *American medicine and the public interest.* New Haven, CT: Yale University Press.

Substance Abuse and Mental Health Services Administration. 2013. *Behavioral health, United States, 2012.* Rockville, MD: Department of Health and Human Services.

Talev, M., et al. 2009, September 9. Obama offers compromises to get health care bill passed. *McClatchy Newspapers.* Available at: http://www.mcclatchydc.com/news/politics-government/article24554320.html. Accessed November 2016.

Turnock, B. J. 1997. *Public health: What it is and how it works.* Gaithersburg, MD: Aspen. pp. 3–38.

Uchida, T., et al. 2013. Global cardiovascular device innovation: Japan-U.S.A synergies. *Circulation Journal* 77, no. 7: 1714–1718.

U.S. Surgeon General. 1999. *Mental health: A report of the Surgeon General. Overview of mental health services.* Available at: http://www.surgeongeneral.gov/library/mentalhealth/chapter2/sec2.html. Accessed February 2011.

Wagner, D. 2005. *The poorhouse: America's forgotten institution.* Lanham, MD: Rowman & Littlefield.

White House, Office of the Press Secretary. 2009. *Weekly address: President Obama calls health insurance reform key to stronger economy and improvement on status quo.* Available at: https://obamawhitehouse.archives.gov/realitycheck/the-press-office/weekly-address-president-obama-calls-health-insurance-reform-key-stronger-economy-a. Accessed June 2017.

Whitted, G. 1993. Private health insurance and employee benefits. In: *Introduction to health services.* 4th ed. S. J. Williams and P. R. Torrens, eds. New York, NY: Delmar. pp. 332–360.

Williams, S. J. 1995. *Essentials of health services.* Albany, NY: Delmar. pp. 108–134.

Wilson, F. A., and D. Neuhauser. 1985. *Health services in the United States.* 2nd ed. Cambridge, MA: Ballinger.

Wright, J. W. 1997. *The New York Times almanac.* New York, NY: Penguin Putnam.

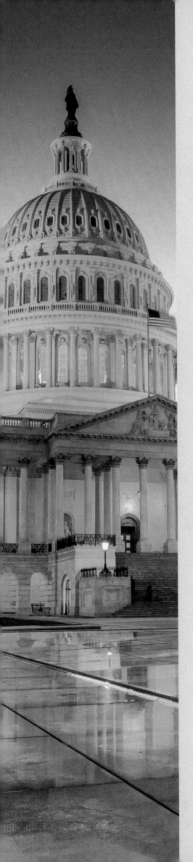

PART II

System Resources

© f11photo/Shutterstock

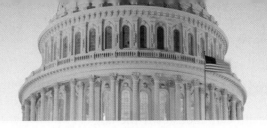

CHAPTER 4

Health Services Professionals

LEARNING OBJECTIVES

- Become familiar with the various types of health services professionals and their training, practice requirements, and practice settings.
- Differentiate between primary care and specialty care, and identify the causes of the imbalance between primary care and specialty care in the United States.
- Learn about the extent of maldistribution in the physician labor force and comprehend the reasons for such maldistribution.
- Outline initiatives under the Affordable Care Act to relieve shortages of primary care providers and to ensure coordinated care delivery in team settings.
- Appreciate the role of midlevel providers in health care delivery.
- Understand the role of allied health professionals in health care delivery.
- Discuss the functions and qualifications of health services administrators.
- Assess global health workforce challenges.

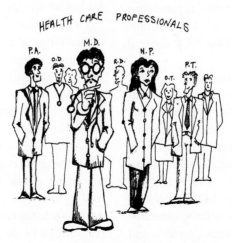

"Hmm, they're all beginning to look like me."

▶ Introduction

The U.S. health care industry is the largest and most powerful employer in the nation, accounting for more than 3% of the total labor force in the United States. In 2014, the health care sector contributed 17.1% of the United States' gross domestic product (World Bank, 2014). Although the number of jobs in many areas of the U.S. economy have decreased since the beginning of the economic recession in December 2007, the health care sector has continued its growth trend. Overall demand for all types of health care services is also expected to continue to increase as the population ages. Hence, substantial growth is anticipated in health care and related occupations. The U.S. Bureau of Labor Statistics (2015a) has projected that "health care occupations" will grow by 19% between 2014 and 2024, whereas the entire U.S. workforce will grow by only 6.5% during the same period.

Health professionals are among the most well-educated and diverse of all labor groups. Almost all of these practitioner groups are now represented by their own professional associations, which are listed in **APPENDIX 4-A** at the end of this chapter.

Health services professionals work in a variety of health care settings, including hospitals, managed care organizations (MCOs), nursing care facilities, mental health institutions, insurance companies, pharmaceutical companies, outpatient facilities, community health centers, migrant health centers, mental health centers, school clinics, physicians' offices, laboratories, voluntary health agencies, professional health associations, colleges of medicine and allied health professions, and research institutions. Most health professionals are employed by hospitals (40.6%), followed by nursing and personal care facilities (10.4%) and physician offices and clinics (9.4%) (**TABLE 4-1**).

The expansion of the number and types of health services professionals is closely related to population trends, advances in research and technology, disease and illness trends, and changes in health care financing and delivery of services. New and complex medical techniques, equipment, and advanced computer-based information systems (ISs) are constantly introduced, and health services professionals must continually learn how to use these innovations. Specialization in medicine has contributed to the proliferation of different types of medical technicians. The shift from acute to chronic disease and a growing emphasis on prevention have created a greater need for professionals who are formally trained to address behavioral risk factors and the delivery of primary care. Increased insurance coverage under the Affordable Care Act (ACA) has also increased the demand for health services professionals.

This chapter provides an overview of the large array of health services professionals employed in diverse health delivery settings. It briefly discusses the training and practice requirements of various health professionals, their major roles, the practice settings in which they are employed, and some critical issues concerning their professions. Emphasis is placed on physicians because they play a leading role in the delivery of health care. At the same time, there has been increased recognition of the role midlevel providers play in boosting the nation's primary care infrastructure.

TABLE 4-1 Persons Employed in Health Service Sites

Site	2000		2016	
	Number of Persons (in thousands)	**Percentage Distribution**	**Number of Persons (in thousands)**	**Percentage Distribution**
All employed civilians	136,891	100.0	151,436	100.0
All health service sites	12,211	100.0	15,442	100.0
Offices and clinics of physicians	1,387	11.4	1,611	9.4
Offices and clinics of dentists	672	5.5	897	5.2
Offices and clinics of chiropractors	120	1.0	135	0.8
Offices and clinics of optometrists	95	0.8	133	0.8
Offices and clinics of other health practitioners	143	1.2	297	1.7
Outpatient care centers	772	6.3	1,603	9.3
Home health care services	548	4.5	1,495	8.7
Other health care services	1,027	8.4	1,417	8.2
Hospitals	5,202	42.6	6,990	40.6
Nursing care facilities	1,593	13.0	1,786	10.4
Residential care facilities, without nursing	652	5.3	846	4.9

Data from Division of Labor Force Statistics, U.S. Bureau of Labor Statistics. 2017. *Labor force statistics from the current population survey.* Available at: https://www.bls.gov/cps/cpsaat18.htm. Accessed April 2017.

▶ Physicians

Physicians play a central role in the delivery of health services by evaluating patients and health conditions, diagnosing abnormalities, and prescribing treatments. Some physicians are engaged in medical education and research to find new and better ways to control and cure health problems. Many are involved in the prevention of illness.

All states require physicians to be licensed to practice. The licensure requirements include graduation from an accredited medical school that awards a Doctor of Medicine (MD) or Doctor of Osteopathic Medicine (DO) degree; successful completion of a licensing examination, governed by either the National Board of

Medical Examiners or the National Board of Osteopathic Medical Examiners; and completion of a supervised internship/residency program (Stanfield et al., 2011) The term **residency** refers to graduate medical education in a specialty that takes the form of paid on-the-job training, usually in a hospital. Before entering a residency, which may last 2 to 6 years, most DOs serve a 12-month rotating internship after graduation.

The number of active physicians, both MDs and DOs, has steadily increased from 14.1 physicians per 10,000 population in 1950 to 29.4 per 10,000 population in 2013 (**TABLE 4-2**). Of the 172 medical schools in the United States, 141 teach allopathic medicine and award a Doctor of Medicine degree;

TABLE 4-2 Active U.S. Physicians According to Type of Physician and Number per 10,000 Population

Year	All Active Physicians	Doctors of Medicine	Doctors of Osteopathy	Active Physicians per 10,000 Population
1950	219,900	209,000	10,900	14.1
1960	259,500	247,300	12,200	14.0
1970	326,500	314,200	12,300	15.6
1980	427,122	409,992	17,130	19.0
1990	567,610	539,616	27,994	22.4
1995	672,859	637,192	35,667	25.0
2000	772,296	727,573	44,723	27.0
2010	865,342	794,862	70,480	27.2
2013	936,844	854,698	82,146	29.4

Data from National Center for Health Statistics. 1996. *Health, United States, 1995.* Hyattsville, MD: U.S. Department of Health and Human Services. p. 220; National Center for Health Statistics. 2002. *Health, United States, 2002.* Hyattsville, MD: U.S. Department of Health and Human Services. p. 274; National Center for Health Statistics. 2006. *Health, United States, 2006.* Hyattsville, MD: U.S. Department of Health and Human Services. p. 358; National Center for Health Statistics. 2016. *Health, United States, 2015.* Hyattsville, MD: U.S. Department of Health and Human Services. p. 283.

31 teach osteopathic medicine and award the Doctor of Osteopathic Medicine degree (National Center for Health Statistics, 2016).

Similarities and Differences Between MDs and DOs

Both MDs and DOs use accepted methods of treatment, including drugs and surgery. The two differ mainly in their philosophies and approaches to medical treatment. **Osteopathic medicine**, practiced by DOs, emphasizes the musculoskeletal system of the body, such as correction of joints or tissues. In their treatment plans, DOs stress preventive medicine and take into account how factors such as diet and environment might influence natural resistance. They take a holistic approach to patient care. In comparison, MDs are trained in **allopathic medicine**, which views medical treatment as an active intervention to counteract and neutralize the effects of disease. MDs, particularly generalists, may also use preventive medicine, along with allopathic treatments.

Approximately 8.8% of all active physicians in the United States are osteopaths (American Osteopathic Association, 2013). Roughly 48% of MDs and more than half of DOs work in primary care settings (National Center for Health Statistics, 2016).

Generalists and Specialists

Most DOs are generalists and most MDs are specialists. In the United States, physicians trained in family medicine/general practice, general internal medicine, and general pediatrics are considered primary care physicians (PCPs) or **generalists** (Rich et al., 1994). Most PCPs provide preventive services (e.g., health examinations, immunizations, mammograms, Papanicolaou smears) and treat frequently occurring and less severe problems. Problems that occur less frequently or that require complex diagnostic or therapeutic approaches are referred to specialists after an initial evaluation.

Physicians in non-primary care specialties are referred to as **specialists**. Specialists must seek certification in an area of medical specialization, which commonly requires additional years of advanced residency training, followed by several years of practice in the specialty. A specialty board examination is often required as the final step in becoming a board-certified specialist. The common medical specialties, along with brief descriptions, are listed in **EXHIBIT 4-1**. Medical specialties may be divided into six major functional groups: (1) the subspecialties of internal medicine; (2) a broad group of medical specialties; (3) obstetrics and gynecology; (4) surgery of all types; (5) hospital-based radiology, anesthesiology, and pathology; and (6) psychiatry. The distribution of physicians by specialty appears in **TABLE 4-3**.

Work Settings and Practice Patterns

Physicians practice in a variety of settings and arrangements. Some work in hospitals as medical residents or staff physicians. Others work in the public sector, such as federal government agencies, public health departments, community and migrant health centers, schools, and prisons. Most physicians, however, are office-based practitioners, and most physician contacts occur in physician offices. An increasing number of physicians are partners or salaried employees, working in both hospitals and various outpatient settings, such as group practices, freestanding ambulatory care clinics, and diagnostic imaging centers.

EXHIBIT 4-1 Definitions of Medical Specialties and Subspecialties

Allergists	Treat conditions and illnesses caused by allergies or related to the immune system
Anesthesiologists	Use drugs and gases to render patients unconscious during surgery
Cardiologists	Treat heart diseases
Dermatologists	Treat infections, growths, and injuries related to the skin
Emergency medicine	Work specifically in emergency departments, treating acute illnesses and emergency situations—for example, trauma
Family physicians	Are prepared to handle most types of illnesses and care for the patient as a whole
General practitioners	Similar to family physicians—examine patients or order tests and have x-rays done to diagnose illness and treat the patient
Geriatricians	Specialize in problems and diseases that accompany aging
Gynecologists	Specialize in the care of the reproductive system of women
Internists	Treat diseases related to the internal organs of the body—for example, conditions of the lungs, blood, kidneys, and heart
Neurologists	Treat disorders of the central nervous system and order tests necessary to detect diseases
Obstetricians	Work with women throughout their pregnancy, deliver infants, and care for the mother after the delivery
Oncologists	Specialize in the diagnosis and treatment of cancers and tumors
Ophthalmologists	Treat diseases and injuries of the eye
Otolaryngologists	Specialize in the treatment of conditions or diseases of the ear, nose, and throat
Pathologists	Study the characteristics, causes, and progression of diseases
Pediatricians	Provide care for children from birth to adolescence
Preventive medicine	Includes occupational medicine, public health, and general preventive treatments
Psychiatrists	Help patients recover from mental illness and regain their mental health
Radiologists	Perform diagnosis and treatment by the use of x-rays and radioactive materials

Surgeons	Operate on patients to treat disease, repair injury, correct deformities, and improve health
General surgeons	Perform many different types of surgery, usually of relatively low difficulty
Neurologic surgeons	Specialize in surgery of the brain, spinal cord, and nervous system
Orthopaedic surgeons	Specialize in the repair of bones and joints
Plastic surgeons	Repair malformed or injured parts of the body
Thoracic surgeons	Perform surgery in the chest cavity—for example, lung and heart surgery
Urologists	Specialize in conditions of the urinary tract in both sexes and of the sexual/reproductive system in males

Data from Stanfield, P. S., et al. 2012. *Introduction to the health professions.* 6th ed. Burlington, MA: Jones & Bartlett Learning.

TABLE 4-3 U.S. Physicians According to Activity and Place of Medical Education, 2013

Activity and Place of Medical Education	Numbers	Percentage	Distribution
Doctors of medicine (professionally active)[1]	854,698	100.0	
Place of Medical Education			
U.S. medical graduates	636,707	74.5	
International medical graduates	217,991	25.5	
Activity			
Patient care	809,845	100.0	
Office-based practice	600,863	74.2	100.0
General and family practice	80,240		13.4
Cardiovascular diseases	17,657		2.9

(continues)

TABLE 4-3 U.S. Physicians According to Activity and Place of Medical Education, 2013 (*continued*)

Activity and Place of Medical Education	Numbers	Percentage	Distribution
Dermatology	9,910		1.6
Gastroenterology	11,322		1.9
Internal medicine	120,439		20.0
Pediatrics	58,719		9.8
Pulmonary diseases	8,870		1.5
General surgery	25,024		4.2
Obstetrics and gynecology	34,780		5.8
Ophthalmology	16,331		2.7
Orthopaedic surgery	20,013		3.3
Otolaryngology	8,136		1.4
Plastic surgery	6,414		1.1
Urological surgery	8,563		1.4
Anesthesiology	33,218		5.5
Diagnostic radiology	18,203		3.0
Emergency medicine	23,414		3.9
Neurology	11,762		2.0
Pathology, anatomic/clinical	10,481		1.7
Psychiatry	26,696		4.4
Radiology	7,527		1.3

Other specialty	43,144		7.2
Hospital-based practice	208,982	25.8	100.0
Residents and interns	117,203		56.1
Full-time hospital staff	91,779		43.9

[1] Excludes inactive, not classified, and address unknown.
Data from National Center for Health Statistics. 2016. *Health, United States, 2015*. Hyattsville, MD: U.S. Department of Health and Human Services. p. 283.

In 2012, physicians in general/family practice accounted for the greatest proportion of ambulatory care visits, followed by those in internal medicine and pediatrics (**FIGURE 4-1**). Physicians in obstetrics and gynecology tend to spend the most hours in patient care per week, even exceeding hours spent by surgeons. Surgeons have the highest average annual net income. Malpractice insurance premiums and operating expenses are the highest in obstetrics/gynecology.

Differences Between Primary and Specialty Care

Primary care can be distinguished from **specialty care** based on the time, focus, and scope of services provided to patients. The five main areas of distinction are as follows:

- In linear time sequence, primary care is first-contact care and is regarded as the entry point to the health care system. Specialty care, when needed, generally follows primary care.
- In a managed care environment where health services functions are integrated, PCPs serve as gatekeepers—an important role in controlling costs, utilization rates, and the rational allocation of resources. In the gatekeeping model, specialty care requires referral from PCPs.

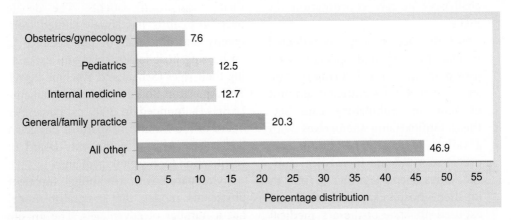

FIGURE 4-1 Ambulatory care visits to physicians according to physician specialty, 2012.

Data from National Center for Health Statistics. 2016. *Health, United States, 2015*. Hyattsville, MD: U.S. Department of Health and Human Services. pp. 268–269.

- Primary care is longitudinal. In other words, primary care providers follow through the course of treatment and coordinate various activities, including initial diagnosis, treatment, referral, consultation, monitoring, and follow-up. PCPs serve as patient advisors and advocates. Their coordinating role is especially important in ensuring continuity of care for chronic conditions. Because specialty care is episodic, it is more focused and intense than primary care.
- Primary care focuses on the person as a whole, whereas specialty care centers on particular diseases or organ systems of the body. Patients often have multiple problems simultaneously, a condition referred to as **comorbidity**. Treating comorbidities requires balancing multiple requirements, addressing changes in health conditions over time, and monitoring drug and disease interactions. Specialty care tends to be limited to illness episodes, the organ system, or the disease process involved. Comorbidities may necessitate referrals to multiple specialists, which present challenges in care coordination for PCPs.
- The difference in scope is reflected in how primary and specialty care providers are trained. Primary care students spend a significant amount of time in ambulatory care settings, familiarizing themselves with a variety of patient conditions and problems. Students in medical subspecialties spend significant time in inpatient hospitals, where they are exposed to state-of-the-art medical technology.

The Expanding Role of Hospitalists

Since the mid-1990s, an increasing amount of inpatient medical care in the United States has been delivered by **hospitalists**, physicians who specialize in the care of hospitalized patients (Schneller, 2006). Hospitalists do not usually have a relationship with the patient prior to hospitalization. Essentially, the patient's primary care provider entrusts the oversight of the patient's care to a hospitalist upon admission, and the patient returns to the regular physician after discharge (Freed, 2004). Approximately 44,000 hospitalists practice in the United States (U.S. Bureau of Labor Statistics, 2015b).

The growth of the number of hospitalists is influenced by the desire of hospital executives, HMOs, and medical groups to reduce inpatient costs and increase efficiency without compromising quality or patient satisfaction. Published research shows that using hospitalists does, in fact, achieve these goals (Wachter, 2004). Research findings have also put to rest initial concerns from PCPs, who were accustomed to the traditional method of rounding on their hospitalized patients. The debate over hospitalists has largely shifted from quality and efficiency of performance to optimizing hospitalists' skills and expanding their roles (Sehgal and Wachter, 2006). The American Board of Hospital Medicine (ABHM), founded in 2009 as a member board of the American Board of Physician Specialists (ABPS), is the only board of certification for hospital medicine.

Compared with traditional inpatient physicians model, the hospitalist model has a number of advantages. The on-site availability of a hospitalist ensures that a dedicated provider is readily available to respond to acute medical crises, manage tests, and answer questions, thereby reducing the time needed for treatments and improving the efficiency of discharge planning. This allows the hospitalist more time to communicate with patients, their families, and patients' PCPs (White and Glazier, 2011). Studies have demonstrated that hospitalist care is associated with shorter lengths of stay, better quality of care, increased patient satisfaction, and lower inpatient costs (Chen et al., 2013; Coffman and Rundall, 2005; Goodwin et al., 2013; White and Glazier, 2011).

▶ Issues in Medical Practice, Training, and Supply

Research has shown that the way physicians practice medicine and prescribe treatments for similar conditions varies significantly. Physicians have at their disposal an increasing number of therapeutic options because of the exponential growth in medical science and technology. Conversely, increasing health care costs continue to threaten the viability of the health care delivery system. The responsibility physicians have to perform difficult balancing acts—simultaneously taking into account the availability of the most advanced treatments, uncertainties about their potential benefits, and whether the higher costs of treatment are justified—contributes to a confusing environment. Hence, support has been growing for the development and refinement of standardized clinical guidelines to streamline clinical decision making and improve quality

of care (discussed in the *Cost, Access, and Quality* chapter). However, there have been some criticisms about the applicability, flexibility, and objectivity of some guidelines. Although the number of conditions for which guidelines are available is steadily increasing, guidelines for *combinations* of conditions (i.e., comorbidity) are not. Furthermore, many of the recommendations incorporated in the most well-accepted clinical guidelines allow for much flexibility, making it difficult to determine whether care provided by physicians complies with recommendations in the guidelines (Garber, 2005). In addition, the changing nature of chronic diseases and comorbidities is creating new challenges in the disease-centered reactive practice patterns (Starfield, 2011). A better care model, such as the chronic care model, requires patient-centered, longitudinal, coordinated, evidence-based, and information system–supported care, which facilitates physician–patient interaction and patient self-management (Coleman et al., 2009).

Medical Training

The principal source of funding for graduate medical education is the Medicare program, which provides explicit payments to teaching hospitals for each resident in training. The government, however, does not mandate how these physicians should be trained. Medical and surgical services furnished by an intern or resident within the scope of his or her training program are covered as provider services, with Medicare paying for these services through Direct Graduate Medical Education (DGME) and Indirect Medical Education (IME) payments. DGME payments offset a portion of the direct costs associated with training physicians (e.g., resident stipends and benefits, supervising physician stipends and benefits). Teaching hospitals depend on IME payments to maintain the state-of-the-art facilities and equipment (such as Level 1 trauma centers), and specialized services (e.g., advanced cancer care) that are critical both for training health professionals and maintaining community health (Association of American Medical Colleges [AAMC], 2014).

Emphasis on hospital-based training in the United States has produced more specialists than PCPs. Meanwhile, the health care delivery system is evolving toward a primary care orientation. The increasing prevalence of chronic diseases further highlights the deficiency of the medical training model in the United States, which focuses mainly on acute interventions. Medical training in primary care needs to be refocused on patient-centered care (as described in the *Outpatient and Primary Care Services* chapter), general internal medicine, and longitudinal clinical experiences.

Supply of Medical Professionals

Aided by tax-financed subsidies, the United States has experienced a steady increase in its physician labor force (Table 4-2; **FIGURE 4-2**). In 2009, for example, there were 273 physicians per 100,000 population (U.S. Census Bureau, 2012). The growth, however, has mainly occurred among specialists. The number of active physicians younger than age 75 is expected to grow from approximately 782,200 in 2014 to 825,200 by 2025 (AAMC, 2016).

A large influx of newly insured individuals seeking care is expected to strain the existing primary care infrastructure and result in personnel shortages in

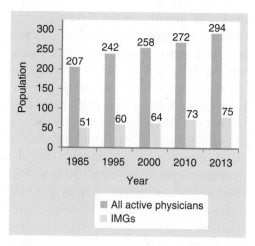

FIGURE 4-2 Supply of U.S. physicians, including international medical graduates (IMGs), per 100,000 population, 1985–2013.

Data from National Center for Health Statistics. 2016. *Health, United States, 2015*. Hyattsville, MD: U.S. Department of Health and Human Services. p. 282.

primary care (Schwartz, 2011). By 2025, an additional 52,000 PCPs would be needed (Petterson et al., 2012). The problem is that the primary care workforce is shrinking. According to a physician workforce report released by the AAMC (2016), primary care specialties are expected to experience a shortfall of between 14,900 and 35,600 physicians by 2025. Physician retirement decisions are also projected to have the greatest impact on supply, and more than one-third of all currently active physicians will be 65 or older within the next decade (AAMC, 2016).

In 2013, $12 million in ACA funding was awarded to train more than 300 new primary care residents during the 2013–2014 academic year; 32 teaching health centers in 21 states received funding (U.S. Department of Health and Human Services [DHHS], 2013a). The ACA also provides for loan repayment for pediatric medical, mental health and surgical subspecialties—specialties known to have shortages—in exchange for professionals in these subspecialties providing care in medically underserved areas (MUAs). Additionally, the law authorizes grants to increase training in geriatrics and behavioral health, and provides incentives for general surgeons who practice in MUAs (Congressional Research Service, 2017). The effects of these initiatives will not be known for several years.

Maldistribution

Maldistribution refers to either a surplus or a shortage of the type of physicians needed to maintain the health status of a given population at an optimal level. Neither shortages nor surpluses are desirable; they result in increased health care expenditures without a positive return in health outcomes. The United States faces maldistributions in terms of both geography and specialty.

Geographic Maldistribution

One of the ironies of excess physician supply is that localities outside metropolitan areas (i.e., counties with fewer than 50,000 residents) continue to have physician shortages. Nonmetropolitan areas have 39.8 PCPs per 100,000 population, compared to 53.3 PCPs per 100,000 population in metropolitan areas (National Center for Health Statistics, 2014). Rural areas, in particular, lack an adequate supply of both PCPs and specialists, even though residents in rural areas are sicker, older, and poorer than those in nonrural areas. Whereas 19.3% of the U.S. population

lives in rural areas, only 11.4% of physicians practice there (National Center for Health Statistics, 2014).

The DHHS designates as Health Professional Shortage Areas (HPSAs) those urban or rural areas, population groups, or medical or other public facilities that have a shortage of providers in primary care, dental care, and mental health care. At the end of 2016, there were 6,626 designated primary care HPSAs, 5,493 dental HPSAs, and 4,627 mental health HPSAs in the United States (DHHS, 2013b).

Several federal programs have demonstrated success in increasing the supply of primary care services in rural areas. Some of these programs, which are discussed in the *Health Services for Special Populations* chapter, include the National Health Service Corps, which makes scholarship support conditional on a commitment to future service in an underserved area; the Migrant and Community Health Center Programs, which provide primary care services to the poor and underserved using federal grants; and support of primary care training programs and Area Health Education Centers.

Specialty Maldistribution

Besides geographic maldistribution of physicians, a considerable imbalance exists between primary and specialty care in the United States. Approximately 47.7% of physicians work in primary care; the remaining 52.3% are specialists (Kaiser Family Foundation, 2016). In other industrialized countries, only 25% to 50% of physicians are specialists (Organization for Economic Cooperation and Development [OECD], 2016).

FIGURE 4-3 illustrates trends in the supply of PCPs. The proportion of active PCPs has been continually declining since 1949 and has reached its lowest point in recent years. Also, the number of physicians entering primary care has been decreasing. According to one study, only 21.5% of third-year internal medicine graduating residents reported general internal medicine as their ultimate career plan. Most of the residents reported subspecialty career plans (West and Dupras, 2012). Moreover, one in six general internists leaves his or her practice by midcareer either due to dissatisfaction or by moving into a subspecialty of internal medicine (Bylsma et al., 2010). The increasing number of international medical graduates (IMGs) practicing in the United States has helped alleviate these PCP shortages to some extent.

Growth of new medical technology is one major driving force behind the increasing number of specialists. Health care is often delivered according to a model that concentrates on diseases and specialist care. Doctors, particularly specialists, increasingly rely on medical technology to diagnose and treat diseases. Most hospitals with the latest medical technologies try to become clinical centers that offer all major specialty fields and employ these specialists. Additionally, medical students may be further attracted to go into subspecialties because their training is organized around medical technologies. This may contribute to the expanding gap between the primary and specialty care workforces.

The higher incomes of specialists relative to PCPs have also contributed to an oversupply of specialists. In recent years, reimbursement systems designed to increase payments to PCPs have been implemented, but wide disparities between the incomes of generalists and specialists persist (**TABLE 4-4**). Specialists also tend to have more predictable work

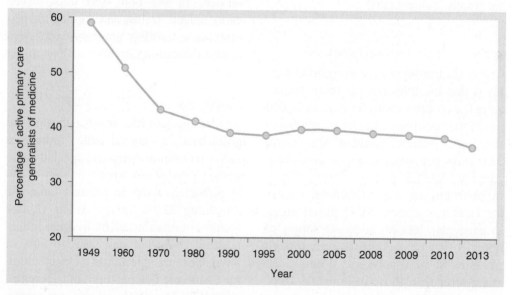

FIGURE 4-3 Trend in U.S. primary care generalists of medicine.

Data from National Center for Health Statistics. 2016. *Health, United States, 2015*. Hyattsville, MD: U.S. Department of Health and Human Services. p. 284.

TABLE 4-4 Mean Annual Compensation for U.S. Physicians by Specialty, May 2016 (in Dollars)

Anesthesiologists	269,600
Family and general practitioners	200,810
Internists, general	201,840
Obstetricians and gynecologists	234,310
Pediatricians, general	184,240
Psychiatrists	200,220
Surgeons	252,910
Physicians and surgeons, all other	205,560

Data from U.S. Bureau of Labor Statistics. 2017. *Occupational employment and wages—May 2016*. Available at: https://www.bls.gov/oes/current/oes_stru.htm. Accessed April 2017.

hours and enjoy higher prestige among their colleagues and the public at large (Rosenblatt and Lishner, 1991; Samuels and Shi, 1993). Higher status and prestige are also accorded to specialties employing the latest advances in medical technology. Unsurprisingly such considerations influence medical students' career decisions.

In terms of racial and ethnic diversity in the health workforce, **TABLE 4-5** shows the percentage of total enrollment of students in programs for selected health occupations by race. This indicates that the trends in racial and ethnic diversity vary considerably by occupation, although minorities tend to be more represented among the lower-skilled occupations.

The medical education environment in the United States is largely organized according to specialties and controlled by those who have achieved leadership positions by demonstrating their abilities in narrow scientific or clinical areas. Medical education in the United States emphasizes technology, intensive procedures, and tertiary care settings, which are generally more appealing to medical students than the more rudimentary field of primary care.

The imbalance between generalists and specialists has several undesirable consequences. Having too many specialists has contributed to the high volume of intensive, expensive, and invasive medical services, and consequently, to the rise in health care costs (Greenfield et al., 1992; Rosenblatt, 1992; Schroeder and Sandy, 1993; Wennberg et al., 1993). Seeking care directly from specialists is often less effective than getting primary care because the latter attempts to provide early intervention before complications develop (Starfield, 1992; Starfield and Simpson, 1993). Higher levels of primary care services are associated with lower overall death and lower mortality rates due to diseases of the heart and cancer (Shi, 1992, 1994). PCPs have been the major providers of care to minorities, the poor, and people living in underserved areas (Ginzberg, 1994; Starr, 1982). They can play a major role in overcoming health disparities (Lee et al., 2016; Shi et al., 2013). However, underserved populations suffer the most from PCP shortages.

▶ International Medical Graduates

The ratio of IMGs to the overall U.S. population has steadily grown over time (Figure 4-2), as has the ratio of IMGs to

TABLE 4-5 Percentage of Total Enrollment of Students in Programs for Selected Health Occupations, by Race, 2008–2009

Race	Allopathic	Osteopathic	Dentistry	Pharmacy
All races	100.0	100.0	100.0	100.0
White, non-Hispanic	61.7	70.0	59.9	58.9
Black, non-Hispanic	7.1	3.5	5.8	6.4
Hispanic	8.1	3.7	6.2	4.1
American Indian	0.8	0.7	0.7	0.5
Asian	21.7	17.1	23.4	22.1

Data from National Center for Health Statistics. 2012. *Health, United States, 2011.* Hyattsville, MD: U.S. Department of Health and Human Services. p. 355.

total active physicians practicing in the United States (**FIGURE 4-4**). Approximately 25.5% of professionally active physicians in the United States are IMGs, also known as foreign medical graduates (National Center for Health Statistics, 2016). This percentage translates into more than 217,000 active IMGs in the U.S. physician workforce (National Center for Health Statistics, 2016). An estimated one-fourth of all residency positions are filled by IMGs (Educational Commission for Foreign Medical Graduates, 2015), and an increasing number of IMGs are filling family practice residency slots (Kozakowski et al., 2016). In 1995, only 6.3% of IMGs

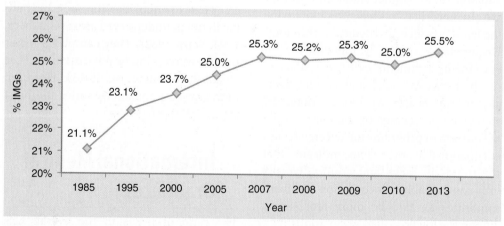

FIGURE 4-4 IMG physicians as a proportion of total active physicians.

Data from National Center for Health Statistics. 2016. *Health, United States, 2015.* Hyattsville, MD: U.S. Department of Health and Human Services. p. 283.

entered family practice residencies; by 2015, that percentage had increased to 11.3% (Boulet et al., 2006; Kozakowski et al., 2016). IMGs account for 51% of all physicians in internal medicine, 7% in pediatrics, and 4.5% in psychiatry (Educational Commission for Foreign Medical Graduates, 2015).

▶ Dentists

Dentists diagnose and treat dental problems related to the teeth, gums, and tissues of the mouth. All dentists must be licensed to practice. The licensure requirements include graduation from an accredited dental school that awards a Doctor of Dental Surgery (DDS) or Doctor of Dental Medicine (DMD) degree and successful completion of both written and practical examinations. Some states require dentists to obtain a specialty license before practicing as a specialist in that state (Stanfield et al., 2012).

Nine specialty areas are recognized by the American Dental Association (ADA): orthodontics (straightening teeth), oral and maxillofacial surgery (operating on the mouth and jaws), oral and maxillofacial radiology (producing and interpreting images of the mouth and jaws), pediatric dentistry (dental care for children), periodontics (treating gums), prosthodontics (making artificial teeth or dentures), endodontics (root canal therapy), public health dentistry (community dental health), and oral pathology (diseases of the mouth). The growth of dental specialties is influenced by technological advances, including implant dentistry, laser-guided surgery, orthognathic surgery (surgery performed on the bones of the jaw) for the restoration of facial form and function, new metal combinations for use in prosthetic devices, new bone graft materials in "tissue-guided regeneration" techniques, and new materials and instruments.

Many dentists are involved in the prevention of dental decay and gum disease. Dental prevention includes regular cleaning of patients' teeth and educating patients on proper dental hygiene. Dentists also spot symptoms that require treatment by a physician. Dentists employ dental hygienists and assistants to perform many of the preventive and routine care services.

Dental hygienists work in dental offices and provide preventive dental care, including cleaning teeth and educating patients on proper dental care. Dental hygienists must be licensed to practice. The licensure requirements include graduation from an accredited school of dental hygiene and successful completion of both a national board written examination and a state or regional clinical examination. Many states require further examination on legal aspects of dental hygiene practice.

Dental assistants work for dentists in the preparation, examination, and treatment of patients. Dental assistants do not have to be licensed to work; however, formal training programs that offer a certificate or diploma are available. Dental assistants typically work alongside dentists.

Most dentists practice in private offices as solo or group practitioners. As such, dental offices operate as private businesses, and dentists often perform business tasks, such as staffing, financing, purchasing, leasing, and work scheduling. Some dentists are employed in clinics operated by private companies, retail stores, or franchised dental outlets. Group dental practices, which offer lower overhead and increased productivity, have grown slowly. The federal government also employs dentists, mainly in the hospitals and clinics of the Department of Veterans Affairs and the U.S. Public Health Service. Mean annual earnings of salaried dentists were $173,860 in 2015 (U.S. Bureau of Labor Statistics, 2017).

The emergence of employer-sponsored dental insurance caused an increased demand for dental care because it enabled a greater segment of the population to afford dental services. The demand for dentists will continue to grow because of the increase in populations, such as the elderly, who have high dental needs, and an increase in public awareness of the importance of dental care to maintain good general health status. Demand will also be affected by the fairly widespread appeal of cosmetic and esthetic dentistry, the prevalence of dental insurance plans, and the inclusion of dental care as part of many public-funded programs, such as Head Start, Medicaid, community and migrant health centers, and maternal and infant care.

▶ Pharmacists

The traditional role of **pharmacists** has been to dispense medicines prescribed by physicians, dentists, and podiatrists, and to provide consultation on the proper selection and use of medicines. All states require a license to practice pharmacy. The licensure requirements traditionally included graduation from an accredited pharmacy program that awards a Bachelor of Pharmacy or Doctor of Pharmacy (PharmD) degree, successful completion of a state board examination, and practical

experience or completion of a supervised internship (Stanfield et al., 2012). Since 2005, the bachelor's degree has been phased out, and a PharmD, requiring 6 years of postsecondary education, has become the standard. The mean annual earnings of pharmacists in 2015 were $120,270 (U.S. Bureau of Labor Statistics, 2017).

Although most pharmacists are generalists who dispense drugs and advise providers and patients, some become specialists. Pharmacotherapists, for example, specialize in drug therapy and work closely with physicians. Nutrition-support pharmacists determine and prepare drugs needed for nutritional therapy. Radiopharmacists, or nuclear pharmacists, produce radioactive drugs used for patient diagnosis and therapy.

Most pharmacists hold salaried positions and work in community pharmacies that are independently owned or are part of a national drugstore, discount store, or department store chain. Pharmacists are also employed by hospitals, MCOs, home health agencies, clinics, government health services organizations, and pharmaceutical manufacturers.

In recent decades, the role of pharmacists has expanded from primarily preparing and dispensing prescriptions to include educating on drug products and serving as experts on specific drugs, drug interactions, and generic drug substitution. For example, under the Omnibus Budget Reconciliation Act of 1990, pharmacists are required to give consumers information about drugs and their potential misuse. This educating and counseling role of pharmacists is broadly referred to as **pharmaceutical care**. The American Council on Pharmaceutical Education (now the Accreditation Council for Pharmacy Education; 1992) defines pharmaceutical care as "a mode of pharmacy practice in which the pharmacist takes an active role on behalf of patients, by assisting prescribers in appropriate drug choices, by effecting distribution of medications to patients, and by assuming direct responsibilities to collaborate with other health care professionals and with patients to achieve the desired therapeutic outcome." This concept entails a high level of drug knowledge, clinical skill, and independent judgment. It also requires that pharmacists share with other health professionals the responsibility for optimizing the outcome of patients' drug therapies, such as health status, quality of life, and satisfaction (Helper and Strand, 1990; Schwartz, 1994; Strand et al., 1991). Physicians often consult pharmacists to identify and prevent potential drug-related problems and resolve actual drug-related problems (Morley and Strand, 1989). Recent studies also indicate that pharmacist-provided medication management can be beneficial for patients, especially those with multiple chronic conditions or complex medication regimens (Carter et al., 2012; Rafferty et al., 2016).

▶ Other Doctoral-Level Health Professionals

In addition to physicians, dentists, and some pharmacists, other health professionals have doctoral education, including optometrists, psychologists, podiatrists, and chiropractors.

Optometrists provide vision care, which includes examination, diagnosis, and correction of vision problems. They must be licensed to practice. The licensure requirements include the possession of a Doctor of Optometry (OD) degree and passing a written and clinical state board examination. Most optometrists work in solo or group practices. Some work for the government, optical stores, or vision care centers as salaried employees.

Psychologists provide patients with mental health care. They must be licensed or certified to practice. The ultimate recognition is the diplomate in psychology, which requires a Doctor of Philosophy (PhD) or Doctor of Psychology (PsyD) degree, a minimum of 5 years' postdoctoral experience, and the successful completion of an examination by the American Board of Examiners in Professional Psychology. Psychologists may specialize in several areas, such as the clinical, counseling, developmental, educational, engineering, personnel, experimental, industrial, psychometric, rehabilitation, school, and social domains (Stanfield et al., 2012).

Podiatrists treat patients with diseases or deformities of the feet, including performing surgical operations, prescribing medications and corrective devices, and administering physiotherapy. They must be licensed to practice. Requirements for licensure include completion of an accredited program that awards a Doctor of Podiatric Medicine (DPM) degree and passing a national examination by the National Board of Podiatric Medical Examiners. Most podiatrists work in private practice, but some are salaried employees of health service organizations.

Chiropractors provide treatment to patients through chiropractic (done by hand) manipulation, physiotherapy, and dietary counseling. They typically help patients with neurologic, muscular, and vascular disturbances. Chiropractic care is based on the belief that the body is a self-healing organism; thus, chiropractors do not prescribe drugs or perform surgery. Chiropractors must be licensed to practice. Requirements for licensure include completion of an accredited program that awards a 4-year Doctor of Chiropractic (DC) degree and passing an examination by the state chiropractic board. Most chiropractors work in private solo or group practice.

Doctoral nursing degrees include the Doctor of Nursing Practice (DNP), Doctor of Nursing Science (DNS), and Doctor of Philosophy in Nursing (PhD) (Ericksen, 2016). The DNS and PhD degrees are research focused, whereas the DNP emphasizes patient care and nursing practice (Ericksen, 2016). A doctoral degree is usually required to become a professor of nursing education or nurse researcher (Ericksen, 2016). Doctoral degrees are also preferred for nurse practitioners, clinical nurse specialists, nurse anesthetists, and nurse-midwives (American Association of Colleges of Nursing [AACN], 2014).

▶ **Nurses**

Nurses constitute the largest group of health care professionals. The nursing profession developed around hospitals after World War I, primarily attracting women. Before that time, more than 70% of nurses worked in private duty, either in patients' homes or hospitals for private-pay patients. Hospital-based nursing flourished after the war as the effectiveness of nursing care became apparent. Federal support of nursing education increased after World War II, with the passage of the Nursing Training Act of 1964, the Health Manpower Act of 1968,

and the Nursing Training Act of 1971. However, despite federal support, state funding remains the primary source of financial support for nursing schools.

Nurses are the major caregivers for sick and injured patients, addressing their physical, mental, and emotional needs. All states require nurses to be licensed to practice. Nurses can be licensed in more than one state through examination or endorsement of a license issued by another state. The licensure requirements include graduation from an approved nursing program and successful completion of a national examination.

Their educational preparation distinguishes the two non-doctoral-degree levels of nurses. **Registered nurses (RNs)** must complete an associate's degree in nursing (ADN), a diploma program, or a baccalaureate degree in nursing (BSN). ADN programs take about 2 to 3 years and are offered by community and junior colleges. Diploma programs take 2 to 3 years and are still offered by a few hospitals. BSN programs take 4 to 5 years and are offered by colleges and universities (Stanfield et al., 2012). **Licensed practical nurses (LPNs)**—called licensed vocational nurses (LVNs) in some states—must complete a state-approved program in practical nursing and a national written examination. Most practical nursing programs last about 1 year and include classroom study, as well as supervised clinical practice. Nurse managers act as supervisors of other nurses; RNs supervise LPNs.

Nurses work in the same variety of settings as other health care professionals. In addition, they work in home health care, hospice care, and long-term care settings. A few work as private-duty nurses in patients' homes. Nurses are often classified according to the settings in which they work—for example, hospital nurses, long-term care nurses, public health nurses, private-duty nurses, office nurses, and occupational health or industrial nurses.

With the remarkable growth in the various types of outpatient settings (see the *Outpatient and Primary Care Services* chapter), hospitals and nursing homes now treat patients who are much sicker than before. This means more patients require a greater amount of care when in residence at these settings. Hence, the ratio of nurses to patients has increased, and nurses' work has become more intensive. The growing number of opportunities for RNs in supportive roles, such as case management, utilization review, quality assurance, and prevention counseling, has also expanded the demand for their services.

Between 2004 and 2014, the total full-time equivalent (FTE) RN workforce increased by 345,200 (American Hospital Association, 2016). In 2016, registered nurses made up one of the largest occupations in the United States, with more than 2.85 million RNs earning an average salary of $72,180 per year (U.S. Bureau of Labor Statistics, 2017). Projections of the future need for nurses indicate there will be a deficit of 918,232 RNs in 2030 (Juraschek et al., 2012). To make the nursing profession more attractive, health services organizations need to initiate measures such as creating incentive packages to attract new nurses, increasing pay and benefits to current nurses, introducing more flexible work schedules, awarding tuition reimbursement for continuing education, and providing on-site daycare assistance.

A nationwide shortage of primary care providers inspired the Advanced Nursing Education Expansion Program, an ACA component that allocated $30 million to support academic training programs for nurse practitioners and certified nurse-midwives. The funds are expected to help pay for instructors and for students' housing and living expenses.

▶ Advanced Practice Nurses

The term **advanced practice nurse (APN)** is a general classification of nurses who have education and clinical experience beyond that required of an RN. APNs include four areas of specialization (Cooper et al., 1998): clinical nurse specialists (CNSs), certified registered nurse anesthetists (CRNAs), nurse practitioners (NPs), and certified nurse-midwives (CNMs). NPs and CNMs are also categorized as midlevel providers and are discussed in the next section. Besides being direct caregivers, APNs perform other professional activities, such as collaborating and consulting with other health care professionals; educating patients and other nurses; collecting data for clinical research projects; and participating in the development and implementation of total quality management programs, critical pathways, case management, and standards of care (Grossman, 1995).

Both CNSs and NPs work at hospitals, primary care, and other settings. Examples of CNS functions in an acute care hospital include taking the patient's social and clinical history at the time of admission, conducting the physical assessment after the patient's admission, adjusting IV infusion rates, managing pain, managing resuscitation orders, removing intracardiac catheters, and ordering routine laboratory tests and radiographic examinations. CNSs generally do not have the legal authority to prescribe drugs. NPs, by comparison, may prescribe drugs in most states. CRNAs are trained to manage anesthesia during surgery, and CNMs deliver babies and manage the care of mothers and healthy newborns before, during, and after delivery.

The requirements for becoming an APN vary greatly from state to state. In general, the designation requires a graduate degree in nursing or certification in an advanced practice specialty area.

▶ Non-physician Providers

Midlevel providers (NPPs) are clinical professionals who practice in many areas similar to those in which physicians practice, but who do not have an MD or a DO degree. NPPs receive less advanced training than physicians but more training than RNs. NPPs, in many instances, can substitute for physicians. Nevertheless, they do not engage in the entire range of primary care or deal with complex cases requiring the expertise of a physician (Cooper et al., 1998). Efforts to formally establish the NPP role began in the late 1960s, in recognition of the fact that they could improve access to primary care, especially in rural areas.

NPPs include physician assistants (PAs), NPs, and CNMs. In the future, the expansion of health insurance coverage and the growth of the U.S. population will continue to drive the demand for NPPs (Jacobson and Jazowski, 2011). As of 2014, the supply of new NPs was increasing at 6.9% per capita, compared to a growth rate of 3.4% for the supply of physicians (National Center for Health Statistics, 2016). Approximately 20,000 NPs and PAs graduated in

2015, up from 11,200 of these NPPs in 2006 (American Hospital Association, 2016).

Roles for these skilled NPPs are expanding as the physician workforce shrinks, the population of seniors expands, and health care becomes accessible to more Americans. NPs, in particular, are assuming a pivotal role in health care. NPPs are capable of providing a large proportion of the primary care services provided by physicians. A substantial body of research evaluating the quality of primary care provided by NPPs shows that these providers perform as well as physicians on important clinical outcome measures, such as mortality, preventable hospitalizations, and improvement of patient health status (Agarwal et al., 2009; Evangelista et al., 2012; Kuo et al., 2015; Laurant et al., 2009). In addition, patients report high levels of satisfaction with care provided by NPPs (Evangelista et al., 2012; Golden, 2014).

Nurse Practitioners

The American Nurses Association (ANA) defines **nurse practitioners (NPs)** as individuals who have completed a program of study leading to competence as RNs in an expanded role. NPs constitute the largest group of NPPs. As of 2016, the United States had approximately 150,230 NPs (U.S. Bureau of Labor Statistics, 2017). Training for NPs covers topics of health promotion, disease prevention, health education, counseling, and disease management. NPs take health histories, provide physical exams and health assessments, and diagnose, treat, and manage patients with acute and chronic health conditions (AACN, 2014).

More than 6,000 new NPs are trained every year in 373 colleges and universities across the United States (AACN, 2016).

The training of NPs may be a certificate program (at least 9 months in duration) or a master's degree program (2 years of full-time study). States vary with regard to licensure and accreditation requirements for these roles. Most NPs are now trained in graduate or postgraduate nursing programs. In addition, NPs must complete clinical training in direct patient care. Certification examinations are offered by the American Nurses Credentialing Center, the American Academy of Nurse Practitioners, and specialty nursing organizations.

One major difference between the training and practice orientation of NPs and PAs is that NPs are oriented toward health promotion and education, whereas PAs are oriented more toward a medical model that focuses on disease (Hooker and McCaig, 2001). NPs spend extra time with patients to help them understand the need to take responsibility for their own health. NP specialties include pediatric, family, adult, psychiatric, and geriatric programs. NPs have statutory prescribing authority in almost all states, and they may serve as independent providers without supervision. NPs can also receive direct reimbursement as providers under the Medicaid and Medicare programs.

Physician Assistants

The American Academy of Physician Assistants (1986) defines **physician assistants (PAs)** as "part of the health-care team . . . [who] work in a dependent relationship with a supervising physician to provide comprehensive care." In 2014, there were approximately 94,400 jobs available for PAs in the United States (U.S. Bureau of Labor Statistics, 2015c).

PAs are licensed to perform medical procedures only under the supervision of a physician who may be on site or off site. Major services provided by PAs include evaluation, monitoring, diagnostics, therapeutics, counseling, and referral (Fitzgerald et al., 1995). In most states, PAs have the authority to prescribe medications.

As of 2017, 218 accredited PA training programs were operating in the United States, with a steady growth in enrollment (The Accreditation Review Commission on Education for the Physician Assistant, 2017). PA programs award bachelor's degrees, certificates, associate degrees, master's degrees, or doctoral degrees. The mean length of the program is 26 months (Hooker and Berlin, 2002). PAs are certified by the National Commission on Certification of Physician Assistants.

Certified Nurse-Midwives

Certified nurse-midwives (CNMs) are RNs with additional training from a nurse-midwifery program, in areas such as maternal and fetal procedures, maternity and child nursing, and patient assessment (Endicott, 1976). CNMs deliver babies, provide family planning education, manage gynecologic and obstetric care, and can substitute for obstetricians/gynecologists in prenatal and postnatal care. They are certified by the American College of Nurse-Midwives (ACNM) to provide care for normal expectant mothers. They refer abnormal or high-risk patients to obstetricians or jointly manage the care of such patients. There are approximately 39 ACNM-accredited nurse-midwifery education programs in the United States (ACNM, 2017).

Midwifery has never assumed the central role in the management of pregnancies in the United States that it has in Europe (Wagner, 1991). Physicians, mainly obstetricians, attend most deliveries in the United States, but some evidence indicates that, for low-risk pregnancies, CNMs are much less likely to use available technical tools to monitor or modify the course of labor. Patients of CNMs are less likely to be electronically monitored, have induced labor, or receive epidural anesthesia. These differences are associated with lower cesarean section rates and less use of resources, such as hospital stays, operating room costs, and use of anesthesia staff (Rosenblatt et al., 1997).

▶ Allied Health Professionals

The term **allied health** is used loosely to categorize several different types of professionals in a vast number of health-related technical areas. Among these professionals are technicians, assistants, therapists, and technologists. These professionals receive specialized training, and their clinical interventions complement the work of physicians and nurses. Certain professionals, however, are allowed to practice independently, depending on state law.

In the early part of the 20th century, the health care provider workforce consisted of physicians, nurses, pharmacists, and optometrists. As knowledge in health sciences expanded and medical care became more complex, physicians found it difficult to spend the necessary time with their patients. Time constraints, as well as the limitations in learning new skills, created a need to train other professionals who could serve as adjuncts to or as substitutes for physicians and nurses.

Section 701 of the Public Health Service Act defines an **allied health professional**

as someone who has received a certificate; associate's, bachelor's, or master's degree; doctoral-level preparation; or post-baccalaureate training in a science related to health care and has responsibility for the delivery of health or related services. These services may include those associated with the identification, evaluation, and prevention of diseases and disorders, dietary and nutritional services, rehabilitation, and health system management.

Allied health professionals can be divided into two broad categories: technicians/assistants and therapists/technologists. **EXHIBIT 4-2** lists the main allied health professions in the United States.

As noted earlier, formal requirements for these professionals range from certificates gained in postsecondary educational programs to postgraduate degrees for some professions. Typically, technicians and assistants receive less than 2 years of postsecondary education. They require supervision from therapists or technologists to ensure that treatment plans are followed. Technicians and assistants include physical therapy assistants (PTAs), certified occupational therapy assistants (COTAs), medical laboratory technicians, radiologic technicians, and respiratory therapy technicians.

Technologists and therapists receive more advanced training. They evaluate patients, diagnose problems, and develop treatment plans. Many technologists and therapists have independent practices. For example, physical therapy is practiced in most U.S. states without the requirement of a prescription or referral from a physician. Many states also allow occupational therapists and speech therapists to see patients without referral from a physician.

EXHIBIT 4-2 Examples of Allied Health Professionals

Activities coordinator	Optician
Audiology technician	Pharmacist
Cardiovascular technician	Physical therapist
Cytotechnologist	Physical therapy assistant
Dental assistant	Physician assistant
Dietary food service manager	Radiology technician
Exercise physiologist	Recreation therapist
Histologic technician	Registered dietitian
Laboratory technician	Registered records administrator
Legal services	Respiratory therapist
Medical records technician	Respiratory therapy technician
Medical technologist	Social services coordinator
Mental health worker	Social worker
Nuclear medicine	Speech therapist
Occupational therapist	Speech therapy assistant
Occupational therapy assistant	

Therapists

Physical therapists (PTs) provide care for patients with movement dysfunction. Educational programs in physical therapy are accredited by the Commission on Accreditation of Physical Therapy Education. As of 2017, there were 236 physical therapy education programs in the United States. Currently, only graduate degree physical therapy programs are accredited. Master's degree programs are typically 2 to 3 years in length, while doctoral degree programs last 3 years. To obtain a license, PTs must also pass the National Physical Therapy Examination or a similar state-administered exam

(Commission on Accreditation in Physical Therapy Education, 2017).

Occupational therapists (OTs) help people of all ages improve their ability to perform tasks in their daily living and working environments. They work with individuals who have conditions that are mentally, physically, developmentally, or emotionally disabling. A master's degree in occupational therapy is the typical minimum requirement for entry into the field. In 2015, 171 master's degree programs or combined bachelor's and master's degree programs were accredited, and 15 doctoral degree programs were accredited by the Accreditation Council for Occupational Therapy Education (ACOTE, 2017).

Speech–language pathologists treat patients with speech and language problems. Audiologists treat patients with hearing problems. The American Speech-Language-Hearing Association is the credentialing association for both audiologists and speech–language pathologists.

Other Allied Health Professionals

Medical dietetics includes dietitians, nutritionists, and dietetic technicians who ensure that institutional foods and diets are prepared in accordance with acceptable nutritional standards. Dietitians are registered by the Commission on Dietetic Registration of the Academy of Nutrition and Dietetics.

Dispensing opticians fit eyeglasses and contact lenses. They are certified by the American Board of Opticianry and the National Contact Lens Examiners.

Social workers help patients and families cope with problems resulting from long-term illness, injury, and rehabilitation. The Council on Social Work Education accredits baccalaureate and master's degree programs in social work in the United States.

Many programs are accredited by the Committee on Allied Health Education and Accreditation under the American Medical Association, including those for the following professionals:

- Anesthesiologist assistants
- Cardiovascular technologists
- Cytotechnologists (study changes in body cells under a microscope)
- Diagnostic medical sonographers (work with ultrasound diagnostic procedures)
- Electroneurodiagnostic technologists (work with procedures related to the electrical activity of the brain and nervous system)
- Emergency medical technician-paramedics (provide medical emergent care to acutely ill or injured persons in prehospital settings)
- Histologic technicians/technologists (analyze blood, tissue, and fluids)
- Medical assistants (perform a number of administrative and clinical duties in physicians' offices)
- Medical illustrators
- Medical laboratory technicians
- Medical record administrators (direct the medical records department)
- Medical record technicians (organize and file medical records)
- Medical technologists (perform clinical laboratory testing)
- Nuclear medicine technologists (operate diagnostic imaging equipment and use radioactive drugs to assist in the diagnosis of illness)
- Ophthalmic medical technicians
- Perfusionists (operate life support respiratory and circulatory equipment)

- Radiologic technologists (perform diagnostic imaging exams, such as x-rays, computed tomography, magnetic resonance imaging, and mammography)
- Respiratory therapists and technicians (treat patients with breathing disorders)
- Specialists in blood bank technology
- Surgeon's assistants
- Surgical technologists (prepare operating rooms and patients for surgery)

Certain health care workers are not required to be licensed, and they usually learn their skills on the job; however, their roles are limited to assisting other professionals in the provision of services. Examples include dietetic assistants, who assist dietitians or dietetic technicians in the provision of nutritional care; electroencephalogram technologists or technicians, who operate electroencephalographs; electrocardiogram (ECG) technicians, who operate electrocardiographs; paraoptometrics, including optometric technicians and assistants, who perform basic tasks related to vision care; health educators, who provide individuals and groups with facts on health, illness, and prevention; psychiatric/mental health technicians, who provide care to patients with mental illness or developmental disabilities; and sanitarians, who collect samples for laboratory analysis and inspect facilities for compliance with public health regulations. Increasingly, these practitioners are seeking their credentials through certifications, registrations, and training programs.

As the number of older people in the United States continues to increase, and as new developments allow for the treatment of more medical conditions, more allied health professionals will be needed. For example, home health aides will be needed as more individuals seek care outside of traditional institutional settings. Jobs for LPNs/LVNs and pharmacy technicians are also expected to increase significantly, to roughly 117,300 and 34,700 positions, respectively by 2024 (U.S. Bureau of Labor Statistics, 2015c).

Allied health professionals represent an important part of the patient care system. They specialize in areas directly related to prevention, wellness, and management of acute and chronic diseases, as well as behavioral health problems. These professionals have a critical role in the health care system and provide comprehensive, patient-centered care to millions of individuals. Studies have affirmed their positive influence on health care services; allied health professionals improve patient access to care, patient volume, and service efficiency, as well as reduce costs of care (American Association of Community Colleges, 2014; Beazoglou et al., 2012; Post and Stoltenberg, 2014).

▶ Health Services Administrators

Health services administrators are employed at the top, middle, and entry levels of various types of organizations that deliver health services. Top-level administrators provide leadership and strategic direction, work closely with the governing boards (see the *Inpatient Facilities and Services* chapter), and are responsible for an organization's long-term success. They are responsible for the operational, clinical, and financial outcomes of their entire organization. Middle-level administrators may have leadership roles for major service centers, such as outpatient, surgical, and nursing services, or they may be departmental managers in charge of single departments, such as diagnostics, dietary, rehabilitation, social services, environmental services, or medical records. Their jobs involve major planning and coordinating functions, organizing human and physical resources, directing and supervising, operational and financial controls, and decision making. They often have direct responsibility for implementing changes, creating efficiencies, and developing new procedures with respect to changes in the health care delivery system. Entry-level administrators may function as assistants to middle-level managers. They may supervise a small number of operatives. For example, their main function may be to oversee and assist with operations critical to the efficient operation of a departmental unit.

Today's medical centers and integrated delivery organizations are among the most complex organizations to manage. Leaders in health care delivery face some unique challenges, including changes in financing and payment structures, as well as having to work with reduced levels of reimbursement. Other challenges include pressures to provide uncompensated care, greater responsibility for quality, accountability for community health, separate contingencies imposed by public and private payers, uncertainties created by new policy developments, changing configurations in the competitive environment, and maintaining the integrity of an organization through the highest level of ethical standards.

Health services administration is taught at the bachelor's and master's levels in a variety of settings, and the programs lead to several different degrees. The settings for such academic programs include schools of medicine, public health, public administration, business administration, and allied health sciences. Bachelor's degrees prepare

students for entry-level positions. Mid- and senior-level positions require a graduate degree. The most common degrees are the Master of Health Administration (MHA) or Master of Health Services Administration (MHSA), Master of Business Administration (MBA, with a health care management emphasis), Master of Public Health (MPH), or Master of Public Administration (or Affairs; MPA). The schools of public health that are accredited by the Council on Education for Public Health (CEPH) play a key role in training health services administrators in their MHA (or MHSA) and MPH programs (CEPH, 2017). Compared to the MPH programs, however, the MHA programs have more course requirements designed to furnish skills in business management (both theory and applied management) and quantitative/analytical areas, which are considered crucial for managing today's health services organizations. This disparity has been viewed as a concern that the schools of public health need to address (Singh et al., 1996).

Educational preparation of nursing home administrators is a notable exception to the MHA model. The training of nursing home administrators has largely been influenced by government licensing regulations. Even though licensure of nursing home administrators dates back to the mid-1960s, regulations favoring a formal postsecondary academic degree are more recent. Passing a national examination administered by the National Association of Boards of Examiners of Long-Term Care Administrators (NAB) is a standard requirement. However, educational qualifications needed to obtain a license vary significantly from one state to another. Although approximately one-third of the states still require less than a bachelor's degree as the minimum academic preparation, an increasing number of practicing nursing home administrators have at least a bachelor's degree. The problem is that most state regulations call for only general levels of education rather than specialized preparation in long-term care administration. General education does not furnish adequate skills in all the domains of practice relevant to nursing home management (Singh et al., 1997). However, various colleges and universities offer specialized programs in nursing home administration.

▶ Global Health Workforce Challenges

A 2006 report issued by the World Health Organization (WHO) identified 57 countries that were facing a health workforce crisis, meaning that each country had fewer than 23 health workers per 10,000 people. Most of these countries are poor, and they are predominately located in sub-Saharan Africa. The report also pointed out that a provider shortage of 4.3 million doctors, midwives, nurses, and support workers existed (WHO, 2006).

Another WHO (2005) publication emphasized that the shift from acute to chronic health problems is placing different demands on the health care workforce, as addressing chronic diseases requires different resources and skill sets. The increased prevalence of chronic conditions globally introduces the need for the workforce to adopt a patient-centered approach, improve communication skills, ensure safety and quality of patient care, monitor patients across time, use available technology, and consider care from a population perspective (WHO, 2005).

A WHO report released in 2014 noted that increasing demands are being put on the health care sector by its aging health workforce. Staff retiring or leaving for better-paying jobs are not being replaced, and not enough young people are entering the profession or being adequately trained to replace them. Moreover, internal and international migration of health workers is also exacerbating regional imbalances (WHO, 2014a).

In Europe, while the number of physicians per capita is increasing, it appears to be insufficient to accommodate the growing needs of an aging population (Lang, 2011). In addition, there have been far more specialists than generalists in recent years; shortages of nurses, physiotherapists, and occupational therapists are predicted to occur in the future (Lang, 2011).

The situation is similar in the United States, where the number of older adults is expected to double between 2005 and 2030 (Institute of Medicine, 2008). This trend will undoubtedly lead to an aging health workforce. On the patient side, the United States is hoping to add new people to the geriatric care-oriented workforce as well as retain the services of existing geriatric specialists (Institute of Medicine, 2008).

Growth in the number of non-MD providers may address these shortages to some extent (Riegel et al., 2012). Evidence supporting the involvement of non-MDs in the prevention and management of chronic health problems continues to grow. For example, integrating non-MDs into multidisciplinary health care teams has emerged as an effective strategy for improving the control of hypertension among high-risk populations (Brownstein et al., 2007; Fleming et al., 2015; Sookaneknun et al., 2004; Walsh et al., 2006). Non-MDs are effective in providing care for patients with chronic conditions, with their care resulting in improvements in patients' ability to keep appointments, better compliance with prescribed regimens, increased risk reduction, and greater engagement of patients in self-monitoring and adherence to medications (Roark et al., 2011).

A growing public health concern across the globe is the migration of health professionals from developing countries to the United States, United Kingdom, Canada, and Australia. For example, IMGs make up 25% of the U.S. physician population, which includes U.S. citizens who go to medical schools abroad (Educational Commission for Foreign Medical Graduates, 2015). To address this migration, WHO has developed the Global Code of Practice on the International Recruitment of Health Personnel, which sets principles and voluntary standards for countries to consider in workforce development and recruitment. This code includes the following components (WHO, 2014b):

- Greater commitment to assist countries facing critical health worker shortages with their efforts to improve and support their health workforce
- Joint investment in research and ISs to monitor the international migration of health workers and develop evidence-based policies
- Commitment of member states to meet their health personnel needs with their own human resources as far as possible, including taking measures to educate, retain, and sustain their health workforces
- Enshrinement of migrant workers' rights and ensuring they are equal to the rights of domestically trained health workers

The migration of health care workers is counterbalanced by another growing trend: medical tourism (see the *Evolution of Health Services in the United States* chapter). The medical tourism industry has undergone significant growth in recent decades, drawing patients from all over the world to medical facilities located in every global region. Medical tourism in the United States has grown steadily, with exports (i.e., travelers coming to the United States) having doubled, and imports (U.S. travelers going abroad) having increased almost nine-fold from a low base in the early 2000s (Chambers, 2015). Approximately 0.5% of all air travelers entering the United States annually—between 100,000 and 200,000 people—list health treatment as a reason for visiting (Chambers, 2015). Foreign patients most often cite access to advanced medical care as their reason for traveling to the United States for treatment. The three largest source markets for foreign travelers visiting the United States for health treatment in 2011 were the Caribbean, Europe, and Central America—accounting for 44%, 24%, and 10% of arrivals, respectively (U.S. Department of Commerce, 2011). U.S. outbound medical tourists are thought to make up approximately 10% of the worldwide total of medical tourists. Data from a U.S. Department of Commerce survey suggest that 150,000 to 320,000 U.S. travelers list health care as a reason for traveling abroad each year, or between 0.2% and 0.6% of all outbound U.S. air travelers (U.S. Department of Commerce, 2011). Americans cite cost savings as the most common reason to go abroad for health treatment.

The market for medical tourism appears poised for further growth, with potentially far-reaching economic impacts on both the source and destination countries. Opportunities for financial benefits from medical tourism include potentially exerting competitive pressure on systems importing health care, which may help drive down the costs of health care services offered in domestic systems. Moreover, medical tourism can be an important source of foreign exchanges, with income being generated both for the health sector in particular and through general increases in tourist income. Some health systems within source countries might even develop relations with off-shore medical tourism facilities in an effort to alleviate their own excessive waiting lists and to lower health care costs (OECD, 2011).

▶ Summary

Health services professionals in the United States constitute the largest labor force within the country. The development of these professionals is influenced by demographic trends, advances in research and technology, disease and illness trends, and the changing environment of health care financing and delivery.

Physicians play a leading role in the delivery of health services in the United States, though the country has a maldistribution of physicians both by specialty and by geography. The current shortages in the health care workforce, especially of PCPs, are likely to continue into the future, given the aging of the population, the growing burden of chronic diseases, and an increased number of insured patients. Various policies and programs have been used or proposed to address both physician imbalance and maldistribution, including regulation of health care professions, reimbursement initiatives targeting suitable incentives, targeted programs for underserved areas, changes in medical school curricula, changes in the financing of medical training, and a more rational referral system.

In addition to physicians, many other health services professionals contribute significantly to the delivery of health care, including nurses, dentists, pharmacists, optometrists, psychologists, podiatrists, chiropractors, midlevel providers, and other allied health professionals. These professionals, who require different levels of training, work in a variety of health care settings as complements to or substitutes for physicians.

Health services administrators face new challenges in the leadership of health care organizations. Meeting these challenges will require reforms in the educational programs designed to train adequate managers for the various sectors of the health care industry.

▶ Test Your Understanding

Terminology

advanced practice nurse (APN)
allied health
allied health professional
allopathic medicine

certified nurse-midwives (CNMs)
chiropractors
comorbidity
dental assistants
dental hygienists

dentists
doctoral nursing degrees
generalists
hospitalists
licensed practical nurses (LPNs)

maldistribution
nurse practitioners (NPs)
occupational therapists (OTs)
optometrists
osteopathic medicine

pharmaceutical care
pharmacists
physical therapists (PTs)
physician assistants (PAs)
podiatrists
primary care

psychologists
registered nurses (RNs)
residency
specialists
specialty care

Review Questions

1. Describe the major types of health services professionals (physicians, nurses, dentists, pharmacists, physician assistants, nurse practitioners, certified nurse-midwives), including their roles, training, practice requirements, and practice settings.

2. Which factors are associated with the development of health services professionals in the United States?

3. What are the major distinctions between primary care and specialty care?

4. Why is there a geographic maldistribution of the physician labor force in the United States?

5. Why is there an imbalance between primary care and specialty care in the United States?

6. Which measures have been or can be employed to overcome problems related to physician maldistribution and imbalance?

7. Who are midlevel providers? What are their roles in the delivery of health care?

8. In general, who are allied health professionals? What role do they play in the delivery of health services?

9. Provide a brief description of the roles and responsibilities of health services administrators.

▶ References

Agarwal, A., et al. 2009. Process and outcome measures among COPD patients with a hospitalization cared for by an advance practice provider or primary care physician. *PLoS One* 24, no. 11: e0148522.

American Academy of Physician Assistants. 1986. *PA fact sheet.* Arlington, VA: Author.

American Association of Colleges of Nursing (AACN). 2014. *Your guide to graduate nursing programs.* Available at: http://www.aacn.nche.edu /publications/brochures/GradStudentsBrochure .pdf. Accessed July 2016.

American Association of Colleges of Nursing (AACN). 2016. *2015–2016 enrollment and graduations in baccalaureate and graduate program in nursing.* Available at: http://www .aacn.nche.edu/leading-initiatives/research-data /employment16.pdf. Accessed February 2017.

American Association of Community Colleges. 2014. *Facts about allied health professionals.* Available at: http://www.aacc.nche.edu/Resources /aaccprograms/health/Documents/rn_lpn_facts .pdf. Accessed February 2017.

American College of Nurse-Midwives (ACNM). 2017. *Midwifery education programs.* Available at: http://www.midwife.org/Education-Programs -Directory. Accessed April 2017.

Accreditation Council for Occupational Therapy Education (ACOTE). 2017. *Occupational therapists accredited programs.* Available at: http://www .aota.org/Education-Careers/Find-School.aspx. Accessed April 2017.

American Council on Pharmaceutical Education (ACPE). 1992. *The proposed revision of accreditation standards and guidelines.* Chicago, IL: National Association of Boards on Pharmacy.

American Hospital Association. 2016. *2016 trend watch chartbook.* Available at: http://www.aha.org/research/reports/tw/chartbook/2016/table5-5.pdf. Accessed February 2017.

American Osteopathic Association. 2013. *Osteopathic medical profession report.* Available at: http://www.osteopathic.org/inside-aoa/about/aoa-annual-statistics/Documents/2013-OMP-report.pdf. Accessed February 2017.

Association of American Medical Colleges (AAMC). 2014. *Graduate medical education: Training tomorrow's physician workforce.* Available at: https://www.aamc.org/download/386374/data/07252014.pdf. Accessed February 2017.

Association of American Medical Colleges (AAMC). 2016. *The complexities of physician supply and demand: Projections from 2014 to 2025.* Available at: https://www.aamc.org/download/458082/data/2016_complexities_of_supply_and_demand_projections.pdf. Accessed February 2017.

Beazoglou, T. J., et al. 2012. Expanded function allied dental personnel and dental practice productivity and efficiency. *Journal of Dental Education* 76: 1054–1060.

Boulet, J. R., et al. 2006. The international medical graduate pipeline: Recent trends in certification and residency training. *Health Affairs* 25, no. 6: 469–477.

Brownstein, J. N., et al. 2007. Effectiveness of community health workers in the care of people with hypertension. *American Journal of Preventive Medicine* 32: 435–447.

Bylsma, W. H., et al. 2010. Where have all the general internists gone? *Journal of General Internal Medicine* 25, no. 10: 1020–1023.

Carter, S. R., et al. 2012. Patients' willingness to use a pharmacist-provided medication management service: The influence of outcome expectancies and communication efficacy. *Research in Social and Administrative Pharmacy* 8, no. 6: 487–498.

Chambers, A. 2015. *Trends in U.S. health travel services trade.* USITC Executive Briefing on Trade. Available at: https://www.usitc.gov/publications/332/executive_briefings/chambers_health-related_travel_final.pdf. Accessed February 2017.

Chen, L. M., et al. 2013. Hospitalist staffing and patient satisfaction in the national Medicare population. *Journal of Hospital Medicine* 8, no. 3: 126–131.

Coffman, J., and T. G. Rundall. 2005. The impact of hospitalists on the cost and quality of inpatient care in the United States: A research synthesis. *Medical Care Research and Review* 62, no. 4: 379–406.

Coleman, K., et al. 2009. Evidence on the chronic care model in the new millennium. *Health Affairs 28*, no. 1: 75–85.

Commission on Accreditation in Physical Therapy Education. 2017. Physical therapist programs. Available at: http://www.capteonline.org/Programs/Developing/PT/. Accessed April 2017.

Congressional Research Service. 2017. *Discretionary spending under the Affordable Care Act (ACA).* Available at: https://fas.org/sgp/crs/misc/R41390.pdf. Accessed February 2017.

Cooper, R. A., et al. 1998. Current and projected workforce of nonphysician clinicians. *Journal of the American Medical Association* 280, no. 9: 788–794.

Council on Education for Public Health (CEPH). 2017. *ASPH graduate training programs.* Available at: http://ceph.org/accredited/. Accessed January 2017.

Division of Labor Force Statistics, U.S. Bureau of Labor Statistics. 2017. *Labor force statistics from the current population survey.* Available at: https://www.bls.gov/cps/cpsaat18.htm. Accessed April 2017.

Educational Commission for Foreign Medical Graduates. 2015. IMG performance in the 2015 match. Available at: http://www.ecfmg.org/news/2015/03/27/img-performance-in-the-2015-match/. Accessed February 2017.

Endicott, K. M. 1976. Health and health manpower. In: *Health in America: 1776–1976.* Health Resources Administration, U.S. Public Health Service. DHEW Pub. No. 76616. Washington, DC: U.S. Department of Health, Education, and Welfare: pp. 138–165.

Ericksen, K. 2016. *Nursing credentials 101: From LPN & LVN to BSN & DNP.* Available at: http://www.rasmussen.edu/degrees/nursing/blog/nursing-credentials-101-from-lpn-lvn-bsn-dnp/. Accessed July 31, 2016.

Evangelista, J. A., et al. 2012. Pediatric nurse practitioner managed cardiology clinics: Patient satisfaction and appointment access. *Journal of Advanced Nursing* 68, no.10: 2165-2174.

Fitzgerald, M. A., et al. 1995. The midlevel provider: Colleague or competitor? *Patient Care* 29, no. 1: 20.

Fleming, S., et al. 2015. Self-screening and non-physician screening for hypertension in communities: A systematic review. *American Journal of Hypertension* 28, no. 11: 1316–1324.

Freed, D. H. 2004. Hospitalists: Evolution, evidence, and eventualities. *Health Care Manager* 23, no. 3: 238–256.

Garber, A. M. 2005. Evidence-based guidelines as a foundation for performance incentives. *Health Affairs* 24, no. 1: 174–179.

Ginzberg, E. 1994. Improving health care for the poor. *Journal of the American Medical Association* 271, no. 6: 464–467.

Golden, J. R. 2014. A nurse practitioner patient care team: Implications for pediatric oncology. *Journal of Pediatric Oncology Nursing* 31, no. 6: 350–356.

Goodwin, J. S., et al. 2013. Variation in length of stay and outcomes among hospitalized patients attributable to hospitals and hospitalists. *Journal of General Internal Medicine* 28, no. 3: 370–376.

Greenfield, S., et al. 1992. Variation in resource utilization among medical specialties and systems of care. *Journal of the American Medical Association* 267, no. 12: 1624–1630.

Grossman, D. 1995. APNs: Pioneers in patient care. *American Journal of Nursing* 95, no. 8: 54–56.

Health Resources and Services Administration (HRSA). 2017. *Designated Health Professional Shortage Areas statistics.* Available at: https://ersrs.hrsa.gov/ReportServer?/HGDW_Reports/BCD_HPSA/BCD_HPSA_SCR50_Qtr_Smry_HTML&rc:Toolbar=false. Accessed April 2017.

Helper, C., and L. Strand. 1990. Opportunities and responsibilities in pharmaceutical care. *American Journal of Hospital Pharmacy* 47, no. 3: 533–543.

Hooker, R. S., and L. E. Berlin. 2002. Trends in the supply of physician assistants and nurse practitioners in the United States. *Health Affairs* 21, no. 5: 174–181.

Hooker, R. S., and L. F. McCaig. 2001. Use of physician assistants and nurse practitioners in primary care, 1995–1999. *Health Affairs* 20, no. 4: 231–238.

Institute of Medicine. 2008. *Retooling for an aging America: Building the health care workforce.* Available at: http://www.nationalacademies.org/hmd/reports/2008/retooling-for-an-aging-america-building-the-health-care-workforce.aspx. Accessed April 2017.

Jacobson, P. D., and S. A. Jazowski. 2011. Physicians, the Affordable Care Act, and primary care: Disruptive change or business as usual? *Journal of General Internal Medicine* 26, no. 8: 934–937.

Juraschek, S. P., et al. 2012. United States registered nurse workforce report card and shortage forecast. *American Journal of Medical Quality* 27, no. 3: 241–249.

Kaiser Family Foundation. 2016. *Total professionally active physicians.* Available at: http://kff.org/other/state-indicator/total-active-physicians. Accessed February 2017.

Kozakowski, S. M., et al. 2016. Entry of US medical school graduates into family medicine residencies: 2015-2016. *Family Medicine* 48, no. 9: 688–695.

Kuo, Y. F., et al. 2015. Potentially preventable hospitalizations in Medicare patients with diabetes: A comparison of primary care provided by nurse practitioners versus physicians. *Medical Care* 53, no. 9: 776–783.

Lang, R. 2011. *Future challenges to the provision of health care in the 21st century. University College London.* Available at: http://www.ucl.ac.uk/lc-ccr/downloads/presentations/R_LANG_COHEHRE_LISBON_PRESENTATION.pdf. Accessed December 2013.

Laurant, M., et al. 2009. The impact of nonphysician clinicians: Do they improve the quality and cost-effectiveness of health care services? *Medical Care Research and Review* 66: 36S–89S.

Lee, D. C., et al. 2016. Insurance-related disparities in primary care quality among U.S. type 2 diabetes patients. *International Journal for Equity in Health* 15, no. 1: 124.

Morley, P., and L. Strand. 1989. Critical reflections of therapeutic drug monitoring. *Journal of Clinical Pharmacy* 2, no. 3: 327–334.

National Center for Health Statistics. 1996. *Health, United States, 1995.* Hyattsville, MD: U.S. Department of Health and Human Services.

National Center for Health Statistics. 2002. *Health, United States, 2002.* Hyattsville, MD: U.S. Department of Health and Human Services.

National Center for Health Statistics. 2006. *Health, United States, 2006.* Hyattsville, MD: U.S. Department of Health and Human Services.

National Center for Health Statistics. 2012. *Health, United States, 2011.* Hyattsville, MD: U.S. Department of Health and Human Services.

National Center for Health Statistics. 2014. *State variability in supply of office-based primary care providers: United States, 2012.* Available at: https://www.cdc.gov/nchs/products/databriefs/db151.htm. Accessed February 2017.

National Center for Health Statistics. 2016. *Health, United States, 2015.* Hyattsville, MD: U.S. Department of Health and Human Services.

Organization for Economic Cooperation and Development (OECD). 2011. *Medical tourism: Treatments, markets and health system implications: A scoping review.* Available at: https://www.oecd.org/els/health-systems/48723982.pdf. Accessed April 2017.

Organization for Economic Cooperation and Development (OECD). 2016. *Health at a glance 2015 database.* Available at: http://stats.oecd.org/index.aspx?DataSetCode=HEALTH_STAT. Accessed February 2017.

Petterson, S. M., et al. 2012. Projecting US primary care physician workforce needs: 2010–2025. *Annals of Family Medicine* 10, no. 6: 503–509.

Post, J. J., and J. L. Stoltenberg. 2014. Use of restorative procedures by allied dental health professionals in Minnesota. *Journal of the American Dental Association* 145, no. 10: 1044–1050.

Rafferty, A., et al. 2016. Pharmacist-provided medication management in interdisciplinary transitions in a community hospital (PMIT). *Annals of Pharmacotherapy* 50, no. 8: 649–655.

Redhead, C. S., and E. D. Williams. 2010. *Public health, workforce, quality, and related provisions in PPACA: Summary and timeline.* Washington, DC: Congressional Research Service.

Rich, E. C., et al. 1994. Preparing generalist physicians: The organizational and policy context. *Journal of General Internal Medicine* 9 (suppl 1): S115–S122.

Riegel, B., et al. 2012. Meeting global needs in primary care with nurse practitioners. *Lancet* 380, no. 9840: 449–450.

Roark, R. F., et al. 2011. The need for transformative innovation in hypertension management. *American Heart Journal* 162, no. 3: 405–411.

Rosenblatt, R. A. 1992. Specialists or generalists: On whom should we base the American health care system? *Journal of the American Medical Association* 267, no. 12: 1665–1666.

Rosenblatt, R. A., et al. 1997. Interspecialty differences in the obstetric care of low-risk women. *American Journal of Public Health* 87: 344–351.

Rosenblatt, R. A., and D. M. Lishner. 1991. Surplus or shortage? Unraveling the physician supply conundrum. *Western Journal of Medicine* 154, no. 1: 43–50.

Samuels, M. E., and L. Shi. 1993. *Physician recruitment and retention: A guide for rural medical group practice.* Englewood, CO: Medical Group Management Press.

Schneller, E. S. 2006. The hospitalist movement in the United States: Agency and common agency issues. *Health Care Management Review* 31, no. 4: 308–316.

Schroeder, S., and L. G. Sandy. 1993. Specialty distribution of U.S. physicians: The invisible driver of health care costs. *New England Journal of Medicine* 328, no. 13: 961–963.

Schwartz, M. 1994. Creating pharmacy's future. *American Pharmacy* NS34: 44–45, 59.

Schwartz, M. D. 2011. Health care reform and the primary care workforce bottleneck. *Journal of General Internal Medicine* 27, no. 4: 469–472.

Sehgal, N. J., and R. M. Wachter. 2006. The expanding role of hospitalists in the United States. *Swiss Medical Weekly* 136: 591–596.

Shi, L. 1992. The relation between primary care and life chances. *Journal of Health Care for the Poor and Underserved* 3, no. 2: 321–335.

Shi, L. 1994. Primary care, specialty care, and life chances. *International Journal of Health Services* 24, no. 3: 431–458.

Shi, L., et al. 2013. Reducing disparities in access to primary care and patient satisfaction with care: The role of health centers. *Journal of Health Care for the Poor and Underserved* 24, no. 1: 56–66.

Singh, D. A., et al. 1996. A comparison of academic curricula in the MPH and the MHA-type degrees in health administration at the accredited schools of public health. *Journal of Health Administration Education* 14, no. 4: 401–414.

Singh, D. A., et al. 1997. How well trained are nursing home administrators? *Hospital and Health Services Administration* 42, no. 1: 101–115.

Sookaneknun, P., et al. 2004. Pharmacist involvement in primary care improves hypertensive patient clinical outcomes. *Annals of Pharmacotherapy* 38: 2023–2028.

Stanfield, P. S., et al. 2012. *Introduction to the health professions.* 6th ed. Burlington, MA: Jones & Bartlett Learning.

Starfield, B. 1992. *Primary care: Concepts, evaluation, and policy.* New York, NY: Oxford University Press.

Starfield, B. 2011. Point: The changing nature of disease implications for health services. *Medical Care* 49, no. 11: 971–972.

Starfield, B., and L. Simpson. 1993. Primary care as part of US health services reform. *Journal of the American Medical Association* 269, no. 24: 3136–3139.

Starr, P. 1982. *The social transformation of American medicine: The rise of a sovereign profession and the making of a vast industry.* New York, NY: Basic Books.

Strand, L. R., et al. 1991. Levels of pharmaceutical care: A needs-based approach. *American Journal of Hospital Pharmacy* 48, no. 3: 547–550.

The Accreditation Review Commission on Education for the Physician Assistant. 2017. *Accredited programs.* Available at: http://www.arc-pa.org/accreditation/accredited-programs/. Accessed April 2017.

U.S. Bureau of Labor Statistics. 2015a. *Employment projections: 2014–24 summary.* Available at: https://www.bls.gov/news.release/ecopro.nr0.htm. Accessed February 2017.

U.S. Bureau of Labor Statistics. 2015b. *Hospitalist: Career outlook.* Available at: https://www.bls.gov/careeroutlook/2015/youre-a-what/hospitalist.htm. Accessed February 2017.

U.S. Bureau of Labor Statistics. 2015c. *Occupational employment and wages—May 2015.* Available at: https://www.bls.gov/ooh/healthcare. Accessed February 2017.

U.S. Bureau of Labor Statistics. 2017. *Occupational employment and wages—May 2016.* Available at: https://www.bls.gov/oes/current/oes_stru.htm. Accessed April 2017.

U.S. Census Bureau. 2012. *Statistical abstract of the United States, 2011.* Washington, DC: Author.

U.S. Department of Commerce, Office of Travel and Tourism Industries. 2011. *Survey of International Air Travelers Program.* Available at: http://travel.trade.gov/research/programs/ifs/index.html. Accessed February 2017.

U.S. Department of Health and Human Services (DHHS). 2013a. *HHS awards $12 million to help teaching health centers train primary care providers.* Available at: http://www.businesswire.com/news/home/20130719005676/en/HHS-awards-12-million-Teaching-Health-Centers. Accessed April 2017.

U.S. Department of Health and Human Services (DHHS). 2013b. *Shortage designation: Health professional shortage areas & medically underserved areas/populations.* Available at: http://www.hrsa.gov/shortage/. Accessed August 2013.

Wachter, R. M. 2004. Hospitalists in the United States: Mission accomplished or work in progress? *New England Journal of Medicine* 350, no. 19: 1935–1936.

Wagner, M. 1991. Maternal and child health services in the United States. *Journal of Public Health Policy* 12, no. 4: 443–449.

Walsh, E., et al. 2006. Quality improvement strategies for hypertension management: A systematic review. *Medical Care* 44: 646–657.

Wennberg, J. E., et al. 1993. Finding equilibrium in U.S. physician supply. *Health Affairs* 12, no. 2: 89–103.

West, C. P., and D. M. Dupras. 2012. General medicine vs subspecialty career plans among internal medicine residents. *Journal of the American Medical Association* 308, no. 21: 2241–2247.

White, H. L., and R. H. Glazier. 2011. Do hospitalist physicians improve the quality of inpatient care delivery? A systematic review of process, efficiency and outcome measures. *BMC Medicine* 9: 58.

White House. 2012. *Fact sheet: Creating health care jobs by addressing primary care workforce needs.* Available at: http://www.whitehouse.gov/the-press-office/2012/04/11/fact-sheet-creating-health-care-jobs-addressing-primary-care-workforce-n. Accessed December 2013.

World Bank. 2014. *Health expenditure, total (% of GDP).* Available at: http://data.worldbank.org/indicator/SH.XPD.TOTL.ZS. Accessed February 2017.

World Health Organization (WHO). 2005. *Preparing a health care workforce for the 21st century: The challenge of chronic conditions.* Available at: http://www.who.int/chp/knowledge/publications/workforce_report.pdf. Accessed December 2013.

World Health Organization (WHO). 2006. *The world health report 2006: Working together for health.* Available at: http://www.who.int/whr/2006/en/index.html. Accessed December 2013.

World Health Organization (WHO). 2014a. *A universal truth: No health without a workforce.* Available at: http://www.who.int/workforcealliance/knowledge/resources/GHWA-a_universal_truth_report.pdf?ua=1. Accessed February 2017.

World Health Organization (WHO). 2014b. *Migration of health workers.* Available at: http://www.who.int/hrh/migration/14075_MigrationofHealth_Workers.pdf. Accessed April 2014.

APPENDIX 4-A

List of Professional Associations

Academy of Nutrition and Dietetics

Accreditation Council for Pharmacy Education

American Academy of Nurse Practitioners

American Academy of Physician Assistants

American Art Therapy Association, Inc.

American Association for Rehabilitation Therapy

American Association for Respiratory Care

American Association of Colleges of Nursing

American Association of Colleges of Osteopathic Medicine

American Association of Colleges of Pharmacy

American Association of Medical Assistants

American Chiropractic Association

American College of Emergency Physicians

American College of Health Care Administrators

American College of Healthcare Executives

American College of Nurse-Midwives

American Dance Therapy Association

American Dental Assistants Association

American Dental Association

American Dental Education Association

American Dental Hygienists' Association

American Health Care Association

American Horticultural Therapy Association

American Hospital Association

American Kinesiotherapy Association

American Medical Association

American Medical Technologists

American Music Therapy Association

American Nurses Association

American Occupational Therapy Association

American Optometric Association

American Organization of Nurse Executives

American Osteopathic Association

American Pharmacists Association

American Physical Therapy Association

American Psychiatric Association

American Psychological Association

American Public Health Association

American Registry of Radiologic Technologists

American School Health Association

American Society of Clinical Pathology

American Society of Health-System Pharmacists

American Society of Radiologic Technologists

American Speech–Language–Hearing Association

American Therapeutic Recreation Association

ASCP Board of Certification

Association of American Medical Colleges

Association of Schools and Colleges of Optometry

Association of Schools and Programs of Public Health

Association of Surgical Technologists

Association of University Programs in Health Administration

Council on Podiatric Medical Education

Council on Social Work Education

Dental Assisting National Board, Inc.

Environmental Management Association

Healthcare Financial Management Association

Institute for Credentialing Excellence

International Society for Clinical Laboratory Technology

LeadingAge

National Academy of Opticianry

National Association for Practical Nurse Education and Service, Inc.

National Association of Boards of Pharmacy

National Association of Chain Drug Stores

National Association of Emergency Medical Technicians

National Association of Social Workers

National Board for Respiratory Care

National Board of Podiatric Medical Examiners

National Council for Therapeutic Recreation Certification

National Environmental Health Association

National League for Nursing

National Nurse-Led Care Consortium

National Registry of Emergency Medical Technicians

National Therapeutic Recreation Society

Opticians Association of America

Physician Assistant Education Association

Society of Nuclear Medicine and Molecular Imaging

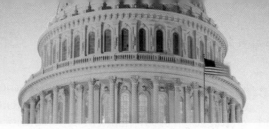

CHAPTER 5

Medical Technology

LEARNING OBJECTIVES

- Understand the meaning and role of medical technology in health care delivery.
- Appreciate the growing applications of information technology and informatics in the delivery of health care.
- Explore the different aspects of telemedicine and telehealth.
- Survey the factors that drive the innovation, dissemination, and utilization of technology.
- Discuss the government's role in technology diffusion.
- Examine the impact of technology on various aspects of domestic and global delivery of health care.
- Study the various facets of health technology assessment, and its current and future directions.
- Summarize the status of medical technology under health care reform.

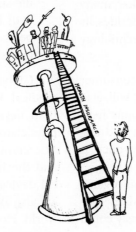

"This must be high technology."

▶ Introduction

Drake and colleagues (1993) labeled technology as "the boon and bane of medicine." In one respect, medical technology has been a great blessing to modern civilization. Sophisticated diagnostic procedures have reduced complications and disability, new medical cures have increased longevity, and new drugs have helped stabilize chronic conditions. However, most new technology comes at a price that society must ultimately pay. A tremendous amount of costly research is necessary to produce most modern breakthroughs. Once technology is developed and put into use, even more costs are generated. Yet, issues surrounding the unrestrained development and use of new technology have received little attention from policymakers.

Historically, developments in science and technology were instrumental in transforming the nature of health care delivery during the postindustrial era in the United States. Since then, the ever-increasing proliferation of new technology has continued to profoundly alter many facets of health care delivery. Besides its role in medical cost inflation, technology has triggered other changes:

- Technology has raised consumer expectations that the latest will also be the best. These expectations have led to increased demand for and utilization of new technology once it becomes available.
- Technology has changed the organization of medical services. Many specialized services that previously could be offered only in hospitals are now available in outpatient settings and patients' homes.

- Technology has driven the scope and content of medical training and the practice of medicine, fueling specialization in medicine.
- Technology has influenced the way status is imputed to various medical workers. Specialization is held in higher regard than primary care and public health.
- Technology assessment is becoming a growing activity because new drugs, devices, and procedures are not always effective or safe. Their effectiveness and potential negative consequences must be evaluated using scientific methods.
- Technology has raised complex social and ethical concerns that defy straightforward answers. Perplexing social and ethical controversies pertaining to modern innovations include the following questions, among others: Who should be subjected to the experimental evaluations of technological breakthroughs to assess their safety and effectiveness? Who should and who should not receive high-tech interventions? To what extent should life-supporting procedures be continued? How can safety and effectiveness be assured for experimental technologies, such as nanomedicine?

Globalization has also enveloped biomedical knowledge and technology. In both developed and developing nations, physicians have access to the same scientific knowledge through medical journals and the Internet. Most drugs and medical devices available in the United States are also available in almost all parts of the world. However, depending on the extent of supply-side rationing, the adoption of new technology often differs widely from one country to another. Thus, even in developed nations, people do not always have adequate access to the latest high-tech therapies. Conversely, in almost all parts of the world, people who possess adequate means can gain access to the latest and best in medicine regardless of the type of health care delivery system in their country.

This chapter discusses medical technology from multiple perspectives. Where appropriate, highlights from other countries are incorporated for comparative purposes.

▶ What Is Medical Technology?

At a fundamental level, **medical technology** is the practical application of the scientific body of knowledge for the purpose of improving health and creating efficiencies in the delivery of health care. Medical science has greatly benefited from rapid developments in other applied sciences, such as chemistry, physics, engineering, and pharmacology. For example, common applications of physics are found in x-ray technology, mammography, ultrasound, use of lasers, and magnetic resonance imaging (MRI). Chemistry has played a critical role in the development of drugs. Computer science and communication technologies have enabled the application of information technology in medicine and telemedicine. Bioengineering is employed in developing robotic systems used in surgery and advanced prostheses.

Nanomedicine is an emerging area, still in its infancy, that involves the application of nanotechnology for medical use. Nanotechnology is not confined to a single field, but rather requires an intense collaboration between disciplines to manipulate materials on the atomic and molecular level—one nanometer is one-billionth of a meter (Taub, 2011). Nano-medicine has potential applications in both diagnostics and therapeutics. For example, a screening test has been developed to identify lung cancer in its very early stages (Taub, 2011). Nanoparticles are being developed as effective carriers of drugs to target regions of the body that have been difficult to reach using traditional drug formulations (Thorley and Tetley, 2013).

Medical technology crosses many facets of health care delivery. **TABLE 5-1** gives examples of some of the main applications of medical technology.

▶ Information Technology and Informatics

Information technology (IT) deals with the transformation of data into useful information. IT involves determining data needs, gathering appropriate data, storing and analyzing the data, and reporting the information in a format desired by its end users. Different types of information are made available for specific uses to health care professionals, managers, payers, patients, researchers, and the government.

IT departments in health care organizations play a critical role in decisions to adopt new information technologies to improve health care delivery, increase organizational efficiency, and comply with various laws and regulations. Health care IT includes medical records systems to collect, transcribe, and store clinical data; radiology and clinical laboratory reporting systems; pharmacy data systems to monitor medication use and avoid

TABLE 5-1 Examples of Medical Technologies

Type	Examples
Diagnostic	Computed tomography (CT) scan Fetal monitor Computerized electrocardiography Automated clinical laboratories Magnetic resonance imaging Blood pressure monitor
Survival (life saving)	Intensive care unit (ICU) Cardiopulmonary resuscitation (CPR) Bone marrow transplant Liver transplant Autologous bone marrow transplant
Illness management	Renal dialysis Pacemaker Percutaneous transluminal coronary angioplasty (PTCA) Stereotactic cingulotomy (psychosurgery)
Cure	Hip joint replacement Organ transplant Lithotripter
Prevention	Implantable automatic cardioverter-defibrillator Pediatric orthopedic repair Diet control for phenylketonuria Vaccines for immunization
Monitoring (body functions, vital signs)	Wearable biosensors
Prosthetics	Electromechanical limbs Artificial heart valves Artificial kidneys Dental implants
Enabling (to assist or extend physical capabilities of medical professionals)	Robotic surgery Cyberknife surgery[1] Nanoknife procedure[2] Laser therapy
Adjunctive therapies	Certain complementary treatments
System management	Health information systems Telemedicine

Facilities and clinical settings	Hospital satellite centers Clinical laboratories Subacute care units Modern home health
Organizational delivery structure	Managed care Integrated delivery networks

[1] A procedure in which high doses of radiation are used with pinpoint accuracy to destroy tumors.

[2] A minimally invasive procedure that uses electric currents to destroy tumors.

Modified from Rosenthal, G. 1979. Anticipating the costs and benefits of new technology: A typology for policy. In: *Medical technology: The culprit behind health care costs?* S. Altman and R. Blendon, eds. Washington, DC: U.S. Government Printing Office. pp. 77–87.

errors, adverse reactions, and drug interactions; scheduling systems for patients, space (such as surgery suites), and personnel; and financial systems for billing and collections, materials management, and many other aspects of organizational management (Cohen, 2004a).

In health care organizations, IT applications fall into three general categories (Austin, 1992):

1. **Clinical information systems** involve the organized processing, storage, and retrieval of information to support patient care delivery. Electronic medical records, for example, provide quick and reliable information necessary to guide clinical decision making and produce timely reports on quality of care delivered. Computerized provider order entry (CPOE) enables clinicians to electronically transmit orders to a recipient—for example, from a physician's office to a pharmacy. The vast majority of hospitals and most outpatient practices now use some form of CPOE (Agency for Healthcare Research and Quality [AHRQ], 2016) with the intent of increasing efficiency and reducing medical errors.

2. **Administrative information systems** assist health care staff in carrying out financial and administrative support activities, such as payroll, patient accounting, billing, materials management, budgeting and cost control, and office automation. In medical clinics, CPOE technology may be set up to interface with the billing system to minimize rejected claims by pinpointing errors in billing codes.

3. **Decision support systems** provide information and analytical tools to support managerial and clinical decision making. *Managerial* decision support systems can be used to forecast patient volume, project staffing requirements, and schedule patients to optimize utilization of patient care and surgical facilities. *Clinical* decision support systems (CDSSs) are designed to improve clinical decision

making. A patient's unique clinical data are matched to a computerized knowledge base, and software algorithms generate patient-specific treatment protocols and recommendations (Haynes and Wilczynski, 2010). CDSSs are meant to help clinicians make better decisions, but not all CDSSs improve the way health care is delivered. One recent study showed that only 58% of CDSSs led to improved care and better patient outcomes (Medlock et al., 2016). Hence, CDSS use is not without challenges that need to be overcome.

Health informatics is broadly defined as the application of information science to improve the efficiency, accuracy, and reliability of health care services. Health informatics requires the use of IT but goes beyond IT by emphasizing the improvement of health care delivery. For example, designing and evaluating the effectiveness of CDSSs are tasks that fall within the domain of health informatics. Applications of informatics are also found in electronic health records and telemedicine.

Electronic Health Records and Systems

Electronic health records (EHRs) are IT applications that enable the processing of any electronically stored information pertaining to individual patients for the purpose of delivering health care services (Murphy et al., 1999). EHRs replace the traditional paper medical records, which document a patient's demographic information, problems and diagnoses, plan of care, progress notes, medications, vital signs, and past medical history, among other items. An EHR system with basic features should incorporate the ability to update patient demographics, view test results, maintain problem lists, compile clinical notes, and manage prescription ordering (Decker et al., 2012).

According to the Institute of Medicine (2003), a fully developed EHR system includes four key components:

- Collection and storage of health information on individual patients over time
- Immediate electronic access to person- and population-level information by authorized users
- Availability of knowledge and decision support that enhances the quality, safety, and efficiency of patient care
- Support of efficient processes for health care delivery

Benefits and Drawbacks of EHRs

It is generally believed that widespread adoption of EHR systems will lead to major savings in health care costs, reduced medical errors, and improved health (Hillestad et al., 2005). Research shows that EHR systems, when properly implemented, can improve quality of health care, promote time efficiencies, support adherence to clinical practice guidelines, and reduce the risk of medication errors and adverse drug effects (Campanella et al., 2015). EHRs have also facilitated access to, retrievability of, and portability of patient data.

Conversely, it has been argued that EHRs have changed the emphasis from patient-centeredness to institutional priorities, serving institutional interests (rather than patient interests) through the documentation process—for example, reimbursement, risk management, quality and work efficiency, and regulatory compliance. Consequently, adoption of EHRs has also increased the time and effort required in documentation (de Ruiter et al., 2016).

EHRs and Quality of Care

Yanamadala and colleagues (2016) found no relationship between EHRs and quality of care as measured by mortality, readmission rates, and clinical complications. These researchers concluded: "To date, we have not yet seen the promised benefits of EHR systems on patient outcomes" in the hospital setting.

In contrast, in a study of at-risk hospital patients, Furukawa and colleagues (2016) found that the occurrence rate of adverse events was less likely among patients with cardiovascular disease, with pneumonia, or undergoing surgery in hospitals with fully electronic EHRs. Clearly, quality of care is multidimensional, and different proxies used for quality are likely to produce different results.

Adler-Milstein and colleagues (2015) also posit that experience with the use of EHRs over time (time-related effects) might show improvement in outcomes in more recent years compared to earlier years. These researchers found a positive association between EHR adoption and performance on process adherence and patient satisfaction, but not on efficiency. Ambulatory care settings that have adopted EHRs might find lowered hospital admission rates but not readmission rates for people with chronic health problems (Lammers et al., 2016).

In conclusion, to date the potential benefits of EHRs have not been fully realized. Future research should shed more light on the magnitude and nature of these benefits.

Interoperability

Interoperability makes it possible to access individual records online from many separate, automated systems within an electronic network, eliminating the need for older methods, such as letters and faxes, for sharing a patient's clinical information among providers. Physicians, for example, need timely information on test results. As a patient transitions from one clinical setting to another, coordination of the patient's care becomes essential.

Health Information Organizations

A **health information organization (HIO)** is an independent organization that brings together health care stakeholders within a defined geographic area and facilitates electronic information exchange among these stakeholders with the objective of improving the delivery of health care in the community. Such stakeholders often include not only health care providers, but also payers, laboratories, and sometimes public health departments. The HIO is managed by a board of directors consisting of representatives from the various stakeholder organizations. Apart from managing the actual exchange of information, HIOs assist providers in setting up protocols for information exchange and in building consensus on which types of information should be exchanged.

In the United States, local or regional systems for the exchange of health information across provider organizations have received support, rather than national systems. HIOs are still at an early stage in their evolution, although there is widespread interest in their development. In 2012, 29% of U.S. hospitals participated in an HIO (Furukawa et al., 2013).

Adoption of EHRs

Both physician clinics and hospitals have been slow to adopt EHRs, mainly because of a lack of capital and the uncertain return on their investment (DesRoches et al., 2008). To promote EHR adoption, the federal government has created financial incentives for various types of providers (discussed in the next subsection). Although EHR adoption increased significantly once these incentives were made available, not all health care organizations have chosen to implement EHRs. On the one hand, the main barriers to EHR adoption are cost (both initial and ongoing costs), technical concerns, technical support, and resistance to change (Kruse et al., 2016a). On the other hand, the main factors that facilitate the adoption of EHRs include efficiency, hospital size, quality, access to data, perceived value, and ability to transfer information (Kruse et al., 2016b).

Purchase and implementation of EHRs in large institutions can take as long as 2 years to complete. Also, implementation is not a one-time event, but rather an ongoing process of testing and modifying the system to make it more effective (Silow-Carroll et al., 2012).

Financial Incentives Under the HITECH Act

To accelerate the adoption of EHRs, some major policy initiatives were launched during the George W. Bush administration. These initiatives culminated in the enactment of the Health Information Technology for Economic and Clinical Health (HITECH) Act, which became part of the American Recovery and Reinvestment Act (ARRA) of 2009—the $787 billion plan to stimulate the economy—passed shortly after the Barack Obama administration took office. The HITECH Act earmarked an estimated $19 billion in direct grants and financial incentives to promote the adoption of EHRs by hospitals and physicians (Wang et al., 2013).

Beginning in 2011, Medicare and Medicaid started offering financial incentives of up to $44,000 for Medicare providers and $63,750 for Medicaid providers for "meaningful use" of health information technology (Centers for Disease Control and Prevention [CDC], 2012). To demonstrate "meaningful use," health care providers have to meet a range of metrics in areas such as quality, safety, efficiency, reduction of health disparities, patient engagement, care coordination, and security of health information (Halamka, 2010). Meaningful use criteria have been phased in over three stages between 2011 and 2015. Starting in 2015, hospitals that fail to meet the meaningful use criteria are subject to financial penalties (DesRoches et al., 2013).

HITECH financial incentives may have had an impact on EHR adoption among small physician-owned practices (Cohen, 2016), but the evidence is weak that the HITECH Act has been instrumental in prompting physicians to adopt EHRs (Mennemeyer et al., 2016). Nevertheless, at least the cost-savings objective of the HITECH Act may have been achieved. Lammers and McLaughlin (2016) have reported overall lower Medicare expenditures for both inpatient and outpatient health care utilization when EHRs are in place.

Confidentiality Under the HIPAA Law

To alleviate concerns by patients and providers about the confidentiality of patient information, the Health Insurance Portability and Accountability Act (HIPAA) of 1996 makes it illegal to gain access to a patient's personal health information (PHI) for reasons other than health care delivery, operations, and reimbursement. The HIPAA legislation mandated strict controls on the transfer of personally identifiable health data between two entities, provisions for disclosure of protected information, and penalties for violation (Clayton, 2001). In January 2013, the U.S. Department of Health and Human Services (DHHS) issued revisions to HIPAA in conjunction with the HITECH Act. More stringent rules now apply to disclosure of breaches of confidential PHI, inclusion of vendors and subcontractors as "business associates" who must comply with HIPAA requirements, restrictions on the use of PHI for marketing purposes, patient authorization related to the use of PHI for research purposes, use of genetic information for underwriting purposes by health insurance companies, and patients' right to receive electronic copies of their PHI (Thompson Coburn LLP, 2013).

Smart Card Technology

Pocket-size smart cards that are embedded with a microchip have found applications in other industries for access control, but adoption of their use in health care delivery has been slow. A **smart card** that is designed for medical use holds personal medical information that can be accessed and updated at hospitals or physicians' offices (Ellis, 2000). The public so far has viewed smart cards with suspicion and distrust. Australians, for example, suspect that smart cards pose problems with information security, personal privacy, and the specter of a national identification card (Martin and Rice, 2010). Americans have similar concerns (Horowitz, 2012).

▶ The Internet, E-Health, M-Health, and E-Therapy

With the growth of the Internet and the proliferation of mobile devices that offer online access, many patients are taking charge of their own health. A number of websites offer physician consultations, and others sell prescription medications. Patients are also forming online support communities to help themselves through discussion groups and bulletin boards. Consequently, patients are becoming active participants in their own health care. Information empowers patients, which leads to changes in the traditional patient–physician dynamics. Even though the vast majority of patients rely on and trust their physicians or other health care professionals for information, care, or support (Fox and Duggan, 2013), the Internet is often the first source of information that patients consult for specific health conditions (Marrie et al., 2013). Indeed, as many as 70% of American adults use the Internet as their first source for health information (Prestin et al., 2015).

Patients who perceive their doctors as less patient centered are more likely to go online for information (Li et al., 2014). Conversely, patients who are satisfied with the care they receive from their physicians tend to rely more on their physician than on the Internet, using the physician as the primary source of health information (Tustin, 2010).

The terms *e-health*, *m-health*, and *e-therapy* are related, and sometimes used interchangeably. There are, however, slight differences between them.

E-Health

"**E-health** refers to all forms of electronic health care delivered over the Internet, ranging from informational, educational, and commercial 'products' to direct services offered by professionals, nonprofessionals, businesses, or consumers themselves" (Maheu et al., 2001). The use of e-health has grown as many providers have created secure Internet portals to enable patients to access their EHRs, allow patient–provider email messaging, and use mobile apps for smartphones and tablets (Ricciardi et al., 2013).

M-Health

The term "mobile health," or **m-health**, refers to "the use of wireless communication devices to support public health and clinical practice" (Kahn et al., 2010). These devices facilitate communication among researchers, clinicians, and patients. Physicians are also recognizing the potential utility of mobile computing. The most common current use is for EHR access (Sclafani et al., 2013).

E-Therapy

E-therapy has emerged as an alternative to face-to-face therapy for behavioral health support and counseling (Skinner and Latchford, 2006). Also referred to as online therapy, e-counseling, teletherapy, or cyber-counseling, **e-therapy** refers to any type of professional therapeutic interaction that makes use of the Internet to connect qualified mental health professionals and their clients (Rochlen et al., 2004). Although e-therapy is not widely used at this point, many Internet mental health interventions have reported promising early results. Both therapist-led and self-directed online therapies can lead to significant alleviation of disorder-related symptomatology (Ybarra and Eaton, 2005). E-therapy has the potential of reaching a significant number of clients who need mental health services yet do not receive them (Wodarski and Frimpong, 2013). Nevertheless, this type of care remains controversial. Issues and problems potentially best suited for online therapy include personal growth and fulfillment; adult children of alcoholics; anxiety disorders, including agoraphobia and social phobias; and body image and shame/guilt issues. Clients who are not appropriate candidates for online therapy include those who have suicidal ideation, thought disorders, borderline personality disorder, or unmonitored medical issues (Stofle, 2001).

Virtual Physician Visits

Another emerging application of communication technology is **virtual physician visits**—that is, online clinical encounters between a patient and a physician. When properly conducted, virtual visits can be quite effective and result in high rates of patient satisfaction, particularly when video technology is incorporated. For example, in one study, such "visits" were effective in improving markers for 76% of the patients with uncontrolled diabetes (Robinson et al., 2016). In another study, patients regarded virtual visits with primary care physicians to be similar to face-to-face visits on measures such as time spent and interaction with the physician. Physicians were also highly satisfied with the virtual visit modality (Dixon and Stahl, 2009). Nevertheless, virtual visits are not appropriate for every type of physician–patient encounter. Virtual visits are a type of telemedicine practice, described in more detail in the next section.

▶ Telemedicine, Telehealth, and Remote Monitoring

The terms "telemedicine" and "telehealth" are often used interchangeably. Both employ telecommunication systems for the purpose of promoting health, but there is a technical difference between the two.

Telemedicine Versus Telehealth

Telemedicine, or distance medicine, employs telecommunications technology for medical diagnosis and patient care when the provider and the client are separated by distance. Similar to a virtual visit, it eliminates the need for face-to-face contact between the examining physician and the patient. Unlike virtual visits, however, telemedicine has applications in the delivery of specialized medical services. Examples include teleradiology, the transmission of radiographic images and scans; telepathology, the viewing of tissue specimens via video-microscopy; telesurgery, controlling robots from a distance to perform surgical procedures; and clinical consultation provided by a wide range of specialists. The use and applications of telemedicine have been expanding, albeit at a slow pace. One example is its use among the prison population: Members of this population tend to be sicker than the general population, and their health care comes at a high cost. According to one analysis, the cost of transporting, guarding, and medically treating an inmate could exceed $2,000 per day (Teichert, 2016).

The term **telehealth** is broader in scope than telemedicine. It encompasses telemedicine, as traditionally known; educational, research, and administrative uses; and clinical applications that involve a variety of caregivers, such as physicians, nurses, psychologists, and pharmacists (Field and Grigsby, 2002).

Characteristics of Telemedicine

Telemedicine can be synchronous or asynchronous. **Synchronous technology** allows telecommunication to occur in real time. For example, interactive video conferencing allows two or more professionals to see and hear each other and even share documents in real time. The technology allows a specialist located at a distance to directly interview and examine a patient. By comparison, **asynchronous technology** employs store-and-forward technology that allows users to review the information later. Interpretation of scans in teleradiology is one example where asynchronous technology is employed.

Newer applications of telemedicine include in-home monitoring of patients. Vital signs, blood pressure, and blood glucose levels can be monitored remotely using video technology—a methodology that has been shown to be effective, well received by patients, capable of maintaining quality of care, and associated with the potential for cost savings (Johnston et al., 2000). Recently, remote monitoring of cardiac implantable electronic devices, such as pacemakers and implantable cardioverter-defibrillators, has been gaining acceptance in the United States and Europe. This technology has been found to be highly effective in managing clinical events, such as arrhythmias, cardiovascular disease progression, and device malfunction, with remarkably few human interventions and low resource use (Ricci et al., 2013; Slotwiner and Wilkoff, 2013).

Rural populations, in particular, face various types of barriers to access of quality health care. These barriers, such as a shortage of providers, long travel distances, physical and social isolation, and weather-related difficulties, can be overcome with appropriate telehealth services. Despite the potential for using telemedicine to deliver services to underserved rural populations, the technology has not yet been widely adopted. One of the main payers for services received by rural populations is Medicare, but its spending on telemedicine is largely reserved for mental health services and represents only a tiny fraction of overall Medicare spending (Neufeld and Doarn, 2015).

Despite the growing interest in telemedicine, its utilization remains limited due to an unclear or unidentified need for certain types of telemedicine services, uncertain reimbursement policies, absence of interstate licensure reciprocity, lack of universal access to necessary technology, concerns about patient confidentiality, and limited precedent regarding liability issues. Such issues are largely eliminated in the Veterans Health Administration (VHA) system. Results from the VHA demonstrate substantial cost savings and patient satisfaction with care delivered through telemedicine (Kahn et al., 2016).

Tele-ICU

Recently, telemedicine has become a subspecialty of critical care practice (tele-intensive care unit, or tele-ICU). Tele-ICU involves a centralized or remotely based critical care team that is networked with the bedside ICU team and patient via advanced audiovisual communication and computer systems. The ICU environment is characterized by numerous distractions and interruptions; while addressing the needs of one patient, the nurse or physician may not be aware of a second patient's change in status that may call for immediate attention. Tele-ICU provides a backup system that can avoid these problems. It operates with the goal of providing additional surveillance and support to hospital-based critical care staff, and ultimately enhancing outcomes for critically ill patients (Goran, 2010).

▶ Innovation, Diffusion, and Utilization of Medical Technology

In the context of medical technology, innovation is the creation of a product, technique, or service perceived to be new by members of a society. The spread of technology into society once it is developed is referred to as **technology diffusion** (Luce, 1993). Rapid diffusion of a technology occurs when the innovation is perceived to be of benefit that can be evaluated or measured, is compatible with the adopter's values and needs, and is covered through third-party payment. Once technology is acquired, its use is almost ensured. Hence, the diffusion and utilization of technology are closely intertwined. The desire to have state-of-the-art technology available and to use it despite its cost or established health benefit is called the **technological imperative**.

High-tech procedures are more readily available in the United States than in most other countries, and little is done to limit the expansion of new medical technology. Compared to most European hospitals, U.S. hospitals perform a far greater number of catheterizations, angioplasties, and bypass heart surgeries. In 2013, the rate of knee replacement in the United States was 87% greater than the median rate in countries belonging to the Organization for Economic Cooperation and Development (OECD, 2015).

The United States also has more high-tech equipment, such as magnetic resonance imaging (MRI) scanners, available to its population than most other countries (**TABLE 5-2**).

TABLE 5-2 MRI Units Available per 1,000,000 Population in Selected Countries, 2014

Japan	51.7
United States	38.1
Germany	30.5
Australia	15.2
France	10.9
United Kingdom	6.1

Data from Organization for Economic Cooperation and Development (OECD). 2016. Magnetic resonance imaging (MRI) units, 2014. Available at: https://data.oecd.org/healtheqt/magnetic-resonance-imaging-mri-units.htm#indicator-chart. Accessed April 2017.

Other nations have tried to limit—mainly through central planning—the diffusion and utilization of high-tech procedures to control medical costs. The U.K. government, for instance, established the National Institute for Health and Clinical Excellence (NICE) in 1999 to decide whether the National Health Service should make select health technologies available (Milewa, 2006). Hence, MRI and computed tomography (CT) scanners are less widely available in the United Kingdom than in most OECD nations. Conversely, in many other European countries, technology diffusion has grown at a rapid pace.

Factors That Drive Innovation and Diffusion

The rate and pattern by which a technology diffuses is often governed by multiple forces (Cohen, 2004b). For example, public and private financing of research and development (R&D) can promote or inhibit innovation. Government regulations, such as the U.S. Food and Drug Administration (FDA) approval process for pharmaceuticals, biological agents, and biomedical devices, can promote or hinder the availability of new drugs and devices. In addition, marketing and promotion by the manufacturers can have an impact on the decisions of both providers and consumers about the adoption and use of technology.

Some of the main forces that have shaped the innovation, diffusion, and utilization of technology in the United States are addressed in the following subsections:

- Anthro-cultural beliefs and values
- Medical specialization
- Financing and payment
- Technology-driven competition
- Expenditures on research and development
- Supply-side controls
- Government policy

Anthro-Cultural Beliefs and Values

Based on their beliefs and values, Americans have much higher expectations of what medical technology can do to cure illness than, for instance, Canadians and Germans. In an opinion survey, a significantly larger number of Americans (35%) than Germans (21%) indicated that it was absolutely essential for them to be able to get the most advanced tests, drugs, medical procedures, and equipment (Kim et al., 2001). In another survey, 91% of Americans indicated that their ability to get the most advanced tests, drugs, medical equipment, and procedures was very important to improving the quality of health care (Schur and Berk, 2008).

As a case in point, in 2007, the Centers for Medicare and Medicaid Services (CMS) proposed to sharply restrict payments for CT angiography for Medicare-insured patients. Even though this newer imaging technology had not been shown to offer any remarkable improvements in diagnosing heart disease, the CMS faced a barrage of criticism over the proposal from radiologists and cardiologists, technology development firms such as General Electric, and 79 members of the U.S. House of Representatives. Ultimately, the CMS announced that it would not impose its proposed determination despite continued uncertainty about the test's usefulness (Appleby, 2008).

The primacy of technology can also be traced to U.S. reliance on the medical model, which is reinforced by American beliefs and values. The emphasis on specialty care in this model, rather than primary care and preventive services, raises the expectations of both physicians and patients that all available technology will be used in every case.

Medical Specialization

Evidence of the technological imperative is most apparent in acute care hospitals, especially those affiliated with medical schools, because they are the main centers for specialty residency training programs in which physicians are trained to use the latest medical advances. Broad exposure to technology early in training affects not only clinical preferences, but also future professional behavior and practice patterns (Cohen, 2004c). Both patients and practitioners also equate high-quality care with high-intensity care.

Financing and Payment

Evidence from several countries suggests that fixed provider payments, such as salaries paid to physicians (rather than fee-for-service arrangements), and strong limits on payments to hospitals, such as stringent use of global budgets, curtail the incentive to use high-tech procedures. Hence, payment incentives can place limitations on how quickly and widely new treatments diffuse into medical practice (McClellan and Kessler, 1999).

Traditionally, the U.S. health care delivery system has lacked internal checks and balances to determine when high-cost services are appropriate. Health insurance promotes the phenomenon referred to as moral hazard and provider-induced demand in the absence of mechanisms to limit utilization of high-cost services. Insurance insulates both patients and providers from any personal accountability for the utilization of high-cost services. Generally, both patients and physicians want to use everything that medical science has to offer as long as out-of-pocket costs are of little concern.

There is likely a two-way relationship between technology diffusion and insurance coverage. Increasingly generous insurance coverage causes increases in spending for new products. Conversely, the development of beneficial but costly new technology puts pressure on insurers to cover those technologies (Danzon and Pauly, 2001). In making their coverage decisions, private insurance companies tend to follow Medicare's lead—Medicare is, by far, the largest and most influential payer in the United States. The current direction in reimbursement decisions is to seek **value**—that is, the most benefits possible for the price paid.

In Europe, research has suggested that higher levels of reimbursement do not always promote technology diffusion there (Cappellaro et al., 2011). This discrepancy with the U.S. experience arises mainly because European national health care programs have the means to suppress unintended diffusion of technology through central planning.

Technology-Driven Competition

Hospitals, as well as outpatient centers, compete to attract insured patients. Well-insured patients look for quality, and institutions create perceptions of higher quality by acquiring and advertising state-of-the-art technology. Specialists have also been responsible for stimulating competition. Many physicians, for example, have opened their own specialty hospitals, diagnostic imaging facilities equipped with next-generation scanners, and same-day surgery centers that offer hotel-like facilities—and these developments have fueled a de facto "medical arms race." In response, hospitals have added new service lines—such as cancer, heart, and brain centers—and acquired costly CT scanners and high-field MRI machines (Kher, 2006), fueling more technology-based competition. To recruit specialists, medical centers often have to obtain new technology and offer high-tech procedures. When hospitals develop new services and invest heavily in modernization programs, other hospitals in the area are often forced to do the same to remain competitive. Such practices result in a tremendous amount of duplication of services and equipment.

Self-Referral and Stark Laws. Investment interests by physicians in various types of facilities prompted Congress to pass regulations against the practice of physician **self-referral**. These laws prohibit physicians from sending patients to facilities in which the referring physician or a family member has an ownership interest or some kind of compensation arrangement. Prohibition of self-referrals is based on the theory of provider-induced demand, which could create overutilization and result in increased health care costs.

The Ethics in Patient Referrals Act of 1989 (commonly known as Stark I after Representative Pete Stark, author of the original bill) prohibited the referral of Medicare patients to laboratories in which the referring physician had an ownership interest. Provisions of this law expanded under the Omnibus Budget Reconciliation Act (OBRA) of 1993. Commonly referred to as Stark II, the statute covers both Medicare and Medicaid referrals. It also expanded the categories of services to include clinical laboratory services; rehabilitation services; radiology services, including MRI, CT scans, and ultrasound; radiation therapy services and supplies; durable medical equipment and supplies; prosthetics, orthotics, and prosthetic devices and supplies; home health services; outpatient prescription drugs; and inpatient and outpatient hospitalization services. Nearly half the states also have self-referral prohibitions that apply to privately insured patients (Mitchell, 2007).

There are some exceptions to the laws, however, such as in-office ancillary services (Wachler and Avery, 2011), which allow physicians to own or lease imaging equipment for their office-based practices. Hence, a significant amount of self-referral still exists (Mitchell, 2007). This is an important exception: Without it, patients would have to seek certain services from a different provider, which would burden them with making additional appointments and having to travel to those facilities to receive recommended services.

Stark Laws have come under heavy criticism from hospital executives, physicians, and some members of Congress. According to these critics, the laws interfere with collaboration and coordination of care between providers ("Hospital Leaders Take Aim at 'Stark' Law," 2016).

Expenditures on Research and Development

Innovation is driven by R&D spending. The ARRA of 2009 allocated $10.4 billion in new funding to the National Institutes of Health (NIH), mainly to support research (Steinbrook, 2009). This funding ended in 2011, with the passage of the Budget Control Act.

Global comparisons of R&D spending on biomedical research are shown in **TABLE 5-3**. Although the United States still leads the world in R&D spending, over a 5-year period, spending on biomedical R&D has declined in the country. Of particular note are the funding cuts within private industry. The same trend is also evident in Europe. The overall spending in the Asia–Oceania region, although still small compared to biomedical R&D spending in the United States, has accelerated at a fast pace from both public and private sources.

TABLE 5-3 Global Biomedical R&D Expenditures[1] in Selected Regions, 2007 and 2012

	2007	2012	Percentage Change
United States	131.3	119.3	−9.1%
Public	48.0	48.9	+1.9%
Industry	83.3	70.4	−15.5%
Europe	83.6	81.8	−2.2%
Public	27.7	28.1	+1.4%
Industry	55.9	53.6	−4.1%
Asia-Oceania[2]	41.1	62.0	+50.9%
Public	13.5	19.3	+43.0%
Industry	27.6	42.7	+54.7%

[1] Expenditures are in billions of dollars. 2007 data are adjusted for inflation to 2012.

[2] The main countries in Asia-Oceania are China, Japan, South Korea, India, and Australia.

Data from Chakma, J., et al. 2014. Asia's ascent—global trends in biomedical R&D expenditures. *New England Journal of Medicine* 370, no. 1: 3–6.

Supply-Side Controls

In the United States, supply-side controls, or explicit rationing, have met with stiff resistance, even though such rationing may be based on certain well-defined criteria. In contrast, other countries have used government policy to control the diffusion of medical technology (see Table 5-2 for an example), which is one way to ration health care. To some extent, the United States also engages in technology rationing through the drug and device approval system of the Food and Drug Administration—discussed later in this chapter.

Rationing curtails costs, but it also restricts access to critically needed care. Canada, which restricts specialist services and limits expensive medical equipment to control health care spending, is a case in point. For several years, the Fraser Institute has researched issues related to access to care in Canada. According to its research, in 2014, patients in that country could expect to wait 9.8 weeks for medically necessary treatment after seeing a specialist—more than 3 weeks longer than the time physicians considered to be clinically reasonable, which is 6.5 weeks (Barua and Ren, 2015). Several studies have reported deaths resulting from delayed heart surgery due to waiting times in Canada, even in cases classified as nonurgent (Sobolev et al., 2013).

Although a full discussion of rationing is beyond the scope of this text, Alexander Friedman (2011) has observed that as we devote more resources to health care, something else of value always emerges. Nevertheless, in the United States, politicians, medical professionals, other experts, and the public have not come to grips with the notion of rationing. Our resources are limited, however, and health care is not the only vital public endeavor. Hence, many experts think that rationing is inevitable, because no modern society has found a way to deliver all the health care that people may desire (see, for example, Churchill, 2011). Rationing inevitably requires controls over the diffusion and utilization of medical technology.

Government Policy

Government policy in the United States plays a significant role in deciding which drugs, devices, and biologics are made available to Americans. The U.S. government is also one of the largest sources of funding for biomedical research. By controlling the amount of funding, public policy indirectly influences medical innovation.

▶ The Government's Role in Technology Diffusion

The growth of technology has been accompanied by issues of cost, safety, benefits, and risks. Federal legislation has been aimed primarily at addressing the concerns related to safety. The government plays a minor role in health care organizations' decisions to acquire new technology. As previously indicated, though, the government is an important source of funding for biomedical research.

Regulation of Drugs, Devices, and Biologics

The FDA is an agency under the DHHS that is responsible for ensuring that drugs and medical devices are safe and effective for their intended use. It also controls access to drugs by deciding whether a certain drug will be available by prescription only or as an over-the-counter purchase.

In addition, the FDA may stipulate how certain over-the-counter products may be purchased and sold. For example, under the Combat Methamphetamine Epidemic Act of 2005 (incorporated into the USA PATRIOT Act and signed by President George W. Bush in March 2006), certain cold and allergy medicines containing pseudoephedrine are required to be kept behind pharmacy counters and sold in only limited quantities to consumers, who must present photo identification and sign a logbook. This action was taken because pseudoephedrine is used in making methamphetamine—a highly addictive drug—in home laboratories.

Regulation of Drugs and Evolution of the Approval Processes

The FDA's regulatory functions have evolved over time (**TABLE 5-4**). The first piece of drug legislation in the United States was the Food and Drugs Act of 1906. The purpose of this law was to prevent the manufacture, sale, or transportation of adulterated, misbranded, poisonous, or deleterious foods, drugs, medicines, and liquors (FDA, 2009a). It authorized the Bureau of Chemistry (the predecessor of the FDA) to take action only after drugs had been marketed to consumers. It was assumed that the manufacturer would conduct safety tests before marketing the product. If innocent consumers were harmed, however, the Bureau of Chemistry could act only after such harm had been done (Bronzino et al., 1990).

Federal law governing drugs was subsequently strengthened by the passage of the Federal Food, Drug, and Cosmetic Act (FD&C Act) of 1938. This legislation was enacted in response to the infamous Elixir Sulfanilamide disaster, in which almost 100

TABLE 5-4 Summary of FDA Legislation

1906	**Food and Drugs Act** The FDA was authorized to take action only after drugs sold to consumers caused harm.
1938	**Food, Drug, and Cosmetic Act** Required premarket notification to the FDA so the agency could assess the safety of a new drug or device.
1962	**Kefauver-Harris Amendments** Premarket notification was inadequate. The FDA took charge of reviewing the efficacy and safety of new drugs, which could be marketed only once approval was granted.
1976	**Medical Devices Amendments** Authorized premarket review of medical devices and classified devices into three classes.
1983	**Orphan Drug Act** Drug manufacturers were given incentives to produce new drugs for rare diseases.
1990	**Safe Medical Devices Act** Health care facilities must report serious or potentially serious device-related injuries, illness, or death of patients and employees.
1992	**Prescription Drug User Fee Act** The FDA received authority to collect application fees from drug companies to provide additional resources to shorten the drug-approval process.
1997	**Food and Drug Administration Modernization Act** Provides for fast-track approvals for life-saving drugs when their expected benefits exceed those of current therapies.
2012	**Food and Drug Administration Safety and Innovation Act** Allows the FDA to use markers that are thought to predict or that are reasonably likely to predict clinical benefit to qualify a drug for accelerated approval if the drug is indicated for a serious condition and fills an unmet medical need.
2013	**Drug Quality and Security Act (renamed as Drug Supply Chain Security Act)** Aimed at the verification, detection, and recall of drugs using an electronic system. A primary goal is to identify counterfeit, unapproved, and potentially dangerous products and to prevent their use.
2016	**21st Century Cures Act** Provides funds to the FDA to shorten the approval time for new drugs and devices.

people died in Tennessee due to poisoning from a toxic solvent used in this liquid's preparation (Flannery, 1986). According to the revised law, a new drug could not be marketed without first notifying the FDA and allowing the agency time to assess the drug's safety (Merrill, 1994).

The drug approval system was further transformed by the drug amendments of 1962, after thalidomide (a sleeping pill that was distributed in the United States as an experimental drug but had been widely marketed in Europe) was shown to cause birth defects (Flannery, 1986). The 1962 amendments (Kefauver-Harris Drug Amendments) essentially stated that premarket notification of drug-related risks was inadequate. The amendments put a premarket approval system in force, giving the FDA authority to review the effectiveness and safety of a new drug before it could be marketed. Its consumer protection role enabled the FDA to prevent harm before it occurred. However, the drug approval process was criticized for slowing down the introduction of new drugs and, consequently, denying patients early benefits from the latest treatments. Drug manufacturers essentially "became prisoners of the agency's [FDA's] indecision, its preoccupation with other issues, or its lack of resources" (Merrill, 1994).

The Orphan Drug Act of 1983 and subsequent amendments were passed to provide incentives for pharmaceutical firms to develop new drugs for rare diseases and conditions. Incentives, such as grant funding to defray the expenses of clinical testing and exclusive marketing rights for 7 years, were necessary because a relatively small number of people are afflicted by rare conditions, creating a relatively small market for drugs treating those conditions. As a result of the

Orphan Drug Act, certain new drug therapies, called **orphan drugs**, have become available for conditions that affect fewer than 200,000 people in the United States.

In the late 1980s, pressure on the FDA from those wanting rapid access to new drugs for the treatment of human immunodeficiency virus (HIV) infection called for a reconsideration of the drug review process (Rakich et al., 1992). For example, saquinavir—a protease inhibitor indicated for patients with advanced HIV infection—received accelerated approval in late 1995; however, its manufacturer, Roche Laboratories, was subsequently required to show that the drug prolonged survival or slowed clinical progression of HIV.

In 1992, Congress passed the Prescription Drug User Fee Act, which authorized the FDA to collect fees from biotechnology and pharmaceutical companies to review their drug applications. The additional funds provided needed resources, and, according to the General Accounting Office (GAO), allowed the FDA to approve new drugs more quickly, thereby enabling them to reach the market in less time. From 1993 to 2001, the median approval time for standard new drugs dropped from 21 months to approximately 14 months. In 2004, the approval time dropped even further to 12.9 months.

In 1997, Congress passed the Food and Drug Administration Modernization Act. This law provides for increased patient access to experimental drugs and medical devices. "Fast-track" approvals are permitted when the potential benefits of new drugs for serious or life-threatening conditions are considered significantly greater than the benefits of current therapies. In addition, the law provides for an expanded database on clinical trials, which is accessible to the public. Under a separate provision, when a manufacturer plans to discontinue a drug, patients who are heavily dependent on the drug receive advance notice.

The Food and Drug Administration Safety and Innovation Act of 2012 allows the FDA to either use a marker that is thought to predict clinical benefit (surrogate endpoint) or use a marker that is considered reasonably likely to predict clinical benefit (intermediate clinical endpoint). These markers allow for faster approval of drugs. For example, the FDA may approve a drug based on evidence that the drug shrinks tumors, because tumor shrinkage is considered reasonably likely to predict a real clinical benefit (FDA, 2013).

Since 1992, when the Prescription Drug User Fee Act was passed, the regulatory focus has been on faster review of new drugs by the FDA. There is no doubt that faster reviews have allowed new drugs to become available more quickly than before this legislation was enacted. Nevertheless, there have been lingering safety concerns, mainly because several years of public use of a drug may elapse before safety problems may emerge. When safety issues do arise, the FDA may issue a "black box warning" that must appear on a prescription drug's label alerting the user to serious or life-threatening risks. In rare cases, the FDA may rescind its approval decision and order that a drug must be withdrawn from the U.S. market. Recent studies have shown that safety risks are often recognized only after the FDA has given approval to market certain drugs. For example, Frank and colleagues (2014) demonstrated that half of all new black box warnings appeared after a drug had been on the market for 12 years; drugs that were withdrawn from the market had been sold for 5 years or longer.

Despite such concerns, the push for faster approvals for drugs and devices does not seem to have changed. The 21st Century Cures Act of 2016 provides funds for the FDA to change its drug and device approval processes with the aim of shortening the period for approving new drugs and devices, especially for life-threatening diseases. Clearly, providing for faster approval of new medical technology while simultaneously ensuring its safety will remain a delicate balancing act.

Drugs from Overseas

The use of foreign-made drug products in the United States has been rapidly increasing. As a safeguard, all drugs approved in the United States must comply with the FD&C Act, regardless of where they are manufactured. To ensure that foreign-made drugs meet this standard, the FDA performs two types of investigations. First, the FDA routinely inspects domestic and foreign drug manufacturing plants. Second, the FDA tests samples of drugs, and bases its surveillance activities on complaints from consumers and health professionals (FDA, 2016a).

Securing the Supply Chain

The U.S. government has taken steps to secure the integrity of the pharmaceutical supply chain, which can be threatened by medication counterfeiting, importation of unapproved and substandard drugs, and grey markets. Such illegal operations often distribute drug products with the potential for serious harm (Brechtelsbauer et al., 2016). The Drug Quality and Security Act of 2013 (renamed as Drug Supply Chain Security Act) was passed to curtail the distribution of unauthorized drug products.

Regulation of Medical Devices and Equipment

The FDA first received jurisdiction over medical devices under the FD&C Act of 1938. However, such jurisdiction was confined to the sale of products believed to be unsafe or that made misleading claims of effectiveness (Merrill, 1994).

In the 1970s, several deaths and miscarriages were attributed to the Dalkon Shield, which had been marketed as a safe and effective contraceptive device (Flannery, 1986). In 1976, the Medical Device Amendments extended the FDA's authority to include premarket review of medical devices divided into three classes. Devices in Class I pose the lowest risk (such as enema kits and elastic bandages). They are subject to general controls regarding misbranding—that is, fraudulent claims regarding their therapeutic effects. Class II devices (such as powered wheelchairs and pregnancy test kits) are subject to special requirements for labeling, performance standards, and postmarket surveillance. The most stringent requirements of premarket approval regarding safety and effectiveness apply to Class III devices, which support life, prevent health impairment, or present an unreasonable risk of illness or injury. For most Class III devices (such as implantable pacemakers and breast implants), premarket approval is required to ensure their safety and effectiveness.

The Safe Medical Devices Act of 1990 strengthened the FDA's hand in controlling the entry of new biomedical devices into the market and in monitoring use of marketed products (Merrill, 1994). Under the Safe Medical Devices Act, health care facilities must report serious or potentially serious device-related injuries or illness of patients and employees to the manufacturer of the device and, if death is involved, to the FDA as well. In essence, this law is intended to serve as an "early warning" system through which the FDA can obtain important information on device problems.

The United States has stricter standards for evaluating the safety and effectiveness of medical devices than are imposed by other countries. Some concern has been expressed that the stricter standards create disincentives for manufacturers to make important medical devices available in the United States (Shuren and Califf, 2016). Ensuring timely access to the new technology while still verifying its safe and appropriate use presents a dilemma. To overcome some of the obstacles, the FDA is building the foundation for a National Evaluation System for health Technology (NEST), which would more efficiently generate better evidence for medical device evaluation and regulatory decision making. The collaborative national evaluation system will link and synthesize data from different sources across the medical device landscape, including clinical registries, EHRs, and medical billing claims (FDA, 2016b).

Regulation of Biologics

Biologics, or biological products, include a wide range of products such as vaccines, blood and blood components, allergenics, somatic cells, gene therapy, tissues, and recombinant therapeutic proteins, particularly when they are used for prevention or treatment of a disease or health condition. Biologics are isolated from a variety of natural sources—human, animal, or microorganism. In contrast to most drugs that are chemically synthesized and have a known chemical structure, most biologics are complex mixtures that are not easily identified or characterized (FDA, 2009b).

The FDA regulates biologics under the Public Health Service Act of 1944; the FD&C Act of 1938; the Biologics Price Competition and Innovation Act of 2009; and the Biosimilar User Fee Act of 2012. The first two acts mainly deal with the safety of biologics by requiring licensing of these products. The last two were part of the ACA and are discussed further in the section "Health Care Reform and Medical Technology."

Certificate of Need

The national Health Planning and Resources Development Act of 1974 required states to enact certificate of need (CON) laws to obtain federal funds to carry out planning functions that would restrict the diffusion of technology. CON laws required hospitals to seek state approval before acquiring major equipment or embarking on new construction or modernization projects (Iglehart, 1982). Effective January 1, 1987, the federal law was repealed, but most states still retain some control over the construction of new health care facilities and acquisition of costly equipment.

States that have retained CON laws have faced controversies and legal challenges (Carlson, 2012). Critics have argued that the CON laws stifle competition. Some evidence also suggests that CON laws may not have been effective in reducing costs, at least for some medical technologies (Ho et al., 2013), nor have they

had a direct effect on reducing per-capita health care expenditures (Hellinger, 2009).

Some states are now ready to abandon the CON laws. The Obama administration weighed in by asserting that CON laws do not conform to the ACA, because they create barriers to entry and expansion, and limit competition and consumer choice (Kirkner, 2016).

Research on Technology

The AHRQ was established in 1989 under the OBRA of 1989 and was originally the Agency for Health Care Policy and Research. AHRQ, a division of the DHHS, is the lead federal agency charged with supporting research that focuses on improving the quality of health care, reducing health care costs, and improving access to essential services. For instance, the agency's Center for Outcomes and Evidence (formerly the Center for Outcomes and Effectiveness Research) conducts and supports studies of the outcomes and effectiveness of diagnostic, therapeutic, and preventive health services and procedures. AHRQ technology assessments are available to medical practitioners, consumers, and others.

Funding for Research

The National Institutes of Health—a division of the DHHS—is the primary agency that both conducts and supports basic and applied biomedical research in the United States. The NIH encompasses 27 different institutes or centers; each has its own research agenda. A large portion of its budget (more than $32 billion in fiscal year 2016) is used for funding extramural research.

NIH's National Institute of General Medical Sciences (NIGMS) is the principal medical research agency. In fiscal year 2016, NIGMS's budget was $2.5 billion. The vast majority of this money funded grants to scientists at universities, medical schools, hospitals, and research institutions throughout the United States (NIGMS, 2016).

The 21st Century Cures Act of 2016 significantly increased funding for the NIH. Approximately $4.8 billion over 10 years has been authorized, part of which is designated for the Cancer Moonshot program championed by former Vice President Joe Biden, which is seeking to find new cures for cancer.

▶ The Impact of Medical Technology

Health care technology involves the practical application of scientific discoveries in many disciplines. The deployment of scientific knowledge has had far-reaching and pervasive effects, as the examples in Table 5-1 suggest. The effects of technology often overlap, making it difficult to pinpoint technology's impact in a single area of health care delivery.

Impact on Quality of Care

When advanced techniques can provide more precise medical diagnoses than before, offer quicker and more complete cures than previously available, or reduce risks in a cost-effective manner, the result is improved quality. Technology can also provide new remedies where none existed before. More effective, less invasive, and safer therapeutic and preventive remedies

can increase longevity and decrease morbidity.

Numerous examples illustrate the role of technology in enhancing the quality of care. Today, coronary angioplasty is commonly performed to open blocked or narrowed coronary arteries. Before this treatment became available, however, patients suffering a heart attack were prescribed prolonged bed rest and treated with morphine and nitroglycerin (Congressional Budget Office [CBO], 2008). Angioplasty has reduced the need for open-heart bypass surgery. The total artificial heart (TAH), approved by the FDA in 2005 for implantation in patients with end-stage heart failure, can be a life-saving medical device for those awaiting heart transplantation. Implantable cardioverter–defibrillators prolong the lives of people who have life-threatening irregular heartbeats.

Laser technology reduces trauma in patients undergoing surgery and shortens the period for postsurgical recovery. These devices are also widely used in medical specialties for both medical and cosmetic procedures. For example, advanced laser procedures are available for high-precision eye surgery.

Robot-assisted surgery has gained significant momentum in several surgical applications. For example, robot-assisted surgery enables minimally invasive techniques to be used for the surgical removal of the prostate, and to surgically treat cancers of the kidney, lung, and thyroid. The robotic approach allows for improved dexterity and precision of the instruments.

Advanced bioimaging methods have created new ways to see the body's inner workings, while minimizing invasive procedures. Modern imaging technologies include MRI, positron emission tomography (PET), single-photon emission computed tomography (SPECT), CT scan, and 3-D fluorescence imaging. PET has important applications in cardiology, neurology, and oncology. For example, it can spot tumors and other problems that may not be detectable with traditional MRI or CT scans. SPECT is of great value in imaging the brain. This type of imaging could also reduce inappropriate use of invasive procedures through a more accurate diagnosis of coronary artery disease (Shaw et al., 2000). Echocardiography and Doppler ultrasound are advanced imaging techniques to study heart function and detect problems. These and other advanced imaging technologies also allow surgeons to perform minimally invasive procedures more precisely (Comaniciu et al., 2016).

Molecular and cell biology has opened a new era in clinical medicine. Screening for genetic disorders, gene therapy, and the introduction of powerful new drugs for cancer and heart disease promise to radically improve the quality of medical care. Genetic research might even help overcome the critical shortage of transplantable organs. On a parallel track, regenerative medicine and tissue engineering hold the promise of creating other biological and bioartificial substitutes that will restore and maintain normal function in a variety of diseased and injured tissues. Products such as bioartificial kidneys, artificial implantable livers, and insulin-producing cells to replace damaged pancreatic cells are examples of what biomedical science might be able to accomplish. Treatment of disease using stem cells that can be derived from discarded human embryos (human embryonic stem cells), fetal

tissue, or adult sources (bone marrow, fat, or skin) is another example of regenerative medicine.

Amid all the enthusiasm that these emerging technologies might generate, some degree of caution must prevail. Experience shows that greater proliferation of technology may not always equate to higher quality. Unless the effect of each individual technology is appropriately assessed, some innovations may be wasteful and others may be harmful.

Impact on Quality of Life

Thanks to new scientific developments, thousands of people are able to live normal lives, which otherwise would not be possible. People with disabling conditions have been able to overcome their limitations in speech, hearing, vision, and movement through prosthetic devices and therapies. Long-term maintenance therapies have enabled people with conditions such as diabetes and end-stage renal disease (ESRD) to engage in activities that they otherwise would not be able to do. Major pharmaceutical breakthroughs have given people with heart disease, cancer, HIV/AIDS, and preterm birth a much longer life expectancy and improved health (Kleinke, 2001). HIV/AIDS is no longer viewed as a killer, but rather as a manageable chronic disease, thanks to new drugs and modern treatments.

Modern technology has also been instrumental in relieving pain and suffering; in fact, pain management has been recognized as a new subspecialty in medicine. For example, in cancer pain management, new opioids have been developed for transdermal, nasal, and nebulized administration, which allow needleless means of controlling pain (Davis, 2006). The technology underlying patient-controlled analgesia allows patients to determine when and how much medication they receive, which gives patients more independence and control.

Development of a substitute for injectable insulin could greatly enhance the quality of life for patients with diabetes—particularly elderly patients, who often require assistance with insulin injections. Uncontrolled diabetes can lead to complications such as heart disease, stroke, kidney failure, and blindness. An inhaled insulin powder product, Afrezza, is now available on the U.S. market, but its long-term acceptance is unknown (Wong et al., 2016). Oral administration of insulin in tablet form is considered more convenient than other methods of delivery, but several barriers still remain to be overcome. Ongoing research in this area appears promising, however.

Impact on Health Care Costs

Technological innovations have been the single most important factor in medical cost inflation. Specifically, during the past several decades, they have accounted for roughly half of the total rise in real (after eliminating the effects of general inflation) health care spending (CBO, 2008; Sorenson et al., 2013). Nevertheless, the impact of technology on costs differs across technologies: Some—such as cancer drugs and invasive medical devices—have significant cost implications, whereas others are cost-neutral or cost-saving (Sorenson et al., 2013).

Three main cost drivers are associated with the adoption of medical technology:

- The cost of acquiring the new technology and equipment
- The need for specially trained physicians and technicians to operate the equipment and to analyze the results, which often leads to increases in labor costs
- Any special housing and setting requirements for the technology, which result in facility costs (McGregor, 1989)

Hence, widespread adoption of technology has a multiplier effect, as costs increase in these three main areas.

A second set of cost drivers is associated with utilization. As discussed previously, perceptions of quality and expectations of better cure, along with insurance coverage, fuel demand for utilization. On the supply side, once technology is adopted by hospitals and physicians, a certain volume of use must be maintained if the organization is to recover its investment. Ultimately, the technology's purchase price has a minimal effect on system-wide health care costs (Littell and Strongin, 1996); instead, the costs associated with utilization of the technology, once it becomes available, become more important. For example, the addition of an MRI unit in a facility leads to approximately 733 more MRI procedures (Baker et al., 2008). Also, many of the most notable medical advances in recent decades involve ongoing treatments for the management of chronic conditions, such as diabetes and coronary artery disease (CBO, 2008), where costs continue to aggregate over time.

Although many new technologies do increase costs, others have been found to actually reduce costs. For example, antiretroviral therapies have been largely credited with the dramatic reductions in hospital stays for patients with AIDS (CDC, 1999). Technology is also credited with driving the overall reduction in the average length of inpatient hospital stays in the United States. Minimally invasive procedures using ultrasound, radio waves, or lasers can be performed in outpatient clinics, thereby reducing the need for hospitalizations.

Moreover, whereas many new technologies may increase labor costs, some actually produce labor cost savings. For example, when Northwestern University Medical Center in Chicago automated its lab, the number of human handling steps decreased from 14 to 1.5, and the turn-around time declined from 8 hours to 90 minutes. Largely because of a significant drop in labor costs, 30% cost savings were realized through the lab automation. Not only that, but the error rate dropped to zero after the system was installed (Flower, 2006).

Instead of focusing solely on the excessive costs that new technologies may produce, attention is now being given to the value or worth of the advances in medical care. In a groundbreaking study, Cutler and colleagues (2006) addressed this issue by examining how medical spending has translated into additional years of life saved, based on the assumption that 50% of the improvements in life expectancy have resulted from medical care. These researchers concluded that the increases in medical spending over the 1960 to 2000 period, in terms of increased life expectancy, have rendered reasonable value for the money spent. For example, for a 45-year-old American who has a remaining life expectancy of 30 years, the value of

remaining life is more than $200,000 per year (Murphy and Topel, 2003). For this 45-year-old person, the average annual spending in health care for each year of life gained was $53,700 (Cutler et al., 2006).

More recently, Chambers and colleagues (2014) evaluated the value offered by the specialty drugs that are produced with advanced biotechnology. These drugs offer treatments for a range of conditions, such as cancer, hepatitis C, and multiple sclerosis, but come at a high cost. The researchers concluded that despite their higher price tags relative to traditional drugs, the specialty drugs confer greater benefits and hence may offer reasonable value for money.

Impact on Access

Geography is an important factor in access to technology. If a technology is not physically available to a patient population living in remote areas, access is limited. Geographic access to many technologies can be improved by providing mobile equipment or by employing new communications technologies to allow remote access to centralized equipment and specialized personnel. For example, GPS (global positioning system) technology significantly improves emergency medical services response time to the scene of motor vehicle crashes and other emergencies (Gonzalez et al., 2009).

Mobile equipment can be transported to rural and remote sites, making it accessible to those populations. Mobile cardiac catheterization laboratories, for example, can provide high technology in rural settings. Cardiac catheterizations can be performed safely in a mobile laboratory at rural hospitals, provided immediate transfer is available for those in need of urgent intervention or revascularization (Peterson and Peterson, 2004). As discussed earlier, access to specialized medical care for rural and other hard-to-reach populations has been transformed through innovations in telemedicine.

Impact on the Structure and Processes of Health Care Delivery

Medical technology has transformed large urban hospitals into medical centers, where the latest diagnostic and therapeutic remedies are offered. Growth in alternative settings (home health and outpatient surgery centers) has also been made possible primarily by technology. For example, numerous surgical procedures are now performed in same-day outpatient settings. In earlier times, many of these patients would have required hospital stays. Extensive home health services have brought many hospital and nursing home services to the patient's home, reducing the need for institutionalization. Apart from telehealth, home care technology includes kidney dialyzers, feeding pumps, ultrasound, ventilators, and pulse oximeters.

The growth of managed care, integrated delivery systems, and emerging accountable care organizations all require robust IT systems and information exchange capabilities. Certain technologies adopted from other industries have improved health care delivery. For example, the ubiquitous bar-coding system has found several new applications in hospitals, including automation of drug dispensing, which drastically reduces medication errors. Scanning of information on nurses' badges, patients' wristbands, and drugs administered ensures that the right drug is given in the right dose to the right patient (Nicol and Huminski, 2006). In some applications, radio-frequency identification (RFID) has started to replace bar-coding technology in the areas of patient identification, equipment management, inventory control, and automatic supply and equipment billing (Roark and Miguel, 2006).

Telecommunications technology used in telemedicine is also used for administrative teleconferencing and continuing medical education. For example, interactive compressed videoconferencing allows for an almost face-to-face meeting in which vendors can demonstrate new products or services and discuss their utilization, costs, and delivery schedules. Eliminating airfares, hotel expenses, and other travel-related costs can achieve significant savings. Interactive videoconferencing is also used for continuing education in the United States and abroad, with participants reporting a high degree of satisfaction with this mode of delivery. Recently, videoconferencing applications have been introduced to provide language interpretation—that is, to translate physician orders and medication regimens for patients who have limited English proficiency (Hamblen, 2006).

Impact on Global Medical Practice

Technology developed in the United States has significantly impacted the practice of medicine worldwide. More than half of the world's leading medical device companies, for example, are based in the United States. In fact, the medical device industry is one of the few American manufacturing industries that consistently exports more than it imports (Holtzman, 2012).

Many nations wait for the United States to develop new technologies, which can then be introduced into their systems in a more controlled and manageable fashion. This process gives them access to high-technology medical care with less national investment. Although the United States is expected to continue to maintain its lead in technological innovation, Europe, Japan, and, more recently, developing nations are also focusing their attention and resources on advances in medical technology (Tripp et al., 2012).

Impact on Bioethics

Increasingly, technological change is raising serious ethical and moral issues. For example, how can medical technology benefit everyone in society? Who should have access to costly new technology? Gene mapping of humans, genetic cloning, stem cell research, and other areas of growing interest to scientists may hold potential benefits, but they also present serious ethical dilemmas. Life support technology raises serious ethical issues, especially in medical decisions regarding continuation or cessation of mechanical support, particularly when a patient exists in a permanent vegetative state. Attention to ethical issues is also critical in medical research involving human subjects and in the evaluation of experimental technologies, such as nanomedicine.

▶ The Assessment of Medical Technology

Technology assessment, or more specifically, **health technology assessment (HTA)**, refers to "any process of examining and reporting properties of a medical technology used in health care, such as safety, effectiveness, feasibility, and indications for use, cost, and cost-effectiveness, as well as social, economic, and ethical consequences, whether intended or unintended" (Institute of Medicine, 1985). HTA seeks to contribute to clinical decision making by providing evidence about the efficacy, safety, and cost-effectiveness of medical technologies. It also informs decision makers, clinicians, patients, and the public about the ethical, legal, and social implications of medical technologies (Lehoux et al., 2009).

Technology assessment can play a critical role in distinguishing between services that are appropriate and those that are not. Unfortunately, the delivery of medical care remains inefficient in many ways. Notably, the U.S. health care system provides incentives for the delivery of care that does not improve health outcomes (Korobkin, 2014). Although HTA presents a tremendous opportunity to reduce waste and improve health outcomes, in the United States it has played only a relatively minor role in coverage and payment decisions, because the resulting decisions would have rationing overtones. The FDA, however, incorporates assessments for efficacy and safety in its decisions to approve or not approve drugs, devices, and medical procedures. Decisions based on HTA have been more commonly adopted in Europe, Canada, and Australia (Sampat and Drummond, 2011).

Efficacy and safety are the basic starting points in evaluating the overall utility of medical technology. Cost-effectiveness and cost-benefit go a step further in evaluating the safety and efficacy in relation to the cost of using the technology.

Efficacy and safety are evaluated through clinical trials. A **clinical trial** is a carefully designed research study in which human subjects participate under controlled observations. Clinical trials are carried out over three or four phases, starting with a small number of subjects to evaluate the safety, dosage range, and side effects of new treatments. Subsequent studies using larger groups of people are carried out to confirm effectiveness and further evaluate safety. Compliance with rigid standards is required under HIPAA to protect the rights of study participants and to ensure that the experimentation protocols are ethical. Every institution that conducts or supports biomedical or behavioral research involving human subjects must establish an institutional review board (IRB), which initially approves and periodically reviews the research.

Efficacy

Efficacy or **effectiveness** is defined simply as the health benefit derived from the use of technology. If a product or service actually produces some health benefit, it can be considered efficacious or effective. Decisions about efficacy require that one ask the right questions. For example, are the current diagnostic capabilities satisfactory? What is the likelihood that the new procedure would result in a better diagnosis? If the problem is more accurately diagnosed, what is the likelihood of a better cure?

The question of evaluating health benefits is not as simple as it may seem. Significant challenges arise in defining and measuring health outcomes. Standardization of the selection of outcomes and outcome measurement instruments is still needed, without which it is difficult to compare the effectiveness of a new technology against an existing one.

It is also recommended that clinical trials include some measure of health-related quality of life (HRQL). HRQL is patients' own subjective perception of the effects of illness and medical intervention on their physical, mental, social, and emotional functioning. For some diseases, such as asthma and psoriasis, survival is not the main issue, but improvement in HRQL is very important. The difficult question is, however, how to measure HRQL (Cleemput and Neyt, 2015). People are also likely to have different opinions about which is better—longer survival time or higher quality of life.

Safety

The assessment of safety is designed to protect patients against unnecessary harm from technology. As a primary benchmark, benefits must outweigh any negative consequences; however, negative consequences cannot always be foreseen. Hence, clinical trials involving patients who may stand to gain the most from a technology are employed to obtain a reasonable consensus on safety. Subsequently, outcomes from wider use of technology are closely monitored to identify any problems related to safety.

Cost-Effectiveness

Cost-efficiency (or cost-effectiveness) goes a step beyond the determination of efficacy. Whereas efficacy is concerned only with the benefit derived from the technology, cost-effectiveness evaluates the additional (marginal) benefits derived in relation to the additional (marginal) costs incurred. Thus, cost-efficiency weighs benefits against costs, which is difficult in actual practice. The difficulty arises from the fact that inputs other than medical care, such as lifestyle factors, affect a person's health. Hence, cost-effectiveness for the vast majority of technologies has not been evaluated.

The traditional view of cost-efficiency is explained by a simplified version of the health production function in which the main input is medical care. Medical treatments and technology utilization are highly cost-effective when medical interventions are initiated. Additional inputs of medical care, however, tend to decrease the benefits in relation to the costs, which continue to rise. At some point in the production of health benefits that are attributable to medical care, the marginal benefits equal the marginal costs. From this point onward, it is highly unlikely that additional technological interventions would result in benefits equal to or in excess of the additional costs. As costs continue to increase, they eventually far exceed the additional health benefit. Economists have labeled this point the **flat of the curve**. It has been suggested that a considerable amount of medical interventions in the United States reach the flat of the curve, referring to a level of intensity of treatment that provides no incremental health benefit (Fuchs, 2004). Hence, high-intensity care is considered wasteful.

More recently, some have argued that flat-of-the-curve medicine is not necessarily wasteful, at least at the aggregate level. For example, increased pharmaceutical consumption in developed countries has helped improve mortality outcomes, especially for people at middle age and older (Miller and Frech, 2000). In other areas, flat-of-the-curve medicine may not be improving physical health outcomes, but it may bring improved mental health (by reducing anxiety and depression, for example), better health maintenance, improved HRQL, or stability in health status, such as reduced variability of age at death (Schoder and Zweifel, 2011).

A **cost-effectiveness analysis** incorporates the elements of both costs and benefits, especially when the costs and benefits are not expressed in terms of dollars (Wan, 1995). If costs cannot be monetarily measured, they may be evaluated in terms of resource inputs, such as staff time, number of service units, space requirements, and degree of specialization needed (specialist versus generalist, physician versus allied health professional). Benefits, which are evaluated in terms of health outcomes, include elements such as efficacy of treatment, prognosis or expected outcomes, number of cases of a certain disease averted, years of life saved, increase in life expectancy, hospitalization and sick days avoided, early return to work, patient satisfaction, and HRQL. Benefits are then evaluated in relation to resource inputs.

Risk is another type of nonmonetary cost. Most medical procedures are not totally safe, and are accompanied by certain levels of risk. Medical care can also result in undesired side effects, iatrogenic illnesses, medical complications, injuries, or death, all of which carry a cost that is often difficult to measure. Hence, the effectiveness of medical interventions should be evaluated not only in terms of costs but also in terms of risks.

Cost-Benefit

In contrast to cost-effectiveness analysis, **cost-benefit analysis** evaluates benefits in relation to costs, when both are expressed in dollar terms (Seidel et al., 1995; Wan, 1995). Hence, cost-benefit analysis is subject to a more rigorous quantitative analysis compared to cost-effectiveness analysis. Cost-benefit analysis is based on four main assumptions: (1) the problem or health condition can be identified or diagnosed; (2) the problem can be controlled or eradicated using an appropriate intervention; (3) the benefit or outcome can be assigned a dollar value; and (4) the cost of the intervention can be determined in dollars.

The same principles that apply to cost-effectiveness are also used for assessing cost-benefit. If the estimated benefits exceed the costs, the additional spending on medical care is worth the extra costs. As a measure of health benefit, the **quality-adjusted life year (QALY)** is commonly used in the United States, Canada, Europe, and Australia; an analysis that includes the use of QALYs is referred to as **cost-utility analysis** (Neumann and Weinstein, 2010). QALY is defined as the value of 1 year of high-quality life. Cutler and McClellan (2001) assigned a value of $100,000 per QALY and demonstrated that, at least in the case of four conditions (i.e., heart attacks, low-birth-weight infants, depression, and cataracts), the estimated benefit of technology was much greater than the cost. For breast cancer treatment, the costs and benefits were found to be equal in magnitude. The value of $100,000 per QALY is debatable, however, and there is no standard method for the calculation of QALY.

In the United States, the use of QALYs remains a theoretical exercise, because it raises both social and ethical concerns. It does not appear that QALY-based cost-effectiveness analyses will be used for making resource allocation, coverage, and payment decisions for some time to come.

▶ Directions and Issues in Health Technology Assessment

Private-Sector Initiatives

In the United States, HTA is conducted predominantly in the private sector, unlike in many European nations that have centralized technology assessment agencies. In the public sector, the Department of Veterans Affairs and the AHRQ mainly conduct clinical trials and other evaluations of technology. Hence, much of the talent needed to assess medical technology is also located, organized, and financed in the private sector. Numerous private agencies, including the Blue Cross and Blue Shield Association, Kaiser Permanente, the American Medical Association, and other professional societies, have undertaken technology assessments.

Need for Coordinated Effort

At present, efforts in HTA remain fragmented and poorly funded, with little or no coordination between public- and private-sector groups to deliberately address the assessment and diffusion of technologies. Also, information garnered from HTA studies is not efficiently shared among medical organizations, health care systems, and policymakers. Consequently, a demand has arisen for broad regional and national HTA programs that would study the effects of health care technology more systematically and involve providers, policymakers, patient advocacy groups, and government representatives (Bozic et al., 2004).

Need for Standardization

HTA methods used by the various organizations still lack standardization, which makes it difficult to compare efficacy and cost-effectiveness results. Once methods are standardized, there will be a need for benchmarking HTA organizations to ensure adherence to the standards (Drummond et al., 2012).

Balance Between Clinical Efficacy and Economic Worth

Achieving a balance between efficacy and cost-effectiveness will require a change in the American mindset, which will not be forthcoming in the near future. Even the CMS does not allow cost-effectiveness to be used in making decisions about care rendered to Medicare- and Medicaid-covered patients. In contrast, European countries, Canada, and Australia use cost-effectiveness openly and explicitly in their centralized health planning decisions (Neumann and Sullivan, 2006). In the United States, the predominant fear is that an organization risks being sued if it denies access to treatments that are known to be medically effective even when their cost-effectiveness is questionable (Bryan et al., 2009). Without malpractice reform, overuse of technology will continue to drive up health care costs. Regardless of

how that discussion is brought about, almost all observers realize that the United States will ultimately have to deal with the parameters of cost and value in an explicit way (Luce and Cohen, 2009).

Ethical Issues

With the rapid pace of innovation, concerns in HTA transcend the traditional questions about safety, effectiveness, and economic value. New technologies also raise social, ethical, and legal concerns. These issues raise complex questions but provide few answers.

How to provide the latest and best in health care within limited resource parameters has become a major concern for all developed countries. In the United States, insurers, pharmaceutical companies, medical device manufacturers, MCOs, and physician advocacy institutions often act and advocate out of their own self-interests. For example, physicians' representatives, such as medical associations, and the medical device and pharmaceutical industries frequently argue in favor of increasing resource inputs in delivering health care (Wild, 2005). They often claim that quality would deteriorate or harm would ensue unless new innovations are funded. When these same groups assume major roles in HTA, a conflict of interest is likely to occur. Biases might also arise in studies funded by sources that have a financial stake in the results. Such concerns have stimulated interest in developing standards for assessments, perhaps under the aegis of a governmental body.

Within social, ethical, and legal constraints, public and private insurers face the problem of deciding whether to cover novel treatments. Recent challenges include, for example, decisions about new reproductive techniques, such as intracytoplasmic sperm injection in vitro fertilization (ICSI IVF); new molecular genetic predictive tests for hereditary breast cancer; and new drugs such as sildenafil (Viagra) for erectile dysfunction (Giacomini, 2005). The introduction of these technologies raises questions about whether society should bear the cost of infertility treatments, genetic tests, and lifestyle remedies that do not affect people's health and longevity—complicated issues that have no easy answers.

Therapies classified as experimental are, in general, not covered by insurance. When new treatments promise previously unattainable health benefits, decisions about assessment of such treatments are often surrounded by controversy. Critical to the debate, but also defying easy answers, is the availability of and payment for treatments considered experimental that may be needed by critically ill patients who could possibly benefit from them (Reiser, 1994). Concerns about withholding treatment from patients are not easily juxtaposed against equally valid concerns about exposing these same patients to unjustified risk.

Ethical issues also surround the conduct of clinical research. Emanuel and colleagues (2000) contended that ethical clinical research must fulfill seven requirements:

1. The research must have social or scientific value for improving health or enhancing knowledge.
2. The study must be scientifically valid and methodologically rigorous.
3. The selection of subjects in clinical trials must be fair.
4. The potential benefits to patients and the knowledge gained for further scientific work must outweigh the risks.
5. Independent review of the research methods and findings must be conducted by unaffiliated individuals.
6. Informed, voluntary consent must be obtained from subjects.
7. The privacy of enrolled subjects must be protected, they must be offered the opportunity to withdraw, and their well-being must be maintained throughout the trial.

▶ Health Care Reform and Medical Technology

Within a relatively short time frame, the United States has experienced the effects of President Barack Obama's Affordable Care Act (ACA) and President Donald Trump's pledge to repeal and replace it. The effects of this transition, if and when it occurs, are not likely to disrupt, in any material way, the innovation, diffusion, and utilization of medical technology. The ACA imposed a 2.3% excise tax on the sale of certain medical devices by manufacturers and importers of these devices. This tax has been passed on to the purchasers of devices, mainly hospitals and physicians, and has filtered down to the consumers through higher health insurance premiums. Trump's executive order signed on January 20, 2017, authorized the Secretary of the DHHS to repeal this tax at his discretion.

When the ACA was passed, it incorporated the provisions of the Price Competition and Innovation Act of 2009. In a nutshell, this law allowed the FDA to approve "biosimilars" under a process similar to the approval of generic drugs. Because of their complexity, the term "generic" cannot apply to biologics; hence, the term "biosimilar" was created to apply to products that are highly similar to, or are interchangeable with, an already approved biological product (referred to as the reference product). Moreover, the Biosimilar User Fee Act of 2012 authorized the FDA to charge biopharmaceutical firms a user fee to pay for the FDA's review of applications for biosimilar products before these products could be marketed. Consumers and policymakers view the introduction of biosimilars as a high priority because they are likely to result in reduced costs (Epstein et al., 2014). Ultimately, the Price Competition and Innovation Act and the Biosimilar User Fee Act may be retained even if the ACA is fully repealed.

Under current law, developers of an original reference product are protected by law, in the sense that no biosimilar license can be granted until the reference product has been licensed for at least 12 years. Also, a biosimilar applicant must disclose to the reference product license holder its application, a description of its manufacturing process, and any other requested information so that the license holder can engage in an efficient process of patent assertion against the biosimilar applicant, if necessary (Johnson, 2010). It is not clear what may transpire in regard to this process under the health care reform efforts.

▶ Summary

Medical technology has produced many benefits by making positive changes in the quality of medical care delivered to patients, who often end up enjoying a better quality of life owing to improved care. Medical technology can be credited with bringing increased longevity and decreased mortality to people around the world. Much of this technology has been developed through the application of scientific knowledge that was discovered in fields other than medicine. For example, applications of computer science and telecommunications have been adapted for use in the delivery of medical services. The application of information technology and informatics is becoming indispensable in efficient delivery of care and in the effective management of modern health care organizations. The fields of e-health, m-health, e-therapy, telemedicine, and telehealth will continue to expand. Nanotechnology is a cutting-edge advancement within the science and engineering fields that is beginning to find applications in health care on an experimental basis.

On the downside, the development and diffusion of technology are closely intertwined with its utilization. Although cost-saving technology is also widely used, the uncontrolled use of most medical technology has prompted deep concerns about rising costs. Unlike other countries, the United States has not found a way to limit the use of high-cost medical technology. However, health policy in the United States does play a role in managing these costs—specifically, through the FDA's drug and device approval process and government funding for biomedical research.

Uncontrolled use of technology also raises bioethical concerns because human lives are involved.

Given the costs and risks associated with the use of technology, its assessment has become an area of growing interest. In the United States, the focus of health technology assessment has traditionally been on safety and efficacy. By comparison, cost-effectiveness is widely used in other countries as a criterion for making coverage decisions. Decisions based on economic worth have not received the same level of support in the United States. As escalating health care expenditures approach a critical point, the appropriateness of medical treatments may be determined based on their incremental health value at a given cost.

New health care reform efforts are likely to change some of the taxation policies established under the ACA. Otherwise, little material change affecting medical technology is expected.

▶ Test Your Understanding

Terminology

administrative information systems
asynchronous technology
biologics
clinical information systems
clinical trial
cost-benefit analysis
cost-effectiveness analysis
cost-efficiency
cost-utility analysis
decision support systems
e-health
e-therapy

effectiveness
efficacy
electronic health records (EHRs)
flat of the curve
health informatics
health information organization (HIO)
health technology assessment (HTA)
information technology (IT)
m-health
medical technology

nanomedicine
orphan drugs
quality-adjusted life year (QALY)
self-referral
smart card
synchronous technology
technological imperative
technology diffusion
telehealth
telemedicine
value
virtual physician visits

Review Questions

1. Medical technology encompasses more than just sophisticated equipment. Discuss.
2. What role does an IT department play in a modern health care organization?
3. Provide brief descriptions of clinical information systems, administrative information systems, and decision support systems in health care delivery.
4. Distinguish between information technology (IT) and health informatics.
5. According to the Institute of Medicine, what are the four main components of a fully developed electronic health record (EHR) system?

6. What are the main provisions of HIPAA with regard to the protection of personal health information? Which provisions were added to HIPAA under the HITECH Act?
7. What is telemedicine? How do the synchronous and asynchronous forms of telemedicine differ in their applications?
8. Which factors have been responsible for the low diffusion and low use of telemedicine?
9. Generally speaking, why is medical technology more readily available and used in the United States than in other countries?
10. How does technology-driven competition lead to greater levels of technology diffusion? How does technological diffusion, in turn, lead to greater competition? How does technology-driven competition lead to duplication of services?
11. Summarize the government's role in technology diffusion.
12. Provide a brief overview of how technology influences the quality of medical care and quality of life.
13. Discuss the relationship between technological innovation and health care expenditures.
14. How has technology affected access to medical care?
15. Discuss the roles of efficacy, safety, and cost-effectiveness in the context of health technology assessment.
16. Why is it important to achieve a balance between clinical efficacy and economic worth (cost-effectiveness) of medical treatments?
17. What are some of the ethical issues surrounding the development and use of medical technology?

▶ References

Adler-Milstein, J., et al. 2015. EHR adoption and hospital performance: Time-related effects. *Health Services Research* 50, no. 6: 1751–1771.

Agency for Healthcare Research and Quality (AHRQ). 2016. *Computerized provider order entry.* Available at: https://psnet.ahrq.gov/primers/primer/6/computerized-provider-order-entry. Accessed November 2016.

Appleby, J. 2008. The case of CT angiography: How Americans view and embrace new technology. *Health Affairs* 27, no. 6: 1515–1521.

Austin, C. J. 1992. *Information systems for health services administration.* 4th ed. Ann Arbor, MI: AUPHA Press/Health Administration Press.

Baker, L. C., et al. 2008. Expanded use of imaging technology and the challenge of measuring value. *Health Affairs* 27, no. 6: 1467–1478.

Barua, B., and F. Ren. 2015. Leaving Canada for medical care, 2015. *Fraser Institute Bulletin.* Available at: https://www.fraserinstitute.org/sites/default/files/leaving-canada-for-medical-care-2015.pdf. Accessed November 2016.

Bozic, K. J., et al. 2004. Health care technology assessment: Basic principles and clinical applications. *Journal of Bone and Joint Surgery* 86A, no. 6: 1305–1314.

Brechtelsbauer, E. D., et al. 2016. Review of the 2015 Drug Supply Chain Security Act. *Hospital Pharmacy* 51, no. 6: 493–500.

Bronzino, J. D., et al. 1990. *Medical technology and society: An interdisciplinary perspective.* Cambridge, MA: MIT Press.

Bryan, S., et al. 2009. Has the time come for cost-effectiveness analysis in U.S. health care? *Health Economics, Policy, and Law* 4, no. 4: 425–443.

Campanella, P., et al. 2015. The impact of electronic health records on healthcare quality: A systematic review and meta-analysis. *European Journal of Public Health* 26, no. 1: 60–64.

Cappellaro, G., et al. 2011. Diffusion of medical technology: The role of financing. *Health Policy* 100, no. 1: 51–59.

Carlson, J. 2012. Targeting constitutionality. Providers going to court over state CON laws. *Modern Healthcare* 42, no. 37: 18.

Centers for Disease Control and Prevention (CDC). 1999. *New data show AIDS patients less likely to be hospitalized.* Available at: http://www.cdc.gov /media/pressrel/r990608.htm. Accessed December 2013.

Centers for Disease Control and Prevention (CDC). 2012. *Meaningful use.* Available at: http://www .cdc.gov/ehrmeaningfuluse/introduction.html. Accessed July 2013.

Chakma, J., et al. 2014. Asia's ascent—global trends in biomedical R&D expenditures. *New England Journal of Medicine* 370, no. 1: 3–6.

Chambers, J. D., et al. 2014. Despite higher costs, specialty drugs may offer value for money comparable to that of traditional drugs. *Health Affairs* 33, no. 10: 1751–1760.

Churchill, L. R. 2011. Rationing, rightness, and distinctively human goods. *American Journal of Bioethics* 11, no. 7: 15–31.

Clayton, P. D. 2001. Confidentiality and medical information. *Annals of Emergency Medicine* 38, no. 3: 312–316.

Cleemput, I., and M. Neyt. 2015. Which quality of life measures fit your relative effectiveness assessment? *International Journal of Technology Assessment in Health* Care 31, no. 3: 147–153.

Cohen, A. B. 2004a. The adoption and use of medical technology in health care organizations. In: *Technology in American health care: Policy directions for effective evaluation and management.* A. B. Cohen and R. S. Hanft, eds. Ann Arbor, MI: University of Michigan Press. pp. 105–147.

Cohen, A. B. 2004b. Critical questions regarding medical technology and its effects. In: *Technology in American health care: Policy directions for effective evaluation and management.* A. B. Cohen and R. S. Hanft, eds. Ann Arbor, MI: University of Michigan Press. pp. 15–42.

Cohen, A. B. 2004c. The diffusion of new medical technology. In: *Technology in American health care: Policy directions for effective evaluation and management.* A. B. Cohen and R. S. Hanft, eds. Ann Arbor, MI: University of Michigan Press. pp. 79–104.

Cohen, M. F. 2016. Impact of the HITECH financial incentives on EHR adoption in small, physician-owned practices. *International Journal of Medical Informatics* 94: 143–154.

Comaniciu, D., et al. 2016. Shaping the future through innovations: From medical imaging to precision medicine. *Medical Image Analysis* 33: 19–26.

Congressional Budget Office (CBO). 2008. *Technological change and the growth of health care spending.* Washington, DC: Congressional Budget Office.

Cutler, D. M., and M. McClellan. 2001. Is technological change in medicine worth it? *Health Affairs* 20, no. 5: 11–29.

Cutler, D. M., et al. 2006. The value of medical spending in the United States, 1960–2000. *New England Journal of Medicine* 355, no. 9: 920–927.

Danzon, P. M., and M. V. Pauly. 2001. Insurance and new technology: From hospital to drugstore. *Health Affairs* 20, no. 5: 86–100.

Davis, M. P. 2006. Management of cancer pain: Focus on new opioid analgesic formulations. *American Journal of Cancer* 5, no. 3: 171–182.

Decker, S. L., et al. 2012. Physicians in nonprimary care and small practices and those age 55 and older lag in adopting electronic health record systems. *Health Affairs* 31, no. 5: 1108–1114.

de Ruiter, H., et al. 2016. Problems with the electronic health record. *Nursing Philosophy* 17, no. 1: 49–58.

DesRoches, C. M., et al. 2008. Electronic health records in ambulatory care: A national survey of physicians. *New England Journal of Medicine* 359, no. 1: 50–60.

DesRoches, C. M., et al. 2013. Some hospitals are falling behind in meeting "meaningful use" criteria and could be vulnerable to penalties in 2015. *Health Affairs* 32, no. 8: 1355–1360.

Dixon, R. F., and J. E. Stahl. 2009. A randomized trial of virtual visits in a general medicine practice. *Journal of Telemedicine and Telecare* 15, no. 3: 115–117.

Drake, D., et al. 1993. *Hard choices: Health care at what cost?* Kansas City, MO: Andrews and McMeel.

Drummond, M., et al. 2012. Can we reliably benchmark health technology assessment organizations? *International Journal of Technology Assessment in Health Care* 28, no. 2: 159–165.

Ellis, D. 2000. *Technology and the future of health care: Preparing for the next 30 years.* San Francisco, CA: Jossey-Bass Publishers.

Emanuel, E. J., et al. (2000). What makes clinical research ethical? *Journal of the American Medical Association* 283, no. 20: 2701–2711.

Epstein, M. S., et al. 2014. Biosimilars: The need, the challenge, the future: The FDA perspective. *American Journal of Gastroenterology* 109, no. 12: 1856–1859.

Field, M. J., and J. Grigsby. 2002. Telemedicine and remote patient monitoring. *Journal of the American Medical Association* 288, no. 4: 423–425.

Flannery, E. J. 1986. Should it be easier or harder to use unapproved drugs and devices? *Hastings Center Report* 16, no. 1: 17–23.

Flower, J. 2006. Imagining the future of health care. *Physician Executive* 32, no. 1: 64–66.

Food and Drug Administration (FDA). 2009a. *Federal Food and Drugs Act of 1906.* Available at: http://www.fda.gov/regulatoryinformation/legislation/ucm148690.htm. Accessed January 2010.

Food and Drug Administration (FDA). 2009b. *What are "biologics" questions and answers.* Available at: http://www.fda.gov/AboutFDA/CentersOffices/OfficeofMedicalProductsandTobacco/CBER/ucm133077.htm. Accessed July 2013.

Food and Drug Administration (FDA). 2013. *Fast track, breakthrough therapy, accelerated approval and priority review.* Available at: http://www.fda.gov/ForConsumers/ByAudience/ForPatientAdvocates/SpeedingAccesstoImportantNewTherapies/ucm128291.htm#fast. Accessed July 2013.

Food and Drug Administration (FDA). 2016a. *National Evaluation System for health Technology.* Available at: http://www.fda.gov/AboutFDA/CentersOffices/OfficeofMedicalProductsandTobacco/CDRH/CDRHReports/ucm301912.htm. Accessed November 2016.

Food and Drug Administration (FDA). 2016b. *How does FDA oversee domestic and foreign drug manufacturing?* Available at: http://www.fda.gov/AboutFDA/Transparency/Basics/ucm194989.htm. Accessed November 2016.

Fox, S., and M. Duggan. 2013. *Health online 2013.* Available at: http://www.pewinternet.org/2013/01/15/health-online-2013/. Accessed April 2017.

Frank, C., et al. 2014. Era of faster FDA drug approval has also seen increased black-box warnings and market withdrawals. *Health Affairs* 33, no. 8: 1453–1459.

Friedman, A. 2011. Rationing and social value judgements. *Journal of Bioethics* 11, no. 7: 28–29.

Fuchs, V. R. 2004. More variation in use of care, more flat-of-the-curve medicine. *Health Affairs* 23 (Variations Suppl): 104–107.

Furukawa, M. F., et al. 2013. Hospital electronic health information exchange grew substantially in 2008–12. *Health Affairs* 32, no. 8: 1346–1354.

Furukawa, M. F., et al. 2016. Electronic health record adoption and rates of in-hospital adverse events. *Journal of Patient Safety.* [Epub ahead of print]. doi: 10.1097/PTS.0000000000000257.

Giacomini, M. 2005. One of these things is not like the others: The idea of precedence in health technology assessment and coverage decisions. *Milbank Quarterly* 83, no. 2: 193–223.

Gonzalez, R. P., et al. 2009. Improving rural emergency medical service response time with global positioning system navigation. *Journal of Trauma* 67, no. 5: 899–902.

Goran, S. F. 2010. A second set of eyes: An introduction to tele-ICU. *Critical Care Nurse* 30: 46–55.

Halamka, J. D. 2010. Making the most of federal health information technology regulations. *Health Affairs* 29, no. 4: 596–600.

Hamblen, M. 2006. Hospitals expand video-conferencing. *Computerworld* 40, no. 23: 21.

Haynes, R. B., and N. L. Wilczynski. 2010. Effects of computerized clinical decision support systems on practitioner performance and patient outcomes: Methods of a decision-maker-researcher partnership systematic review. *Implementation Science* 5: 12.

Hellinger, F. J. 2009. The effect of certificate-of-need laws on hospital beds and healthcare expenditures: An empirical analysis. *American Journal of Managed Care* 15, no. 10: 737–744.

Hillestad, R., et al. 2005. Can electronic medical record systems transform health care? Potential health benefits, savings, and costs. *Health Affairs* 24, no. 5: 1103–1117.

Ho, V., et al. 2013. State deregulation and Medicare costs for acute cardiac care. *Medical Care Research & Review* 70, no. 2: 185–205.

Holtzman, Y. 2012. *The U.S. medical device industry in 2012: Challenges at home and abroad.* Available at: http://www.mddionline.com/article/medtech-2012-SWOT. Accessed July 2013.

Horowitz, B. T. 2012, March 28. Smart card use surging in health care, government. *eWeek.* p. 7.

Hospital leaders take aim at "Stark" Law in a Senate Finance Committee hearing. 2016. *AHA News* 52, no. 15: 7.

Iglehart, J. K. 1982. The cost and regulation of medical technology: Future policy directions. In: *Technology and the future of health care.* J. B. McKinlay, ed. Cambridge, MA: MIT Press. pp. 69–103.

Institute of Medicine. 1985. *Assessing medical technologies.* Washington, DC: National Academies Press.

Institute of Medicine. 2003. *Key capabilities of an electronic health records system.* Washington, DC: National Academies Press.

Johnson, C. 2010. *Generic biologics: A regulatory pathway, but who can afford the tolls?* Available at: http://wtnnews.com/articles/7486/. Accessed July 2013.

Johnston, B., et al. 2000. Outcomes of the Kaiser Permanente tele-home health research project. *Archives of Family Medicine* 9: 40–45.

Kahn, E. N., et al. 2016. Neurosurgery and telemedicine in the United States: Assessment of the risks and opportunities. *World Neurosurgery* 89: 133–138.

Kahn, J. G., et al. 2010. "Mobile" health needs and opportunities in developing countries. *Health Affairs* 29, no. 2: 252–258.

Kher, U. 2006. The hospital wars. *Time* 168, no. 24: 64–68.

Kim, M., et al. 2001. How interested are Americans in new medical technologies? A multicountry comparison. *Health Affairs* 20, no. 5: 194–201.

Kirkner, R. M. 2016. Certificate of need: '70s remnant shows its age. *Managed Care* 25, no. 3: 11–12.

Kleinke, J. D. 2001. The price of progress: Prescription drugs in the health care market. *Health Affairs* 20, no. 5: 43–60.

Korobkin, R. 2014. Relative value health insurance. *Journal of Health Politics, Policy and Law* 39, no. 2: 417–440.

Kruse, C. S., et al. 2016a. Adoption factors of the electronic health record: A systematic review. *Journal of Medical Systems* 40, no. 12: 1–7.

Kruse, C. S., et al. 2016b. Barriers to electronic health record adoption: A systematic literature review. *JMIR Medical Informatics* 4, no. 2: e19.

Lammers, E. J., and C. G. McLaughlin. 2016. Meaningful use of electronic health records and Medicare expenditures: Evidence from a panel data analysis of U.S. health care markets, 2010–2013. *Health Services Research.* [Epub ahead of print]. doi: 10.1111/1475-6773.12550.

Lammers, E. J., et al. 2016. Physician EHR adoption and potentially preventable hospital admissions among Medicare beneficiaries: Panel data evidence 2010–2013. *Health Services Research.* [Epub ahead of print]. doi: 10.1111/1475-6773.12586.

Lehoux, P., et al. 2009. What medical specialists like and dislike about health technology assessment reports. *Journal of Health Services Research & Policy* 14, no. 4: 197–203.

Li, N., et al. 2014. Reasons for and predictors of patients' online health information seeking following a medical appointment. *Family Practice* 31, no. 5: 550–556.

Littell, C. L., and R. J. Strongin. 1996. The truth about technology and health care costs. *IEEE Technology and Society Magazine* 15, no. 3: 10–14.

Luce, B. R. 1993. Medical technology and its assessment. In: *Introduction to health services.* 4th ed. S. J. Williams and P. R. Torrens, eds. Albany, NY: Delmar Publishers. pp. 245–268.

Luce, B., and R. S. Cohen. 2009. Health technology assessment in the United States. *International Journal of Technology Assessment in Health Care* 25 (Supplement 1): 33–41.

Maheu, M. M., et al. 2001. *E-health, telehealth, and telemedicine: A guide to start-up and success.* San Francisco, CA: Jossey-Bass.

Marrie, R. A., et al. 2013. Preferred sources of health information in persons with multiple sclerosis: Degree of trust and information sought. *Journal of Medical Internet Research* 15, no. 4: e67.

Martin, N. J., and J. L. Rice. 2010. Building better government IT: Understanding community beliefs and attitudes toward smart card technologies. *Behavior & Information Technology* 29, no. 4: 433–444.

McClellan, M., and D. Kessler. 1999. A global analysis of technological change in health care: The case of heart attacks. *Health Affairs* 18, no. 3: 250–257.

McGregor, M. 1989. Technology and the allocation of resources. *New England Journal of Medicine* 320, no. 2: 118–120.

Medlock, S., et al. 2016. Modeling information flows in clinical decision support: Key insights for enhancing system effectiveness. *Journal of the American Medical Informatics Association* 23, no. 5: 1001–1006.

Mennemeyer, S. T., et al. 2016. Impact of the HITECH Act on physicians' adoption of electronic health records. *Journal of the*

American Medical Informatics Association 23, no. 2: 375–379.

Merrill, R. A. 1994. Regulation of drugs and devices: An evolution. *Health Affairs* 13, no. 3: 47–69.

Milewa, T. 2006. Health technology adoption and the politics of governance in the UK. *Social Science and Medicine* 63, no. 12: 3102–3112.

Miller, R. D., Jr., and H. E. Frech III. 2000. Is there a link between pharmaceutical consumption and improved health in OECD countries? *Pharmacoeconomics* 18 (Supplement 1): 33–45.

Mitchell, J. M. 2007. The prevalence of physician self-referral arrangements after Stark II: Evidence from advanced diagnostic imaging. *Health Affairs* 26, no. 3: w415–w424.

Murphy, G. F., et al. 1999. EHR vision, definition, and characteristics. In: *Electronic health records: Changing the vision.* G. F. Murphy, et al., eds. Philadelphia, PA: Saunders. pp. 3–26.

Murphy, K. M., and R. H. Topel. 2003. The economic value of medical research. In: *Measuring the gains from medical research: An economic approach.* K. M. Murphy and R. H. Topel, eds. Chicago, IL: University of Chicago Press. pp. 41–73.

National Institute of General Medical Sciences (NIGMS). 2016. *Budget, financial management & congressional material.* Available at: https://www.nigms.nih.gov/About/Budget/Pages/default.aspx. Accessed November 2016.

Neufeld, J. D., and C. R. Doarn. 2015. Telemedicine spending by Medicare: A snapshot from 2012. *Telemedicine Journal and E-Health: The Official Journal of the American Telemedicine Association* 21, no. 8: 686–693.

Neumann, P. J., and S. D. Sullivan. 2006. Economic evaluation in the US: What is the missing link? *Pharmacoeconomics* 24, no. 11: 1163–1168.

Neumann, P. J., and M. C. Weinstein. 2010. Legislation against use of cost-effectiveness information. *New England Journal of Medicine* 363, no. 16: 1495–1497.

Nicol, N., and L. Huminski. 2006. How we cut drug errors. *Modern Healthcare* 36, no. 34: 38.

Organization for Economic Cooperation and Development (OECD). 2016. Magnetic resonance imaging (MRI) units, 2014. Available at: https://data.oecd.org/healtheqt/magnetic-resonance-imaging-mri-units.htm#indicator-chart. Accessed April 2017.

Organization for Economic Cooperation and Development (OECD). 2015. *Health at a glance 2015: OECD indicators.* Available at: http://www.keepeek.com/Digital-Asset-Management/oecd/social-issues-migration-health/health-at-a-glance-2015/knee-replacement-surgery-2013-or-nearest-year_health_glance-2015-graph87-en#.WB5vNCTAq9U. Accessed November 2016.

Peterson, L. F., and L. R. Peterson. 2004. The safety of performing diagnostic cardiac catheterizations in a mobile catheterization laboratory at primary care hospitals. *Angiology* 55, no. 5: 499–506.

Prestin, A., et al. 2015. Is online health activity alive and well or flatlining? Findings from 10 years of the Health Information National Trends Survey. *Journal of Health Communication* 20, no. 7: 790–798.

Rakich, J. S., et al. 1992. *Managing health services organizations.* Baltimore, MD: Health Professions Press.

Reiser, S. J. 1994. Criteria for standard versus experimental therapy. *Health Affairs* 13, no. 3: 127–136.

Ricci, R. P., et al. 2013. Effectiveness of remote monitoring of CIEDs in detection and treatment of clinical and device-related cardiovascular events in daily practice: The HomeGuide Registry. *Europace* 15, no. 7: 970–977.

Ricciardi, L., et al. 2013. A national action plan to support consumer engagement via e-health. *Health Affairs* 32, no. 2: 376–384.

Roark, D. C., and K. Miguel. 2006. Replacing bar coding: Radio frequency identification. *Nursing* 36, no. 12: 30.

Robinson, M. D., et al. 2016. Measuring satisfaction and usability of facetime for virtual visits in patients with uncontrolled diabetes. *Telemedicine & e-Health* 22, no. 2: 138–143.

Rochlen, A. B., et al. 2004. Online therapy: Review of relevant definitions, debates, and current empirical support. *Journal of Clinical Psychology* 60, no. 3: 269–283.

Rosenthal, G. 1979. Anticipating the costs and benefits of new technology: A typology for policy. In: *Medical technology: The culprit behind health care costs?* S. Altman and R. Blendon, eds. Washington, DC: U.S. Government Printing Office. pp. 77–87.

Sampat, B., and M. Drummond. 2011. Another special relationship? Interactions between health technology policies and health care systems in the United States and the United Kingdom. *Journal of Health Politics, Policy and Law* 36, no. 1: 119–139.

Schoder, J., and P. Zweifel. 2011. Flat-of-the-curve medicine: A new perspective on the production of health. *Health Economics Review* 1, no. 1: 1–10.

Schur, C. L., and M. L. Berk. 2008. Views on health care technology: Americans consider the risks and sources of information. *Health Affairs* 27, no. 6: 1654–1664.

Sclafani, J., et al. 2013. Mobile tablet use among academic physicians and trainees. *Journal of Medical Systems* 37, no. 1: 1–6.

Seidel, L. F., et al. 1995. *Applied quantitative methods for health services management.* Baltimore, MD: Health Professions Press.

Shaw, L. J., et al. 2000. Clinical and economic outcomes assessment in nuclear cardiology. *Quarterly Journal of Nuclear Medicine* 44, no. 2: 138–152.

Shuren, J., and R. M. Califf. 2016. Need for a national evaluation system for health technology. *Journal of the American Medical Association* 316, no. 11: 1153–1154.

Silow-Carroll, S., et al. 2012. *Using electronic health records to improve quality and efficiency: The experiences of leading hospitals.* New York, NY: Commonwealth Fund.

Skinner, A. E. G., and G. Latchford. 2006. Attitudes to counselling via the Internet: A comparison between in-person counselling client and Internet support group users. *Counseling and Psychotherapy Research* 6, no. 3: 92–97.

Slotwiner, D., and B. Wilkoff. 2013. Cost efficiency and reimbursement of remote monitoring: A US perspective. *Europace* 15 (Supplement 1): i54–i58.

Sobolev, B. G., et al. 2013. The occurrence of adverse events in relation to time after registration for coronary artery bypass surgery: A population-based observational study. *Journal of Cardiothoracic Surgery* 8, no. 1 (Special Section): 1–14.

Sorenson, C., et al. 2013. Medical technology as a key driver of rising health expenditures: Disentangling the relationship. *ClinicoEconomics and Outcomes Research* 5: 223–234.

Steinbrook, R. 2009. The NIH stimulus: The Recovery Act and biomedical research. *New England Journal of Medicine* 360, no. 15: 1479–1481.

Stofle, G. S. 2001. *Choosing an online therapist.* Harrisburg, PA: White Hat Communications.

Taub, J. 2011. The smallest revolution: 5 recent breakthroughs in nanomedicine. *Scientific American.* Available at: http://blogs.scientific american.com/guest-blog/2011/09/30/the -smallest-revolution-five-recent-breakthroughs -in-nanomedicine. Accessed July 2013.

Teichert, E. 2016. Putting telemedicine behind bars. *Modern Healthcare* 46, no. 43: 22.

Thompson Coburn LLP. 2013. *2013 HIPAA changes.* Available at: http://www.jdsupra.com /legalnews/2013-hipaa-changes-59764/. Accessed April 2017.

Thorley, A. J., and T. D. Tetley. 2013. New perspectives in nanomedicine. *Pharmacology & Therapeutics* 140, no. 2: 176–185.

Tripp, S., et al. 2012. *The economic impact of the U.S. advanced medical technology industry.* Cleveland, OH: Battelle Technology Partnership Practice.

Tustin, N. 2010. The role of patient satisfaction on online health information seeking. *Journal of Health Communication* 15, no. 1: 3–17.

Wachler, A. B., and P. A. Avery. 2011. *Stark II proposed regulations: Rule offers additional guidance while regulators seek more input from health care community.* Available at: http://www .wachler.com/CM/Publications/Publications17 .asp. Accessed January 2011.

Wan, T. T. H. 1995. *Analysis and evaluation of health care systems: An integrated approach to managerial decision making.* Baltimore, MD: Health Professions Press.

Wang, T., et al. 2013. Funding alternatives in EHR adoption beyond HITECH incentives and traditional approaches. *Healthcare Financial Management* 67, no. 5: 86–91.

Wild, C. 2005. Ethics of resource allocation: Instruments for rational decision making in support of a sustainable health care. *Poiesis & Praxis* 3, no. 4: 296–309.

Wodarski, J., and J. Frimpong. 2013. Application of e-therapy programs to the social work practice. *Journal of Human Behavior in the Social Environment* 23, no. 1: 29–36.

Wong, C. Y., et al. 2016. Oral delivery of insulin for treatment of diabetes: Status quo, challenges and opportunities. *Journal of Pharmacy and Pharmacology* 68, no. 9: 1093–1108.

Yanamadala, S., et al. 2016. Electronic health records and quality of care: An observational study modeling impact on mortality, readmissions, and complications. *Medicine* 95, no. 19: e3332.

Ybarra, M. L., and W. W. Eaton. 2005. Internet-based mental health interventions. *Mental Health Services Research* 7, no. 2: 75–87.

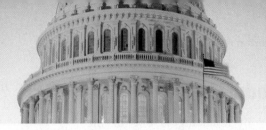

CHAPTER 6
Health Services Financing

LEARNING OBJECTIVES

- Study the role of health care financing and its impact on the delivery of health care.
- Understand the basic concept of insurance and how general insurance terminology applies to health insurance.
- Differentiate among group insurance, self-insurance, individual health insurance, managed care, high-deductible plans, and Medigap plans.
- Explore trends in employer-based health insurance.
- Examine the distinctive features of public insurance programs, such as Medicare, Medicaid, the Children's Health Insurance Program, the Department of Defense's programs, the Veterans Health Administration, and the Indian Health Service.
- Understand the various methods of reimbursement and developing trends in reimbursement.
- Discuss national health care and personal health care expenditures and trends in private and public financing.
- Explore the effects of the Affordable Care Act on financing and insurance.
- Assess current directions and issues in health care financing.

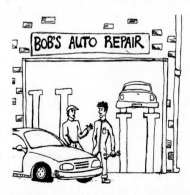

"I have comprehensive insurance."

▶ Introduction

Complexity of financing is one of the primary characteristics of medical care delivery in the United States. Single-payer systems in countries such as Australia, Canada, and the United Kingdom simplify health care financing: Taxes are raised by the government to provide health insurance to the citizens, and private financing plays a minor role for those who want more extensive coverage than what the government offers. In the United States, both public and private financing play substantial roles. In the public sector, the government has created a multitude of tax-financed programs; each program serves a defined category of citizens provided they meet the established qualifications. Insurance overlap is also relatively common. For example, a significant number of Medicare beneficiaries either qualify for Medicaid or have purchased private supplementary insurance to pay for expenses not covered by Medicare. In the private sector, financing for health insurance is shared between the employer and the employee; the employer provides the bulk of financing. Self-employed people purchase health insurance in the open market. For the unemployed, the underemployed (those working part-time who do not qualify for employer-sponsored health insurance), and those who had lost their private insurance due to the original formulation of the Affordable Care Act (ACA), the government attempted to facilitate the purchase of health insurance starting in 2014.

The actual payments to providers of care are handled in numerous ways. Patients generally pay a portion of the costs directly, but the bulk of these costs are paid through a variety of insurance plans and government programs. The government and some large employers use the services of third-party administrators to process payment claims from providers.

In this chapter, financing is discussed in broad terms that include the concepts of financing, insurance, and payment. This does not mean, however, that the three functions are structurally integrated. For example, government-financed programs, such as Medicare and Medicaid, integrate the functions of financing and insurance, but contracted third-party administrators make the actual payments to the providers after services have been delivered. Traditional insurance plans integrate the functions of insurance and payment, whereas both employers and employees provide the financing. Managed care has gone one step further in integrating all four functions of health care delivery—financing, insurance, delivery, and payment.

This chapter focuses on financing for both private and public health insurance, points out trends, discusses health care expenditures, explains various payment methods to reimburse providers, and provides glimpses into what the ACA was able to achieve and where it fell short. The chapter concludes with current directions and issues in health insurance and financing.

▶ The Role and Scope of Health Services Financing

As its central role, health services financing pays for health insurance premiums. Providers generally rely on the patients' insurance to get paid for the services they deliver. The various methods used to determine how much providers should be paid (i.e., reimbursement) for their services are also closely intertwined with the broad financing function.

To a large extent, financing determines who has access to health care and who does not, although many uninsured people have access to charitable care, and charity will continue to play a noteworthy role for a sector of the population in the United States. Regardless of which health care reform initiatives are eventually passed in President Donald Trump's administration, there always will be uninsured people in America—such as illegal immigrants, young healthy individuals who choose not to buy insurance, and those who do not qualify for Medicaid based on income—just as there were still a sizable number of uninsured people under the ACA.

The demand for health care greatly influences its financing. Health insurance increases the demand for covered services; the demand would be less if those same services were paid out of pocket. Increased demand means greater utilization of health services, given adequate supply. According to economic theory, insurance lowers the out-of-pocket cost of medical care to consumers; hence, they will consume more medical services than if they had to pay the entire price out of their own pockets. Consumer behavior that leads to a higher utilization of health care services when the services are covered by insurance is referred to as **moral hazard** (Feldstein, 1993).

Financing also exerts powerful influences on supply-side factors, such as how much health care is produced in the private sector. Health care services and technology proliferate when services are covered by insurance. Even new services and technologies may start emerging, and new models of organization may form. Conversely, when reimbursement is cut, supply of health care services can also be curtailed.

Issues pertaining to reimbursement for services are critical in health services management decision making. Demand-side factors, including reimbursement, typically guide health services managers in evaluating the type and extent of services to offer. The amount of reimbursement needed to recoup capital costs over time also heavily influences decisions such as acquisition of new equipment, renovation or expansion of facilities, and launching of new services.

Similarly, financing can influence the supply and distribution of health care professionals. As an example, employer financing for dental insurance spawned the growth of dentists and dental hygienists. Mechanisms for reimbursing physicians, such as the resource-based relative value scale (RBRVS) used by Medicare, directly affect physicians' incomes. One of the main goals of RBRVS, implemented in 1992, was to entice more medical residents into general practice by increasing the reimbursement for services provided by generalists. Due to other factors, however, the imbalance between generalists and specialists has persisted.

Financing eventually affects—both directly and indirectly—the total health care expenditures incurred by a health care delivery system. The next section discusses the relationship between financing and health care expenditures and provides a general framework for controlling health care costs.

▶ Financing and Cost Control

Health care financing and cost control are closely intertwined. **FIGURE 6-1** presents a conceptual model of cost control. In the U.S. health care delivery system, insurance is the main factor that determines the level of demand for medical services. Restricting financing for health insurance—as occurs with demand-side rationing—eventually controls total health care expenditures. Conversely, extension of health insurance to the uninsured, without supply-side rationing, increases total health care expenditures (E). Apart from the extent of insurance coverage, the cost of health insurance also affects system-wide health care expenditures.

Insurance, along with payment (price = P), influences the supply or availability of health services. Reducing reimbursement for providers has a direct influence on E, as well as an indirect influence through shrinkage in supply. Cuts in reimbursement have been used in the United States, as well as in other countries, as a primary strategy to contain the growth of health care expenditures.

Diffusion of technology and other types of services can be directly restricted through health planning, which is commonly used in countries that have national health insurance. When supply of technology is rationed, people may be insured but do not have free access to those services. Reduced utilization of expensive technology results in direct savings. Countries that have national health care also achieve indirect savings by having fewer specialist physicians and specialized technicians and by spending less on research and development (R&D).

Insurance and supply of health care services together determine access and, ultimately, the utilization of services (quantity of services consumed = Q). Utilization can also be directly controlled. For example, private health insurance, as well as Medicare and Medicaid, try to exert some limits on utilization by specifying which services are not covered.

Because E = P × Q, rising health care costs can be controlled by managing the numerous factors that influence P and Q. Many of these factors are external to the health care delivery system. The P component, for example, includes general economy-wide inflation, as well as medical

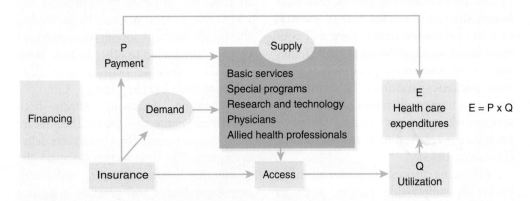

FIGURE 6-1 Influence of financing on the delivery of health services.

inflation that exceeds general inflation. In addition to being influenced by the intrinsic factors discussed in this section, the Q component is a function of changes in the size and demographic composition (i.e., age, sex, and racial mix) of the population (Levitt et al., 1994).

▶ The Insurance Function

Insurance is a mechanism for protection against risk; that is its primary purpose. In this context, **risk** refers to the possibility of a substantial financial loss from an event of which the probability of occurrence is relatively small (at least in a given individual's case). For example, even though auto accidents are common in the United States, the likelihood is quite small that a specific individual will have an auto accident in a given year. Even when the risk is small, people buy insurance to protect their assets against catastrophic loss.

The insuring agency that assumes risk is called the **insurer**, or underwriter. **Underwriting** is a systematic technique for evaluating, selecting (or rejecting), classifying, and rating risks. Medical underwriting, for example, takes into account the health status of people to be insured. Four fundamental principles underlie the concept of insurance (Health Insurance Institute, 1969; Vaughn and Elliott, 1987):

- Risk is unpredictable for the individual insured.
- Risk can be predicted with a reasonable degree of accuracy for a large group or a population.
- Insurance provides a mechanism for transferring or shifting risk from the individual to the group through the pooling of resources.
- All members of the insured group share actual losses on some equitable basis.

Technically, health care services for all Americans 65 and older (the elderly population) are provided through Medicare. For those younger than age 65, private insurance—either employment based or self-financed—is the predominant avenue for receiving health care. Medicaid and the Children's Health Insurance Program (CHIP) cover many of the poor, including children in low-income households. Other public programs cover defined groups of people, such as the insurance program offered by the Department of Veterans Affairs (VA) and the military health system. The remainder of the population, without any coverage, are the uninsured.

Because of some overlap in coverage, it is almost impossible to neatly fit people into categories based on specific types of health insurance. **FIGURE 6-2** provides broad approximations of the proportion of the U.S. population covered through private and public sources of health insurance. Under the ACA, coverage under both private and public sources increased between 2013 and 2015, and the proportion of uninsured dropped from 13.3% to 9.1% (Barnett and Vornovitsky, 2016).

Health insurance, particularly private health insurance, comes in the form of a **plan**, which specifies, among other details, information pertaining to costs, covered services, and ways to obtain health care when needed. Numerous plans are available. Anyone covered by health insurance is called the **insured** or a **beneficiary**. Two types of employer-sponsored plans are single coverage plans and family coverage plans; the latter cover the spouse

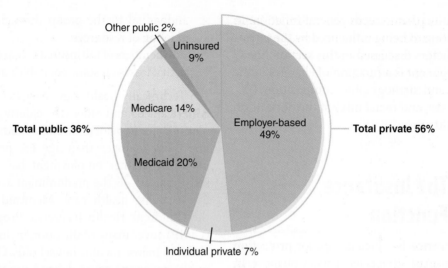

FIGURE 6-2 Health insurance status of the total U.S. population, 2015.

Note: Numbers may not add to 100 because of rounding.

Data from Kaiser Family Foundation. 2017. *Health insurance coverage of the total population. Timeframe: 2015.* Available at: http://kff.org/other/state -indicator/total-population/?currentTimeframe=0. Accessed January 2017.

and dependent children of the working employee. Medicare and Medicaid plans recognize only individual beneficiaries. In the case of married couples, for instance, Medicare and Medicaid recognize each spouse as an independent beneficiary.

▶ Private Health Insurance

Private health insurance has also been called "voluntary health insurance." Most private health insurance is employment based, but workers are not mandated to buy it. Private insurance includes many different types of health plan providers, such as commercial insurance companies (e.g., United Health Group, Well Point, Cigna, and Aetna), Blue Cross/Blue Shield, and managed care organizations (MCOs). The nonprofit Blue Cross and Blue Shield Associations are similar to private health insurance companies, and the

companies named here operate their own MCOs. Many businesses are self-insured, using insurance companies for stop-loss coverage.

Basic Health Insurance Terminology

Premiums

A **premium** is the amount charged by the insurer to insure against specified risks. An employer may offer more than one health insurance plan, in which case premiums can vary depending on the plan selected by the employee. Employment-based health insurance is heavily subsidized by the employer, and the employee is asked to share in the cost of premiums. Cost trends are discussed later in this chapter.

Risk Rating

Premiums are determined by the actuarial assessment of risk, or **risk rating**, that adjusts premiums to reflect health status. Three different methods have been used to determine premiums: experience rating, community rating, and adjusted community rating.

Experience rating is based on a group's own medical claims experience. Under this method, premiums differ from group to group because different groups have different risks. For example, people working in various industries are exposed to various levels and types of hazards, people in certain occupations are more susceptible to certain illnesses or injuries, and older groups represent higher risks than younger groups. High-risk groups are expected to incur high utilization of medical care services, so these groups are charged higher premiums compared to preferred or favorable risk groups. The main issue with experience rating is that it makes premiums unaffordable for high-risk groups.

Community rating spreads the risk among members of a larger population. Premiums are based on the utilization experience of the entire population covered by the same type of health insurance. Under pure community rating, the same rate applies to everyone regardless of age, gender, occupation, or any other indicator of health risk (Goodman and Musgrave, 1992). For example, a person who is employed in a hazardous occupation would pay the same premium as someone who does not. When premiums are based on community rating, the good risks—that is, healthy people—actually subsidize the insurance cost for the poor risks (Somers and Somers, 1977). In other words, costs shift from people in poor health to people in good health and make health insurance less affordable for those who are healthy.

Adjusted community rating, also known as modified community rating, is a middle-of-the road approach that overcomes the main drawbacks of experience rating and pure community rating. Under this method, price differences take into account demographic factors such as age, gender, geography, and family composition, while ignoring other risk factors. The ACA required the use of adjusted community rating to determine premiums for individuals and small groups.

Cost Sharing

In addition to paying a share of the cost of premiums through payroll deductions, insured individuals pay a portion of the actual cost of medical services out of their own pockets. These out-of-pocket expenses take the form of deductibles and copayments and are incurred only if and when medical services are used. A **deductible** is the amount the insured must first pay each year before any benefits are payable by the plan. For example, suppose a plan requires the insured to pay a $1,000 deductible. When the insured receives medical care, the plan starts paying only after the cost of medical services received by the insured has exceeded $1,000 in a given year. Many plans now allow the insured to use primary care and wellness services without having to pay a deductible.

The second type of cost sharing is a **copayment**, which is a flat amount the insured must pay each time health services are received. Health plans may also use **coinsurance**, which is a set proportion of the medical costs that the insured must pay out of pocket. As an example, for a certain health care product or service covered by a health plan, a copayment of $30 or an 80/20 coinsurance may be required. In the latter case, once the deductible has been met, the plan pays 80% of the costs; the insured pays the remaining 20%.

In case of a catastrophic illness or injury, the deductible and copayment/coinsurance amounts can add up to a substantial sum. Hence, health plans generally have an annual maximum limit on out-of-pocket cost sharing. Once the maximum cost sharing amount has been reached, the plan pays 100% of any additional expenses.

The rationale for cost sharing is to control utilization of health care services. Since insurance creates moral hazard by insulating the insured against the cost of health care, making the insured share in the cost promotes more responsible behavior in health care utilization. A comprehensive study employing a controlled experimental design conducted in the 1970s, commonly referred to as the Rand Health Insurance Experiment, demonstrated that cost sharing had a material impact on lowering utilization, without any significant negative health consequences. Experts now generally agree that cost sharing reduces utilization. It should be noted, however, that even though moral hazard does exist, and it results in frivolous and inefficient services, expensive health care procedures in case of serious illness become affordable only with insurance (Nyman and Trenz, 2016).

Covered Services

Services covered by an insurance plan are referred to as **benefits**. Each health insurance plan spells out in a contract both the type of medical services it covers and the services it does not cover. A typical disclaimer included in most contracts states that only "medically necessary" services are covered, regardless of whether such services are provided by a physician. Almost all plans include medical and surgical services, hospitalizations, emergency services, prescriptions, maternity care, and delivery of a baby. Within specified limits, most plans also provide mental health services, substance abuse services, home health care, skilled nursing care, rehabilitation, supplies, and equipment. Services such as eyeglasses and dental care are generally not covered by health insurance; vision and dental insurance plans can be purchased separately. Services most commonly excluded are those not ordered by a physician, such as self-care and over-the-counter products. Other services commonly excluded from health insurance coverage are cosmetic and reconstructive surgery, work-related illness and injury (covered under workers' compensation), rest cures, genetic counseling, and the like.

Types of Private Insurance

Group Insurance

Group insurance can be obtained through an employer, a union, or a professional organization. A **group insurance** program anticipates that a substantial number of people in the group will purchase insurance through its sponsor. Because risk is spread out among the many insured, group insurance provides the advantage of lower costs than if the same type of coverage was purchased in the individual insurance market.

Unlike monetary wages, health insurance benefits provided through an employer are not subject to income tax. Consequently, a dollar of health insurance received from the employer is worth more than the same amount received in taxable wages or an after-tax dollar spent out of pocket for medical care. The tax policy provides an incentive to obtain health insurance as a benefit that is largely paid by the employer.

Starting in the 1950s, major medical insurance became widely available. This type of insurance was designed to cover catastrophic situations that could subject families to substantial financial hardships, such as hospitalization, extended illness, and expensive surgery. Since the 1970s, health insurance plans have become comprehensive in coverage, and include basic and routine physician office visits and diagnostic services. Hence, health insurance today is an anomaly to the fundamental concept behind insurance. Comprehensive coverage has also increased the cost of health insurance.

Self-Insurance

In a **self-insured plan**, the employer acts as its own insurer instead of obtaining insurance through an insurance company. Rather than pay insurers a dividend to bear the risk, many employers simply assume the risk by budgeting a certain amount to pay medical claims incurred by their employees. In 2016, 61% of all covered workers in private and public organizations were enrolled in self-insured plans; 94% of workers employed in businesses with 5,000 or more employees were in self-insured plans (Kaiser Family Foundation, and Health Research and Educational Trust [Kaiser/HRET], 2016, p. 188).

Both large and small employers can self-insure, but most that choose this route are large businesses. Self-insured employers can protect themselves against any potential risk of high losses by purchasing **reinsurance**, also called stop-loss coverage, from a private insurance company. Being self-insured gives employers a greater degree of control, and costs are contained through a slower rise in premiums during periods of rapid inflation (Gabel et al., 2003).

The movement toward self-insurance by large employers was spurred by government policies. Self-insured employers are exempt from a premium tax that insurance companies must pay, the cost of which is passed on to customers through higher premiums. Further, the Employee Retirement Income Security Act (ERISA) of 1974 exempts self-insured plans from certain mandatory benefits that regular health insurance plans are required to provide in many states. Self-insured plans also avoid other types of state insurance regulations, such as reserve requirements and consumer protection requirements. Because of these plans' many advantages, employers that are large enough to make it feasible for themselves have viewed self-insurance as a better economic alternative. Notably, the ACA did not affect self-insured plans, so they have remained immune from certain ACA mandates, such as the one requiring health plans to include "essential health benefits" (Noble and Chirba, 2013).

Individual Private Health Insurance

Individually purchased private health insurance (nongroup plans) has been a relatively small, but important source of coverage for some Americans. In 2015, approximately 7% of the U.S. population had nongroup private insurance (Kaiser, 2017). The family farmer, the early retiree, the self-employed person, and the employee of a business that does not offer health insurance—all of these people tend to rely on individual health insurance. For underwriting purposes, the risk indicated by each individual's health status and demographics are taken into account. Consequently, high-risk individuals are often unable to obtain privately purchased health insurance. This barrier was eliminated by provisions in the ACA that required health insurers to cover anyone regardless of pre-existing medical conditions.

Managed Care Plans

MCOs, such as health maintenance organizations (HMOs) and preferred provider organizations (PPOs), emerged in the 1980s in response to the rapid escalation of health care costs. At first, managed care plans differed from and were less expensive than the plans offered by traditional insurance companies. However, several factors over time converged on MCOs, and traditional insurance companies eventually began offering managed care plans. Today, the vast majority of health insurance takes the form of managed care plans.

High-Deductible Health Plans and Savings Options

High-deductible health plans (HDHPs) combine a savings option with a health insurance plan that carries a high deductible. HDHPs have shown significant growth in recent years. In 2016, HDHPs covered 29% of all workers in employment-based plans, up from just 4% in 2006 (Kaiser/HRET, 2016, p. 3). Because of their high deductibles, premiums for HDHPs are generally lower than those for other types of health plans.

Savings options give consumers greater control over how to use the funds. Hence, these plans are also referred to as **consumer-directed health plans**. There are two main types of HDHPs/savings options, which are subject to different guidelines under U.S. tax law (**EXHIBIT 6-1**).

Short-Term Stop-Gap Coverage

People often leave an employer for various reasons. Leaving an employer means loss of health insurance coverage, at least temporarily. For example, when people move to a different employer, they may encounter a waiting period before their new health insurance starts. The waiting period was limited to 90 days or less under the ACA. Other individuals may face temporary unemployment after separating from a job. Some people leave the workforce before age 65, so they do not qualify for Medicare. To address short-term coverage gaps, Congress passed the Consolidated Omnibus Budget Reconciliation Act (COBRA) of 1985, which allows workers to keep their employer's group coverage for 18 months after leaving a job. The individuals are required to pay 102% of the group rate to continue health benefits, but because the employer subsidy is no longer available, the high cost of premiums prevents many from keeping their health insurance during periods of insurance gap.

The Health Insurance Portability and Accountability Act (HIPAA) of 1996 provided for continued coverage beyond the original COBRA provisions. Extended coverage of up to 29 months is available if the insured or a family member is determined by the Social Security Administration to be disabled at any time during the first 60 days of COBRA coverage. Extended coverage of up to 36 months is available to the spouse and dependent children if the

EXHIBIT 6-1 Key Differences Between a Health Reimbursement Arrangement and a Health Savings Account[1]

Health Reimbursement Arrangement (HRA)	Health Savings Account (HSA)
Established solely by the employer. Self-employed individuals cannot establish an HRA. The account is owned by the employer.	Established by the individual. The employer can assist in establishing an HSA. The account is owned by the employee.
Having an HDHP is not mandatory. Employers may offer HRAs in addition to or in place of health insurance, which may include an HDHP. Funds are used for deductibles, copayments, insurance premiums, and other medical and related expenses authorized by the Internal Revenue Service.	The individual must have a "qualified health plan" that meets federal standards and is an HDHP. The minimum annual deductible for 2017 was $1,300 for a single plan ($2,600 for a family plan). In 2017, the maximum annual out-of-pocket expenses for deductibles and copayments were capped at $6,550 for a single plan ($13,100 for a family plan). Funds cannot be used for HDHP premiums.
Funded solely by the employer; employees are not allowed to contribute. There is no limit on the amount of contribution. Contributions are tax free.	The individual must fund the HSA. Employers may contribute, but are not required to do so. The maximum contribution for 2017, which is fully tax deductible, was $3,400 for a single plan ($6,750 for a family plan). Enrollees who are 55 years and older can contribute an extra $1,000 to either plan.
An employer may offer an HRA to a retiree even after age 65, or allow a retiree or terminated employee to keep an existing HRA. Conversely, an employer may terminate the account.	The individual must be younger than age 65 and not have any other health insurance (dental, vision, and long-term care insurance do not count). When a person becomes eligible for Medicare at age 65, the remaining balance in an HSA can be used, but no funds can be added.

[1] An employer may offer an HRA and an HSA. In this case, funds from the HRA can be used to pay the premiums for an HDHP, which is required with the HSA.

former employee dies, enrolls in Medicare, or gets divorced or legally separated.

Medigap

Medigap, also called Medicare Supplement Insurance, is private health insurance that can be purchased only by those enrolled in the original Medicare program—a program that has high out-of-pocket costs (discussed later in the "Medicare" section). It is illegal for an insurance company to sell a Medigap plan to someone who is covered by Medicaid or Medicare Advantage. Medigap plans cover all or a portion of Medicare deductibles and copayments/coinsurance.

Federal law requires the sale of only standardized plans, each containing uniform benefits to help consumers decide which plan would best suit their needs. There are 10 federally approved standard plans, but not all states have all the plans available. These plans are labeled A through D, F, G, and K through N. The out-of-pocket costs most commonly covered by the plans include hospital deductibles and copayments, skilled nursing facility copayments, and Part B deductibles and copayments/coinsurance. Medigap plans do not cover extended long-term care, vision care, dental care, hearing aids, or private-duty nursing. Premiums vary according to the plan selected and the insurance company selling the plan.

Trends in Private Health Insurance

Until recently, private health insurance coverage (both employer based and individually purchased) among Americans had been steadily declining for several years. For example, in 2000, 75.1% of the U.S. population younger than age 65 (those older than age 65 are covered by Medicare) was covered by private health insurance. By 2010, that proportion had dropped to 61.7%. A small uptick in coverage occurred between 2013 and 2014, from 61.8% to 63.7% covered (National Center for Health Statistics [NCHS], 2016, p. 313). It is very likely that this increase reflects some of the effects of the ACA. Although the ACA may have increased privately purchased health insurance, it has not really had a positive effect on overall employment-based coverage, as pointed out in the next section.

Trends in Employment-Based Health Insurance

The ACA's employer mandate for providing job-based health insurance went into effect in 2015. This mandate applied to employers with 50 or more full-time equivalent (FTE) workers. Often referred to as a **play-or-pay** mandate, it required employers to either provide their employees with health insurance (play) or pay a penalty for not doing so.

Almost 93% of all employers in the United States, however, employ fewer than 50 FTE employees. Only 1.6% of employers had 200 or more workers in 2016—yet those large employers employed 62% of the workforce (Kaiser/HRET, 2016, p. 19).

TABLE 6-1 shows, by employer size, the percentage of employers that offer health insurance and the percentage of workers covered by health benefits. There was clearly an upward trend in both the offer and coverage rates among small employers (3–49 workers) between 2005 and 2010. Surprisingly, after 2010, when the ACA was passed, both offer and coverage rates declined. The rates dropped even further in 2016, after the employer mandate took effect in 2015. Clearly, the ACA had a negative effect on workers employed by small businesses.

Among large employers (200 or more workers), even though the offer rates have remained relatively stable over time, worker coverage has slowly declined, reaching its lowest point of 61% in 2016. Whether these effects are attributable to the ACA is not clear. In fact, the downward trend has been occurring for several years. For example, among large employers, 69% of the workers were covered under their employer's health plan in 2001. The offer rates since then have not changed—so we must look

TABLE 6-1 Trends in Employment-Based Health Insurance, Selected Years

	Workforce Size	2005	2010	2015	2016
Percentage of employers offering health insurance	3–9 workers	47	59	47	46
	10–24 workers	72	76	63	61
	25–49 workers	87	92	82	80
	≥ 200 workers	97	99	98	98
Percentage of covered workers	3–24 workers	41	44	35	32
	25–49 workers	55	59	49	47
	≥ 200 workers	66	63	63	61

Data from Kaiser Family Foundation, and Health Research and Educational Trust (Kaiser/HRET). 2016. *Employer health benefits: 2016 annual survey.* Menlo Park, CA: Author.

to structural changes within the American industry for possible answers as to why the worker coverage rates have decreased.

In recent years, many large corporations have folded their manufacturing operations in the United States and moved those operations overseas. Consequently, employment in the United States has shifted toward lower-paying jobs in the service industries. For example, among businesses that offer health insurance, 77% of the employees in the manufacturing sector obtained coverage, compared to only 37% in the retail sector (Kaiser/HRET, 2016, p. 61). Even though their employers might offer health insurance benefits, the premiums are too expensive for many of these workers. In addition, more workers have moved (willingly or unwillingly) into part-time jobs. Those who decide not to be covered under their employer's plans may have either paid the penalty under the ACA's individual mandate or purchased insurance through government-sponsored exchanges, especially if they qualified for tax subsidies.

Premium Costs in Employment-Based Plans

Businesses, mainly the smaller ones, that do not offer health insurance to their employees continue to cite cost as the most important reason for not doing so (Kaiser/HRET, 2016, p. 42). During the 5-year period of 2011 to 2016, the average premium costs for employers rose 18.5% for an individual plan, from $5,429 to $6,435 per year, and the average premium costs rose a little more than 20% for a family plan, from $15,073 to $18,142 per year (Kaiser/HRET, 2011; 2016). During this same period, the employee share of the premiums rose by 22% for single coverage and by 28% for family coverage, while the overall inflation rate rose by 6% and workers' earnings rose by 11% (Kaiser/ HRET, 2016, pp. 38, 88). Employers have increasingly shifted the burden of health insurance costs to their workers, and workers have spent more of their earnings on health insurance because their wages have not increased at the same rate as the cost of insurance. Before the ACA was implemented, rising cost of health insurance was the most cited reason by workers who did not purchase employment-based health insurance (Employee Benefit Research Institute [EBRI], 2013). In 2014, they were mandated to purchase health insurance either from their employers or through the government exchanges. The ACA, however, was not effective in making health insurance more affordable.

Trends in Utilization Costs: Cost Sharing

Between 2011 and 2016, the average annual deductible rose from $991 to $1,478 for an individual plan, an increase of almost 50%. The lowest deductible in PPO plans ($1,028 in 2016) rose by 52%. PPO plan deductibles for family coverage ($2,147 in 2016) rose by 41% during the same period (Kaiser/HRET, 2016, pp. 128, 140).

As for copayments/coinsurance, only 7% of employer-sponsored plans did not require these employee payments for primary care visits in 2016. The average copayment was $24 for primary care and $38 for specialty care office visits (Kaiser/ HRET, 2016, p. 147). The ACA placed limits on total out-of-pocket cost sharing for deductibles and copayments/coinsurance.

In 2017, these limits were $7,150 and $14,300 for single and family plans, respectively.

▶ Private Coverage and Cost Under the Affordable Care Act

The ACA segmented the individual health insurance market into two groups: those who bought coverage through the government-established exchanges (also called "marketplaces") to benefit from federal premium subsidies, and those who did not qualify for premium subsidies and bought health insurance outside the exchanges. To help them purchase health insurance through the exchanges, premium subsidies were made available to people with incomes between 100% and 400% of the federal poverty level (FPL), provided these people did not qualify for Medicaid or employment-based coverage.

The number of Americans who gained health insurance under the various provisions of the ACA has been estimated to be approximately 20 million (Jost and Pollack, 2016), or an estimated 7.3% of the nonelderly U.S. population. Of these people, almost 44% were enrolled in Medicaid, 23% in exchange-based plans (with premium subsidies), and 8.8% in other privately purchased health plans (without premium subsidies). Approximately 28.2 million people remained uninsured (Blumberg and Holahan, 2016).[1]

---

[1] Blumberg and Holahan estimated that almost 5 million people gained health insurance through their employers subsequent to the implementation of the ACA. However, data from the Employer Health Benefits Survey (Kaiser/HRET, 2016), as discussed previously, do not bear this contention out.

In the context of coverage and cost, six main provisions of the ACA are noteworthy. First, effective September 2010, insurers were mandated to enroll young adults until the age of 26 under their parents' plans. Prior to this law, coverage for young adults typically ended at age 19, or at age 23 in case of full-time students (Shane et al., 2016). Between the pre-ACA period of 2007–2009 and the post-ACA period of 2011–2013, uninsurance among young adults declined by 5 percentage points (Berger, 2015). The law helped mainly nonpoor young adults in gaining insurance coverage (Berger, 2015; Han et al., 2016). The pool of young adults covered as a result of the mandate increased by 2.1% and, as expected, the mandate resulted in an increase in insurance premiums. Instead of passing the higher costs to the employees through higher employee contributions, it is likely that employers may have increased the amount of cost sharing in family plans (Depew and Bailey, 2015), as detailed in the previous section. Despite the additional cost, the mandate did not lead to any significant increase in preventive care utilization (Barbaresco et al., 2015), or use of other key services such as doctor visits and prescription drug fills (Shane et al., 2016). This outcome is not surprising given that this age group is generally healthy. Most of them very likely would not have purchased insurance on their own.

Second, in 2014, the ACA made it illegal to charge more or to refuse coverage for people who had **preexisting conditions**, such as diabetes, cancer, heart disease, and HIV/AIDS. Even though charging more or refusing insurance to people with poor health status can be criticized on equity grounds, a disregard of insurance underwriting principles makes premiums increase for everyone, and healthy people end up subsidizing health insurance for the unhealthy. As would be expected, the ACA improved access to health care for high-cost individuals who had preexisting conditions (Jost and Pollack, 2016).

Third, all health plans had to include certain "essential health benefits" and meet certain requirements. Only "qualified health plans" could be sold through the exchanges. Among other benefits, health plans were required to include preventive and wellness care. Of special note was coverage for contraceptives with no cost sharing—a benefit designed to help, in particular, low-income women. Coverage for abortion remained tied to complex rules, and states were given the authority to ban such coverage (Sonfield and Pollack, 2013).

Fourth, a fee was imposed on insurers for the privilege of selling plans through the exchanges. Such costs would normally be passed on to the consumers in the form of higher premiums (Mulvany, 2013).

Fifth, the ACA required a minimum medical loss ratio of 85% for large-group insurance plans and 80% for individual or small-group plans to pay medical claims. The percentage of premium revenue spent on medical expenses is termed the **medical loss ratio (MLR)**. Insurers use the remainder of the money obtained through premiums for administration, marketing, and profits. Health plans that did not meet the mandates were required to give rebates to the enrollees. These rebates amounted to less than 1% of the premiums in 2011 (Hall and McCue, 2013), and, therefore, had a miniscule effect on savings by consumers.

Sixth, an individual mandate went into effect in 2014; it required all legal residents of the United States to have health insurance, or else pay a penalty tax. Those without coverage under an employer's plan had the option to buy insurance through the exchanges. Many did forego the purchase of health insurance because the penalties were not regarded as severe enough.

The ACA provisions made health coverage more secure and effective for people who actually became sick or injured. These same provisions increased premiums, particularly for those in the individual and small-group markets who did not qualify for ACA's tax subsidies. Based on data from the early implementation of the ACA in 2014, Kowalski (2014) estimated that premiums in the individual health insurance market increased by 24.4% beyond what they would have if they had simply followed previous trends. In 2017, premiums for people who bought insurance on their own increased by an average of 25% from what they were in 2016 (Herron, 2016). In many states, these increases were much higher—for example, 43% in Mississippi and 62% in Tennessee (Radnofsky and Armour, 2016). Most of the premium hikes were offset by more generous government subsidies for marketplace plans, but ultimately these increases were paid by taxpayers and by those who did not qualify for subsidies.

Deductibles also reached often-unaffordable levels in 2017. For the mid-level plan ("silver" plan), the annual deductible reached $3,572 for individuals and $7,474 for families, meaning that these amounts had to be first paid out of pocket before insurance would pay anything. The deductibles were substantially higher than what they were in employment-based plans (see the "Trends in Utilization Costs: Cost Sharing" section).

On top of the vastly increased costs of health insurance in the nonemployer market, some of the largest insurers, such as United Health and Aetna, pulled out of the ACA exchanges, citing huge losses for their decision to pull out. Consequently, many parts of the country were left with only one insurer for purchasing health insurance through the exchanges, with roughly 19% of exchange-based enrollment being affected by these changes (Cox and Semanskee, 2016). Many people had to switch insurers.

President Trump has promised health insurance for all Americans. It remains to be seen how the "new" system would cover the large number of Americans left uninsured despite the ACA, and how cost of health insurance and other inequities within the system would be addressed.

▶ Public Health Insurance

Since 1965, government financing has played a significant role in expanding health care services, mainly to those who otherwise would not be able to afford them. Today, a significant proportion of health care services in the United States are supported through public programs. More than one-third of the U.S. population is covered under various public insurance programs (see Figure 6-2), an increase from previous years. This section discusses the financing, eligibility requirements, and services covered under the various public health insurance programs and the effects of the ACA on these services.

Public financing supports **categorical programs**, each of which is designed to benefit a certain category of people. Examples are Medicare for the elderly and certain disabled individuals, Medicaid for the indigent, Department of Defense programs for active service members and their families, and Department of Veterans Affairs (VA) health care for war veterans. Even though the government finances public insurance, for the most part, health care services are obtained through the private sector. An exception is the VA program, in which the financing, insurance, delivery, and payment functions are largely integrated.

Medicare

The Medicare program, also referred to as Title 18 of the Social Security Act, finances medical care for three groups of people: (1) persons 65 years and older, (2) disabled individuals who are entitled to Social Security benefits, and (3) people who have end-stage renal disease (ESRD—permanent kidney failure, requiring dialysis or a kidney transplant). People in these three categories can enroll regardless of their income status.

Shortly after its creation in 1967, the Medicare program had 19.5 million beneficiaries (NCHS, 1996, p. 263). In 2015, Medicare covered 55.3 million beneficiaries. The number of beneficiaries has continued to increase because of the aging of the U.S. population. Although the vast majority of Medicare beneficiaries are 65 years and older, 16% were younger disabled individuals in 2015 (Centers for Medicare and Medicaid Services [CMS], 2016a).

Medicare is a federal program operated under the administrative oversight of the Centers for Medicare and Medicaid Services, a branch of the Department of Health and Human Services (DHHS). Because it is a federal program, eligibility criteria and benefits are consistent throughout the United States.

The Balanced Budget Act (BBA) of 1997 established an independent federal agency, the Medicare Payment Advisory Commission (MedPAC), to advise the U.S. Congress on various issues affecting the Medicare program. MedPAC's statutory mandate includes analysis of payments to health care providers participating in Medicare, access to care, and quality of care.

For almost 30 years after its inception, Medicare had a dual structure comprising two separate insurance programs referred to as Part A and Part B. It has since become a four-part program.

Part A: Hospital Insurance

Part A, the Hospital Insurance (HI) portion of Medicare, is a true **entitlement** program. Throughout their working lives, people contribute to Medicare through special payroll taxes; hence, they are entitled to Part A benefits regardless of the amount of income and assets they may have. The employer and the employee share equally in financing the HI trust fund. All working individuals, including those who are self-employed, pay the mandatory taxes. Since 1994, all earnings have been subject to Medicare tax.

To qualify for Part A, a person or the person's spouse must have worked, earned a minimum specified amount, and paid Medicare taxes for at least 40 quarters (10 years) to earn at least 40 credits. People who have earned less than 40 credits can get Part A by paying a monthly premium.

Part A covers inpatient services for acute-care hospitals, psychiatric hospitals, inpatient rehabilitation facilities, skilled nursing facility (SNF) services, home health visits, and hospice care. Following is an overview of the type of benefits provided under Part A:

1. A maximum of 90 days of inpatient hospital care is allowed per benefit period. Once the 90 days are exhausted, a lifetime reserve of 60 additional hospital inpatient days remains. A **benefit period** is a spell of illness beginning with hospitalization and ending when a beneficiary has not been an inpatient in a hospital or an SNF for 60 consecutive days. The number of benefit periods is unlimited. These rules apply to acute-care hospitals and inpatient rehabilitation facilities.

2. A total of 90 days of care per spell of illness is allowed for treatment in a psychiatric inpatient facility, with a 60-day lifetime reserve. Lifetime use is limited to 190 days of treatment.

3. Medicare pays for up to 100 days of care in a Medicare-certified SNF, subsequent to inpatient hospitalization for at least 3 consecutive days, not including the day of discharge. Admission to the SNF must occur within 30 days of hospital discharge.

4. Medicare pays for home health care obtained from a Medicare-certified home health agency when a person is homebound and requires intermittent or part-time skilled nursing care or rehabilitation. Payment is made for 60-day episodes of care. A beneficiary can have unlimited episodes.

5. For terminally ill patients, Medicare pays for care provided by a Medicare-certified hospice.

A deductible applies to each benefit period (except to home health and hospice), and copayments are based on the duration of services (except for home health). **EXHIBIT 6-2** gives specific details on the Part A program for 2017.

Part B: Supplementary Medical Insurance

Part B, the supplementary medical insurance (SMI) portion of Medicare, is a voluntary program financed partly by general tax revenues and partly by required premium contributions. It is estimated that the beneficiaries bear approximately 25% of the cost of premiums. Since 2007, Part B premiums have been income based, as required by the Medicare Prescription Drug, Improvement, and Modernization Act (MMA) of 2003. Those beneficiaries whose incomes exceed a threshold amount pay a higher premium—known as the Income-Related Monthly Adjustment Amount (IRMAA). For 2017, the income threshold that triggered IRMAA was $85,000 per year ($170,000 per couple). The intent of the MMA legislation was to reduce tax-financed premium subsidies for higher-income individuals. Hence, for example, an individual earning more than $214,000 in 2017 paid $428.60 in monthly premiums, whereas someone earning less than or equal to $85,000 paid $134.

EXHIBIT 6-2 Medicare Part A Financing, Benefits, Deductible, and Copayments for 2017

Financing

The Hospital Insurance trust fund is financed by a payroll tax of 1.45% from the employee and 1.45% from the employer on all income. Self-employed individuals must pay the full 2.9%. As of 2013, single taxpayers earning $200,000 or more and married couples earning $250,000 or more were required to pay an additional 0.9%, as mandated by the ACA.

Premiums   None
(Those who do not qualify for premium-free coverage can buy coverage at a monthly premium of up to $413.)

Deductible $1,316 per benefit period

Benefits	Copayments
Inpatient hospital (room, meals, nursing care, operating room services, blood transfusions, special care units, drugs and medical supplies, laboratory tests, rehabilitation therapies, and medical social services)	None for the first 60 days [benefit period] $329 per day for days 61–90 [benefit period or spell of illness in psychiatric facilities] $658 per day for days 91–150 [nonrenewable lifetime reserve days] 100% of costs after 150 days
Skilled nursing facility (after a 3-day hospital stay)	None for the first 20 days in a benefit period $164.50 per day for days 21–100 in a benefit period
Home health services (part-time skilled nursing care, home health aide, rehabilitation therapies, medical equipment, social services, and medical supplies)	None for home health visits 20% of approved amount for medical equipment
Hospice care	A small copayment for drugs
Inpatient psychiatric care (190-day lifetime limit)	Same as for inpatient hospital

Noncovered Services

Long-term care
Custodial services
Personal convenience services (televisions, telephones, private-duty nurses, private rooms when not medically necessary)

Data from Centers for Medicare and Medicaid Services and Social Security Administration.

Almost all persons entitled to HI also choose to enroll in SMI because they cannot get similar coverage at the same price from private insurers. The main services covered by SMI in 2017 are listed in **EXHIBIT 6-3**. Part B also covers limited home health services under certain conditions.

Effective January 2011, the ACA provided for an annual physical exam (called a wellness exam) for all Part B enrollees, without any cost sharing. The main purpose of the wellness exam is to do a risk assessment and develop an individualized prevention plan.

Part C: Medicare Advantage

Part C is, in reality, not a new benefit program because it does not add specifically defined new services. Instead, it provides some additional choices of health plans, with the objective of channeling a greater number of beneficiaries into managed care plans. The BBA of 1997 authorized the Medicare+Choice program, which took effect on January 1, 1998. Medicare+Choice was renamed Medicare Advantage (MA) under the MMA of 2003. Beneficiaries have the option to remain in the original Medicare fee-for-service program, and if the CMS has contracted with an MCO that serves a beneficiary's geographic area, the beneficiary has the option to join the Medicare Advantage plan. If they join the plan, the beneficiaries receive both Part A and Part B services through the MCO. Prescription drugs under Part D are also included if offered by the MCO.

Enrollment in Medicare Advantage plans has steadily increased since 2004, when only 5.3 million beneficiaries used this option (Gold et al., 2013). More recently, enrollment has climbed from 11.1 million (24% of all Medicare beneficiaries) in 2010 to 17.6 million (31% of beneficiaries) in 2016 (Jacobson et al., 2016).

Premiums for Medicare Advantage are in addition to those paid to Medicare for Part B coverage. As a trade-off, the beneficiary gets additional benefits that are not available in the original Medicare plan, and there is no need to purchase Medigap coverage. Part C enrollees also have lower out-of-pocket costs. Hence, Part C is a cost-effective option for many beneficiaries. Research suggests that, on average, MA plans offer care of equal or higher quality and for less cost than traditional Medicare. Thus, MA plans may be offering better value than traditional Medicare (Newhouse and McGuire, 2014).

The MMA of 2003 required that Medicare Advantage include special needs plans. These plans were first offered in 2005 to meet the special needs of people who were institutionalized, enrolled in both Medicare and Medicaid, or had chronic or disabling conditions. Medicare Advantage Special Needs Plans (MA-SNP) are available in limited areas, and not all plans cover all special needs situations.

The ACA aimed to reduce payments to MA plans, with the goal of achieving some level of parity between the expenditures for Part C and the expenditures under the original Medicare program, in which spending per beneficiary had been less. Payments have also been risk adjusted and include incentives for quality. MA plans have responded by raising premiums and out-of-pocket costs for the enrollees. However, at least through 2016, enrollments in MA plans have continued to rise.

EXHIBIT 6-3 Medicare Part B Financing, Benefits, Deductible, and Coinsurance for 2017

Financing

The general tax revenues of the federal government support approximately 75% of the program costs. The remaining 25% is financed through monthly premiums paid by persons enrolled in Part B.

Standard premium	$134 per month (less for people receiving Social Security)
Income-adjusted premium[1]	$187.50 to $428.60 per month
Deductible	$183 annually
Coinsurance	80/20

Main Benefits

Physician services
Emergency department services
Outpatient surgery
Diagnostic tests and laboratory services
Outpatient physical therapy, occupational therapy, and speech therapy
Outpatient mental health services
Limited home health care under certain conditions
Ambulance
Renal dialysis
Artificial limbs and braces
Blood transfusions and blood components
Organ transplants
Medical equipment and supplies
Rural health clinic services
Annual physical exam

- Wellness exam
- Preventive services (as medically needed): alcohol misuse screening and counseling, bone mass measurement, mammography, cardiovascular screening, Pap smears, colorectal cancer screening, depression screening, diabetes screening, glaucoma tests, HIV screening, nutritional counseling for diabetes and renal disease, obesity screening and counseling, prostate cancer screening, sexually transmitted infections screening, shots (flu, pneumococcal, hepatitis B), and tobacco use cessation counseling

Noncovered Services

Dental services
Hearing aids
Eyeglasses (except after cataract surgery)
Services not related to treatment or injury

[1] For single beneficiaries whose annual incomes exceed $85,000.
Data from Centers for Medicare and Medicaid Services.

Part D: Prescription Drug Coverage

Part D was added to the existing Medicare program under the MMA of 2003 and was fully implemented in January 2006. Part D is available to anyone who has coverage under Part A or Part B. The prescription drug program requires payment of a monthly premium to Medicare, which is in addition to the premium for Part B. Certain low-income beneficiaries are automatically enrolled without having to pay a premium. As of January 2011, the ACA imposed an IRMAA, such that people in certain income categories pay higher premiums.

Coverage is offered through two types of private plans approved by Medicare. Stand-alone prescription drug plans (PDPs) that offer only drug coverage are used mainly by those who want to stay in the original Medicare fee-for-service program. In contrast, Medicare Advantage Prescription Drug plans (MA-PDs) are available to those persons who are enrolled in Part C if the MCO provides prescription drug coverage—and most do.

The national average for monthly premiums in 2017 was expected to be $42.17, an increase of 9% over the average monthly premium in 2016 (Hoadley et al., 2016). The Part D program also requires payment of a deductible, following which a basic level of coverage becomes available. After that, a coverage gap, or "doughnut hole," requires the beneficiary to pay the full cost of drugs (at a discount) until a defined level of spending is reached. This gap is then followed by a catastrophic level of coverage (**EXHIBIT 6-4**). Special provisions in the program are designed to help low-income enrollees by keeping their out-of-pocket costs to a minimum.

Under the ACA, all Part D drugs must be covered under a manufacturer discount agreement with the CMS. The beneficiaries receive discounts on drugs while in the coverage gap.

Medicare Out-of-Pocket Costs

Medicare carries relatively high deductibles, copayments, and premiums (see Exhibits 6-2, 6-3, and 6-4). Eyeglasses, dental care, and many long-term care services are not covered, and there is no limit on out-of-pocket expenses, except that all Medicare Advantage plans have cost sharing limits ($6,700 when in-network providers are used). The traditional Medicare program has no out-of-pocket maximums. Hence, most Medicare beneficiaries are left with high out-of-pocket costs, which represent an important share of their incomes. Medicaid (provided the beneficiary qualifies), employer retirement benefits, and purchase of private supplement insurance plans (Medigap) are some of the ways to pay for most of these out-of-pocket costs.

Medicare Enrolled Population and Total Expenditures

Medicare consumes more than one-fifth of the United States' national health expenditures. Data on enrolled population and expenditures appear in **TABLE 6-2**. Compared to previous years, Medicare spending growth was remarkably slow during the 2010 to 2015 period. While the Medicare population grew by 3%, expenditures grew by 4.4%—a vast improvement over

EXHIBIT 6-4 Medicare Part D Benefits and Individual Out-of-Pocket Costs for 2017

Premiums	$42.17 per month (estimated national average)[1]
	IRMAA ranging from $13.30 to $76.20
Deductible	$400 annually

Three levels of benefits and out-of-pocket costs beyond the $400 deductible:

Initial coverage	Medicare pays 75% of the cost of drugs until the combined total payments by the plan and the beneficiary reach $3,700.
Coverage gap	Beneficiary pays 40% of the cost for brand-name drugs, and 51% of the cost for generic drugs.
	Coverage gap ends when the beneficiary has spent $4,950 out of pocket (for brand-name drugs, the manufacturer's discount also counts toward out-of-pocket spending).
Catastrophic level	Beneficiary pays a small coinsurance (about 5%) or copayment.

The Extra Help Program

A special part of the Medicare drug coverage program called Extra Help is designed to serve people who have low incomes and savings. This group of beneficiaries includes those who receive Medicaid or Supplemental Security Income. For those who qualify, the out-of-pocket costs are minimal.

[1] Actual premium varies according to income and the plan selected by the beneficiary.
Data from Centers for Medicare and Medicaid Services (CMS). 2017. *Costs for Medicare drug coverage.* Available at: https://www.medicare.gov/part-d /costs/part-d-costs.html. Accessed May 2017.

the 9% growth rate during the decade of 2000 to 2010. Policies driven by the ACA have been largely credited with this improvement.

Medicare Financing and Spending for Services

Data on financing and spending appear in **FIGURE 6-3** and **FIGURE 6-4**. General taxes fund most of the Medicare expenditures, followed by payroll taxes. Most benefit payments go to hospitals, with private

Medicare Advantage plans being the next largest funding recipients.

Medicare Trust Funds

Medicare has established two main trust funds: The HI trust fund provides the money pool for Part A services, and the SMI trust fund provides the money pool for Parts B and D. Each trust fund accounts for its own incomes and expenditures. Taxes, premiums, and other revenues are credited to the respective trust funds, and

TABLE 6-2 Medicare: Enrolled Population and Expenditures in Selected Years

1970	1980	1990	2000	2010	2015
Population Covered (in Millions)					
20.4	28.4	34.3	39.7	47.7	55.3
Expenditures (in Billions)					
$7.5	$36.8	$111.00	$221.8	$522.9	$647.6
Proportion of Total U.S. Health Care Expenditures					
10.0%	14.5%	15.5%	16.4%	20.2%	20.2%
Average Annual Increase in Expenditures from the Previous Year Shown					
	17%	12%	7%	9%	4.4%

Data from National Center for Health Statistics (NCHS). 2012. *Health, United States, 2012.* Hyattsville, MD: U.S. Department of Health and Human Services. pp. 323, 356; Centers for Medicare and Medicaid Services (CMS). 2016a. *2016 Annual report of the boards of trustees of the federal hospital insurance and federal supplementary medical insurance trust funds.* Available at: https://www.cms.gov/Research-Statistics-Data-and-Systems/Statistics-Trends-and-Reports /ReportsTrustFunds/downloads/tr2016.pdf. Accessed January 2017.

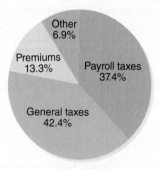

FIGURE 6-3 Sources of Medicare financing, 2015.

Data from Centers for Medicare and Medicaid Services (CMS). 2016a. *2016 Annual report of the boards of trustees of the federal hospital insurance and federal supplementary medical insurance trust funds.* Available at: https:// www.cms.gov/Research-Statistics-Data-and-Systems/Statistics-Trends-and -Reports/ReportsTrustFunds/downloads/tr2016.pdf. Accessed January 2017.

benefit payments and administrative costs are the only purposes for which disbursements from the funds can be made.

TABLE 6-3 compares the trust fund results for 2012 and 2015. Deficit spending (expenditures exceeding revenues) by the trust funds greatly decreased between 2012 and 2015. This positive change is very likely attributable to the many provisions contained in the ACA to reduce Medicare costs and increase revenues. Despite these gains, however, the Medicare trustees project that deficit financing will return: By 2028, HI revenues are anticipated to cover only 87% of program costs, compared to almost 99% of program costs in 2015. The trustees project depletion of HI funds by 2028, and recommend further legislation to address this issue; such legislation must be enacted sooner rather than later to minimize the impact on beneficiaries, providers, and taxpayers (CMS, 2016a).

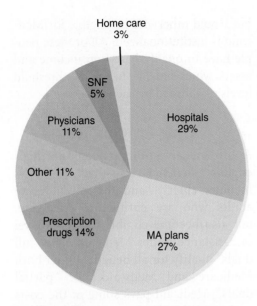

FIGURE 6-4 Medicare spending for services, 2015.

Data from Centers for Medicare and Medicaid Services (CMS). 2016a. *2016 Annual report of the boards of trustees of the federal hospital insurance and federal supplementary medical insurance trust funds.* Available at: https:// www.cms.gov/Research-Statistics-Data-and-Systems/Statistics-Trends-and -Reports/ReportsTrustFunds/downloads/tr2016.pdf. Accessed January 2017.

The SMI trust fund is adequately financed through 2026 because premium income and general revenue income for Parts B and D are reset each year to cover expected costs. Such financing, however, would have to increase faster than the general economy to cover expected expenditure growth (CMS, 2016a).

A combination of three main factors raises concerns about the future solvency of Medicare:

- The cost of delivering health care continues to grow at a rate faster than the rate of inflation in the general economy.
- An aging population will consume a greater quantity of health care services.
- The workforce has been shrinking, and wage increases to support payroll tax revenues have been smaller than the rise in medical inflation.

TABLE 6-3 Status of HI and SMI Trust Funds (Billions of Dollars), 2012–2015

	HI		SMI	
	2012	**2015**	**2012**	**2015**
Assets at the beginning of year	$244.2	$197.3	$80.7	$69.2
Revenues	243.0	275.4	293.9	369.0
Expenditures	266.8	278.9	307.4	368.8
Difference between revenues and expenditures	−23.8	−3.5	−13.5	0.2
Assets at the end of year	220.4	193.8	67.2	69.5

Data from Centers for Medicare and Medicaid Services (CMS). 2013. *2013 Annual report of the boards of trustees of the federal hospital insurance and federal supplementary medical insurance trust funds.* Available at: https://downloads.cms.gov/files/tr2013.pdf. Accessed April 2017; Centers for Medicare and Medicaid Services (CMS). 2016a. *2016 Annual report of the boards of trustees of the federal hospital insurance and federal supplementary medical insurance trust funds.* Available at: https://www.cms.gov/Research-Statistics-Data-and-Systems/Statistics-Trends-and-Reports/ReportsTrustFunds /downloads/tr2016.pdf. Accessed January 2017.

Medicaid

Medicaid, also referred to as Title 19 of the Social Security Act, was originally designed to finance health care services for the indigent. Hence, Medicaid is almost entirely a taxpayer-financed program. Since its inception, Medicaid has been a **means-tested program** in which eligibility depends on people's financial resources. Each state administers its own Medicaid program under federal guidelines.

Medicaid is jointly financed by the federal and state governments. The federal government provides matching funds to the states based on the per capita income in each state. By law, federal matching—known as the Federal Medical Assistance Percentage (FMAP)—cannot be less than 50% or more than 83% of total state Medicaid program costs. Wealthier states have a smaller share of their costs reimbursed by the federal government.

Rules for Medicaid Eligibility

Three main categories of people are automatically eligible for Medicaid: (1) families with children receiving support under the Temporary Assistance for Needy Families (TANF) program; (2) people receiving Supplemental Security Income (SSI), which includes many of the elderly, the blind, and the disabled with low incomes; and (3) children and pregnant women whose family income is at or below 133% of the FPL. States, at their discretion, have defined other "medically needy" categories based on people's income and assets. The most important of these are individuals who are institutionalized in nursing or psychiatric facilities and individuals who are receiving community-based services but would otherwise be eligible for Medicaid if institutionalized. All of these people have to qualify based on income and assets, which must be below the threshold levels established by each state.

Dual-Eligible Beneficiaries

Approximately 9 million people are dual-eligible beneficiaries—that is, low-income elderly and disabled young adults who are entitled to Medicare, but also become eligible for some level of assistance under Medicaid. The "full duals" qualify for all benefits under both Medicare and Medicaid. For "partial duals," Medicaid pays some of the costs such as Medicare premiums, deductibles, and copayments. Dual-eligible beneficiaries generally have extensive health care needs because of chronic conditions, disability, or need for long-term care services.

Medicaid Experiences Under the ACA

Under financial penalties, the ACA had mandated all states to cover any legal U.S. resident younger than age 65 with income up to 138% of the FPL (after an adjustment of 5 percentage points applied to 133% of FPL based on modified adjusted gross income), starting January 2014. Federal matching funds at 100% for newly eligible individuals were authorized for 3 years (2014–2016), with a gradual reduction of this rate each year to 90% in 2020. The U.S. Supreme Court then struck down the mandate, giving states the option to either expand or not expand their Medicaid programs without any penalty from the federal government. As of 2016, 31 states and the District of Columbia had expanded their Medicaid programs, and 19 states had not.

Medicaid expansion has helped a significant number of low-income people gain health coverage. Under federal law, access to emergency departments (EDs) does not require insurance coverage. Yet, in the post-ACA era, Medicaid-paid use of hospital EDs increased by 27% (Pines et al., 2016). This is not surprising given the shortage of primary care physicians in the United States, combined with the low participation rates in Medicaid by many physicians. Indeed, research shows—based on the experience in Oregon, where Medicaid expansion began in the late 1980s—that Medicaid expansion results in increased use of EDs, even over time after the new enrollees have had the opportunity to seek alternative sources of care (Finkelstein et al., 2016). The main beneficiaries of higher ED use are the hospitals, which get at least some payment for Medicaid-insured patients. Previously, a large portion of such care would have been written off as uncompensated. Given the enormous expansion of Medicaid managed care, one might expect that MCOs would provide better access to services for the enrollees. Medicaid managed care penetration in a geographic market, however, is associated with increased probability of ED use, difficulty seeing a specialist, and unmet need for prescription drugs, without a reduction in expenditures (Caswell and Long, 2015).

Based on their research, Roberts and Gaskin (2015) concluded that Medicaid expansion under the ACA would require more than 2,000 additional primary care providers. Nevertheless, a comprehensive literature review suggests that, overall, the ACA-linked Medicaid expansion resulted in better access to care and utilization (Antonisse et al., 2016). Still other studies have pointed to challenges that may make it difficult to meet the increased demand for care among the newly eligible Medicaid population.

Although Medicaid beneficiaries express a relatively high level of satisfaction with their access to care, on closer examination it appears that this access comes from visiting hospital EDs and community health centers (Goozner, 2015). Unfortunately, community health centers are not available everywhere in the United States.

Issues with Medicaid

The main problem with Medicaid is lack of reimbursement for providers. Hence, many physicians and some other providers do not serve Medicaid-covered patients. Medicaid reimbursement is a fraction of what is paid by Medicare and private insurers. Despite this discrepancy, the U.S. Supreme Court ruled in *Armstrong v. Exceptional Child Center, Inc.* that Medicaid providers do not have the right to seek relief in federal courts to force states to pay higher reimbursement (Huberfeld, 2015). Under the ACA, payments were brought up to Medicare levels only temporarily. Hence, the issue of physician participation is an ongoing one.

Another critical issue with Medicaid is **churning**—that is, the constant exit and reentry of beneficiaries in this system as their eligibility changes. Churning occurs because many beneficiaries have incomes that may fluctuate from one month to another. Data suggest that 30% of Medicaid beneficiaries lose their eligibility within 6 months of enrollment (Sommers and Rosenbaum, 2011), and approximately half lose it within 12 months (Sommers et al., 2014). Churning often disrupts access and continuity of care. Moreover, under the ACA mandate that all persons have health insurance, those bumped from Medicaid must find new coverage—typically through the government-sponsored exchanges.

Given the issues discussed here and in the previous section, most Americans would not be satisfied with Medicaid as their source of health insurance. Indeed, since its inception, the presence of Medicaid has resulted in a two-tier health care system in the United States, with one branch serving the poor and the other branch reserved for the nonpoor.

Medicaid Enrollment and Spending

Just before 2014, Medicaid enrollment stood at approximately 60 million. During the first half of 2014, after the ACA was implemented, 6 million people gained coverage through Medicaid (Haislmaier and Gonshorowski, 2014). Federal spending on Medicaid, attributed to the ACA, increased by $36 billion in 2014 (Medicaid and CHIP Payment and Access Commission [MACPAC], 2016).

Because of the churning phenomenon discussed in the previous section, the enrollment figures do not remain stable. Hence, the CMS furnishes quarterly reports on enrollments. As of February 2016, Medicaid enrollment had grown to a little more than 74 million (CMS, 2016b), a 23% growth since late 2013, much of which may be attributable to the ACA. Hence, Medicaid has become the second largest source

of insurance coverage, second only to employer-based coverage (see Figure 6-2).

In 2014, Medicaid spending amounted to approximately 16% of total U.S. health care expenditures, or $498 billion (MACPAC, 2016). By comparison, Medicare accounts for 20% of total expenditures. Over the next several years, Medicaid is projected to grow at a rate that is comparable to or slower than Medicare. **FIGURE 6-5** summarizes the spending on the various Medicaid-covered services.

Children's Health Insurance Program

The Children's Health Insurance Program (CHIP), codified as Title 21 of the Social Security Act, was initiated under the BBA of 1997 in response to the plight of uninsured children whose families' incomes

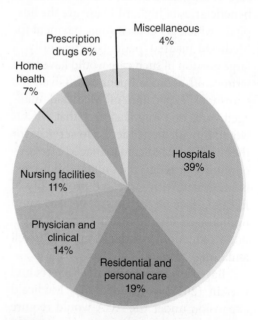

FIGURE 6-5 Medicaid spending for services, 2014.

Data from Medicaid and CHIP Payment and Access Commission (MACPAC). 2016. *Report to Congress on Medicaid and CHIP, June 2016*. Washington, DC: Author.

exceeded the Medicaid threshold levels, which made them ineligible for Medicaid coverage. These children were estimated to number 10.1 million—nearly one-fourth of all uninsured persons—in 1996.

The program offers federal funds in the form of set block grants to states. To cover children up to 19 years of age, a state can expand its existing Medicaid program, establish a separate program for children, or use a combined approach. Federal law requires that ineligibility for Medicaid be established before approval for CHIP coverage. Each state establishes its own eligibility criteria for CHIP, which must comply with the federal guidelines. There is no federal income threshold, but many states cover children in families with incomes up to 200% of the FPL, provided the children are not covered under another private or public health insurance program. Several states have established income criteria above 200% of FPL. CHIP does not cover parents or adults.

Similar to the case with Medicaid, CHIP financing is shared between the federal and state governments. In an effort to strengthen CHIP, federal matching funds are 15 percentage points higher than what they are for Medicaid.

Research has shown that CHIP has had a significant impact in reducing the number of uninsured children (Hudson, 2005). CHIP has also been credited with improving access, continuity of care, and quality of care for children in all racial/ethnic groups, as well as reducing racial/ethnic disparities in access, unmet need, and continuity of care (Shone et al., 2005).

Health Care for the Military

The U.S. Department of Defense (DOD) operates a large and complex health care program, known as the Military Health System, that provides medical services to active duty and retired members of the armed forces, their dependents, survivors, and former spouses. This program has also been extended to National Guard/Reserve members. The Military Health System has a global scope. Approximately 150,000 military, civilian, and contract personnel are employed in hospitals and clinics operated by the military. Each of the military departments—Army, Navy, and Air Force—operates its own medical facilities. DOD's health care budget exceeds $50 billion, and it provides services to 9.6 million beneficiaries (DOD, 2014).

TRICARE is the insurance arm of the military health care system. Beneficiaries may obtain health care either through DOD's medical facilities or through services purchased from civilian providers.

TRICARE offers several different health insurance plans, including managed care and fee-for-service options, and different options depending on whether the eligible beneficiaries live in the United States or overseas. For retirees age 65 and older, TRICARE offers a plan that works in conjunction with Medicare—the enrollee must enroll in Parts A and B. Service members who separate from service due to a service-connected injury or illness may be eligible for VA benefits and certain TRICARE benefits. TRICARE- and VA-eligible beneficiaries can choose to use either their TRICARE or VA benefits for each separate episode of care.

Veterans Health Administration

The Veterans Health Administration (VHA), the health services branch of the U.S. Department of Veterans Affairs (VA), operates the largest integrated health services system in the United States. The system encompasses more than 1,700 sites of care that include hospitals, outpatient clinics, community living centers (nursing homes), and various other facilities. Each year, VHA provides medical services to 8.76 million veterans (VHA, 2017). Its Office of Research and Development focuses its research activities on health issues that affect veterans. The system actively engages in medical education through affiliations with academic health systems.

VHA was originally established to treat veterans with war-related injuries and to help rehabilitate past service members with war-related disabilities. This original mission was later expanded. Today, non-service-related conditions account for the bulk of the care provided, as poor veterans with medical conditions unrelated to military combat increasingly use the system. More than half of the veterans served by VHA have no service-connected disabilities (NCHS, 2012). Congress requires VHA to provide services on a priority basis to veterans with service-connected illnesses and disabilities, low incomes, or special health care needs.

Funding for the VHA program is appropriated in the annual national budget approved by Congress. The structure of VHA funding is patterned after the global budget model, in which budget appropriations are determined in advance for the entire system. The VHA then distributes these funds to its organizational units having oversight for the delivery of health care.

The organizational units comprise 23 geographically distributed Veterans Integrated Service Networks (VISNs). Each VISN is responsible for coordinating the activities of the hospitals, outpatient clinics, nursing homes, and other facilities located within its jurisdiction.

The VHA also operates the Civilian Health and Medical Program of the Department of Veterans Affairs (CHAMPVA), which covers dependents of permanently and totally disabled veterans. The VHA shares the cost of covered health care services and supplies with eligible beneficiaries.

Despite its many successes, the VHA system suffers from capacity and financing constraints, which result in lack of access and timely care for many veterans. In 2014, highly publicized reports described lack of access to care, preventable deaths that occurred while veterans were waiting for care, and falsification of lists to make waiting times appear shorter (Giroir and Wilensky, 2015). In response, Congress passed the Veterans Access, Choice, and Accountability Act of 2014. A Veterans Choice Program was created to allow certain veterans who experience lengthy wait times and live 40 or more miles away from a VA facility to be able to obtain care from community-based providers. President Trump has promised to further bolster the health care system for the nation's veterans.

Indian Health Service

The federal program administered by the Indian Health Service (IHS), a division of the DHHS, provides comprehensive health care services directly to members of federally recognized American Indian and Alaska Native (AIAN) tribes and their descendants. AIANs, as citizens of the United States, are eligible to participate in all public, private, and state health programs available to the general population. However, for many Indians, IHS-supported programs are the only source of health care because no alternative sources of medical care are available, especially in isolated areas. IHS programs serve almost 2.2 million AIANs residing on or near reservations and in rural communities. Services are provided in more than 883 IHS-owned or -leased and tribal health care facilities. These facilities include hospitals, health centers, school centers, health stations, and Alaska village clinics. Delivery of services is organized through 12 area offices.

▶ The Payment Function

Insurance companies, MCOs, Blue Cross/Blue Shield, and the government (for Medicare and Medicaid) are referred to as **third-party payers**, with the other two parties being the patient and the provider. The payment function has two main facets: (1) the determination of the methods and amounts of reimbursement for the delivery of services and (2) the actual payment after services have been rendered. The set fee for each type of service is commonly referred to as a charge or rate. Technically, a **charge** is a fee set by the provider, which is akin to price in general commerce. A **rate** is a price set by a third-party payer. An index of charges listing individual fees for each type of service is referred to as a **fee schedule**. In general, to receive payment for services rendered, the provider must file a **claim** with the third-party payer. For the sake of simplicity, in this section, we refer to the determination of rates as "reimbursement" and to the payment of claims as "disbursement."

Historically, providers have preferred the fee-for-service method, but it has now largely fallen out of favor with payers because it leads to cost escalations. The Medicare program, in particular, has been at the forefront of devising innovative reimbursement methods; private payers often follow suit. Today, numerous reimbursement methods exist and are used for different types of services. Physicians, dentists, optometrists, therapists, hospitals, nursing facilities, and so on may be paid according to different reimbursement mechanisms.

Fee for Service

Fee for service is the oldest method of reimbursement and is still in existence, although its use has been greatly reduced. Fee for service is based on the assumption that health care is provided in a set of identifiable and individually distinct units of services, such as examination, x-ray, urinalysis, and a tetanus shot, in the case of physician services. For surgery, such individual services may include an admission kit, numerous medical supplies (each accounted for separately), surgeon's fees, anesthesia, anesthesiologist's fees, recovery room charges, and so forth. Each of these services is separately itemized on one bill, and there can be more than one bill. For example, the hospital, the surgeon, the pathologist, and the anesthesiologist bill for their services separately.

Initially, providers established their own fee-for-service charges and insurers passively paid the claims. Later, insurers started to limit reimbursement to a usual, customary, and reasonable (UCR) amount. Each insurer determined on its own what the UCR charge should be, through community or statewide surveys of what providers were charging. If the actual charges exceeded the UCR amount, then reimbursement from insurers was limited to the UCR amount. Providers would then **balance bill**—that is, ask the patients to pay the difference between the actual charges and the payments received from third-party payers.

The main problem under fee-for-service arrangements is that providers have an incentive to deliver additional services that are not always essential. Providers can increase their incomes by increasing the volume of services. However, dentists, therapists, and some physicians continue to receive payment according to the fee-for-service model.

Bundled Payments

Fee for service essentially pays for unbundled services. A bundled fee, also referred to as package pricing, includes a number of related services in one price. For example, optometrists sometimes advertise package prices that include the charges for eye exams, frames for eyeglasses, and corrective lenses. The various prospective payment methods of reimbursement are also examples of payments for bundled services. Package pricing reduces the incentive for providing nonessential services. Some evidence indicates that

bundled payment methods, especially when they are prospectively set, are effective in reducing health care spending without significantly affecting quality of care (Hussey et al., 2012).

Medicare has pioneered a bundled payment mechanism that pays providers a single sum for a given episode. Some episodic models are still being explored, but the most extensive one includes all services during hospitalization and subsequent delivery of post-acute services, such as rehabilitation and nursing home care. Incentives to share cost savings with Medicare are also incorporated (Tanenbaum, 2017). The theory behind episodic payments is that various providers collaborating to deliver services to a patient through an entire episode will result in coordinated care, improved quality, and lesser cost.

Resource-Based Relative Value Scale

Under the Omnibus Budget Reconciliation Act (OBRA) of 1989, Medicare developed a reimbursement mechanism to pay physicians according to a "relative value" assigned to each physician service. The resource-based relative value scale (RBRVS) was implemented in 1992. Subsequently, third-party payers adopted the RBRVS system.

RBRVS incorporates **relative value units (RVUs)** based on the time, skill, and intensity (physician work) it takes to provide a service. Hence, RVUs reflect resource inputs—time, effort, and expertise—to deliver a service. RVUs are established for different types of services that are identified by codes. The Healthcare Common Procedures Coding System (HCPCS) includes the Current Procedural

Terminology (CPT) codes (Level I) and Level II codes for services, such as supplies, equipment, and devices.

In addition to RVUs associated with physician work, separate RVUs are included for the cost of practice (overhead costs), malpractice insurance, and geographic cost variations. Then, a standard dollar amount, called a conversion factor (CF), is used and a sustainable growth rate (SGR) factor is applied to establish a **Medicare Physician Fee Schedule (MPFS)**—a price list for physician services, based on which individual payments are made when physicians file their claims. Other factors, such as involvement of nonphysician practitioners and reporting of quality measures, can also come into play (MedPAC, 2016a).

In essence, RBRVS is a variation of fee for service, so it has not addressed the issue of volume-driven payment. The number of RVUs can be increased by increasing the volume of services delivered, thereby increasing practice throughput and boosting the number of billable services per patient (Jessee, 2011). The controversial SGR formula has gone through several "doc fixes" in Congress, with the goal of averting severe payment cuts for physicians. These "fixes" have resulted in increased overall expenditures for physician services.

Value-Based Reimbursement

Medicare has continued to innovate in regard to its reimbursement methodologies so as to give more emphasis to improved quality and reduced cost. Under the Medicare Access and CHIP Reauthorization Act (MACRA) of 2015, Medicare implemented a quality payment program.

For physician services, the new law repealed the SGR formula and some of the other adjustments to the MPFS. The quality payment program will start payment adjustments in January 2019 based on performance. These adjustments will reflect performance data collected as of January 2017. MACRA streamlines the reporting of previously used quality measures into one composite performance score.

MACRA makes available two different tracks in which clinicians can opt to participate. The first option, known as the Merit-based Incentive Payment System (MIPS), ties payment bonuses or penalties to quality measures, resource use (input costs) compared to similar care episodes and clinical conditions, care coordination and shared decision making, and use of electronic health records. The second option, known as Advanced Alternative Payment Models (APMs), applies to clinicians who participate in accountable care organizations (ACOs) and patient-centered medical homes.

ACOs—groups of providers, such as physicians and hospitals, that have agreed to be held accountable for the cost and quality for a group of beneficiaries—are paid mainly through the Medicare Shared Savings Program (MSSP). Under the ACA, any cost savings achieved through these arrangements are shared in the form of bonuses between participating ACOs and Medicare. Beneficiaries do not enroll in ACOs, but are assigned to ACOs by Medicare. The beneficiaries are free to obtain services outside the ACO; if they choose to go outside the ACO, the ACO remains responsible for the spending. This provides an incentive to the ACO providers to keep their enrollees satisfied so they will stay with the ACO providers (MedPAC, 2016b).

Medicare has also enforced a quality reporting program for certain types of facilities, such as ambulatory surgical centers, home health agencies, and hospices. Facilities that do not submit quality data to the CMS are assessed a penalty in the form of reduced reimbursement.

Managed Care Approaches

MCOs have concentrated on three main approaches to payment. The first is the preferred-provider approach, which may be regarded as a variation of fee for service. The main distinction is that an MCO contracts with certain "preferred providers" and negotiates discounts off the charges to establish fee schedules.

In the second approach, which is called **capitation**, the provider is paid a set monthly fee per enrollee, which is sometimes referred to as a per member per month (PMPM) rate. The fixed monthly fee (PMPM rate × number of enrollees) is paid to the provider regardless of how often the enrollees receive medical services from the provider. Capitation removes the incentive for providers to increase the volume of services to generate additional revenues. It also makes providers prudent in providing only necessary services.

Salary, combined with productivity-related bonuses, is the third payment method used by some MCOs that employ their own physicians.

Cost-Plus Reimbursement

Cost-plus reimbursement was the traditional method used by Medicare and Medicaid to establish per diem (daily) rates for inpatient stays in hospitals, nursing homes, and other institutions. Under the cost-plus method, reimbursement rates for institutions are based on the total costs incurred in operating the institution. The institution is required to submit a cost report to the third-party payer. Complex formulas are developed, designating certain costs as "nonallowable" and placing cost ceilings in other areas. The formulas are used to calculate the per diem reimbursement rate, also referred to as a per patient-day (PPD) rate. The method is called cost-plus because, in addition to the total operating costs, the reimbursement formula takes a portion of the capital costs into account in arriving at the PPD rate. Because the reimbursement methodology sets rates after evaluating the costs retrospectively (by looking back), this mechanism is broadly referred to as **retrospective reimbursement**.

Under the cost-plus system, total reimbursement is directly related to length of stay, services rendered, and cost of providing the services. Providers have an incentive to provide services indiscriminately, which in turn drives up costs. There is little motivation for efficiency and cost-containment in the delivery of services. Paradoxically, health care institutions can increase their profits by increasing costs under such a system.

Because of the perverse financial incentives inherent in retrospective cost-based reimbursement, this approach has been largely replaced by various prospective reimbursement methods. An exception is the federal critical access hospital program, which continues to allow certain rural hospitals to be paid under the cost-plus reimbursement system. Medicare-certified hospices are also reimbursed based on per diem rates that are intended to cover the costs of services.

Prospective Reimbursement

In contrast to retrospective reimbursement, in which historical costs are used to determine the amount to be paid, **prospective reimbursement** is forward-looking, and uses certain established criteria to determine the amount of reimbursement in advance, before services are delivered. Prospective reimbursement not only minimizes some of the abuses inherent in cost-plus approaches, but also enables providers, such as Medicare, to better predict future health care spending. In addition, it provides strong incentives to health care organizations to reduce costs. The organization makes a profit only if it can keep its costs below the prospective reimbursement amount. Inability to control costs jeopardizes the organization's financial health.

Medicare has been using the prospective payment system (PPS) to reimburse inpatient hospital acute care services under Medicare Part A since 1983. Subsequently, the BBA of 1997 mandated implementation of a PPS for hospital outpatient services and post-acute-care providers, such as SNFs, home health agencies, and inpatient rehabilitation facilities.

Depending on the type of service setting, the prospective reimbursement methods discussed in the subsequent sections are based on diagnosis-related groups (DRGs), ambulatory payment classification (APC), case-mix methods, and home health resource groups (HHRGs).

Diagnosis-Related Groups

Overview of DRG-Based Reimbursement. The PPS for acute-care hospital inpatient reimbursement was enacted under the Social Security Amendments of 1983. The predetermined reimbursement amount is set according to DRGs. Each DRG groups together principal diagnoses that are expected to require similar amounts of hospital resources in the delivery of care.

The primary factor governing the amount of reimbursement is the type of case (a DRG classification), but additional factors can create differences in reimbursement for the same DRG. DRG-based rates are adjusted for geographic differences (wage levels in various areas and location of the hospital in an urban versus rural area); whether the institution is a teaching hospital (i.e., has residency programs for medical graduates); and whether a hospital treats a disproportionate share of low-income patients. The last provision was authorized by Congress to give extra financial support to "safety net" hospitals (called disproportionate share hospitals), which are mainly located in inner cities and rural areas, and serve a large number of poor people. Additional payments are also made for cases that involve extremely long hospital stays or are extremely expensive, which are referred to as **outliers**.

The hospital receives a predetermined fixed rate per discharge (i.e., per case) based on the patient's DRG classification and adjustment factors just pointed out. The bundle of services consists of whatever medical care the patient requires for a given principal diagnosis. The fixed payment rates give providers financial incentives to reduce costs.

Refined Medicare Severity DRGs. In 2007, the CMS adopted a refined DRG-based PPS method that includes patient severity to better reflect hospital resource use. The new system has 335 base DRGs, most of which are further split into two or three Medicare severity diagnosis-related groups

(MS-DRGs) based on comorbidities (secondary conditions) or complications (developed during hospital stay). This new payment system had 756 MS-DRGs in use in 2016. Each MS-DRG carries a relative weight that reflects how costly it would be to take care of a patient in a given MS-DRG category relative to other categories. A new type of adjustment to the reimbursement method is for the use of certain technologies. Also added to the reimbursement is 65% of bad debts resulting from nonpayment of deductibles and copayments.

Because DRG-based payments have a financial incentive for hospitals to keep the length of stay as short as possible, the ACA required reduction in payments to hospitals that incurred excessive Medicare readmissions for selected conditions. The objective is to prevent discharging a patient too soon, and there is a penalty for patients who develop hospital-acquired preventable medical conditions (MedPAC, 2016c).

Psychiatric DRG-Based Payment

On average, Medicare beneficiaries account for approximately one-fourth of discharges in inpatient psychiatric facilities. These facilities are paid a per diem rate rather than a case-specific rate, based on psychiatric MS-DRGs. Base rates are established by using national average daily costs for routine, ancillary, and capital costs, updated for inflation. The base rates are adjusted for certain factors, similar to the adjustments for acute-care hospitals. (MedPAC, 2016d).

Long-Term Care Hospital Payment System

Long-term care hospitals (LTCHs) are paid in three different ways. For post-acute care following stay in an intensive care unit (ICU)

and for ventilator-dependent patients, Medicare uses a PPS system. Per-discharge payment rates are set according to Medicare severity long-term care diagnosis-related groups (MS-LTC-DRGs). For patients who do not meet the preceding criteria, the reimbursement is the lower of the acute-care rate under hospital PPS or the cost of caring for the patient. The MS-LTC-DRGs use the same groups as for acute-care PPS, but have specific weights applicable to patients receiving care in LTCHs (MedPAC, 2016e).

Outpatient Prospective Payment System

In August 2000, Medicare's Outpatient Prospective Payment System (OPPS) was implemented to pay for services provided by hospital outpatient departments. The ambulatory payment classification (APC) divides all outpatient services into groups based on clinical and cost similarity. With few exceptions, all services within an APC have the same payment rate. In addition, the CMS has created new technology APCs that cover these technologies until enough data become available to establish payment rates for them. Expensive drugs and biologicals also have separate APCs. The reimbursement rates are adjusted for factors such as geographic variations in wages. Adjustments are also made for outpatient services delivered by certain cancer centers and children's hospitals. APC reimbursement is in the form of a bundled rate that includes services such as anesthesia, certain drugs, supplies, and recovery room charges in a packaged price established by Medicare.

In January 2008, Medicare implemented an OPPS to pay for facility services, such as nursing, recovery care, anesthetics, drugs, and other supplies, in ambulatory surgery centers (freestanding or hospital based). The most common procedures performed in these centers include cataract removal and lens replacement, upper gastrointestinal endoscopy, and colonoscopy. Physician services are reimbursed separately under the physician fee schedule based on RBRVS (MedPAC, 2009).

Case-Mix Methods

Case mix is an aggregate of the severity of conditions requiring clinical intervention. Case-mix categories are mutually exclusive and differentiate patients according to the extent of resource use. On a case-mix index, higher score categories include patients who have more severe conditions than those in lower score categories. A comprehensive assessment of each patient's condition determines the case mix for an inpatient facility. Patients who require similar levels of services are then categorized into groups that are relatively uniform according to resource consumption.

Resource Utilization Groups. The case-mix method is used for paying SNFs. Implemented in 1998, the PPS provides for a per diem prospective rate based on the intensity of care needed by patients in an SNF. The Minimum Data Set (MDS) is the instrument used for a comprehensive assessment of each patient. It consists of a core set of screening elements used to assess the clinical, functional, and psychosocial needs of each patient admitted to an SNF. A patient's day of care is assigned to one of 66 resource utilization groups (RUGs). The RUG categories differentiate between patients according to expected resource use. Among the variables used to identify resource utilization are patient characteristics, such as principal diagnosis, functional limitations, cognitive patterns, psychological condition, skin problems, bladder and bowel function, nutritional status, and special treatments and procedures needed.

The aim of RUG-based PPS is to ensure that Medicare payments are related to the care requirements of the patient and are made equitably to SNFs with different patient caseloads. The per diem rate is all-inclusive, meaning it includes payment for all covered SNF services, such as nursing care and rehabilitation. Adjustments to the PPS rate are made for differences in wages prevailing in various geographic areas and for facility location in an urban versus rural area.

Case-Mix Groups. Since 2002, inpatient rehabilitation facilities (rehabilitation hospitals and distinctly certified rehabilitation units in general hospitals) have been reimbursed according to case-mix groups (CMGs). Each patient must undergo a patient assessment at admission and discharge. Based on information from the assessment, the patient is assigned to one of the intensive rehabilitation categories, based on the primary reason for rehabilitation, such as stroke or hip fracture, age, functional level, or cognitive impairment. Patients are further categorized into one of four tiers, based on any comorbidities; each tier adjusts the base payment either up or down.

The primary function of inpatient rehabilitation is to provide intensive rehabilitation therapy. Hence, Medicare rules require that no less than 60% of the total patient population in such units have one of 13 specified conditions that require intensive rehabilitation (MedPAC, 2016f).

Home Health Resource Groups

Implemented in 2000, the PPS for home health pays a fixed, predetermined rate for each 60-day episode of care regardless of the specific services delivered, which can be skilled nursing care, rehabilitation, medical social work, and/or home health aide services. All services provided by a home health agency are bundled under one payment made on a per-patient basis, except that the costs of any durable medical equipment (DME) are not included in the bundled rate. To capture the expected resource use, patients are assigned to one of the 153 HHRGs, based on clinical and functional status and service use, which is measured by the Outcome and Assessment Information Set (OASIS). The HHRGs range from groups of relatively uncomplicated patients to those who have severe medical conditions, have severe functional limitations, or need extensive therapy. If a patient received fewer than five visits during a 60-day episode, the home health agency is paid per visit based on the type of visit (MedPAC, 2016g).

Disbursement of Funds

After services have been delivered, some agency must perform the administrative task of verifying and paying the claims received from the providers. Disbursement of funds (claims processing) is carried out in accordance with the reimbursement policy adopted by the particular program. Commercial insurance companies and MCOs may either have their own claims departments to process payments to providers or outsource this function. Self-insured employers typically contract with a **third-party administrator (TPA)** to process and pay claims. The TPA may also monitor utilization and perform other oversight functions. The government contracts with third parties in the private sector to process Medicare claims. These so-called Medicare Administrative Contractors are private insurers. For Medicaid, each state has established billing codes and claim submission procedures.

▶ National Health Care Expenditures

In 2015, national health expenditures (NHE)—also referred to as health care spending—in the United States amounted to a little more than $3.2 trillion, or an average per-capita spending of $9,990 for each American. **TABLE 6-4** provides NHE data for selected years. NHE represented 17.8% of the U.S. **gross domestic product (GDP)**, where the GDP is the total value of goods and services produced in the United States and is an indicator of total economic production, or total consumption (CMS, 2016c). Hence, 17.8% of GDP refers to the share of the total economic output consumed by health care products and services in 2015. Because of the 2007–2009 recession and a slow economic growth since then, the share of GDP is somewhat higher than would otherwise be expected. Nevertheless, the data leave little doubt that health care continues to consume an ever-rising share of the United States' total economic production.

Total spending grew at an average annual rate of 6.7% from 1990 to 2000, at 7.3% from 2000 to 2010, and at 4.3%

TABLE 6-4 U.S. National Health Expenditures in Selected Years			
Year	**Amount (in Billions)**	**Percentage of GDP**	**Amount per Capita**
1960	$27.2	5.0	$146
1970	74.6	6.9	355
1980	255.3	8.9	1,108
1990	721.4	12.1	2,843
2000	1,369.7	13.3	4,857
2010	2,596.4	17.4	8,404
2015	3,205.6	17.8	9,990
2020 (projected)	4,198.3	18.7	12,490

Data from Centers for Medicare and Medicaid Services (CMS). 2016c. *National health expenditure data: Historical.* Available at: https://www.cms.gov /research-statistics-data-and-systems/statistics-trends-and-reports/nationalhealthexpenddata/nationalhealthaccountshistorical.html. Accessed January 2017.

from 2010 to 2015. However, in 2015 alone, NHE grew by 5.8%. Nevertheless, the slower growth of NHE in recent years compared to previous decades no doubt reflects cost-containment efforts undertaken by various payers, notably the federal government for Medicare spending.

According to projections made by CMS's Office of the Actuary, the annual rate of NHE increase from 2015 to 2020 is expected to be 5.6%. NHE is expected to surpass $4 trillion by 2020, when it will consume 18.7% of GDP. This prediction reflects the expectation that the NHE rate of increase will be faster than the GDP rate of increase.

Differences Between National and Personal Health Expenditures

National health expenditures are an aggregate of the amount a nation spends for all health services and supplies, public health services, health-related research, administrative costs, and investment in structures and equipment during a calendar year. The proportional distribution of NHE into the various categories of health services in the United States appears in **TABLE 6-5**.

Personal health expenditures, which are a component of national health expenditures, comprise the total spending for services and goods related directly to patient

TABLE 6-5 Percentage Distribution of U.S. National Health Expenditures, 2010 and 2015		
	2010	2015
NHE	100.0	100.0
Personal health care	84.5	84.8
Hospital care	31.7	32.3
Physician and clinical services	19.8	19.8
Dental services	4.0	3.7
Nursing home care	5.4	4.9
Other professional services	2.7	2.7
Home health	2.7	2.8
Prescription drugs	9.7	10.1
Other personal health care	5.0	5.1
Other medical products	3.5	3.4
Government administration and net cost of private health insurance	7.1	7.9
Government public health activities	2.9	2.5
Investment	5.5	4.8
Noncommercial research	1.9	1.5
Structures and equipment	3.6	3.4
Total NHE (billions)	$2,596.4	$3,205.6
Personal health expenditures (billions)	$2,194.6	$2,717.2

Data from Centers for Medicare and Medicaid Services (CMS). 2016c. *National health expenditure data: Historical.* Available at: https://www.cms.gov
/research-statistics-data-and-systems/statistics-trends-and-reports/nationalhealthexpenddata/nationalhealthaccountshistorical.html. Accessed
January 2017.

care. Personal health expenditures constitute the amount remaining after subtracting
from NHE all of the spending for research,
structures (e.g., construction, additions,
alterations) and equipment, administrative
expenses incurred in private and public
health insurance programs, and costs of
government public health activities. In 2015,
84.8% of U.S. NHE was attributed to the
various services classified under personal
health expenditures. As a share of NHE in
percentage terms, the biggest rise between
2010 and 2015 was experienced by the government administration and net cost of private health insurance category, which reflects
the administrative costs of health insurance
under the ACA. Other areas with notable
increases included prescription drugs and
hospital services (see Table 6-5).

Trends in Private and Public Expenditures

Since 1987, CMS's Office of the Actuary
has used a standard format to compile
data separated between private and public health care expenditures. Results for
selected years are shown in **FIGURE 6-6**.
Notice the gradual decline in private
expenditures and proportional increases
in public expenditures over time. Clearly,
proportional increases in Medicare, Medicaid, and CHIP programs continue to
outpace expenditure from private sources
of health care.

The Nation's Health Care Dollar

FIGURE 6-7 provides a comprehensive picture of where U.S. national health care dollars come from (revenues), including both

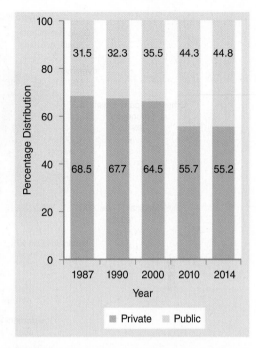

FIGURE 6-6 Proportional distribution of U.S. private
and public shares of national health expenditures.

Data from National Center for Health Statistics (NCHS). 2016. *Health, United
States, 2015.* Hyattsville, MD: U.S. Department of Health and Human
Services. pp. 310–311.

private and public sources, and how they
are spent (expenditures). Between 2011
and 2015, the most notable changes were an
increase in federal funding of Medicaid (up
from 9% in 2011) and a slight drop in Medicare funding (down from 21% in 2011). A
difference of one percentage point may
appear small, but it amounts to $27 billion
in terms of NHE for 2011. Both changes
in public financing could be attributed to
the ACA, which authorized federal dollars
for Medicaid expansion and cuts to private insurers participating in the Medicare
Advantage program. As discussed previously, private health insurance revenues did
not have a notable effect on NHE.

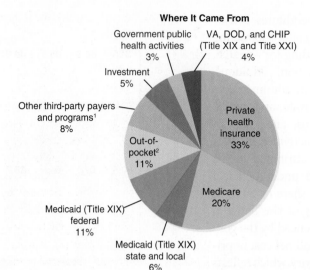

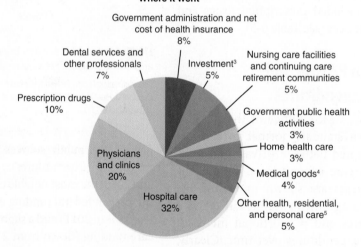

Total National Health Expenditures = $3,205.6 Billion

FIGURE 6-7 The U.S. health dollar, 2015.

[1] Includes work-site health care, other private revenues, Indian Health Service, workers' compensation, general assistance, maternal and child health, vocational rehabilitation, Substance Abuse and Mental Health Services Administration, school health, and other federal and state local programs.

[2] Includes copayments, deductibles, and any amounts not covered by health insurance.

[3] Includes research and structures and equipment.

[4] Includes durable and nondurable goods.

[5] Includes expenditures for residential care facilities, ambulance providers, medical care delivered in nontraditional settings (such as community centers, senior citizens centers, schools, and military field stations), and expenditures for Home and Community Waiver programs under Medicaid.

Note: Numbers may not add to 100 because of rounding.

Data from Centers for Medicare and Medicaid Services (CMS). 2016c. National health expenditure data: Historical. Available at: https://www.cms.gov/research-statistics -data-and-systems/statistics-trends-and-reports/nationalhealthexpenddata/nationalhealthaccountshistorical.html. Accessed January 2017. See NHE Tables.

On the expenditures side, the main changes were increases in the administration of private and public health insurance (up from 7% in 2011) and hospital care (up from 31% in 2011). There were slight drops in investments in research, structures, and equipment, as well as in payments to nursing care facilities.

▶ Current Directions and Issues

On the issue of health insurance and access to health care, significant ambiguity existed when this manuscript was prepared. As a broad undertaking to transform U.S. health care, the ACA had made major changes that spanned almost the full spectrum of health care, not just insurance. Undoing some of the changes will be a complex task, especially to avoid disruptions in coverage and to keep costs under control. In the meantime, President Trump signed an executive order on his first day in office that provides remedies for the collection of various penalties under the ACA. Subsequently, on May 5, 2017, the congressional House of Representatives passed the American Health Care Act (AHCA). This bill will undergo changes and be passed by the Senate before it reaches the President for his signature.

Value and Affordability

Whether the ACA has been a good value for consumers can be disputed. The answer actually depends on how the question is phrased—that is, for whom it has been a good value.

Certainly, those persons covered under Medicaid, those who received tax subsidies to buy health insurance, and those with preexisting health conditions and poor health status would have found the cost of health insurance to be a good value. The purpose of health insurance, however, is to ensure that the insured can gain access to health care services as and when needed. As discussed previously, conclusions about how access has been affected will remain rather sketchy until more data become available. It seems that the use of EDs for routine care has not abated, especially for Medicaid enrollees.

Under the ACA, those who did not qualify for subsidies did not get a good value if their premiums increased substantially or if they could not use their insurance to obtain routine health care services because of high deductibles. Likewise, for taxpayers, the ACA has not been a good value because of the higher taxes needed to support Medicaid expansion and subsidies. The cost of these subsidies is likely hidden under the spending category "other third-party payers and programs" (see Figure 6-7), which increased from 7% to 8% between 2011 and 2015. The cost of net subsidies, after taking into account the penalties paid by the uninsured, was estimated to be $660 billion, or 3.6% of GDP (Congressional Budget Office, 2016). For any future health reform under the Trump administration, affordability of health care for the consumers will be the most pressing issue (Jost and Pollack, 2016).

Adverse Selection

Adverse selection occurs when high-risk individuals—that is, people who are likely to use more health care services than others because of their poor health status—enroll in health insurance plans in greater numbers, compared to people who are healthy. Conversely, a health plan may face lower enrollments of young and healthy people, whose utilization of services would be much lower than the rate for people in poor health. When adverse selection occurs, premiums must be raised for everyone, which makes health insurance less affordable for those in good health.

Experience under the ACA demonstrated that adverse selection occurred in the individual health insurance market. Overall enrollments through the exchanges have fallen short of the initial projections, leaving more high-risk people in the individual insurance market. The tax penalties were apparently not harsh enough to push healthy people into buying insurance. Previously, high-risk individuals got their insurance through state-based high-risk pools. The ACA, in effect, abolished the high-risk pools and mandated that insurers cover all individuals regardless of health status. Because enough healthy individuals did not sign up, premium costs became unaffordable for many insureds.

Cost Shifting

When the amount of reimbursement from some payer becomes inadequate or when uncompensated services are rendered without payment from some source, **cost shifting** is a mechanism used to make up for revenue shortfalls. In cost shifting, providers charge extra to payers who do not exercise strict cost controls. A study on cost shifting by hospitals reported that hospitals in less competitive markets raised prices to private insurers when faced with shortfalls between Medicare payments and their projected costs (Robinson, 2011). Conversely, in competitive markets, hospitals focus on cutting costs when faced with reimbursement shortfalls from public payers.

The expansion of coverage under the ACA will be paid for in part by reducing payments to hospitals and other providers. In response, hospitals and other providers have consolidated, eroding competition. For example, the number of hospitals in highly integrated health systems grew at twice the rate from 2014 to 2015 compared to the rate of growth from 2013 to 2014 (Sanofi-Aventis, 2016). These large providers have been able to devise new ways to shift costs.

Fraud and Abuse

Health care fraud and program abuse are troubling aspects of health care financing. The Government Accountability Office (GAO) has designated Medicare and Medicaid as high-risk programs that are particularly vulnerable to fraud and abuse. Although some people have been convicted of engaging in multimillion-dollar schemes that defrauded health care programs, the full extent of the problem remains unknown (GAO, 2016) because health care fraud is almost impossible to measure.

Fraud can take several forms, and a single case can involve more than one fraud scheme. Examples of fraud include billing for services not provided, delivery of unnecessary services, providing compensation to others or receiving kickbacks for participating in a fraud scheme, and misrepresentation of services to receive higher reimbursement (GAO, 2016).

Several different laws—such as the False Claims Act, Social Security Act, and the Anti-Kickback statute—apply to health care fraud and abuse. Under the HIPAA legislation, a national Health Care Fraud and Abuse Control Program was established to coordinate federal, state, and local law enforcement activities with respect to health care fraud and abuse. This collaborative approach resulted in identifying and prosecuting the most egregious instances of health care fraud. During fiscal year 2014, the federal government recovered approximately $3.3 billion in health care fraud judgments and settlements (GAO, 2016).

▶ Summary

Financing is the lifeblood of any health care delivery system. At its most fundamental level, it determines who pays for health care services and for whom. At a secondary level, financing determines who produces which types of health care services. Hence, financing affects both the demand and supply sides of the health care equation.

A significant amount of financing is attributed to the government, mainly to provide health insurance or direct services to defined categories of people. Because most publicly financed services are obtained in the private sector, the government has a sizable interest in setting the amount of reimbursement to providers.

The ACA significantly reduced the number of uninsured Americans, mainly through the expansion of Medicaid (even though some states did not implement it) and, to a lesser extent, by facilitating the creation of health insurance marketplaces, known as exchanges, for the private purchase of health insurance. Federal subsidies were made available to people with incomes between 100% and 400% of the FPL. Even so, the largest source of health insurance in the United States remains employer-based programs, which did not show any growth in coverage. Job-based coverage had been declining for several years before the ACA was enacted, but the ACA did not seem to help this situation.

The financial stability of Medicare trust funds has improved somewhat, but they are still headed toward insolvency unless the trend can be reversed. To reduce costs and improve quality, the ACA implemented cuts to insurers participating in Medicare Advantage and established value-based reimbursement programs.

On a national level, U.S. health care expenditures have continued to shift from the private sector to the public sector. Current issues affecting financing include affordability of health care, adverse selection (which has raised premiums in the individual insurance market), cost shifting (promoted by reduced competition), and fraud and abuse (which principally affects public programs).

▶ Test Your Understanding

Terminology

adjusted community rating
adverse selection
balance bill
beneficiary
benefit period
benefits
capitation
case mix
categorical programs
charge
churning
claim
coinsurance
community rating
consumer-directed health
    plans
copayment
cost shifting
cost-plus reimbursement
deductible

entitlement
experience rating
fee schedule
gross domestic product
    (GDP)
group insurance
high-deductible health
    plans (HDHPs)
insurance
insured
insurer
means-tested program
medical loss ratio (MLR)
Medicare Physician Fee
    Schedule (MPFS)
Medigap
moral hazard
national health
    expenditures
outliers

personal health
    expenditures
plan
play-or-pay
preexisting conditions
premium
prospective
    reimbursement
rate
reinsurance
relative value units (RVUs)
retrospective
    reimbursement
risk
risk rating
self-insured plan
third-party administrator
    (TPA)
third-party payers
underwriting

Review Questions

1. What is meant by health care financing in its broad sense? How does financing affect the health care delivery system?

2. Discuss the general concept of insurance and its general principles. Describe the various types of private health insurance options, pointing out the differences among them.

3. Discuss how the concepts of premium, covered services, and cost sharing apply to health insurance.

4. What is the difference between experience rating and community rating?

5. What is Medicare Part A? Discuss the financing and cost-sharing features of Medicare Part A. Which benefits does Part A cover? Which benefits are not covered?

6. What is Medicare Part B? Discuss the financing and cost-sharing features of Medicare Part B. Which main benefits are covered under Part B? Which services are not covered?

7. Briefly describe the Medicare Advantage program.

8. Briefly explain the prescription drug program under Medicare Part D.

9. What are Medicare trust funds? Discuss the current state and the future challenges faced by the Medicare

trust funds. Which main factors pose these challenges?

10. How did the Supreme Court's ruling on the ACA affect Medicaid? How did the ACA affect the Medicaid program in terms of coverage and cost?

11. What provisions has the federal government made for providing health care to military personnel and to veterans of the U.S. armed forces?

12. What are the major methods of reimbursement for outpatient services?

13. What are the differences between the retrospective and prospective methods of reimbursement?

14. Discuss the concept of value-based purchasing, as required by the ACA.

15. Discuss the prospective payment system under DRGs.

16. Distinguish between national health expenditures and personal health expenditures.

17. What is adverse selection? What are its consequences?

18. What is the relationship between reimbursement cuts and cost shifting? How do hospitals react in different markets to cuts in reimbursement?

19. Which type of illegal activities constitute health care fraud and abuse?

▶ References

Antonisse, L., et al. 2016. *The effects of Medicaid expansion under the ACA: Findings from a literature review.* Henry J. Kaiser Family Foundation. Available at: http://files.kff.org/attachment/Issue -brief-The-Effects-of-Medicaid-Expansion -under-the-ACA-Findings-from-a-Literature -Review. Accessed January 2017.

Barbaresco, S., et al. 2015. Impacts of the Affordable Care Act dependent coverage provision on health-related outcomes of young adults. *Journal of Health Economics* 40: 54–68.

Barnett, J. C., and M. S. Vornovitsky. 2016. *Health insurance coverage in the United States: 2015: Current population reports.* Washington, DC: U.S. Government Printing Office.

Berger, A. 2015. *Did the Affordable Care Act affect insurance coverage for young adults?* Data Brief No. 2. IHIS project at the Minnesota Population Center, University of Minnesota. Available at: https://ihis.ipums.org/ihis/resources/IHIS_Data _Brief_No_2.pdf. Accessed January 2017.

Blumberg, L. J., and J. Holahan. 2016. Early experience with the ACA: Coverage gains, pooling of risk, and Medicaid expansion. *Journal of Law, Medicine & Ethics* 44, no. 4: 538–545.

Caswell, K. J., and S. K. Long. 2015. The expanding role of managed care in the Medicaid program:

Implications for health care access, use, and expenditures for nonelderly adults. *Inquiry* 52. PMID: 25882616.

Centers for Medicare and Medicaid Services (CMS). 2013. *2013 Annual report of the boards of trustees of the federal hospital insurance and federal supplementary medical insurance trust funds.* Available at: https://downloads.cms.gov /files/tr2013.pdf. Accessed April 2017.

Centers for Medicare and Medicaid Services (CMS). 2016a. *2016 Annual report of the boards of trustees of the federal hospital insurance and federal supplementary medical insurance trust funds.* Available at: https://www.cms.gov/Research -Statistics-Data-and-Systems/Statistics-Trends -and-Reports/ReportsTrustFunds/downloads /tr2016.pdf. Accessed January 2017.

Centers for Medicare and Medicaid Services (CMS). 2016b. *Total Medicaid enrollees: VIII group break out report.* Available at: https://www .medicaid.gov/medicaid/program-information /downloads/cms-64-enrollment-report-jan -mar-2016.pdf. Accessed January 2017.

Centers for Medicare and Medicaid Services (CMS). 2016c. *National health expenditure data: Historical.* Available at: https://www.cms.gov /research-statistics-data-and-systems/statistics

-trends-and-reports/nationalhealthexpend
data/nationalhealthaccountshistorical.html.
Accessed January 2017.

Centers for Medicare and Medicaid Services (CMS). 2017. *Costs for Medicare drug coverage.* Available at: https://www.medicare.gov/part-d /costs/part-d-costs.html. Accessed May 2017.

Congressional Budget Office. 2016. *Federal subsidies for health insurance coverage for people under age 65: 2016 to 2026.* Available at: https://www.cbo.gov/sites/default/files/114th -congress-2015-2016/reports/51385-Health InsuranceBaseline_OneCol.pdf. Accessed January 2017.

Cox, C., and A. Semanskee. 2016. *Preliminary data on insurer exits and entrants in 2017 Affordable Care Act marketplaces.* Kaiser Family Foundation. Available at: http://kff.org/health-reform/issue -brief/preliminary-data-on-insurer-exits -and-entrants-in-2017-affordable-care-act -marketplaces. Accessed January 2017.

Depew, B., and J. Bailey. 2015. Did the Affordable Care Act's dependent coverage mandate increase premiums? *Journal of Health Economics* 41: 1–14.

Employee Benefit Research Institute (EBRI). 2013. *Fast facts: Why uninsured? Most workers cite cost.* No. 243. Washington, DC: Employee Benefit Research Institute.

Feldstein, P. J. 1993. *Health care economics.* 4th ed. New York, NY: Delmar Publishers.

Finkelstein, A. N., et al. 2016. Effect of Medicaid coverage on ED use: Further evidence from Oregon's experiment. *New England Journal of Medicine* 375, no. 16: 1505–1507.

Gabel, J. R., et al. 2003. Self-insurance in times of growing and retreating managed care. *Health Affairs* 22, no. 2: 202–210.

Giroir, B. P., and G. R. Wilensky. 2015. Reforming the Veterans Health Administration: Beyond palliation of symptoms. *New England Journal of Medicine* 373, no. 18: 1693–1695.

Gold, M., et al. 2013. *Medicare Advantage 2013 spotlight: Enrollment market update.* Issue Brief. Menlo Park, CA: Kaiser Family Foundation.

Goodman, J. C., and G. L. Musgrave. 1992. *Patient power: Solving America's health care crisis.* Washington, DC: CATO Institute.

Goozner, M. 2015. Medicaid's enduring pay problem. *Modern Healthcare* 45, no. 22: 24.

Government Accountability Office (GAO). 2016. *Health care fraud: Information on most common schemes and the likely effect of smart cards.* Available at: http://www.gao.gov /assets/680/674771.pdf. Accessed May 2017.

Haislmaier, E. F., and D. Gonshorowski. 2014. *Obamacare's enrollment increase: Mainly due to Medicaid expansion.* Heritage Foundation. Available at: http://www.heritage.org/research /reports/2014/10/obamacares-enrollment -increase-mainly-due-to-medicaid-expansion. Accessed January 2017.

Hall, M. A., and M. J. McCue. 2013. *Insurers' medical loss ratios and quality improvement spending in 2011.* Issue Brief, March 2013. Washington, DC: Commonwealth Fund.

Han, X., et al. 2016. Characteristics of young adults enrolled through the Affordable Care Act dependent coverage expansion. *Journal of Adolescent Health* 59, no. 6: 648–653.

Health Insurance Institute. 1969. *Modern health insurance.* New York, NY: Author.

Herron, J. 2016, November 1. Here's how much Obamacare premiums are rising in all 50 states. *Fiscal Times.* Available at: http://www .thefiscaltimes.com/2016/11/01/Here-s-How -Much-Obamacare-Premiums-Are-Rising-All -50-States. Accessed January 2017.

Hoadley, J., et al. 2016. *Medicare Part D: A first look at prescription drug plans in 2017.* Available at: http://files.kff.org/attachment/Issue -Brief-Medicare-Part-D-A-First-Look-at -Prescription-Drug-Plans-in-2017. Accessed January 2017.

Huberfeld, N. 2015. The Supreme Court ruling that blocked providers from seeking higher Medicaid payments also undercut the entire program. *Health Affairs* 34, no. 7: 1156–1161.

Hudson, J. L. 2005. The impact of SCHIP on insurance coverage of children. *Inquiry* 42, no. 3: 232–254.

Hussey, P. S., et al. 2012. *Bundled payment: Effects on health care spending and quality.* Rockville, MD: Agency for Healthcare Research and Quality.

Jacobson, G., et al. 2016. *Medicare Advantage 2016 spotlight: Enrollment market update.* Henry J. Kaiser Family Foundation. Available at: http://kff.org/medicare/issue-brief/medicare -advantage-2016-spotlight-enrollment-market -update. Accessed January 2017.

Jessee, W. F. 2011. Is there an ACO in your future? *MGMA Connexion* 11, no. 1: 5–6.

Jost, T. S., and H. A. Pollack. 2016. Making health care truly affordable after health care reform. *Journal of Law, Medicine & Ethics* 44, no. 4: 546–554.

Kaiser Family Foundation. 2017. *Health insurance coverage of the total population. Timeframe: 2015.* Available at: http://kff.org/other/state-indicator /total-population/?currentTimeframe=0. Accessed January 2017.

Kaiser Family Foundation, and Health Research and Educational Trust (Kaiser/HRET). 2011. *Employer health benefits: 2011 annual survey.* Menlo Park, CA: Author.

Kaiser Family Foundation, and Health Research and Educational Trust (Kaiser/HRET). 2016. *Employer health benefits: 2016 annual survey.* Menlo Park, CA: Author.

Kowalski, A. E. 2014. *The early impact of the Affordable Care Act, state by state.* Brookings Papers on Economic Activity. Available at: https://www.brookings.edu/wp-content /uploads/2016/07/Fall2014BPEA_Kowalski.pdf. Accessed January 2017.

Levitt, K. R., et al. 1994. National health spending trends, 1960–1993. *Health Affairs* 13, no. 5: 14–31.

Medicaid and CHIP Payment and Access Commission (MACPAC). 2016. *Report to Congress on Medicaid and CHIP, June 2016.* Washington, DC: Author.

Medicare Payment Advisory Commission (MedPAC). 2009. *Ambulatory surgical centers payment system.* Available at: http://www .medpac.gov/documents/MedPAC_Payment _Basics_09_ASC.pdf. Accessed January 2011.

Medicare Payment Advisory Commission (MedPAC). 2016a. *Physician and other professional payment system.* Available at: http://www .medpac.gov/docs/default-source/payment -basics/medpac_payment_basics_16_physician _final.pdf?sfvrsn=0. Accessed January 2017.

Medicare Payment Advisory Commission (MedPAC). 2016b. *Accountable care organization payment systems.* Available at: http://www .medpac.gov/docs/default-source/payment -basics/medpac_payment_basics_16_aco_final .pdf?sfvrsn=0. Accessed January 2017.

Medicare Payment Advisory Commission (MedPAC). 2016c. *Hospital acute inpatient services payment system.* Available at: http://www

.medpac.gov/docs/default-source/payment -basics/medpac_payment_basics_16_hospital _finalecfc0fadfa9c665e80adff00009edf9c .pdf?sfvrsn=0. Accessed January 2017.

Medicare Payment Advisory Commission (MedPAC). 2016d. *Inpatient psychiatric facility services payment system.* Available at: http:// www.medpac.gov/docs/default-source /payment-basics/medpac_payment_basics_16 _psych_final.pdf?sfvrsn=0. Accessed January 2017.

Medicare Payment Advisory Commission (MedPAC). 2016e. *Long-term care hospitals payment system.* Available at: http://www .medpac.gov/docs/default-source/payment -basics/medpac_payment_basics_16_ltch_final .pdf?sfvrsn=0. Accessed January 2017.

Medicare Payment Advisory Commission (MedPAC). 2016f. *Inpatient rehabilitation facilities payment system.* Available at: http://www.medpac.gov /docs/default-source/payment-basics/medpac _payment_basics_16_irf_final.pdf?sfvrsn=0. Accessed January 2017.

Medicare Payment Advisory Commission (MedPAC). 2016g. *Home health care services payment system.* Available at: http://www .medpac.gov/docs/default-source/payment -basics/medpac_payment_basics_16_hha _final.pdf?sfvrsn=0. Accessed January 2017.

Mulvany, C. 2013. Insurance market reform: The grand experiment. *Healthcare Financial Management* 67, no. 4: 82–86, 88.

National Center for Health Statistics (NCHS). 1996. *Health, United States, 1995.* Hyattsville, MD: U.S. Department of Health and Human Services.

National Center for Health Statistics (NCHS). 2012. *Health, United States, 2012.* Hyattsville, MD: U.S. Department of Health and Human Services.

National Center for Health Statistics (NCHS). 2016. *Health, United States, 2015.* Hyattsville, MD: U.S. Department of Health and Human Services.

Newhouse, J. P., and T. G. McGuire. 2014. How successful is Medicare Advantage? *Milbank Quarterly* 92, no. 2: 351–394.

Noble, A., and M. A. Chirba. 2013. Individual and group coverage under the ACA: More patches to the federal-state crazy quilt. *Health Affairs Blog.* Available at: http://healthaffairs

.org/blog/2013/01/17/individual-and-group
-coverage-under-the-aca-more-patches-to-the
-federal-state-crazy-quilt. Accessed February
2017.

Nyman, J. A., and H. M. Trenz. 2016. Affordability
of the health expenditures of insured Americans
before the Affordable Care Act. *American
Journal of Public Health* 106, no. 2: 264–266.

Pines, J. M., et al. 2016. Medicaid expansion in 2014
did not increase emergency department use but
did change insurance payer mix. *Health Affairs*
35, no. 8: 1480–1486.

Radnofsky, L., and S. Armour. 2016, August 24.
States start to approve steep increases in health
premiums. *Wall Street Journal: Online Edition*,
p. 1.

Roberts, E. T., and D. J. Gaskin. 2015. Projecting
primary care use in the Medicaid expansion
population: Evidence for providers and policy
makers. *Medical Care Research and Review* 72,
no. 5: 515–561.

Robinson, J. 2011. Hospitals respond to Medicare
payment shortfalls by both shifting costs and
cutting them, based on market concentration.
Health Affairs 30, no. 7: 1265–1271.

Sanofi-Aventis. 2016. *Managed care digest series:
Hospital/systems digest, 2016.* Bridgewater, NJ:
Author.

Shane, D. M., et al. 2016. Continued gains in health
insurance but few signs of increased utilization:
An update on the ACA's dependent coverage
mandate. *Medical Care Research and Review* 73,
no. 4: 478–492.

Shone, L. P., et al. 2005. Reduction in racial and
ethnic disparities after enrollment in the State
Children's Health Insurance Program. *Pediatrics*
115, no. 6: e697–e705.

Somers, A. R., and H. M. Somers. 1977. *Health and
health care: Policies in perspective.* Germantown,
MD: Aspen Systems.

Sommers, B. D., and S. Rosenbaum. 2011. Issues in
health reform: How changes in eligibility may
move millions back and forth between Medicaid
and insurance exchanges. *Health Affairs* 30, no.
2: 228–236.

Sommers, B. D., et al. 2014. Medicaid and
marketplace eligibility changes will occur often
in all states: Policy options can ease impact.
Health Affairs 33, no. 4: 700–707.

Sonfield, A., and H. A. Pollack. 2013. The Affordable
Care Act and reproductive health: Potential
gains and serious challenges. *Journal of Health
Politics, Policy and Law* 38, no. 2: 373–391.

Tanenbaum, S. J. 2017. Can payment reform be
social reform? The lure and liabilities of the
"triple aim." *Journal of Health Politics, Policy and
Law* 42, no. 1: 53–71.

U.S. Department of Defense (DOD). 2014. *Final
report to the secretary of defense: Military Health
System review.* Available at: http://archive.
defense.gov/pubs/140930_MHS_Review_Final
_Report_Main_Body.pdf. Accessed January
2017.

Vaughn, E. J., and C. M. Elliott. 1987. *Fundamentals
of risk and insurance.* New York, NY: John Wiley
& Sons.

Veterans Health Administration (VHA). 2017.
Veterans Health Administration. Available at:
https://www.va.gov/health. Accessed January
2017.

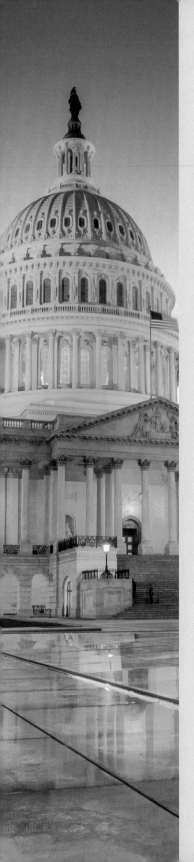

PART III

System Processes

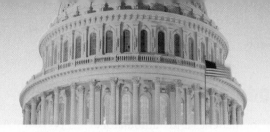

CHAPTER 7

Outpatient and Primary Care Services

LEARNING OBJECTIVES

- Understand the meanings of outpatient, ambulatory, and primary care.
- Explore the main principles behind patient-centered medical homes and community-based primary care.
- Identify the reasons for the dramatic growth in outpatient services.
- Survey the various types of outpatient settings and services.
- Describe the role of complementary and alternative medicine in health care.
- Describe primary care delivery in other countries.
- Assess the impact of the Affordable Care Act on primary care.

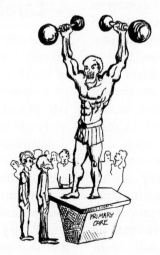

"I suppose a system based on primary care is more robust."

▶ Introduction

The terms "outpatient" and "ambulatory" have often been used interchangeably. Historically, outpatient care has been independent from services provided in health care institutions. In earlier days, physicians saw patients in their clinics, and most physicians also made home visits to treat patients within the limitations of medical science prevalent in those days. Institutions for inpatient care, such as hospitals and nursing homes, developed later. With advances in medical science, the locus of health care delivery coalesced around the institutional setting of community hospitals. As the range of services that could be provided on an outpatient basis continued to expand, hospitals gradually became the dominant players in providing the vast majority of outpatient care, with the exception of basic diagnostic care provided in physicians' offices (Barr and Breindel, 2004). Hospitals were better equipped to provide outpatient services because they had the resources necessary to capitalize on technological innovation. For example, hospital laboratories and diagnostic units were better equipped to perform most tests and diagnostic procedures than independent providers. In comparison, independent providers faced greater capital constraints and competitive pressures in the health care marketplace.

Later, health care delivery increasingly grew beyond expensive acute care hospitals to various alternative outpatient settings. Although basic primary care has traditionally been the foundation of outpatient services, some intensive procedures are also increasingly being performed on an outpatient basis. Additionally, consumer demand has fueled the growth of complementary and alternative medicine.

Today, a large variety of outpatient services are available in the United States, yet many Americans do not have adequate access to health care because of maldistribution or shortages of providers and services. Hospital emergency care and community health centers constitute the main safety net for primary care services, particularly for uninsured individuals. Delivery of outpatient care by public agencies has been limited in scope and detached from the dominant private system of health services delivery. State and local government agencies sponsor limited outpatient services such as child immunizations, maternal and infant care, health screenings in public schools, monitoring of certain contagious diseases (e.g., tuberculosis), family planning, and prevention of sexually transmitted diseases. The Affordable Care Act includes provisions to address some of the issues of access for poor and vulnerable populations.

▶ What Is Outpatient Care?

Outpatient services do not require an overnight inpatient stay in an institution of health care delivery, such as a hospital or long-term care facility. Many hospitals, in addition to admitting patients for overnight or longer stays, have emergency departments (EDs) and other outpatient service centers, such as outpatient surgery, rehabilitation, and specialized clinics.

Outpatient services are also referred to as **ambulatory care**. Strictly speaking, ambulatory care constitutes diagnostic and therapeutic services and treatments provided to the "walking" (ambulatory) patient. Hence, in a restricted sense, the term "ambulatory care" refers to care rendered to patients who come to physicians' offices, hospital outpatient departments, and health centers to receive care. This term is also used synonymously with "community medicine" (Wilson and Neuhauser, 1985) because the geographic location of ambulatory services is intended to serve the surrounding community, providing convenience and easy accessibility to health care services for the members of that community.

However, patients do not always walk or drive their personal vehicles to the service centers to receive ambulatory care. For example, in a hospital ED, patients may arrive by land or air ambulance. EDs, in most cases, are equipped to provide secondary and tertiary care services rather than primary care. In other instances, such as with mobile diagnostic units and home health care, services are transported to the patient, instead of the patient coming to receive the services. Hence, the terms

"outpatient" and "inpatient" are more precise, with the term **outpatient services** referring to any health care services that are not provided on the basis of an overnight stay in which room and board are incurred.

▶ The Scope of Outpatient Services

Since the 1980s, extraordinary growth has occurred in the volume and variety of outpatient services, and new settings have emerged for delivering outpatient services. **TABLE 7-1** provides some examples. Hospital-based medical systems and integrated delivery organizations now offer a range of health care services that include a variety of outpatient services. In some areas, the growth of non-hospital-based ambulatory services has intensified the competition between hospitals and community-based providers over patients

TABLE 7-1 Owners, Providers, and Settings for Ambulatory Care Services	
Past	**Present**
Owners/Providers	
■ Independent physician practitioners ■ Hospitals ■ Community health agencies ■ Home health agencies	■ Independent physician practitioners ■ Hospitals ■ Community health agencies ■ Managed care organizations ■ Insurance companies ■ Corporate employers ■ Group practices ■ National physician chains ■ Home health companies ■ National diversified health care companies

(continues)

TABLE 7-1 Owners, Providers, and Settings for Ambulatory Care Services (*continued*)	
Past	**Present**
Service Settings	
<ul><li>Hospital outpatient departments</li><li>Physicians' offices</li><li>Outpatient surgery centers</li><li>Hospital emergency departments</li><li>Home health agencies</li><li>Neighborhood health centers</li></ul>	<ul><li>Physicians' offices</li><li>Walk-in clinics/urgent care centers</li><li>Retail clinics</li><li>Outpatient surgery centers</li><li>Chemotherapy and radiation therapy centers</li><li>Dialysis centers</li><li>Community health centers</li><li>Diagnostic imaging centers</li><li>Mobile imaging centers</li><li>Fitness/wellness centers</li><li>Occupational health centers</li><li>Psychiatric outpatient centers</li><li>Rehabilitation centers</li><li>Sports medicine clinics</li><li>Hand injury rehabilitation clinics</li><li>Women's health clinics</li><li>Wound care centers</li></ul>

Data from Barr, K. W., and C. L. Breindel. 2004. Ambulatory care. In: *Health care administration: Planning, implementing, and managing organized delivery systems.* L. F. Wolper, ed. 4th ed. Burlington, MA: Jones & Bartlett Learning. pp. 507–546.

seeking outpatient care. Examples of such competitors in the outpatient services market include home health care, freestanding clinics for routine and urgent care, retail clinics, outpatient rehabilitation, and freestanding imaging centers. Other services, such as dental care and optometric services, remain independent of other types of health care services. Financing is the main reason for their independent nature: Medical insurance plans are generally separate from dental and vision care plans. Philosophical and technical differences account for other variations. Chiropractic care, for instance, is generally covered by most health plans but remains isolated from the mainstream practice of medicine. Complementary and alternative therapies as well as self-care are not covered by insurance, yet the products and services in these categories continue to experience remarkable growth.

Primary care is the foundation of ambulatory health services, but not all ambulatory care is primary care. For example, hospital ED services are not intended to be primary in nature. Conversely, services other than primary care have now become an integral part of outpatient services. Thanks to the technological advances in medicine, many advanced treatments are now provided in ambulatory care settings. Examples include conditions requiring urgent treatment, outpatient surgery, renal dialysis, and chemotherapy.

▶ Primary Care

Primary care plays a central role in a health care delivery system. Other essential levels of care include secondary and tertiary care (distinct from the primary, secondary, and tertiary prevention discussed in the *Beliefs, Values, and Health* chapter). Compared to primary care, secondary and tertiary care services are more complex and specialized.

Primary care is distinguished from secondary and tertiary care according to its duration, frequency, and level of intensity. **Secondary care** is usually short term, involving sporadic consultation from a specialist to provide expert opinion and surgical or other advanced interventions that primary care physicians (PCPs) are not equipped to perform. It includes hospitalization, routine surgery, specialty consultation, and rehabilitation.

Tertiary care is the most complex level of care, which is provided for relatively uncommon conditions. Typically, tertiary care is institution based, highly specialized, and technology driven. Much of tertiary care is rendered in large teaching hospitals, such as university hospitals. Examples include trauma care, burn treatment, neonatal intensive care, tissue transplants, and open heart surgery. In some instances, tertiary treatment may be extended, and the tertiary care physician may assume long-term responsibility for the bulk of the patient's care.

It has been estimated that 75% to 85% of people in the general population require only primary care services in a given year, 10% to 12% require referrals to short-term secondary care services, and 5% to 10% use tertiary care specialists (Starfield, 1994). These proportions vary in populations with special health care needs.

Definitions of primary care often focus on the type or level of services, such as prevention, diagnostic and therapeutic services, health education and counseling, and minor surgery. Although primary care specifically emphasizes these services, many specialists also provide the same spectrum of services. For example, the practice of most ophthalmologists has a large element of prevention, as well as diagnosis, treatment, follow-up, and minor surgery. Similarly, most cardiologists are engaged in health education and counseling. Hence, primary care should be more appropriately viewed as an approach to providing health care rather than as a set of specific services (Starfield, 1994).

World Health Organization Definition

Traditionally, primary care has been the cornerstone of ambulatory care services. The World Health Organization (WHO, 1978) describes **primary health care** as follows:

> Essential health care based on practical, scientifically sound, and socially acceptable methods and technology made universally accessible to individuals and families in the community by means acceptable to them and at a cost that the community and the country can afford to maintain at every stage of their development in a spirit of self-reliance and self-determination. It forms an integral part of both the country's health system of which it is the central function and the main focus of the overall social and economic development of the community. It is the first level of contact of individuals, the family, and the community with the national health system, bringing health care

as close as possible to where people live and work and constitutes the first element of a continuing health care process.[1]

Three elements in this definition are particularly noteworthy for an understanding of primary care: point of entry, coordination of care, and essential care.

Point of Entry

Primary care is the point of entry into the health services system in which health care delivery is organized around primary care (Starfield, 1992). Primary care is the first contact a patient makes with the health care delivery system. This first contact feature is closely associated with the "gatekeeper" role of the primary care practitioner. **Gatekeeping** implies that patients do not visit specialists and are not admitted to a hospital without first being referred by their PCPs. The interposition of primary care protects patients from undergoing unnecessary procedures and overtreatment (Franks et al., 1992).

The United Kingdom's National Health Service (NHS) is an example of a health care delivery system founded on the principles of gatekeeping. In the NHS, primary care is the single portal of entry to secondary care and acts as a filter so that 90% of care is provided outside hospitals in ambulatory care settings (Orton, 1994). General practitioners (GPs) are primary care gatekeepers in the U.K. system. In the United States, under certain managed care, such as most Kaiser Health Plans, patients initiate care with their PCPs and obtain authorization when specialized services are needed.

Coordination of Care

One of the main functions of primary care is to coordinate the delivery of health services between the patient and the myriad of delivery components of the system. Hence, in addition to providing basic services, primary care professionals serve as patient advisors and advocates. Coordination of an individual's total health care needs is meant to ensure continuity and comprehensiveness. These desirable goals of primary care are best achieved when the patient and the provider have formed a close mutual relationship over time. Primary care can be regarded as the hub of the health care delivery system wheel. The various components of the health care delivery system are located around the rim of this wheel, and the spokes signify the coordination of continuous and comprehensive care (**FIGURE 7-1**).

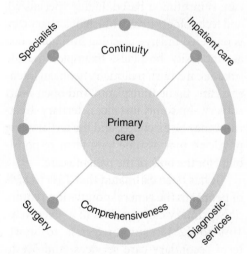

FIGURE 7-1 The coordination role of primary care in health care delivery.

---

[1] Reproduced from World Health Organization (WHO). 1978. *Primary health care*. Geneva, Switzerland: WHO.

Countries whose health systems are oriented more toward primary care achieve better health levels, higher satisfaction with health services among their citizens, and lower expenditures for the overall delivery of health care (Starfield, 1994, 1998). Even in the United States, better health outcomes are achieved in states with higher ratios of PCPs and better availability of primary care (Shi, 1994; Shi and Starfield, 2000, 2001; Shi et al., 2002). Higher ratios of family and general physicians in the population are associated with lower hospitalization rates for conditions that can be successfully treated with good primary care (Chang et al., 2011; Parchman and Culler, 1994). Having a regular source of primary care also leads to fewer ED visits and inappropriate specialty consults. The primary care setting is the ideal place to manage chronic conditions so individuals can stay healthier over time (Rubin et al., 2015; Sepulveda et al., 2008). Adults who have PCPs as their regular source of care experience lower mortality (Franks et al., 1998; Jerant et al., 2012). Research has also shown that primary care may play an important role in mitigating the adverse health effects of income inequality (Jones et al., 2013; Shi et al., 1999). A higher proportion of PCPs in a given area has been shown to lead to lower spending on health care (Chernew et al., 2009).

Coordination of health care has definite advantages. Studies have shown that both the appropriateness and the outcomes of health care interventions are better when PCPs refer patients to specialists, as opposed to patients self-referring to specialists (Bakwin, 1945; Roos, 1979).

Essential Care

Primary health care is regarded as essential health care. The goal of the health care delivery system is to optimize population health, not just the health of individuals who have the means to access health services. Achieving this goal requires that disparities across population subgroups be minimized to ensure equal access. Because financing of health care is a key element in determining access, universal access to primary care services is better achieved under a national health care program.

Institute of Medicine Definition

The Institute of Medicine's (IOM) Committee on the Future of Primary Care recommends that primary care be the usual and preferred, though not the only, route of entry into the health care system. To emphasize this point, the IOM has defined primary care as "the provision of integrated, accessible health care services by clinicians who are accountable for addressing a large majority of personal health care needs, developing a sustained partnership with patients, and practicing in the context of family and community" (Vanselow et al., 1995, p. 192).

The term "integrated" in this definition embodies the concepts of comprehensive, coordinated, and continuous services that provide a seamless process of care. Primary care is *comprehensive* because it addresses any health problem at any given stage of a patient's life cycle. *Coordination* ensures the provision of a combination of health services to best meet the patient's needs. *Continuity* refers to care administered over time by a single provider or a team of health care professionals.

The IOM definition also emphasizes accessibility and accountability as key characteristics of primary care. *Accessibility* refers to the ease with which a patient can initiate an interaction with a clinician for any health problem. It includes efforts to eliminate barriers, such as those posed by geography, financing, culture, race, and language. Both clinicians and patients have **accountability**. The clinical system is accountable for providing quality care, producing patient satisfaction, using resources efficiently, and behaving in an ethical manner. Patients are responsible for their own health to the extent that they can influence it, as well for judicious use of resources when they need health care. The partnership between a patient and a clinician is based on mutual trust, respect, and responsibility.

Various countries have established policies that hold primary care practices accountable for managing chronic conditions and meeting clinical standards. These policies tend to include financial incentives and primary care practice redesign, with an emphasis on information technology (IT) and use of interdisciplinary teams to support effective, safe, patient-centered, coordinated, and efficient care.

The IOM definition of primary care recognizes that primary care clinicians must consider the influence of the family on a patient's health status and be aware of the patient's living conditions, family dynamics, and cultural background. In addition, exemplary primary care requires an understanding of and a responsibility for the community's health (Vanselow et al., 1995).

▶ Primary Care and the Affordable Care Act

The Affordable Care Act (ACA) included four major provisions related to primary care:

- Increased Medicare and Medicaid payments to primary care providers
- New incentives such as funding for scholarships and loan repayment for primary care providers working in underserved areas
- Expansion of the health center program and strengthening of health center capacity
- Creation of additional training programs, such as 11 Teaching Health Centers to train primary care providers

These measures were aimed at enhancing the primary care workforce and strengthening the primary care system, especially in underserved areas (Ku et al., 2011).

On the surface, these measures appear to be steps in the right direction. Unfortunately, given the critical shortages in primary care (see the *System Resources* chapter), building a workforce cannot be accomplished in a short period of time. Current and prospective physicians will also evaluate factors other than the proposed incentives when determining whether they will become PCPs or specialists. For example, physicians may feel burdened and frustrated by new regulatory demands if they have to spend a large share of their time complying with added regulations instead of seeing patients. In addition, because the increased reimbursement for PCPs under the ACA was temporary, this may not turn out to be a significant factor in providers' decisions to leave or stay in practice or influencing medical students to enter primary care.

As a result of the ACA, the primary care system in the United States is expected to experience an influx of newly insured patients. However, if PCPs become overburdened, many of the goals of primary care may remain unrealized for a large segment of the U.S. population.

The ACA also eliminated out-of-pocket costs for preventive services such as immunizations, certain cancer screenings, contraception, reproductive counseling, obesity screening, and behavioral assessments for children. This coverage is guaranteed for more than 137 million Americans, including 55 million women. Approximately 39 million Medicare beneficiaries have received preventive services such as cancer screenings, bone-mass measurements, annual physical examinations, and smoking cessation assistance due to the elimination of out-of-pocket costs for this care.

On another front, the ACA allocated $1.5 billion to National Health Service Corps, a training program, which for decades has offered scholarships and loan forgiveness to young primary care clinicians who volunteer to practice in underserved areas. As of September 30, 2015, there were 9,600 Corps clinicians providing primary care services, more than twice the number of these clinicians in 2008 (White House, 2016).

▶ New Directions in Primary Care

Patient-Centered Medical Homes

The term "medical home" was first coined in 1967 to describe the team-oriented approaches developed for special-needs children whose health care needs require constant coordination. A **medical home** consists of an interdisciplinary team of physicians and allied health professionals who partner with patients and their families, taking responsibility for ongoing patient care using a team approach, technology, and evidence-based protocols to deliver and coordinate care. PCPs serve as advocates for patients to help them access services across the wide variety of health care services, ensuring that the patient's values, wishes, and directives are honored (Caudill et al., 2011).

The patient-centered medical home (PCMH) has emerged as a promising solution to address the significant fragmentation, poor quality, and high costs that afflict the U.S. health care system. With regard to PCMH and service utilization, evaluations of appropriate care have typically focused on greater use of preventive services, immunizations, and well-care visits, whereas evaluations of inappropriate use of services have examined outcomes such as ED visits, rates of hospitalization for preventable ambulatory conditions, and use of high-cost or inefficient procedures. Findings from these evaluations provide considerable support for the value of PCMHs, as they promote appropriate care and reduce inappropriate care (Christensen et al., 2013; Ferrante et al., 2010; Rosenthal et al., 2015; Shi et al., 2015; Shi et al., 2016).

In terms of the impact of a PCMH on the patient's experience and quality of care, studies suggest that both adult patients and parents of pediatric patients who go to a PCMH-designated primary care practice are satisfied with the care that they and their children receive and likely to perceive these health care interactions as positive experiences (Christensen et al., 2013; Rosenthal et al., 2015); however, evidence for the associations between PCMH and some other quality indicators remains mixed (Christensen et al., 2013; Rosenthal et al.,

2015; Stevens et al., 2010). Likewise, findings regarding PCMH and health care costs are inconsistent (Christensen et al., 2013; Gao et al., 2016; Gilfillan et al., 2010; Reid et al., 2009).

In terms of the impact of PCMHs and clinical outcomes, several studies have demonstrated a positive impact of PCMHs on clinical measures at the practice level (Gao et al., 2016; Shi et al., 2015; Shi et al., 2016), but insufficient evidence is available to determine the effect of PCMH implementation at the patient level. More rigorous evaluations and standardization of key outcomes are needed to strengthen the empirical basis for the medical home concept and to assess the viability of implementation (Mulvihill et al., 2007).

A number of tools are used to assess important aspects of the PCMH. For example, the National Committee for Quality Assurance's (NCQA) Physician Practice Connections—Patient-Centered Medical Home (PPC-PCMH) tool is a practice self-report measure that has become the de facto standard used to judge "medical homeness." It assesses nine standards: access and communication, patient tracking and registries, care management, patient self-management support, electronic prescribing, test tracking, referral tracking, performance reporting and improvement, and advanced electronic communications. The three-level scoring system implicitly acknowledges that, for most practices, meeting these reporting standards will be a staged process (NCQA, 2008).

Unlike the NCQA, the Accreditation Association for Ambulatory Health Care (AAAHC) conducts mandatory site visits to all applicants for its PCMH recognition program. AAAHC's recognition program involves the largest number of survey items by far (238 items), and AAAHC is unique in that it allows applicants to apply for either "accreditation" (which involves obtaining the base AAAHC accreditation in addition to meeting AAAHC's medical home standards) or a less burdensome option called "certification" (which does not require the base AAAHC accreditation). The AAAHC's Medical Home tool measures a practice's performance in regard to patient rights and responsibilities; organizational governance and administration; the patient-care team relationship; comprehensiveness, continuity, and accessibility of care; clinical records and health information; and quality of care (AAAHC, 2009).

Other PCMH assessment tools include the Joint Commission's Primary Care Medical Home Designation Standards (Joint Commission, 2011), URAC's Patient-Centered Health Care Home (PCHCH) Program Toolkit, TransforMED's Medical Home Implementation Quotient, and the Center for Medical Home Improvement's Medical Home Index. State-level tools are also available, including BlueCross BlueShield of Michigan's PCMH Designation standards, Minnesota's statewide multipayer Health Care Home Certification standards, and Oklahoma's SoonerCare (Medicaid) PCMH standards, among others (Burton et al., 2012).

Most of the PCMH assessment tools cover several key content domains: access to care, comprehensiveness of care, continuity of care, culturally competent communication, patient engagement and self-management, coordination of care, care plan, population management, team-based care, evidence-based care, quality measurement and improvement, community resources, medical records, health IT, standardized care, adherence to current law, and congruence between practice and patient (Burton et al., 2012).

Community-Oriented Primary Care

Current thoughts about primary care delivery have extended beyond the traditional biomedical paradigm, which focuses on medical care for the individual in an encounter-based system. The broader biopsychosocial paradigm emphasizes the health of the population, as well as that of the individual. **Community-oriented primary care (COPC)** emphasizes the relations between the population and community, on the one hand, and personal health care, on the other hand (van Weel et al., 2008). COPC incorporates the elements of good primary care delivery and adds a population-based approach to identifying and addressing community health problems. The main challenge has been bringing together individual health needs in the larger context of community health needs.

COPC incorporates the ideals espoused by both WHO and IOM in the delivery of primary care. The 1978 International Conference on Primary Health Care (held at Alma-Ata in the former Soviet Union, under the auspices of WHO) declared a philosophical vision of an affordable community-based primary health care system (WHO, 1978). More recently, WHO (2010) has offered some additional guidelines that encompass five key elements: (1) reducing exclusion and social disparities in health through universal coverage reforms, (2) organizing health services around people's needs and expectations, (3) integrating health into all sectors, (4) pursuing collaborative models of policy dialogue, and (5) increasing stakeholder participation. IOM (2012) has endorsed COPC as a dynamic, interdisciplinary model that integrates primary care and public health creating significant improvements in primary care delivery.

The application and adoption of COPC principles in actual practice, however, has not materialized in the United States. One fundamental problem is a lack of consensus on what a "community" is or should be. Assuming that consensus on the definition of a community can be reached, technological advances have reached a stage of development at which they can adequately reflect a community's health. Information technology can also assist in prioritizing and developing a course of action. Perhaps the biggest hurdles to COPC in the United States are workforce shortages and financial incentives. COPC requires a major transformation of the current system and faces the same implementation problems as medical homes.

▶ Primary Care Providers

Physicians in general family practice are most commonly the providers of primary care in Europe. In the United States, primary care practitioners are not restricted to physicians trained in general and family practice, but also include physicians trained in internal medicine, pediatrics, and obstetrics and gynecology. One cannot assume, however, that these various types of practitioners are equally skilled in rendering primary care services (Starfield, 1994). Unless a medical training program is dedicated to providing instruction in primary care, significant differences are likely to exist between its graduates and other PCPs. In fact, some controversy and competition have arisen among practitioners as to which specialists should be providing primary care. The specialty of family practice, in particular, represents a challenge to internal medicine in providing adult primary care and to pediatrics in providing child primary care.

Nonphysician practitioners (NPPs) are also playing a larger role in the delivery of primary care in the United States. In light of the increasing emphasis on health care cost containment, NPPs—who include nurse practitioners (NPs), physician assistants (PAs), and certified nurse-midwives (CNMs), among others—are in great demand in primary care delivery settings, particularly in medically underserved area (MUAs). Data from Medicaid managed care organizations (MCOs) demonstrate that patients receiving care from NPs at nurse-managed health centers experience significantly fewer emergency room visits, hospital inpatient days, and specialist visits, and female patients are at a significantly lower risk of giving birth to low-birth-weight infants, compared to patients in conventional health care (National Nursing Centers Consortium, 2003).

A recent retrospective cross-sectional analysis of national administrative data from Veterans Health Administration (VHA) primary care encounters showed NPs and PAs attended approximately 30% of all VHA primary care encounters, and NPs, PAs, and physicians fill similar roles in VHA primary care (Morgan et al., 2012). Similar results were also found in a study conducted in community health centers, with NPs and PAs providing 21%

and 10%, respectively, of care for vulnerable populations (Morgan et al., 2015). Nevertheless, PCPs continue to fill an expert role that NPPs cannot match.

▶ Growth in Outpatient Services

In the United States, the proportion of total surgeries performed in outpatient departments of community hospitals increased from 16.3% in 1980 to 65.6% in 2013 (**FIGURE 7-2**). This decline in inpatient procedures has actually been outweighed by the growth of ambulatory procedures. Moreover, for patients older than 65 years, the rate of inpatient surgeries has not decreased (Kozak et al., 1999; National Center for Health Statistics, 2010). In a study performed by Wier et al. (2015), the 10 most common ambulatory surgeries performed in community hospitals in 28 states were lens and cataract procedures (9.3% of all ambulatory surgeries), other therapeutic procedures on muscles and tendons (5.8%), other operating room therapeutic procedures on joints (4.5%), cholecystectomy and common duct exploration (4.0%), excision of semilunar cartilage of the knee (3.6%), inguinal and femoral hernia repair (2.8%), other operating room therapeutic procedures on the skin and breast (2.5%), lumpectomy and quadrantectomy of the breast (2.4%), decompression peripheral nerve (2.4%), and other hernia repair (2.3%).

Over the years, several noteworthy changes have been instrumental in shifting the delivery of health care from inpatient to outpatient settings. These changes can be broadly classified as reimbursement, technological factors, utilization

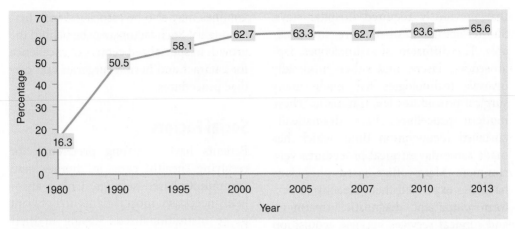

FIGURE 7-2 Percentage of total surgeries performed in outpatient departments of U.S. community hospitals, 1980–2013.

Data from National Center for Health Statistics. 2016. *Health, United States, 2015.* Hyattsville, MD: U.S. Department of Health and Human Services. p. 281.

control factors, physician practice factors, and social factors.

Reimbursement

Until the 1980s, health insurance coverage was usually more generous for inpatient services than for outpatient services. For years, many interventions that could have been performed safely and effectively on an outpatient basis remained inpatient procedures because third-party reimbursement for outpatient care was limited. These payment policies began to change during the 1980s. In response, hospitals aggressively developed outpatient services to offset their declining revenues from inpatient care.

In the mid-1980s, Medicare substituted a prospective payment system (PPS) for its traditional cost-plus system to reimburse inpatient hospital services (see the *Health Services Financing* chapter). PPS reimbursement, which is based on diagnosis-related groups (DRGs), provides fixed case-based payments to hospitals.

In contrast, the outpatient sector was not subject to payment restrictions. Therefore, hospitals had a strong incentive to minimize inpatient lengths of stay and to provide continued treatment in outpatient settings—which led to mushrooming costs in the outpatient sector. In 2000, Medicare implemented prospective reimbursement mechanisms in an effort to contain these costs, such as the Medicare Outpatient Prospective Payment System (OPPS) for services provided in hospital outpatient departments and home health resource groups (HHRGs) for home health care (see the *Health Services Financing* chapter). Cost-containment strategies adopted by managed care also stress lower inpatient use, with a corresponding emphasis on outpatient services.

Technological Factors

The development of new diagnostic and treatment procedures and less invasive surgical methods has made it possible to provide services in outpatient settings that previously required hospital stays. Shorter-acting anesthetics are now available. The diffusion of arthroscopes, laparoscopes, lasers, and other minimally invasive technologies has made many surgical procedures less traumatic. These modern procedures have dramatically curtailed recuperation time, which has made same-day surgical procedures very common. Many office-based physicians have also expanded their capacity to perform outpatient diagnostic, treatment, and surgical services because acquisition of technology has become more feasible and cost-effective.

Utilization Control Factors

To discourage lengthy hospital stays, payers have instituted prior authorization policies for inpatient admission as well as close monitoring during hospitalization. The *Managed Care and Integrated Organizations* chapter discusses the most widely adopted utilization control methods.

Physician Practice Factors

The growth of managed care and the consolidation trend associated with large hospital-centered institutions weakened physician autonomy and professional control over the delivery of medical care. Physicians also lost income. To counter these forces, an increasing number of physicians have broken their ties with hospitals and started their own specialized care centers, such as ambulatory surgery centers and cardiac care centers. In these kinds of specialized ambulatory care centers, physicians often find that they can perform more procedures in less time and earn higher incomes (Jackson, 2002). Higher

volumes may also be associated with better quality. Such factors may be behind the growth in specialized centers of excellence for cataract and hernia surgeries and cardiac procedures.

Social Factors

Patients have a strong preference for receiving health care in home- and community-based settings. Unless absolutely necessary, most patients do not want to be institutionalized. Staying in their own homes gives people a strong sense of independence and control over their lives—elements considered important for better quality of life.

Large hospitals have traditionally been located in congested urban centers, but increasing numbers of suburbanites now perceive these locations as inconvenient. Hence, many freestanding outpatient centers and satellite clinics operated by inner-city hospitals are now located in the suburbs.

▶ Types of Outpatient Care Settings and Methods of Delivery

The services described in this section are not always operated independently of each other. For example, a hospital may operate physician clinics in addition to some of the freestanding facilities described here. Also, in a constantly evolving system, new settings and methods are likely to emerge. However, in general, the various settings for outpatient service delivery found in the U.S. health care delivery system can be grouped as follows:

- Private practice
- Hospital-based services
- Freestanding facilities
- Retail clinics
- Mobile medical, diagnostic, and screening services
- Home health care
- Hospice services
- Ambulatory long-term care services
- Public health services
- Community health centers
- Free clinics
- Telephone access
- Complementary and alternative medicine

Private Practice

Physicians, as office-based practitioners, are the backbone of ambulatory care and constitute the vast majority of primary care services. Most visits entail relatively limited examination and testing, and encounters with the physician are generally brief. Office waiting time is typically longer than the actual time spent with the physician.

In the past, the solo practice of medicine and small partnerships attracted the large numbers of practitioners. Self-employment offered a degree of independence not generally available in large organizational settings. Today, however, most physicians are affiliated with group practices or institutions, such as hospitals and MCOs. Several factors account for this shift: uncertainties created by rapid changes in the health care delivery system, contracting by MCOs with consolidated organizations rather than solo entities, competition from large health care delivery organizations, the high cost of operating a solo practice, complexity of billings and collections in a multiple-payer system,

and increased external demands, such as the necessity of having up-to-date IT systems. Group practice and other organizational arrangements offer the benefits of a patient referral network, negotiated leverage with MCOs, sharing of overhead expenses, ease of obtaining coverage from colleagues for personal time off, and attractive starting salaries, with benefits and profit-sharing plans.

Group practice of medicine in the United States has experienced a sharp increase in recent years (**FIGURE 7-3**). An estimated 59.3% of physicians are now in solo or single-specialty group practices, whereas 24.7% are in multispecialty group practices (American Medical Association,

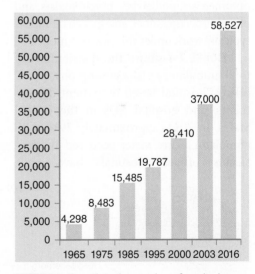

FIGURE 7-3 Growth in the number of medical group practices in the United States.

Data from Medical Group Management Association. *Medical group fast facts.* Available at: http://www.mgma.com/uploadedFiles/Store_Content /Surveys_and_Benchmarking/8523-Table-of-Content-MGMA -Performance-and-Practices-of-Successful-Medical-Groups.pdf; SK&A. 2016. *Medical group practice list.* http://www.skainfo.com/databases /medical-group-practice-list. Accessed January 2016; VHA Inc. and Deloitte & Touche. 1997. *Environmental assessment: Redesigning health care for the millennium.* Irving, TX: VHA Inc.; SMG Solutions. 2000. *Report and directory: Medical group practices.* Chicago, IL: SMG Solutions.

2015). Most of these groups are small, with 40.9% having no more than 4 physicians. By comparison, 31.9% have 5 to 24 physicians, and only 19.8% have 25 or more physicians.

Group practice clinics also offer important advantages to patients. In many instances, patients can receive up-to-date diagnostic, treatment, pharmaceutical, and certain surgical services in the same location. All but the most advanced secondary and tertiary procedures can be performed within these large clinics. Patients also often see cross-referrals among partner physicians located near each other as an added convenience.

Apart from physicians, other private practitioners often work in solo or group practice settings. For example, dentists, optometrists, podiatrists, psychologists, and physical, occupational, and speech therapists typically work under this practice model.

FIGURE 7-4 shows the distribution of total ambulatory visits among physicians' offices, hospital-based outpatient departments, and hospital EDs in the United States. In 2011, approximately 79% of all ambulatory care visits occurred in physicians' offices. Hospitals have made substantial strides in gaining market share through their outpatient services.

Hospital-Based Outpatient Services

A few years ago, hospital administrators regarded the outpatient departments of urban hospitals with a certain level of contempt. The outpatient department was often viewed as the "stepchild" of the institution and the least popular area of the hospital in which to work. Even today, some hospital outpatient clinics in inner-city areas may function as the community's safety net, providing primary care to medically indigent and uninsured populations. For the most part, however, outpatient services are now a key source of profit for hospitals. Consequently, hospitals have expanded their outpatient departments, and utilization of these services has grown (see Figure 7-4). This trend is the result of fierce competition in the health care industry; as MCOs emphasize preventive and outpatient care, there has been a relentless drive to cut costs. To compensate for the steady erosion in inpatient revenues

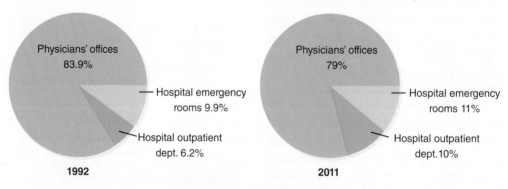

Total visits in 1992 = 908,446,000
Total visits in 2011 = 1,257,000,000

FIGURE 7-4 Ambulatory care visits in the United States.

Data from National Center for Health Statistics. 2016. *Health, United States, 2015.* Hyattsville, MD: U.S. Department of Health and Human Services. p. 265.

stemming from MCO frugality, hospitals have begun sprucing up and expanding their outpatient services.

A hospital-developed continuum of inpatient and outpatient services offers opportunities for cross-referrals among services that keep patients within the same delivery system. For example, a hospital that provides both inpatient and outpatient services can enhance its revenues by referring postsurgical cases to its affiliated units for rehabilitation and home care follow-up. Patients receiving various types of outpatient services constitute an important source of referrals back to hospitals for inpatient care. By offering both inpatient and outpatient services, hospitals can also expand their patient base.

Prior to 1985, outpatient care accounted for less than 15% of the total gross patient revenues for all U.S. hospitals. This share has now grown to 46% (American Hospital Association, 2016). As part of the growing competition in delivery of outpatient services, hospitals and hospital systems have launched specialized services, such as sports medicine, women's health, and renal dialysis. Many hospitals have also developed health promotion/disease prevention and health fitness programs as outreach efforts to the communities they serve.

Most hospital-based outpatient services can be broadly classified into five main types: clinical, surgical, emergency, home health, and women's health.

Clinical Services

Acquisition of group practices has enabled hospitals to increase their market share for outpatient clinical care. Referrals for inpatient, surgical, and other specialized services have generated additional revenues

for these hospitals. Both public and private nonprofit hospitals located in inner-city locations provide uncompensated clinical services through their outpatient settings to patients who do not have access to private practitioner offices for routine care. Teaching hospitals operate various clinics, offering highly specialized, research-based services.

Surgical Services

Hospital-based ambulatory surgery centers provide same-day surgical care; patients are sent home after a few hours of recovery time following surgery. Follow-up care generally continues in the physician's office. In outpatient medical procedures, hospitals have the upper hand over freestanding centers due to their advances in medical technology, pain management, and prompt responses to emergent conditions (**FIGURE 7-5**).

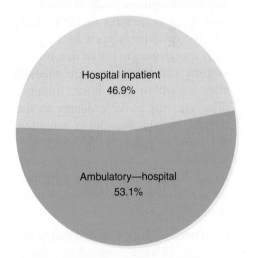

Total procedures (2010) = 51.4 million

FIGURE 7-5 Medical procedures by location.

Data from Wier, L. M., et al. 2015. *Surgeries in hospital-owned outpatient facilities, 2012.* Available at: https://www.hcup-us.ahrq.gov/reports /statbriefs/sb188-Surgeries-Hospital-Outpatient-Facilities-2012.pdf. Accessed January 2017.

Emergency Services

The ED has long been a vital outpatient component of many community hospitals. The main purpose of this department is to have services available around the clock for patients who are acutely ill or injured, particularly those with serious or life-threatening conditions requiring immediate attention. When deemed medically appropriate, prompt hospitalization can occur directly from the ED. This department has various specialists on call and is commonly staffed by physicians who have specialized training in emergency medicine. In small hospitals, the staff may be members of the regular medical staff in rotation. Another option is to contract ED staffing to physician groups specializing in emergency medicine.

Weinerman and colleagues (1966) defined three categories of conditions for which patients present themselves to the ED:

- **Emergent conditions** are critical and require immediate medical attention; time delay is harmful to the patient, and the disorder is acute and potentially threatening to life or function.
- **Urgent conditions** require medical attention within a few hours; a longer delay presents possible danger to the patient, and the disorder is acute but not severe enough to be life threatening.
- **Nonurgent conditions** do not require the resources of an emergency service, and the disorder is nonacute or minor in severity.

It has been well documented that in the United States, EDs are overused for nonurgent or routine care that could be more appropriately addressed in a primary care setting. Of the 136.3 million ED patient visits reported to the National Ambulatory Medical Care Survey in 2011, for example, 1.2% were triaged as needing immediate attention, 10.7% as emergent, 42.3% as urgent, 35.5% as semi-urgent, and 8% as nonurgent (National Center for Health Statistics, 2011). Reasons for nonurgent use of ED include unavailability of primary care, erroneous self-assessment of severity of ailment or injury, the 24-hour open-door policy, convenience, socioeconomic stress, psychiatric comorbidities, and a lack of social support (Hummel et al., 2014; Liggins, 1993; Padgett and Brodsky, 1992). Moreover, because the Emergency Medical Treatment and Active Labor Act (EMTALA) of 1986 requires screening and evaluation of every patient, necessary stabilizing treatment, and admitting when necessary regardless of ability to pay, EDs often function as a public "safety net" for the uninsured.

The uninsured and people on Medicaid use disproportionately more ED services than people who have private insurance coverage (Capp et al., 2015; McCaig and Burt, 2002; Meisel et al., 2011). Many private physicians do not provide services to Medicaid enrollees because of low reimbursement, which often leaves people on Medicaid without a regular source of primary care (Hing et al., 2015; McNamara et al., 1993).

Crowding in EDs has also been exacerbated by hospital and ED closings nationwide. In 1992, approximately 6,000 hospitals had EDs; fewer than 5,000 remain today (Morganti et al., 2013). Yet, the demand for ED visits has increased considerably, as reflected by the growth in the annual number of ED visits—up from 93.4 million to 130.4 million between 1994 and 2013 (McCaig and Newar, 2006; National Center for Health Statistics, 2013). Because of overcrowding, EDs must use triage mechanisms to screen patients according to their level of severity.

Because EDs require high-tech facilities, necessitate highly trained personnel, and must be accessible 24 hours a day, their costs are high and their services are not designed for nonurgent care. Inappropriate use of emergency services wastes precious resources. Hence, alternatives to the ED for nonurgent and routine care are critically needed—a problem that can be traced back to the United States' inadequate primary care infrastructure. Precisely for this reason, the ACA did not have any material impact on the overuse of EDs for nonurgent conditions (Searing and Cantlin, 2016).

Home Health Care

Many hospitals have opened separate home health departments, which provide mainly postacute care and rehabilitation therapies. Hospitals have entered the home health business to keep discharged patients within the hospital system. Hospitals operate approximately 7.4% of all Medicare-certified home health agencies in the United States (Centers for Medicare and Medicaid Services [CMS], 2016a). Home health care is discussed in detail later in this chapter.

Women's Health Centers

Emerging recognition in the 1980s of the prominence of women as a major health market led medical institutions to develop specialized women's health centers in hospital-based and/or hospital-affiliated settings. Following are some of the reasons behind the growth of women's centers:

- Recognition that women are the major users of health care. They seek health care more often than men do. Morbidity is greater among women than among men, even after adjusting data for childbearing-related conditions.
- A change in philosophy in American culture toward women, as the idea of gender equality becomes more popular.
- Recognition that the female majority in the United States will continue to grow, as the aging population includes more females. **TABLE 7-2** shows current population trends.

TABLE 7-2 Growth in Female U.S. Resident Population by Age Groups Between 1980 and 2014 (in Thousands)

	Age Groups (in Years)						
	< 15	*15–44*	*45–64*	*65–74*	*75–84*	*≥ 85*	*Total*
1980	25,073	52,833	23,342	8,824	4,862	1,559	116,493
2014	29,882	63,356	42,790	14,049	7,789	4,053	161,921
Growth	4,809	10,523	19,448	5,225	2,927	2,494	45,428

Data from National Center for Health Statistics. 2016. *Health, United States, 2015*. Hyattsville, MD: U.S. Department of Health and Human Services. p. 65.

Hospital-sponsored women's health centers rely on a variety of service delivery models. These models exist on a continuum that includes telephone information and referral, educational programs, health screening and diagnostics, comprehensive primary care for women, and mental health services. In addition to services in obstetrics, gynecology, and primary care, women's health centers offer mammography, ultrasound, osteoporosis screening, and other health screenings. Women's health is discussed in greater detail in the *Health Services for Special Populations* chapter.

Freestanding Facilities

Freestanding medical clinics include walk-in clinics, urgent care centers, surgicenters, and other outpatient facilities, such as outpatient rehabilitation centers, optometric centers, and dental clinics. These clinics, which are often owned or controlled by private corporations, commonly employ practitioners on salary.

Walk-in clinics provide ambulatory services, ranging from basic primary care to urgent care, but they are used on a nonroutine, episodic basis. The main advantages of these clinics are convenience of location, evening and weekend hours, and availability of services on a "walk-in" (no appointment) basis.

Urgent care centers offer extended hours; many are open 24 hours a day, 7 days a week and accept patients with no appointments. These centers offer a wide range of routine services for basic and acute conditions on a first-come, first-served basis, but they are not comparable to hospital EDs.

Surgicenters are freestanding ambulatory surgery centers independent of hospitals. They usually provide a full range of services for the types of surgery that can be performed on an outpatient basis and do not require overnight hospitalization.

Outpatient rehabilitation centers provide physical therapy, occupational therapy, and speech pathology services. In the past, generous Medicare reimbursement attracted various operators to open outpatient rehabilitation centers, but caps were instituted under the Balanced Budget Act of 1997. The therapy reimbursement caps are determined on a calendar year basis. For physical therapy and speech–language pathology services combined, the annual cap per patient was $1,940 for 2016. For occupational therapy services, the cap was $1,940 for 2016. Deductible and coinsurance amounts applied to therapy services count toward the amount accrued before a cap is reached (CMS, 2016b).

In recent years, neighborhood optical centers providing vision services have replaced many office-based opticians. Other freestanding facilities include audiology clinics, dental centers, hemodialysis centers, pharmacies, and suppliers of **durable medical equipment (DME)**. DME suppliers furnish ostomy supplies, hospital beds, oxygen tanks, walkers, wheelchairs, and many other types of supplies and equipment. A growing number of the various types of freestanding facilities are part of large regional and nationwide chains, which are opening new facilities at an unprecedented rate in new geographic locations.

Retail Clinics

The introduction of small clinics, staffed mostly by nonphysician practitioners, in shopping malls and large retail stores has been a relatively recent phenomenon.

Once viewed as a threat to PCPs, retail clinics are now increasingly viewed as complementary services that are conveniently available to people for minor ailments. Because of their low cost of operation, even most uninsured people can pay for their services out of pocket. In turn, payers have also started to establish contracts with retail clinics. The number of retail clinics in the United States was expected to double to more than 2,800 by 2017 (RAND Corporation, 2016).

Mobile Medical, Diagnostic, and Screening Services

Ambulance service and first aid treatment provided to the victims of severe illness, accidents, and disasters by trained emergency medical technicians (EMTs) are the most commonly encountered mobile medical services. Such services are also referred to as prehospital medicine.

Early attention following traumatic injury is often lifesaving. EMTs are specially trained to provide such attention at the site and in transit to the hospital. Most ambulance personnel have a Basic-EMT rating, but advanced training can lead to EMT-Paramedic certification. Paramedics are trained to administer emergency drugs and provide advanced life support (ALS) emergency medical services. Examples include intravenous administration of fluids and drugs, treatment for shock, electrocardiograms (ECGs), electrical interventions to support cardiac function, and endotracheal intubation (insertion of a tube as an air passage through the trachea).

To provide a speedy response to emergencies, most urban centers have developed formal emergency medical systems that incorporate all area hospital EDs,

along with transportation and communication systems. These communities typically establish 911 emergency phone lines to provide immediate access to services for those persons needing emergency care. When the system receives a 911 call, an ambulance is dispatched by a central communications center, which also identifies and alerts the hospital most appropriately equipped to deal with the type of emergency and located closest to the site where the emergency has occurred. Specialized ambulance services or advanced life support ambulances include mobile coronary care units, shock-trauma vans, and disaster relief vans, all of which are staffed by paramedics and EMTs who have advanced training.

Mobile medical services also constitute an efficient and convenient way to provide certain types of routine health services. Mobile eye care, podiatric care, and dental care units, for example, can be brought to a nursing home or retirement center where they can efficiently serve many patients residing in the facility. They are a convenient service for the patients, many of whom include the frail and elderly, patients who can then avoid an often difficult and tiring trip to a regular clinic.

Mobile diagnostic services include mammography and magnetic resonance imaging (MRI). Such mobile units take advanced diagnostic services to small towns and rural communities. They offer the advantages of convenience to patients and cost-efficiency in the delivery of diagnostic care.

Health screening vans, staffed by volunteers who are trained professionals and operated by various nonprofit organizations, are often seen at malls and fair sites. Various types of health education and health promotion services and screening checks, such as blood pressure and cholesterol screening, are commonly performed for anyone who walks in.

Home Health Care

Home health care brings certain types of services to patients in their own homes. Without home services, the only alternative for most such patients would be institutionalization in a hospital or nursing home. Home health is consistent with the philosophy of maintaining people in the least restrictive environment possible.

Home health care encompasses a wide range of services and supplies that a person receives at home under a plan of care established by a doctor. It can include skilled nursing and home health aide services, physical therapy, occupational therapy, speech-language pathology services, medical social services, DME (e.g., wheelchairs, hospital beds, oxygen, and walkers), medical supplies, and other services provided in the individual's home (National Council on Aging, 2016). Home health is delivered in the United States by a combination of large and small home health providers, both for-profit and nonprofit. More than 12,400 home health agencies serve patients across the United States, with approximately 12,100 of those agencies being certified to treat Medicare patients (CMS, 2015b; National Council on Aging, 2016). The total number of home health aides employed in the home health care services industry increased from 208,130 in 2004 to 348,740 in 2014 (Alliance for Home Health Quality and Innovation, 2015).

Growth in expenditures going to freestanding home health care agencies

(additional services of home health care are provided in hospital-based facilities and are considered hospital care) accelerated from 2014 to 2015, with this spending increasing 6.3% to reach $88.8 billion in 2015; by comparison, the growth rate was 4.5% from 2013 to 2014. Stronger growth in spending by both Medicare (2.6%) and Medicaid (6.0%)—the two largest payers, which collectively accounted for 76% of U.S. home health spending—along with faster growth in private health insurance and out-of-pocket spending drove the overall acceleration of home health expenditures in 2015 (CMS, 2016a).

According to publicly available data published in 2015 by "Home Health Compare," patient outcomes improve after receiving home health care. These data show that, after receiving home health care, 89% of wounds improved or healed after an operation, 68% of patients had less pain when moving around, 68% got better at bathing, and 65% had improved breathing (Alliance for Home Health Quality and Innovation, 2015; CMS, 2015b). A patient being discharged to home health care immediately following hospitalization is generally the least costly setting in which to deliver care, compared to discharging patients to skilled nursing facilities, inpatient rehabilitation facilities, or long-term acute care hospitals as the first setting post discharge. For example, Medicare expenditures for a patient treated in the home after hospital discharge average $20,345, compared to an average of $28,294 for post-discharge care across all settings (Dobson, 2012).

Home health providers often leverage technology to enable the provision of care at home. In varying degrees, these providers use a diverse array of technologies ranging from remote monitoring, including phone calls (including the growing array of mobile technologies and applications), to health information technology, to in-home therapeutic and diagnostic technologies. Such technologies are often key tools that enable home health providers to improve quality and reduce the cost of care delivered to patients (Alliance for Home Health Quality and Innovation, 2014).

FIGURE 7-6 shows the demographic characteristics of patients who received home health care in 2013. According to the Alliance for Home Health Quality and Innovation (2015), 3.4 million patients received home health care in the United States in that year. Home health care patients tended to be age 65 or older (85%), female (61.5%), and white (79%).

Because of variations in data sources, national expenditures for home health care are difficult to calculate. The CMS (2015a) estimates that total expenditures for home health amounted to $88.8 billion in 2015. Medicare and Medicaid accounted for 76% of home health spending (CMS, 2015a). Payments to home health agencies were sharply cut under the Balanced Budget Act of 1997. As a result, home health expenditures accounted for only 2.6% of total Medicare spending in 2015, compared to 9% in 1997 (CMS, 2015a; National Association for Home Care and Hospice, 2010).

FIGURE 7-7 shows revenue sources for home health care providers and the average distribution of revenues from these sources. **TABLE 7-3** and **TABLE 7-4** provide additional statistics on home health.

Gender

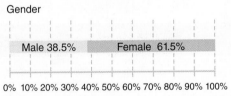

Age

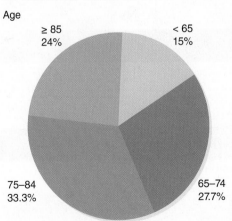

FIGURE 7-6 Demographic characteristics of U.S. home health patients, 2013.

Data from Alliance for Home Health Quality and Innovation. 2015. *Home health chartbook* 2015. Available at: http://ahhqi.org/images/uploads /AHHQI_2015_Chartbook_FINAL_October_Aug2016Update.pdf. Accessed February 2017.

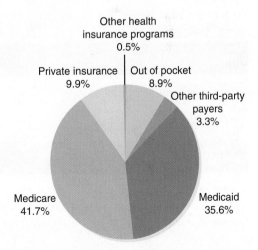

Total payments = $83.2 billion

FIGURE 7-7 Estimated payments for home care by payment source, 2014.

Data from National Center for Health Statistics. 2016. *Health, United States, 2015.* Hyattsville, MD: U.S. Department of Health and Human Services. p. 298.

TABLE 7-3 Selected Organizational Characteristics of U.S. Home Health and Hospice Care Agencies in the United States, 2014

Characteristic	Home Health Care[1]	Hospice Care[1]
	Number (Standard Error)	
All agencies[2]	12,400	4,000
	Percentage Distributions (Standard Error)	
All agencies[2]	100.0	100.0
Ownership		
Proprietary	80.0	60.2
Voluntary nonprofit	15.0	25.9
Government and other	5.0	13.9
Medicare Certification Status		
Certified as home health care agency	98.7	NA
Certified as hospice care agency	NA	NA
Medicaid Certification Status		
Certified as home health care agency	78.0	NA
Certified as hospice care agency	NA	NA
Geographic Region		
Northeast	8.1	11.3
Midwest	22.8	22.8
South	46.6	41.2
West	17.3	24.8

Location		
Metropolitan statistical area (MSA)[3]	84.6	76.6
Micropolitan statistical area[4]	8.1	14.0
Neither	7.3	9.4

[1] Include agencies that provide both home health and hospice care services (mixed).

[2] Include agencies that provide home health care services, hospice care services, or both types of services and currently or recently served home health and/or hospice care patients. Agencies that provided only homemaker services or housekeeping services, assistance with instrumental activities of daily living (IADLs), or durable medical equipment and supplies were excluded from the survey.

[3] A metropolitan statistical area is a county or group of contiguous counties that contains at least one urbanized area of 50,000 or more population. It may also contain other counties that are economically and socially integrated with the central county as measured by commuting.

[4] A micropolitan statistical area is a nonmetropolitan county or group of contiguous nonmetropolitan counties that contains an urban cluster of 10,000 to 49,999 persons. It may include surrounding counties if there are strong economic ties among the counties, based on commuting patterns.

Note: Numbers may not add to totals because of rounding and/or because estimates and percentage distributions include a category of unknowns not reported in the table. Percentages are based on the unrounded numbers.

Data from Harris-Kojetin, L., et al. 2016. Long-term care providers and services users in the United states: Data from the National Study of Long-Term Care Providers, 2013-2014. *Vital & Health Statistics* 3, no. 38.

TABLE 7-4 Home Health and Hospice Care Patients Served at the Time of the Interview, by Agency Type and Number of Patients in the United States, 2007

Number of Patients	Home Health Care Only	Home Health and Hospice Care (Mixed)
Mean (Standard Error)		
Number of home health care patients	109.0 (9.2)	177.7 (17.7)
Percentage Distributions (Standard Error)		
Total	100.0	100.0
0–25	16.0 (4.3)[1]	9.8 (2.4)[1]
26–50	21.3 (4.2)[1]	25.1 (6.4)[1]
51–100	29.0 (4.0)	18.4 (3.1)

(continues)

TABLE 7-4 Home Health and Hospice Care Patients Served at the Time of the Interview, by Agency Type and Number of Patients in the United States, 2007 (*continued*)

Number of Patients	Home Health Care Only	Home Health and Hospice Care (Mixed)
101–150	10.8 (2.3)[1]	9.4 (1.9)[1]
151 or more	23.0 (3.5)	37.4 (4.8)

Number of Patients	Hospice Care Only	Home Health and Hospice Care (Mixed)
	Mean (Standard Error)	
Number of hospice care patients	78.1 (6.4)	39.1 (5.7)
	Percentage Distributions (Standard Error)	
Total	100.0	100.0
0–25	29.5 (5.4)	57.6 (5.6)
26–50	22.1 (4.9)	24.5 (5.9)
51–100	21.2 (4.0)	6.3 (1.4)[1]
101–150	9.9 (2.5)[1]	[2]
151 or more	11.6 (2.3)[1]	[2]

[1] Estimate does not meet standards of reliability or precision because the sample size is between 30 and 59 or the sample size is greater than 59 but has a relative standard error of 30% or more.

[2] Estimate does not meet standards of reliability or precision because the sample size is fewer than 30.

Note: Unknowns are excluded when calculating estimates. There was 1 (unweighted) case with an unknown number of home health care patients and 19 (unweighted) cases with an unknown number of hospice care patients. Percentages are based on the unrounded numbers.

Reproduced from Park-Lee E.Y., and F. H. Decker. 2010. Comparison of home and hospice care agencies by organizational characteristics and services provided: United States, 2007. *National Health Statistics Reports* no. 30: 1–23.

Hospice Services

The term **hospice** refers to a cluster of comprehensive services for terminally ill persons with a medically determined life expectancy of 6 months or less. More than half of all patients in hospice programs are diagnosed with cancer upon admission. Hospice, whose programs provide services that address the special needs of dying persons and their families. It is a method of care, not a location, and services are

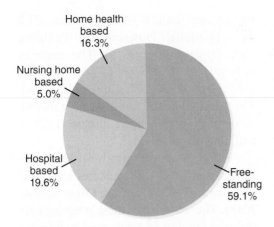

FIGURE 7-8 Types of hospice agencies, 2014.

Data from National Hospice and Palliative Care Organization. 2015. *NHPCO facts and figures: Hospice care in America.* Available at: http://www.nhpco .org/sites/default/files/public/Statistics_Research/2015_Facts_Figures.pdf. Accessed February 2017. p. 8.

taken to patients and their families wherever they are located. Thus, hospice can be a part of home health care when the services are provided in the patient's home. In other instances, hospice services are taken to patients in nursing homes, retirement centers, or hospitals. Services can be organized out of a hospital, nursing home, freestanding hospice facility, or home health agency (**FIGURE 7-8**).

Hospice regards the patient and family as the unit of care. This special kind of care includes the following considerations:

- Meeting the patient's physical needs, with an emphasis on pain management and comfort
- Meeting the patient's and family's emotional and spiritual needs
- Providing support for the family members before and after the patient's death
- Focusing on maintaining quality of life rather than prolonging life (Miller, 1996)

The two primary areas of emphasis in hospice care are: (1) pain and symptom management, which is referred to as **palliation**, and (2) psychosocial and spiritual support according to the holistic model of care (see the *Beliefs, Values, and Health* chapter). Counseling and spiritual help are made available to relieve anguish and help the patient deal with his or her death. Social services include help with arranging final affairs. Apart from medical, nursing, and social services staff, hospice organizations rely heavily on volunteers.

The idea of providing comprehensive care to terminally ill patients was first promoted by Dame Cicely Saunders in the 1960s in England. In the United States, the first hospice was established in 1974 by Sylvia Lack in New Haven, Connecticut (Beresford, 1989). Hospice organizations expanded after Medicare extended hospice benefits in 1983. Hospice is a cost-effective option for both private and public payers. It is estimated that for every $1 spent on hospice, Medicare saves $1.52 in Part A and Part B expenditures (National Hospice Organization, 1995). Hospice enrollment has been found to save money for Medicare to improve care quality for patients across a number of different lengths of service (Kelly et al., 2013). The difference in costs mainly reflects services that are not medically intensive. Many states now provide hospice benefits under Medicaid. **FIGURE 7-9** shows the sources of coverage for hospice services.

To receive Medicare certification, a hospice must meet these basic conditions:

- Provide physician certification that the patient's prognosis is for a life expectancy of 6 months or less
- Make nursing services, physician services, and drugs and biologics available on a 24-hour basis

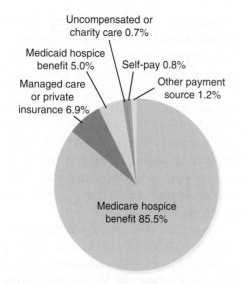

FIGURE 7-9 Coverage of patients for hospice care at the time of admission, 2014.

Note: Numbers may not add to 100% because of rounding.

Data from the National Hospice and Palliative Care Organization. 2015. NHPCO facts and figures: Hospice care in America. Available at: http://www .nhpco.org/sites/default/files/public/Statistics_Research/2015_Facts _Figures.pdf. Accessed February 2017. p. 10.

- Provide nursing services under the supervision of a registered nurse
- Make arrangements for inpatient care when necessary
- Provide social services by a qualified social worker under the direction of a physician
- Make counseling services available to both the patient and the family, including bereavement support after the patient's death
- Provide needed medications, medical supplies, and equipment for pain management and palliation
- Provide physical, occupational, and speech therapy services when necessary
- Provide home health aide and home-maker services when needed

In 2014, 1.66 million patients in the United States received hospice services;

the average length of service was 71.3 days (National Hospice and Palliative Care Organization, 2015). The majority of hospice patients were 65 years or older (83.9%), female (53.7%), and white (76%). The top diagnoses were cancer (36.6%), dementia (14.8%), heart disease (14.7%), and lung disease (9.3%).

There are approximately 6,100 hospice programs in the United States (National Hospice and Palliative Care Organization, 2015). The majority of these programs are independent (59.1%), followed by hospital based (19.6%), home health agency based (16.3%), and nursing home based (5.0%).

Medicare is the largest source of financing for hospice. In terms of levels of hospice care, the Medicare Hospice Benefit affords patients four levels of care to meet their needs: routine home care, continuous home care, inpatient respite care, and general inpatient care. In 2014, 93.8% of care was provided at the routine home care level (National Hospice and Palliative Care Organization, 2015). Tables 7-3 and 7-4 provide additional statistics on hospice care.

The U.S. hospice movement was founded by volunteers, and there is a continued commitment to volunteer service in this movement. In fact, hospice is unique in that it is the only provider whose Medicare conditions of participation requires volunteers to provide at least 5% of total patient-care hours. In 2014, approximately 430,000 hospice volunteers provided 19 million hours of service (National Hospice and Palliative Care Organization, 2015).

Ambulatory Long-Term Care Services

Long-term care has typically been associated with inpatient care provided in nursing homes, but providers in two main types of settings—case management and adult day care—deliver outpatient services. **Case management** provides coordination and referral among a variety of health care services. The objective is to find the most appropriate setting to meet a patient's health care needs. **Adult day care** complements informal care provided at home by family members with professional services available in adult day care centers during the normal workday. The *Long-Term Care* chapter discusses both services in more detail.

Public Health Services

Public health services in the United States are typically provided by local health departments, and the range of services offered varies greatly by locality. Generally, public health services are limited to well-baby care, sexually transmitted disease clinics, family planning services, screening and treatment for tuberculosis, and ambulatory mental health. Inner-city, poor, and uninsured populations are the main beneficiaries of these services. Health programs delivered in public schools fall under the public health domain and are limited to vision and hearing screening and assistance with dysfunctions that impede learning. Ambulatory clinics in prisons also fall in the public health domain.

The public school setting is a growing area of practice for physical therapists, occupational therapists, and speech–language pathologists. These professionals help children with special physical and emotional dysfunctions. The Individuals with Disabilities Education Act (IDEA) of 1975 (which is subject to reauthorization every 3 years) has been instrumental in enabling children with special needs to receive services in public schools so that they can obtain optimal access to education.

Community Health Centers

Creation of community health centers (CHCs)—formerly called neighborhood health centers (NHCs)—was authorized during the 1960s as part of the Johnson administration's War on Poverty campaign, mainly to address health care needs in medically underserved regions of the United States. The federal government's application of the **medically underserved** designation signals that a community has a dearth of primary care providers and delivery settings, as well as poor health indicators for the populace. Such areas are often characterized by economic, geographic, or cultural barriers that limit access to primary health care for a large segment of the population. CHCs are required by law to locate in MUAs and provide services to anyone seeking care, regardless of insurance status or ability to pay. Hence, CHCs are a primary care safety net for the nation's poor and uninsured in both inner-city and rural areas.

CHCs are private, nonprofit organizations, but they operate under the auspices of the federal government. Section 330 of the Public Health Service Act provides federal grant funding for CHCs. These centers also heavily depend on funding through the Medicaid program. Private-pay patients are charged on sliding-fee scales, determined by the patient's income.

CHCs tailor their services to family-oriented primary and preventive health care and dental services (Shi et al., 2007).

These centers have developed considerable expertise in managing the health care needs of underserved populations. Many have established systems of care that include outreach programs, case management, transportation, translation services, alcohol and drug abuse screening and treatment, mental health services, health education, and social services.

In 2015, CHCs served 24.3 million patients in the United States, who collectively made more than 96 million patient visits. Most patients who utilize CHCs are members of vulnerable populations—92% of the patients were below the 200% federal poverty level and 24% were uninsured in 2015. Among special populations, approximately 1.2 million homeless individuals, 910,172 agricultural workers, and 1,510,842 residents from public housing received services under this program (Health Resources and Services Administration [HRSA], 2015). From 2008 to 2015, the number of new health centers supported by HRSA increased by 27%, and the total number of patients served increased by 42%—that is, by more than 7.2 million additional patients. In 2015 alone, HRSA provided funding for almost 430 new health center sites and increased access to care for more than 1.8 million additional patients (HRSA, 2016).

Despite serving a population that is often sicker and at greater risk for poor health outcomes than the general population, the quality of care provided at CHCs is equivalent and often surpasses care provided by other primary care providers. More than 93% of HRSA-funded health centers met or exceeded at least one *Healthy People 2020* goal for clinical performance in 2015. More than 68% of these centers are recognized by national accrediting organizations

as patient-centered medical homes. More than 92% of CHCs have electronic health records (EHRs) installed and in use at all sites and for all providers (HRSA, 2016).

Health centers also meet or exceed nationally accepted practice standards for treatment of chronic conditions. In fact, the Institute of Medicine and the Government Accountability Office have recognized health centers as models for screening, diagnosing, and managing chronic conditions such as diabetes, cardiovascular disease, asthma, depression, cancer, and human immunodeficiency virus (HIV) disease. Health centers have improved health outcomes for their patients and have lowered the cost of treating patients with chronic illness (National Association of Community Health Centers [NACHC], 2016a).

Studies have shown that CHCs provide accessible, cost-effective, and quality care (NACHC, 2015, 2016b, 2016c). Because the majority of the patients they serve are members of vulnerable groups (i.e., low income, minorities, homeless), CHCs play an important role in reducing health disparities among these populations (NACHC, 2013). CHCs are key partners for Medicaid, as Medicaid seeks to accelerate practice innovations that drive savings while also improving outcomes (NACHC, 2016d).

A unique quality of health center programs is the emphasis placed on both primary care services and enabling services—that is, nonclinical services intended to eliminate geographic, linguistic, cultural, and socioeconomic barriers to care, such as transportation, interpretation, case management, and health education, among others. To care for the diverse nonclinical needs of their patients, health centers have increased their enabling services staff by 40% since 2010 (HRSA, 2014).

In 2011, the ACA provided $1 billion to CHCs to expand primary care to nearly 11 million underserved Americans who did not have a regular source of care. Under the ACA, access to health center services increased, particularly for Medicaid patients. Moreover, increased direct investment in health centers led to expanded primary care capacity (Kaiser Family Foundation, 2017).

Free Clinics

Modeled after the 19th-century dispensary, the **free clinic** is a general ambulatory care center, serving primarily the poor, the homeless, and the uninsured. Free clinics have three main characteristics:

- Services are provided at no charge or at a very nominal charge.
- The clinic is not directly supported or operated by a government agency or health department.
- Services are delivered mainly by trained volunteer staff.

Free clinics focus on the delivery of primary care. Other services offered by these facilities vary, depending on the number and training of their volunteer staff.

The number of free clinics has continued to grow nationally and is estimated at more than 1,200 across the United States (National Association of Free and Charitable Clinics [NAFC], 2016). Although mainly a voluntary effort, care delivery through free clinics has taken on the form of an organized movement. The NAFC focuses on the issues and needs of the free clinics and the people they serve in the United States.

Other Clinics

Federal funding is used to operate migrant health centers that serve transient farmworkers in agricultural communities and rural health centers that serve populations in isolated underserved rural areas. The Community Mental Health Center program was established to provide ambulatory mental health services in underserved areas.

Telephone Access

Telephone access is a means of bringing expert opinion and advice to the patient, especially during the hours when physicians' offices are closed. Referred to as **telephone triage**, this type of access has expanded under managed care.

The Park Nicollet Clinic of the Minneapolis, Minnesota Health System illustrates how such a system functions. Their telephone call-in system operates 7 days a week, 24 hours a day. The system is staffed by specially trained nurses who receive patients' calls. Using a computer-based clinical decision support system (see the *Medical Technology* chapter), the nurse can access the patient's medical history and view the most recent radiology and laboratory test results. The decision support system enables the nurse to give instructions on how to deal with the patient's problem. Consultation with a primary care physician is done when necessary (Appleby, 1995). The nurse can direct patients to appropriate medical services, such as an ED or a physician's office.

The URAC Organization accredits telephone triage and health information programs.

▶ Complementary and Alternative Medicine

Because of the tremendous growth of this part of the health care spectrum, the role of complementary and alternative medicine (CAM)—also referred to as "nonconventional therapies" or "natural medicine"—in the delivery of health care cannot be ignored. Although the terms "complementary medicine" and "alternative medicine" are often used synonymously, technically there is a distinction between the two: Complementary treatments are used *together with* conventional medicine, whereas **alternative medicine** is used *instead of* conventional medicine (Barnes et al., 2008).

In the United States, the dominant health care practice is biomedicine-based allopathic medicine, also referred to as conventional medicine. Complementary and alternative medicine refers to the broad domain of all health care resources other than those intrinsic to biomedicine (CAM Research Methodology Conference, 1997) and covers a heterogeneous spectrum of ancient to new approaches that purport to prevent or treat disease (Barnes et al., 2008).

CAM therapies include a wide range of treatments, such as homeopathy, herbal formulas, use of other natural products as preventive and treatment agents, acupuncture, meditation, yoga exercises, biofeedback, and spiritual guidance or prayer. Chiropractic is also largely regarded as a CAM treatment.

No particular settings of health care delivery are involved in CAM treatments. With few exceptions, most therapies are self-administered or at least require active patient participation. The types of trained and licensed health care professionals discussed in the *System Resources* chapter are rarely involved in the delivery of unconventional care. A doctor of naturopathic medicine (ND) degree and Diplomate of the Homeopathic Academy of Naturopathic Physicians (DHANP) are offered in the United States. Also, natural medicine–based private clinics are emerging across the United States.

Even though the efficacy of most CAM treatments has not been scientifically established, their use has exploded. CAM's growth has happened mainly for the following reasons:

- Most people who seek CAM therapies believe that they have already explored conventional Western treatments but have not been helped. Most of these patients have chronic disorders, such as persistent pain, for which Western medicine can usually offer only symptomatic relief rather than definitive treatment.
- People who want to avoid or delay certain complex surgeries or toxic allopathic treatments are persuaded that at least there is no harm in trying alternative treatments first.
- Most people feel empowered by access to a vast amount of medical and health-related information available through the Internet and feel in control to pursue what they think is best for their own health.
- Many patients report that they seek alternative therapies and individuals who practice them because they want practitioners to take the time to listen to them, understand them, and deal with their personal life as well as their pathology. They believe that alternative practitioners will meet those needs (Gordon, 1996).

According to the 2012 National Health Interview Survey (NHIS), 33.2% of adults in the United States age 18 years and older and 11.6% of children age 4 to 17 years used some form of complementary health approach in the previous 12 months (CMS, 2012). Although people of all backgrounds use CAM, its use among adults is greater among women and those with higher levels of education and higher incomes (National Center for Complementary and Integrative Health [NCCIH], 2016a). In a 2010 survey of people age 50 years and older, conducted by the NCCIHI and AARP, 33% of respondents reported that they had discussed CAM with a health care provider (NCCIH, 2016b).

People use CAM for a wide array of diseases and conditions. American adults are most likely to use CAM for musculoskeletal problems such as back, neck, or joint pain (NCCIH, 2016a).

Effective coordination of conventional medical services and CAM has the potential to save money and improve quality because, for some chronic problems, conventional medicine offers few proven benefits. Examples include psychosomatic ailments and cases in which patients have recurring complaints of unexplained painful symptoms or spells of dizziness. Such nagging complaints can cause the patient to rack up high medical costs and compromise the individual's quality of life. Lower-cost therapies, such as stress management and meditation classes, can save numerous trips to physicians and costly diagnostic tests.

One study found median expenditures to be $39 for CAM care, compared to $74.40 for conventional outpatient care (Lafferty et al., 2006). In 2012, Americans spent $30.2 billion out-of-pocket on complementary health approaches—$28.3 billion for adults and $1.9 billion for children—during the 12 months prior to the survey. This equates to 1.1% of total health care expenditures in the United States ($2.82 trillion) and to 9.2% of total out-of-pocket health care spending ($328.8 billion). Americans spent $14.7 billion out-of-pocket on visits to complementary practitioners, which is almost 30% of what they spent out-of-pocket on services received from conventional physicians ($49.6 billion). They spent $12.8 billion out-of-pocket on natural product supplements, which was approximately one-fourth of what they spent out-of-pocket on prescription drugs ($54.1 billion) (Nahin et al., 2016; NCCIH, 2016a).

CAM also appears to be popular in Europe, Canada, and other industrialized countries. Even though most of these countries provide universal access to medical care, a significant number of people try alternative treatments.

Given the growing public demand for complementary medicine and its claims for health promotion, disease prevention, and promise for certain chronic conditions, mainstream medicine has shown a growing interest in better understanding the value of alternative treatments. Even so, skepticism is justifiable because alternative medicine is predominantly unregulated. Also, the efficacy of most treatments and the safety of some have not been scientifically evaluated. Some recent findings suggest that cranberry juice cocktail has no effect on preventing recurrent urinary tract infections (Barbosa-Cesnik et al., 2011), but white tea extract has potential anticancer benefits (Mao et al., 2010), and Echinacea does not reduce the duration and severity of the common cold (Barrett et al., 2010). Only rigorous scientific inquiry and research-based evidence will bring about a genuine integration of alternative therapies into the conventional practice of medicine. A 2013 publication in the *Natural Medicine Journal* noted that published research studies have revealed that CAM therapies are cost-effective and may present cost savings, but more research is necessary on individual treatments (Tais and Zoberg, 2013).

Nevertheless, some developments are noteworthy. In 1993, Congress established the Office of Alternative Medicine (OAM), which became the National Center for Complementary and Alternative Medicine (NCCAM) in 1998. Budget allocations for the center have increased from $2 million in 1993 to $128.3 million in 2012 (NCCAM, 2013). The center has three main objectives: (1) explore complementary and alternative healing practices in the context of rigorous science, (2) train complementary and alternative medicine researchers, and (3) disseminate authoritative information to the public and professionals. A few U.S. medical schools now include instruction in alternative medicine.

▶ Utilization of Outpatient Services

In 2010, Americans made approximately 922,596 million visits, or three visits per person, to office-based physicians (**TABLE 7-5**). Physicians in general and family practice accounted for the largest

TABLE 7-5 U.S. Physician Characteristics, 2013

Physician Characteristics	Number of Visits (in Thousands)
All visits	922,596
Physician Specialty[1]	
General and family practice	210,771
Internal medicine	125,776
Pediatrics	102,172
Obstetrics and gynecology	59,402
Orthopedic surgery	47,858
Ophthalmology	43,168
Dermatology	25,157
Cardiovascular diseases	36,722

Psychiatry	38,062
Otolaryngology	16,225
Urology	20,741
General surgery	17,892
Neurology	14,376
All other specialties	164,274
Professional Degree	
Doctor of medicine	860,503
Doctor of osteopathy	62,094
Specialty Type[1]	
Primary care	490,831
Medical specialty	252,615
Surgical specialty	179,150
Geographic Region	
Northeast	196,630
Midwest	179,358
South	332,422
West	214,186
Metropolitan Status	
Metropolitan statistical area	841,369
Non-metropolitan statistical area	81,227

[1] Physician specialty and specialty type are defined in the "Technical Notes" of the source document.

Note: Numbers may not add to totals because of rounding.

Reproduced from Centers for Disease Control and Prevention (CDC). 2013. *National Ambulatory Medical Care Survey: 2013 summary tables.* Available at: https://www.cdc.gov/nchs/data/ahcd/namcs_summary/2013_namcs_web_tables.pdf. Accessed April 2017.

share of these visits (22.8%), followed by physicians in internal medicine (13.6%), pediatrics (11.1%), and obstetrics and gynecology (6.4%). Doctors of osteopathy accounted for 6.7% of the visits. The South led the United States in the proportion of physician visits (36.0%), followed by the West (23.2%), the Northeast (21.3%), and the Midwest (19.4%). Most physician office visits (91.2%) took place in metropolitan areas.

TABLE 7-6 presents the most frequently mentioned principal reasons for visiting a physician in 2007. The top 10 reasons were progress visit, general medical examination, postoperative visit, cough, medication, hypertension, prenatal examination, for other and unspecified test results, counseling not otherwise specific, and diabetes mellitus. **TABLE 7-7** shows the most frequent principal diagnoses cared for by office-based physicians.

TABLE 7-6 Principal Reason for Visiting a Physician

Principal Reason for Visit	Number of Visits
All visits	922,596
Progress visit, not otherwise specified	81,738
General medical examination	74,062
Postoperative visit	30,472
Cough	25,061
Medication, other and unspecified kinds	20,930
Hypertension	16,049
Prenatal examination, routine	16,032
For other and unspecified test results	15,817
Counseling, not otherwise specific	14,649
Diabetes mellitus	14,127
Knee symptoms	13,892
Back symptoms	13,655
Stomach pain, cramps, and spasms	13,011

Gynecologic examination	12,158
Well-baby examination	11,879
Skin rash	10,825
Shoulder symptoms	10,745
Symptoms referable to throat	10,328
All other reasons	496,051

Note: Numbers may not add to totals because of rounding.

Modified from Centers for Disease Control and Prevention (CDC). 2013. *National Ambulatory Medical Care Survey: 2013 summary tables.* Available at: https://www.cdc.gov/nchs/data/ahcd/namcs_summary/2013_namcs_web_tables.pdf. Accessed April 2017.

TABLE 7-7 Primary Diagnosis Group

Primary Diagnosis Group[1]	Number of Visits	Percentage Distribution
All visits	922,596	100.0
Essential hypertension	39,879	4.3
Routine infant or child health check	35,200	3.8
Spinal disorders	34,109	3.7
Arthropathies and related disorders	33,849	3.7
Diabetes mellitus	27,326	3.0
General medical examination	27,016	2.9
Acute upper respiratory infections, excluding pharyngitis	24,139	2.6
Malignant neoplasms	22,048	2.4
Rheumatism, excluding back	18,932	2.1

(continues)

TABLE 7-7 Primary Diagnosis Group (*continued*)

Primary Diagnosis Group[1]	Number of Visits	Percentage Distribution
Heart disease, excluding ischemic	18,578	2.0
Normal pregnancy	14,601	1.6
Follow-up examination	14,565	1.6
Specific procedures and aftercare	14,190	1.5
Gynecologic examination	11,495	1.3
Psychoses, excluding major depressive disorder	11,437	1.2
Disorders of lipoid metabolism	11,124	1.2
Attention-deficit disorder	10,881	1.2
Benign neoplasms	10,791	1.2
Anxiety states	10,197	1.1
Abdominal pain	9,687	1.1
All other diagnoses[2]	522,553	56.6

[1] Based on the *International Classification of Diseases, Ninth Revision, Clinical Modification* (ICD-9-CM).
[2] Includes all other diagnoses not listed above, as well as unknown and blank diagnoses.
Note: Numbers may not add to totals because of rounding.

Modified from Centers for Disease Control and Prevention (CDC). 2013. *National Ambulatory Medical Care Survey: 2013 summary tables.* Available at: https://www.cdc.gov/nchs/data/ahcd/namcs_summary/2013_namcs_web_tables.pdf. Accessed April 2017.

▶ **Primary Care in Other Countries**

Around the world, there is little consistency in how primary care services are accessed and how physicians get paid. In the United Kingdom, Netherlands, and New Zealand, patients register with a primary care doctor.

In Australia, the Netherlands, New Zealand, Norway, Sweden, Iceland, Italy, Denmark, and the United Kingdom, patients go through primary care for referrals to specialists and are often required to register with primary care practices (except in Australia). Canada, France, and Germany use financial incentives to encourage registration with primary care practices and coordinated referrals (Schoen et al., 2012; Thomson et al., 2012). The German "sickness funds" (insurance plans) offer an enrollment option.

The United Kingdom offers the most comprehensive coverage with little or no patient cost sharing. Canada covers physician visits in full, but medication coverage varies by province. Australia, New Zealand, and Germany include varying degrees of cost sharing (Schoen et al., 2012). Other countries may use moderate cost sharing (Schoen et al., 2012).

In Australia, Canada, France, Germany, Switzerland, and the United States, payers typically use fee-for-service payments and employ performance incentives (Schoen et al., 2012; Thomson et al., 2012). Conversely, the Netherlands, New Zealand, Norway, Denmark, and the United Kingdom use a combination of capitation, fee for service, and incentives (Schoen et al., 2012; Thomson et al., 2012).

Approximately 59% of doctors in France, the Netherlands, New Zealand, and Switzerland report that their patients can get same- or next-day appointments when sick, compared to only 22% in Canada. In Australia, Canada, France, Germany, New Zealand, and Norway, more than 60% of providers report long waits to see specialists. In the United States, physicians complain that they spend a significant amount of time with insurance-related issues, which limits access to care for their patients (Schoen et al., 2012).

Primary care is mostly privatized in all the countries mentioned earlier, with the exception of Iceland (mostly public) and Sweden (mixed). Physicians in Australia, Canada, Norway, the United Kingdom, and the United States are more likely to work in group practices of five or more doctors. Physicians in the Netherlands, France, Germany, and Switzerland are more likely to work in smaller practices.

In the 2015 International Health Policy Survey of Primary Care Physicians survey conducted by the Commonwealth Fund (2016), doctors in 10 countries reported that their practices struggle to coordinate care and communicate with other health and social services providers, and also questioned their preparedness to care for patients with challenging issues. There has been conceptual convergence in recent years on the need to redesign primary care to meet the health care needs of aging populations and address the increased prevalence of chronic disease around the world (Schoen et al., 2012).

▶ Summary

In the history of health care delivery, the main settings for ambulatory services have come full circle. First came a shift from outpatient settings to hospitals. Now, ambulatory services delivered outside the hospital have mushroomed. The reasons for this shift are mainly economic, social, and technological. Many physicians have broken their ties with hospitals and started their own specialized care centers, such as ambulatory surgery centers and cardiac care centers. A variety of general medical and surgical interventions are provided in ambulatory care settings. Thus, ambulatory services now transcend basic and routine primary care services. Conversely, primary care itself has become "specialized." Primary care is no longer concerned simply with the treatment of simple ailments; primary care physicians must coordinate a plethora of services to maintain the long-term viability of their patients' health. Application of principles to establish patient-centered medical homes and delivery of community-based primary care is slow in taking shape.

In response to the changing economic incentives within the health care delivery system, numerous types of outpatient services have emerged, and a variety of settings for the delivery of services have developed.

The growing interest in complementary and alternative medicine is largely consumer driven. Compared to the conventional Western medicine found in the United States, alternative medicine, with its emphasis on self-care, is an area where many patients feel more in control of their own destiny.

▶ Test Your Understanding

Terminology

accountability	emergent conditions	palliation
adult day care	free clinic	primary health care
alternative medicine	gatekeeping	secondary care
ambulatory care	home health care	surgicenters
case management	hospice	telephone triage
community-oriented primary care (COPC)	medical home	tertiary care
	medically underserved	urgent care centers
durable medical equipment (DME)	nonurgent conditions	urgent conditions
	outpatient services	walk-in clinic

Review Questions

1. Describe how some of the changes in the health services delivery system have led to a decline in hospital inpatient days and a growth in ambulatory services.
2. What implications has the decline in hospital occupancy rates had for hospital management?
3. All primary care is ambulatory, but not all ambulatory services represent primary care. Discuss.
4. What are the main characteristics of primary care?
5. Critique the gatekeeping role of primary care.
6. Discuss how the patient-centered medical home advances primary care.

7. What is community-oriented primary care? Explain.
8. Discuss the two main factors that determine what should be an adequate mix of generalists and specialists.
9. What are some of the reasons why solo practitioners are joining group practices?
10. Why is it important for hospital administrators to regard outpatient care as a key component of their overall business strategy?
11. Discuss the main hospital-based outpatient services.
12. What are some of the social changes that led to the creation of specialized health centers for women?

13. Why do patients sometimes use the hospital emergency department for nonurgent conditions? What are the consequences?
14. What are mobile health care services? Discuss the various types of mobile services.
15. What is the basic philosophy of home health care? Describe the services it provides.
16. What are the conditions of eligibility for receiving home health services under Medicare?
17. Explain the concept of hospice care and the types of services a hospice provides.
18. What are some of the main requirements for Medicare certification of a hospice program?
19. Describe the scope of public health ambulatory services in the United States.
20. Describe the main public and voluntary outpatient clinics and the main problems they face.
21. What is complementary and alternative medicine? What role does it play in the delivery of health care?
22. Briefly explain how a telephone triage system functions.
23. Discuss the global trends in primary care.

▶ References

Accreditation Association for Ambulatory Health Care (AAAHC). 2009. *AAAHC standards.* Available at: http://www.aaahc.org/en/accreditation/primary-care-medical-home/. Accessed February 2017.

Alliance for Home Health Quality and Innovation. 2014. *The Future of Home Health Care Project.* Available at: http://www.ahhqi.org/images/pdf/future-whitepaper.pdf. Accessed February 2017.

Alliance for Home Health Quality and Innovation. 2015. *Home health chartbook 2015.* Available at: http://ahhqi.org/images/uploads/AHHQI_2015_Chartbook_FINAL_October_Aug2016Update.pdf. Accessed February 2017.

American Hospital Association. 2016. *TrendWatch chartbook.* Washington, DC: Author.

American Medical Association. 2015. *Updated data on physician practice arrangements: Inching toward hospital ownership.* Available at: https://www.ama-assn.org/sites/default/files/media-browser/premium/health-policy/prp-practice-arrangement-2015.pdf. Accessed January 2017.

Appleby, C. 1995. Boxed in? *Hospitals and Health Networks* 69, no. 18: 28–34.

Bakwin, H. 1945. Pseudodoxia pediatrica. *New England Journal of Medicine* 232: 691–697.

Barbosa-Cesnik, C., et al. 2011. Cranberry juice fails to prevent recurrent urinary tract infection: Results from a randomized placebo-controlled trial. *Clinical Infectious Diseases* 52: 23–30.

Barnes, P. M., et al. 2008. *Complementary and alternative medicine use among adults and children: United States, 2007.* Hyattsville, MD: National Center for Health Statistics.

Barr, K. W., and C. L. Breindel. 2004. Ambulatory care. In: *Health care administration: Planning, implementing, and managing organized delivery systems.* L. F. Wolper, ed. 4th ed. Sudbury, MA; Jones and Bartlett Publishers. pp. 507–546.

Barrett, B., et al. 2010. Echinacea for treating the common cold. *Annals of Internal Medicine* 153: 769–777.

Beresford, L. 1989. *History of the National Hospice Organization.* Arlington, VA: National Hospice Organization.

Burton, R. A., et al. 2012. *Patient-centered medical home recognition tools: A comparison of ten surveys' content and operational details.* Available at: http://web.pdx.edu/~nwallace/CRHSP/PCMHTools.pdf. Accessed February 2017.

CAM Research Methodology Conference. 1997. Defining and describing complementary and alternative medicine. *Alternative Therapies* 3, no. 2: 49–56.

Capp, R., et al. 2015. Characteristics of Medicaid-covered emergency department visits made by nonelderly adults: A national study. *Journal of Emergency Medicine* 49, no. 6: 984–989.

Caudill, T., et al. 2011. Health care reform and primary care: Training physicians for tomorrow's challenges. *Academic Medicine* 86, no. 2: 158–160.

Centers for Disease Control and Prevention (CDC). 2013. *National Ambulatory Medical Care Survey: 2013 summary tables.* Available at: https://www.cdc.gov/nchs/data/ahcd/namcs_summary/2013_namcs_web_tables.pdf. Accessed April 2017.

Centers for Medicare and Medicaid Services (CMS). 2012. *National health expenditure data for 2012.* Available at: https://www.cms.gov/Research-Statistics-Data-and-systems/Statistics-Trends-and-reports/NationalHealthExpendData. Accessed February 2017.

Centers for Medicare and Medicaid Services (CMS). 2015a. *National health expenditures 2015 highlights.* Available at: https://www.cms.gov/research-statistics-data-and-systems/statistics-trends-and-reports/nationalhealthexpenddata/downloads/highlights.pdf. Accessed February 2017.

Centers for Medicare and Medicaid Services (CMS). 2015b. *Home health care agencies.* Available at: https://data.medicare.gov/Home-Health-Compare/Home-Health-Care-Agencies/6jpm-sxkc/data. Accessed February 2017.

Centers for Medicare and Medicaid Services (CMS). 2016a. *Home Health Compare datasets.* Available at: https://data.medicare.gov/data/home-health-compare. Accessed February 2017.

Centers for Medicare and Medicaid Services (CMS). 2016b. *Therapy cap.* Available at: https://www.cms.gov/Research-Statistics-Data-and-Systems/Monitoring-Programs/Medicare-FFS-Compliance-Programs/Medical-Review/TherapyCap.html. Accessed February 2017.

Chang, C. H., et al. 2011. Primary care physician workforce and Medicare beneficiaries' health outcomes. *Journal of the American Medical Association* 25, no. 20: 2096–2104.

Chernew, M. E., et al. 2009. Would having more primary care doctors cut health spending growth? *Health Affairs* 28: 1327–1335.

Christensen, E. W., et al. 2013. Impact of a patient-centered medical home on access, quality, and cost. *Military Medicine* 178, no. 2: 135–141.

Commonwealth Fund. 2016. *International profiles of health care systems, 2015.* Available at: http://www.commonwealthfund.org/~/media/files/publications/fund-report/2016/jan/1857_mossialos_intl_profiles_2015_v7.pdf. Accessed January 2017.

Dobson, A., et al. 2012. *Improving health care quality and efficiency: Clinically Appropriate and Cost-Effective Placement (CACEP) Project.* Available at: http://ahhqi.org/images/pdf/cacep-report.pdf. Accessed February 2017.

Ferrante, J. M., et al. 2010. Principles of the patient-centered medical home and preventive services delivery. *Annals of Family Medicine* 8: 108–116.

Franks, P., et al. 1992. Gatekeeping revisited: Protecting patients from overtreatment. *New England Journal of Medicine* 327, no. 4: 424–429.

Franks, P., et al. 1998. Primary care physicians and specialists as personal physicians: Health care expenditures and mortality experience. *Journal of Family Practice* 47: 105–109.

Gao, Y., et al. 2016. Characteristics associated with patient-centered medical home capability in health centers: A cross-sectional analysis. *Journal of General Internal Medicine* 31, no. 9: 1041–1051.

Gilfillan, R. J., et al. 2010. Value and the medical home: Effects of transformed primary care. *American Journal of Managed Care* 16: 607–614.

Gordon, J. S. 1996. Alternative medicine and the family practitioner. *American Family Physician* 54, no. 7: 2205–2212.

Harris-Kojetin, L., et al. 2016. Long-term care providers and services users in the United States: Data from the National Study of Long-Term Care Providers, 2013-2014. *Vital & Health Statistics* 3, no. 38.

Health Resources and Services Administration (HRSA). 2014. *Uniform data system.* Available at: https://bphc.hrsa.gov/uds/datacenter.aspx. Accessed May 2017.

Health Resources and Services Administration (HRSA). 2015. *Health center data.* Available at: https://bphc.hrsa.gov/uds/datacenter.aspx. Accessed February 2017.

Health Resources and Services Administration (HRSA). 2016. *Health center program: Impact and growth.* Available at: https://bphc.hrsa.gov/about/healthcenterprogram/index.html. Accessed February 2017.

Hing, E., et al. 2015. Acceptance of new patients with public and private insurance by office-based physicians: United States, 2013. *NCHS Data Brief* 195: 1–8.

Hummel, K., et al. 2014. Why parents use the emergency department during evening hours for nonemergent pediatric care. *Clinical Pediatrics* 53, no. 11: 1055–1061.

Institute of Medicine (IOM). 2012. *Primary care and public health: Exploring integration to improve population health.* Washington, DC: National Academies Press.

Jackson, C. 2002. Cutting into the market: Rise of ambulatory surgery centers. *American Medical News.* Available at: http://www.amednews.com/2002/bisa0415. Accessed December 2002.

Jerant, A., et al. 2012. Primary care attributes and mortality: A national person-level study. *Annals of Family Medicine* 10, no. 1: 34–41.

Joint Commission. 2011. Optional self-assessment for Primary Care Medical Home (PCMH) certification for ambulatory health care centers. Available at: http://www.jointcommission.org/assets/1/18/AHC_PCMH_SAT.pdf. Accessed February 2017.

Jones, E., et al. 2013. Access to oral health care: The role of federally qualified health centers in addressing disparities and expanding access. *American Journal of Public Health* 103, no. 3: 488–493.

Kaiser Family Foundation. 2017. *Community health centers: Recent growth and the role of the ACA.* Available at: http://files.kff.org/attachment/Issue-Brief-Community-Health-Centers-Recent-Growth-and-the-Role-of-the-ACA. Accessed February 2017.

Kelley, A. S., et al. 2013. Hospice enrollment saves money for Medicare and improves care quality across a number of different lengths-of-stay. *Health Affairs (Millwood)* 32, no. 3: 552–561.

Kozak, L. J., et al. 1999. Changing patterns of surgical care in the United States, 1980–1995. *Health Care Financing Review* 21, no. 1: 31–49.

Ku, L., et al. 2011. The states' next challenge: Securing primary care for expanded Medicaid populations. *New England Journal of Medicine* 364: 493–495.

Lafferty, W. E., et al. 2006. Insurance coverage and subsequent utilization of complementary and alternative medicine providers. *American Journal of Managed Care* 12, no. 7: 397–404.

Liggins, K. 1993. Inappropriate attendance at accident and emergency departments: A literature review. *Journal of Advanced Nursing* 18, no. 7: 1141–1145.

Mao, J. T., et al. 2010. White tea extract induces apoptosis in non-small cell lung cancer cells: The role of PPAR-γ and 15-lipoxygenases. *Cancer Prevention Research* 3, no. 9: 1132–1140.

McCaig, L. F., and C. W. Burt. 2002. *National Hospital Ambulatory Medical Care Survey: 1999 emergency department summary.* Atlanta, GA: Centers for Disease Control and Prevention/National Center for Health Statistics.

McCaig, L. F., and E. W. Newar. 2006. *National Hospital Ambulatory Medical Care Survey: 2004 emergency department summary.* Atlanta, GA: Centers for Disease Control and Prevention/National Center for Health Statistics.

McNamara, P., et al. 1993. Pathwork access: Primary care in EDs on the rise. *Hospitals* 67, no. 10: 44–46.

Medical Group Management Association. *Medical group fast facts.* Available at: http://www.mgma.com/uploadedFiles/Store_Content/Surveys_and_Benchmarking/8523-Table-of-Content-MGMA-Performance-and-Practices-of-Successful-Medical-Groups.pdf.

Meisel, Z. F., et al. 2011. Variations in ambulance use in the United States: The role of health insurance. *Academic Emergency Medicine* 18, no. 10: 1036–1044.

Miller, G. 1996. Hospice. In: *The continuum of long-term care: An integrated systems approach.* C. J. Evashwick, ed. Albany, NY: Delmar Publishers. pp. 98–108.

Morgan, P., et al. 2012. Characteristics of primary care office visits to nurse practitioners, physician assistants and physicians in United States Veterans Health Administration facilities, 2005 to 2010: A retrospective cross-sectional analysis. *Human Resources for Health* 13, no. 10: 42. doi: 10.1186/1478-4491-10-42.

Morgan, P., et al. 2015. Nurse practitioners, physician assistants, and physicians in community health centers, 2006–2010. *Healthcare* 3, no. 2: 102–107.

Morganti, K. G., et al. 2013. *The evolving role of emergency departments in the United States.* Available at: http://www.rand.org/content/dam/rand/pubs/research_reports/RR200/RR280/RAND_RR280.pdf. Accessed February 2017.

Mulvihill, B. A., et al. 2007. Does access to a medical home differ according to child and family characteristics, including special-health-care-needs status, among children in Alabama? *Pediatrics* 119: 107–113.

Nahin, R. L., et al. 2016. *Expenditures on complementary health approaches: United States, 2012.* National Health Statistics Reports. Hyattsville, MD: National Center for Health Statistics.

National Association for Home Care and Hospice. 2010. *Basic statistics about home care.* Available at: http://www.nahc.org/assets/1/7/10hc_stats .pdf. Accessed May 2017.

National Association of Community Health Centers (NACHC). 2013. *Studies on health centers and disparities.* Available at: http://www.nachc.org /client/documents/HC%20Disparities%20 Studies%2006.13.pdf. Accessed August 2013.

National Association of Community Health Centers (NACHC). 2015. *Studies on health centers improving access to care.* Available at: http://nachc.org/wp-content/uploads/2015/06 /HC_Access_0415.pdf. Accessed February 2017.

National Association of Community Health Centers (NACHC). 2016a. *America's health centers.* Available at: http://nachc.org/wp-content /uploads/2015/06/Americas-Health-Centers -March-2016.pdf. Accessed February 2017.

National Association of Community Health Centers (NACHC). 2016b. *Studies of health center quality of care.* Available at: http:// nachc.org/wp-content/uploads/2016/06/HC _Quality_06.16.pdf. Accessed February 2017.

National Association of Community Health Centers (NACHC). 2016c. *Studies of health center cost effectiveness.* Available at: http://nachc.org /wp-content/uploads/2016/06/HC_CE_06.16 .pdf. Accessed February 2017.

National Association of Community Health Centers (NACHC). 2016d. *Health centers and Medicaid.* Available at: http://nachc.org/wp-content /uploads/2016/12/Medicaid-FS_12.16.pdf. Accessed February 2017.

National Association of Free and Charitable Clinics (NAFC). 2016. *Free and charitable clinic health care reform talking points.* Available at: http://www.nafcclinics.org/sites/default/files /NAFC%20ACA%20Related%20Talking%20 Points%202015.pdf. Accessed January 2017.

National Center for Complementary and Alternative Medicine (NCCAM). 2013. *Appropriations history.* Available at: http://nccam.nih.gov/about /budget/congressional/2014#His. Accessed January 2014.

National Center for Complementary and Integrative Health (NCCIH). 2016a. *2016 strategic plan.* Available at: https://nccih.nih.gov/sites/nccam .nih.gov/files/NCCIH_2016_Strategic_Plan .pdf. Accessed February 2017.

National Center for Complementary and Integrative Health (NCCIH). 2016b. *Complementary and alternative medicine: What people aged 50 and older discuss with their health care providers.* Available at: https://nccih.nih.gov/sites/nccam .nih.gov/files/news/camstats/2010/NCCAM _aarp_survey.pdf. Accessed February 2017.

National Center for Health Statistics. 2010. *National Hospital Discharge Survey.* Available at: https:// www.cdc.gov/nchs/nhds/nhds_publications .htm. Accessed January 2017.

National Center for Health Statistics. 2011. *National Hospital Ambulatory Medical Care Survey: 2011 emergency department summary tables.* Available at: https://www.cdc.gov/nchs/data /ahcd/nhamcs_emergency/2011_ed_web _tables.pdf. Accessed February 2017.

National Center for Health Statistics. 2013. *National Hospital Ambulatory Medical Care Survey: 2013 emergency department summary tables.* Available at: https://www.cdc.gov/nchs/data /ahcd/nhamcs_emergency/2013_ed_web _tables.pdf. Accessed February 2017.

National Center for Health Statistics. 2016. *Health, United States, 2015.* Hyattsville, MD: U.S. Department of Health and Human Services.

National Committee for Quality Assurance (NCQA). 2008. *Physician Practice Connections: Patient-Centered Medical Home.* Available at: https://www.nmms.org/files/uploaded/files /NCQA%20Stds%20&%20Guidelines%20 for%20PCMH.pdf. Accessed February 2017.

National Council on Aging. 2016. *Home health care vs. custodial care.* Available at: https:// www.ncoa.org/wp-content/uploads/home-vs -custodial.pdf. Accessed February 2017.

National Hospice and Palliative Care Organization. 2015. *NHPCO facts and figures: Hospice care in America.* Available at: http://www.nhpco .org/sites/default/files/public/Statistics_Research /2015_Facts_Figures.pdf. Accessed February 2017.

National Hospice Organization. 1995. *An analysis of the cost savings of the Medicare hospice benefit (National Hospice Organization Item Code 712901).* Miami, FL: Lewin-VHI Inc.

National Nursing Centers Consortium. 2003. *Nurse-managed health centers briefing.* pp. 1–4.

Orton, P. 1994. Shared care. *Lancet* 344, no. 8934: 1413–1415.

Padgett, D. K., and B. Brodsky. 1992. Psychosocial factors influencing non-urgent use of the emergency room: A review of the literature and recommendations for research and improved service delivery. *Social Science & Medicine* 35, no. 9: 1189–1197.

Parchman, M., and S. Culler. 1994. Primary care physicians and avoidable hospitalization. *Journal of Family Practice* 39: 123–128.

Park-Lee E.Y., and F. H. Decker. 2010. Comparison of home and hospice care agencies by organizational characteristics and services provided: United States, 2007. *National Health Statistics Reports* no. 30: 1–23.

RAND Corporation. 2016. *The evolving role of retail clinics.* Available at: http://www.rand.org/pubs/research_briefs/RB9491-2.html. Accessed February 2017.

Reid, R. J., et al. 2009. Patient-centered medical home demonstration: A prospective, quasi-experimental, before and after evaluation. *American Journal of Managed Care* 27: 362–367.

Roos, N. 1979. Who should do the surgery? Tonsillectomy and adenoidectomy in one Canadian province. *Inquiry* 16, no. 1: 73–83.

Rosenthal, M. B., et al. 2015. Impact of the Rochester Medical Home Initiative on primary care practices, quality, utilization, and costs. *Medical Care* 53, no. 11: 967–973.

Rubin, G., et al. 2015. The expanding role of primary care in cancer control. *Lancet Oncology* 16, no. 12: 1231–1272.

Schoen, C., et al. 2012. A survey of primary care doctors in ten countries shows progress in use of health information technology, less in other areas. *Health Affairs* 31, no. 12: 2805–2816.

Searing, L. M., and K. A. Cantlin. 2016. Nonurgent emergency department visits by insured and uninsured adults. *Public Health Nursing* 33, no. 2: 93–98.

Sepulveda, M.-J., et al. 2008. Primary care: Can it solve employers' health care dilemma? *Health Affairs* 27: 151–158.

Shi, L. 1994. Primary care, specialty care, and life chances. *International Journal of Health Services* 24, no. 3: 431–458.

Shi, L., and B. Starfield. 2000. Primary care, income inequality, and self-related health in the US: Mixed-level analysis. *International Journal of Health Services* 30: 541–555.

Shi, L., and B. Starfield. 2001. Primary care physician supply, income inequality, and racial mortality in US metropolitan areas. *American Journal of Public Health* 91: 1246–1250.

Shi, L., et al. 1999. Income inequality, primary care, and health indicators. *Journal of Family Practice* 48: 275–284.

Shi, L., et al. 2002. Primary care, self-rated health care, and reduction in social disparities in health. *Health Services Research* 37, no. 3: 529–550.

Shi, L., et al. 2007. Health center financial performance: National trends and state variation, 1998–2004. *Journal of Public Health Management and Practice* 13, no. 2: 133–150.

Shi, L., et al. 2015. Patient-centered medical home capability and clinical performance in HRSA-supported health centers. *Medical Care* 53, no. 5: 389–395.

Shi, L., et al. 2016. Patient-centered medical home recognition and clinical performance in U.S. community health centers. *Health Service Research.* doi: 10.1111/1475-6773.12523.

SK&A. 2016. *Medical group practice list.* Available at: http://www.skainfo.com/databases/medical-group-practice-list. Accessed January 2016.

SMG Solutions. 2000. *Report and directory: Medical group practices.* Chicago, IL: SMG Solutions.

Starfield, B. 1992. *Primary care: Concept, evaluation, and policy.* New York, NY: Oxford University Press.

Starfield, B. 1994. Is primary care essential? *Lancet* 344, no. 8930: 1129–1133.

Starfield, B. 1998. *Primary care: Balancing health needs, services and technology.* New York, NY: Oxford University Press.

Stevens, G. D., et al. 2010. National disparities in the quality of a medical home for children. *Maternal Child Health* 14: 580–589.

Tais, S., and E. Zoberg. 2013. The economic evaluation of complementary and alternative medicine. *Natural Medicine Journal* 5, no. 2. Available at: http://www.naturalmedicinejournal.com/journal/2013-02/economic-evaluation-complementary-and-alternative-medicine. Accessed May 2017.

Thomson, S., et al., eds. 2012. *International profiles of health care systems.* New York, NY: Commonwealth Fund. Available at: http://www.commonwealthfund.org/~/media/Files/Publications/Fund%20Report/2012/Nov/1645_Squires_intl_profiles_hlt_care_systems_2012.pdf. Accessed January 2014.

Vanselow, N. A., et al. 1995. From the Institute of Medicine. *Journal of the American Medical Association* 273, no. 3: 192.

van Weel, C., et al. 2008. Integration of personal and community health care. *Lancet* 372, no. 9642: 871–872.

VHA Inc. and Deloitte & Touche. 1997. *Environmental assessment: Redesigning health care for the millennium.* Irving, TX: VHA Inc.

Weinerman, E. R., et al. 1966. Yale studies in ambulatory medical care. V. Determinants of use of hospital emergency services. *American Journal of Public Health* 56, no. 7: 1037–1056.

White House. 2016. *Fact sheet: Health care accomplishments.* Available at: https://obamawhitehouse .archives.gov/the-press-office/2016/03/22/fact -sheet-health-care-accomplishments. Accessed January 2017.

Wier, L. M., et al. 2015. *Surgeries in hospital-owned outpatient facilities, 2012.* Available at: https:// www.hcup-us.ahrq.gov/reports/statbriefs/sb188 -Surgeries-Hospital-Outpatient-Facilities-2012 .pdf. Accessed January 2017.

Wilson, F. A., and D. Neuhauser. 1985. *Health services in the United States.* 2nd ed. Cambridge, MA: Ballinger Publishing.

World Health Organization (WHO). 1978. *Primary health care.* Geneva, Switzerland: WHO.

World Health Organization (WHO). 2010. *Primary health care.* Geneva, Switzerland: WHO.

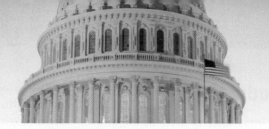

CHAPTER 8

Inpatient Facilities and Services

LEARNING OBJECTIVES

- Get a functional perspective on the evolution of hospitals.
- Survey the factors that contributed to the growth of hospitals prior to the 1980s.
- Understand the reasons for the subsequent decline of hospitals and their utilization.
- Describe some key measures pertaining to hospital operations and inpatient utilization.
- Compare utilization measures in U.S. hospitals to those in other countries.
- Differentiate among various types of hospitals.
- Describe how the Affordable Care Act affected physician-owned specialty hospitals and nonprofit hospitals.
- Comprehend some basic concepts in hospital governance.
- Understand and differentiate between licensure, certification, and accreditation and the Magnet Recognition Program of the American Nurses Credentialing Center.
- Get a perspective on some key ethical issues.

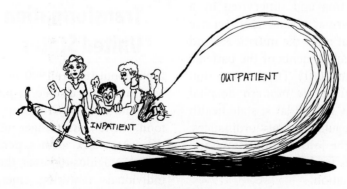

"We have the inpatient sector under control."

▶ Introduction

The term **inpatient** is used in conjunction with an overnight stay in a health care facility, such as a hospital, whereas *outpatient* refers to services provided while the patient is not lodged in a health care facility. Although the primary function of hospitals is to deliver inpatient acute care services, many hospitals have expanded their scope of services to include nonacute and outpatient care.

According to the American Hospital Association (AHA), a **hospital** is an institution with at least six beds whose primary function is "to deliver patient services, diagnostic and therapeutic, for particular or general medical conditions" (AHA, 1994). In addition, a hospital must be licensed, have an organized physician staff, and provide continuous nursing services under the supervision of registered nurses. Other characteristics of a hospital include an identifiable governing body that is legally responsible for the conduct of the hospital, a chief executive with continuous responsibility for the operation of the hospital, maintenance of medical records on each patient, pharmacy services maintained in the institution and supervised by a registered pharmacist, and food service operations that meet the nutritional and therapeutic requirements of the patients (Health Forum, 2001). The construction and operation of the modern hospital is governed by federal laws; state health department regulations; city ordinances; standards of the Joint Commission; and national codes for building, fire protection, and sanitation.

In the past 200 years or so, hospitals have gradually evolved from ordinary institutions of refuge for the homeless and poor to ultramodern facilities that provide technologically advanced services to the critically ill and injured. The term "medical center" is used by some hospitals, reflecting their high level of specialization and wide scope of services, which may include teaching and research. Growth of multihospital chains, especially those providing a variety of health care services in addition to acute care, has led to the nomenclature "hospital system" or "health system."

Hospital care consumes the biggest share of national health care spending. To date, efforts to control rising hospital costs in the United States have met with little success.

This chapter describes institutional care delivery with specific reference to acute care—mostly characterized by secondary and tertiary levels of care—in community hospitals. It also discusses various ways to classify hospitals and points out important trends and critical issues that will continue to shape the delivery of inpatient services.

▶ Hospital Transformation in the United States

From about 1840 to 1900, hospitals underwent a drastic change in purpose, function, and number. From supplying merely food, shelter, and meager medical care to the pauper sick, armies, persons infected with contagious diseases, the insane, and individuals requiring emergency treatment, they began to provide skilled medical and surgical attention and nursing care to all classes of people (Raffel, 1980). Subsequently, hospitals became centers of medical training and research. More recent transformations have been mainly organizational in nature, as hospitals have consolidated into medical systems, delivering a broad range of health care services. These transformations can be neatly categorized according to five significant functions in the evolution of hospitals:

1. Primitive institutions of social welfare
2. Distinct institutions of care for the sick
3. Organized institutions of medical practice
4. Advanced institutions of medical training and research
5. Consolidated systems of health services delivery

Primitive Institutions of Social Welfare

Except for a few hospitals that were located in some of the major U.S. cities, during the 1800s, most locations in the country had municipal almshouses (or poorhouses) and pesthouses. Financed through charitable gifts and local government funds, these institutions essentially performed a social welfare function. Almshouses served primarily the destitute of society who needed food and shelter. They also took care of the sick, who received limited nursing care as needed. People generally stayed in these institutions for months, rather than days. Pesthouses were used to quarantine people who were sick with contagious diseases, such as smallpox and yellow fever, so the rest of the community would be protected.

Distinct Institutions of Care for the Sick

Not until the late 1800s did infirmaries or hospital departments of city poorhouses break away to become independent medical care institutions. These were the first public hospitals (Haglund and Dowling, 1993), in this case operated by local governments. For example, the Kings County Almshouse and Infirmary, organized in Brooklyn in 1830, later became the Kings County Hospital (Raffel, 1980). Nevertheless, these first public hospitals still served mainly the indigent. Hospitals at this stage often had poor hygiene, inadequate ventilation, and care provided by untrained nurses.

In Europe, the first hospitals were established predominantly by religious orders. Nurses, who were primarily monks and nuns, attended to both the physical and spiritual needs of the patients. Later, many of these hospitals became tax-financed public institutions as less church money became available for hospitals and monasteries. In England, private donations and taxes supported the "royal hospitals." Other British hospitals were nonprofit (or voluntary) hospitals, which served as a model for such hospitals in the United States (Raffel and Raffel, 1994). Later, creation of the National Health Service in 1948 brought the British nonprofit hospitals under public (government) ownership.

In the United States, the founding of **voluntary hospitals**—nonprofit community hospitals financed through local philanthropy as opposed to taxes— was often inspired by influential physicians, with the financial backing of local donors and philanthropists. These hospitals accepted both indigent and paying patients, but to cover their operating expenses, they required charitable contributions from private citizens.

The first voluntary hospital in the United States established specifically to care for the sick was the Pennsylvania Hospital in Philadelphia, which opened in 1752. At the time, the city already had an almshouse. However, Dr. Thomas Bond, a London-trained physician, brought to prominence the need for a hospital to care for the sick poor of the city. Benjamin Franklin, who was a friend and advisor of Dr. Bond, was instrumental in promoting the idea and in raising voluntary contributions. According to the hospital's charter, the contributors had the right to make all laws and regulations relating to the hospital's operation. The contributors also elected members to form the governing board, or the board of trustees. Thus, the control of voluntary hospitals was in the hands of influential community laypeople rather than physicians (Raffel and Raffel, 1994).

Other prominent voluntary hospitals included the New York Hospital in New York, which was completed in 1775 but, due to the Revolutionary War, was not opened to civilian patients until 1791. The Massachusetts General Hospital in Boston was incorporated in 1812 and opened in 1821. During this period, the almshouses continued to serve an important function by receiving overflow patients who could not be admitted to the hospitals because of the unavailability of beds or who had to be discharged from hospitals because they were declared incurable (Raffel and Raffel, 1994). Later hospitals in the United States were modeled after the Pennsylvania, New York, and Massachusetts General hospitals.

Organized Institutions of Medical Practice

Social and demographic change, but above all advances in medical science and technology, transformed hospitals into institutions of medical practice. Beginning in the latter half of the 19th century, new medical technology, facilities, and personnel training all became centered in the hospital.

Improvements in hygiene, advanced medical care, and surgical services made hospitals more acceptable to the middle and upper classes. Hospitals actually began to attract affluent patients who could afford to pay privately. Thus, the hospital was transformed from a charitable institution into one that could generate a profit. In many instances, physicians started opening small hospitals, financed by wealthy and influential sponsors. These facilities were the first proprietary (for-profit) hospitals.

In the early 20th century, the field of hospital administration became a discipline in its own right. Hospitals needed administrators with expertise in financial management and organizational skills to manage them. The administrative structure of the hospital was organized into departments, such as food service, pharmacy, x-ray, and laboratory. It became necessary to employ professional staff to manage the delivery of services. Efficiency began to emerge as an important element in the management of hospitals. This early emphasis on efficiency foreshadowed two main issues that continue to affect health policy and hospital management: the pressure on hospitals to introduce new technology while containing costs and the assumption that hospitals should operate like businesses (Arndt and Bigelow, 2006).

Pressure to control costs, along with the availability of advanced medical care in outpatient settings, forced hospitals to limit care to more acute periods of illness rather than the full course of a disease.

Hospital accreditation was another notable development in the early 20th century. The American College of Surgeons (ACS) began inspecting hospitals in 1918 and developed standards for hospital equipment and hospital wards. Until 1951, the ACS single-handedly worked to improve hospital-based medical practice. This effort evolved into the formation of the Joint Commission on Accreditation of Hospitals, a private nonprofit body formed in 1951 through the joint efforts of the ACS, the American College of Physicians, the AHA, and the American Medical Association (AMA). The organization changed its name in 1987 to the Joint Commission on Accreditation of Healthcare Organizations, which more accurately describes the variety of health facilities it accredits. Since 2007, its official name has been The Joint Commission.

Advanced Institutions of Medical Training and Research

Advances in biomedical knowledge made it necessary for physicians to receive most of their training in hospitals. This led to collaborations between hospitals and universities. Pennsylvania Hospital, for example, taught courses required by the College of Philadelphia's medical school, which later became the University of Pennsylvania School of Medicine. Similarly, New York Hospital served as a teaching hospital for medical students of Columbia Medical School, and Massachusetts General Hospital provided practical clinical

instruction for students of Harvard Medical School (Raffel and Raffel, 1994). To complete one's medical training, internships and residencies became necessary.

The Johns Hopkins Hospital (opened in 1889), with its adjoining medical school (opened in 1893), inaugurated a new era during which teaching was combined with clinical practice and scientific inquiry in medicine. In affiliation with university-based medical schools, many hospitals became centers of medical research. The vast number of clinical records and a large array of medical conditions among hospital patients provided a wealth of data that informed investigative studies to advance medical knowledge. Even today, large hospitals play an important role in clinical studies. To a lesser extent, some aspects of medical training have shifted to outpatient settings, such as nursing homes, hospices, and community health centers.

Consolidated Systems of Health Services Delivery

Hospitals have been the major cost centers in the health care delivery system. During the 1980s and 1990s, concerns over rising costs prompted introduction of prospective and capitated payment methods and aggressive utilization review practices that brought about drastic reductions in the length of inpatient stays. The declining utilization of acute care beds had left most hospitals with excess capacity in the form of empty beds. As the acute inpatient care sector of health care delivery became less profitable, hospitals adopted a number of consolidation strategies. Multihospital systems formed through mergers and acquisitions; hospital systems diversified into nonacute services, such as outpatient centers, home health care, long-term care, and subacute care; and some hospitals affiliated with networks through contractual arrangements.

Intense consolidation in certain hospital markets diluted competition, which benefited hospitals. Research suggests that hospital consolidation in the 1990s raised prices by at least 5% as competition eroded (Vogt and Town, 2006).

▶ The Expansion Phase: Late 1800s to Mid-1980s

Hospitals grew in numbers when they became a necessary local adjunct of medical practice. Growth in medical technology increased the volume of surgical procedures, almost all of which were performed in hospitals. The number of U.S. hospitals grew from 178 (35,604 beds) in 1872 to 4,359 (421,065 beds) in 1909. By 1929, 6,665 hospitals provided 907,133 beds in the United States (Haglund and Dowling, 1993). As new beds were built, their availability almost ensured that they would be used. This phenomenon led Milton Roemer (1916–2001) to proclaim, "a built bed is a filled bed"—an assertion known popularly as Roemer's law (Roemer, 1961).

Haglund and Dowling (1993) identified six significant factors in the growth of hospitals: advances in medical science, development of specialized technology, advances in medical education, development of professional nursing, growth of health insurance, and the role of government. The first three factors were discussed in the previous section; this section covers the last three.

Development of Professional Nursing

During the latter half of the 19th century, Florence Nightingale was instrumental in transforming nursing into a recognized profession in Great Britain. Following the founding of the Nightingale School of Nursing in England, nursing schools in the United States were established at Bellevue Hospital (New York City), New Haven Hospital (New Haven, Connecticut), and Massachusetts General Hospital (Boston). The benefits of having trained nurses in hospitals became apparent as the increased efficacy of treatment and hygiene associated with such care improved patient recovery (Haglund and Dowling, 1993). As a result, hospitals increasingly came to be regarded as places of healing, and found acceptance with the middle and upper classes.

Growth of Private Health Insurance

Private health insurance in the United States first began as a hospital insurance plan to protect both patients and hospitals against financial instability. During and after the Great Depression of the 1930s, many hospitals were forced to close, and the financial solvency of many more was threatened. Consequently, the number of hospitals in the United States dropped from 6,852 in 1928 to 6,189 in 1937. The growth of private health insurance subsequently became a vehicle for enabling people to pay for hospital services, and the flow of insurance money helped revive the financial stability of hospitals. Historically, insurance plans provided generous coverage for inpatient care, placing few restrictions on patients and physicians who opted for care consisting of more expensive hospital services (Feldstein, 1971).

Role of Government

Government funding for hospital construction perhaps played the most important role in the expansion of hospitals in the 20th century. Subsequently, Medicare and Medicaid provided indirect funding to the hospital industry by vastly expanding public-sector health insurance.

The Hill-Burton Act

Relatively little hospital construction took place during the Great Depression and World War II, so, by the end of the war, there was a severe shortage of hospital beds. The Hospital Survey and Construction Act of 1946, commonly referred to as the Hill-Burton Act, provided federal grants to states for the construction of new community hospitals (nonfederal, short-stay hospitals). This legislation required that each state develop and upgrade, annually, a plan for health facility construction based on bed-to-population ratios, which became the basis for the allocation of federal construction grants to the states (Raffel, 1980).

In 1946, after World War II ended, 3.2 community hospital beds were available per 1,000 civilian population in the United States. The objective of Hill-Burton was to reach 4.5 beds per 1,000 population (Teisberg et al., 1991). The Hill-Burton program assisted in the construction of nearly 40% of the beds in the nation's short-stay general hospitals and was the greatest single factor that increased the U.S. bed supply during the 1950s and 1960s (Haglund

and Dowling, 1993). The Hill-Burton Act made it possible for even small, remote communities to have their own hospitals (Wolfson and Hopes, 1994). By 1980, the United States had reached its goal of 4.5 community hospital beds per 1,000 civilian population (National Center for Health Statistics, 2002) even though the Hill-Burton program ended in 1974.

The Hill-Burton Act was instrumental in promoting the growth of nonprofit community hospitals because it required hospitals constructed with federal funds to provide a certain amount of charitable care. Competition from these new hospitals led to the closure of many smaller proprietary, for-profit hospitals. Thanks to the Hill-Burton Act, nonprofit community hospitals in the United States far outnumber all other types of hospitals even today.

Public Health Insurance

The creation of the Medicare and Medicaid programs in 1965 also had a significant—albeit indirect—impact on the increase in the number of hospital beds and their utilization (Feldstein, 1993), as government-funded health insurance became available to a large number of elderly and poor Americans. Between 1965 and 1980, the number of community hospitals in the United States increased from 5,736 (741,000 beds) to 5,830 (988,000 beds); total admissions per 1,000 population increased from 130 to 154; and total inpatient days per 1,000 population increased from 1,007 to 1,159. The percentage of occupied beds also remained relatively stable at around 76% (AHA, 1990). **FIGURE 8-1** shows trends from 1940 to 2013 in the number of beds per 1,000 resident population.

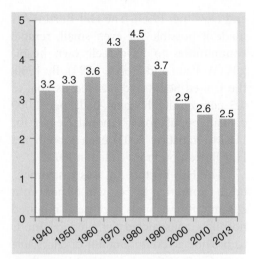

FIGURE 8-1 Trends in the number of U.S. community hospital beds per 1,000 resident population.

Data from National Center for Health Statistics. 2002. *Health, United States, 2002.* Hyattsville, MD: U.S. Department of Health and Human Services. p. 281; National Center for Health Statistics. 2016. *Health, United States, 2015.* Hyattsville, MD: U.S. Department of Health and Human Services. p. 289.

▶ The Downsizing Phase: Mid-1980s Onward

The mid-1980s marked a turning point in the growth and use of hospital beds. After a sharp decline in 1985, the number of community hospitals and the total number of beds have continued to decline (**FIGURE 8-2**). Note that the slight uptick in hospital beds since 2005 reflects an increase in for-profit hospitals, as shown in Table 8-5. The average bed capacity of a community hospital also declined from 169.5 beds in 1980 to 160 beds in 2013 (National Center for Health Statistics, 2016), which means that the average hospital has become smaller in size.

Even as the numbers of hospitals and beds have contracted, further declines have occurred in the actual utilization of the shrunken capacity. Occupancy rates

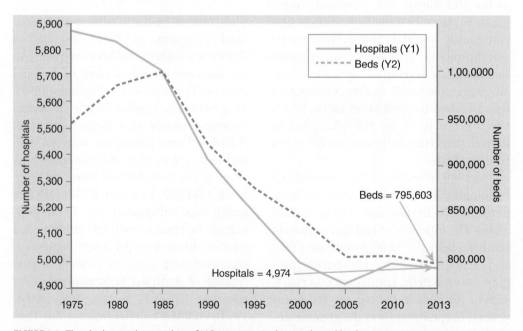

FIGURE 8-2 The decline in the number of U.S. community hospitals and beds.

Data from National Center for Health Statistics. 2002. *Health, United States, 2002.* Hyattsville, MD: U.S. Department of Health and Human Services. p. 279; National Center for Health Statistics. 2016. *Health, United States, 2015.* Hyattsville, MD: U.S. Department of Health and Human Services. p. 289.

(percentage of beds occupied) in community hospitals declined from 75.2% in 1980 to 62.9% in 2013 (National Center for Health Statistics, 2016). Similarly, the average length of stay in community hospitals has declined from 7.6 days in 1980 to 5.4 days and has remained constant at this level since 2010 (National Center for Health Statistics, 2016).

The main reasons for the decline in hospital capacity and utilization are a shift from inpatient to outpatient care, changes in reimbursement, impact of managed care, and hospital closures.

Shift from Inpatient to Outpatient Care

Within hospitals, a dramatic shift from inpatient to outpatient utilization has occurred, as illustrated by the increasing ratios between hospital outpatient visits and inpatient days (**FIGURE 8-3**). Along with this shift in the use of hospital services, the share of personal health expenditures for hospital care had declined until 2005, but has slowly crept up since then (**TABLE 8-1**).

Changes in Reimbursement

The Tax Equity and Fiscal Responsibility Act (TEFRA) of 1982 required the conversion of hospital Medicare reimbursement from cost-plus to a prospective payment system (PPS) based on diagnosis-related groups (DRGs). Under PPS, hospitals are paid a fixed amount per admission according to the patient's principal diagnosis, regardless of how long the patient stays in the hospital. To make a profit, the hospital must keep its costs below the fixed reimbursement amount, which creates an incentive to minimize the patient's length of stay. Following Medicare's lead, other

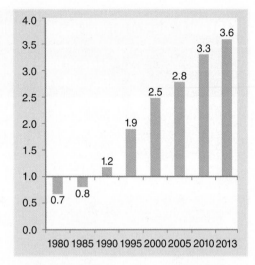

FIGURE 8-3 Ratio of hospital outpatient visits to inpatient days for all U.S. hospitals, 1980–2013 (selected years).

Note: For 2005, 2010, and 2013 data, inpatient days were estimated from hospital admissions and average length of stay.

Data from National Center for Health Statistics. 2002. *Health, United States, 2002.* Hyattsville, MD: Department of Health and Human Services. p. 110; National Center for Health Statistics. 2013. *Health, United States, 2012.* Hyattsville, MD: Department of Health and Human Services. p. 307; National Center for Health Statistics. 2016. *Health, United States, 2015.* Hyattsville, MD: Department of Health and Human Services. p. 281.

payers soon adopted prospective methods to reimburse hospitals. Private payers also resorted to competitive pricing and discounted fees and closely monitored when patients would be hospitalized and for how long. As PPS reimbursement exerted pressure on hospitals to reduce the length of stay after admission, early discharge from hospitals became practical only as alternative services, such as home health care and subacute long-term care, were developed to deliver postacute continuity of care.

The effect of PPS reimbursement on hospitals was dramatic. In the 1980s, 550 hospitals closed and 159 mergers and acquisitions occurred (Balotsky, 2005). Since then, the number of community hospital beds per 1,000 resident population has continued to decline, reaching 2.5

TABLE 8-1 Share of Personal Health Expenditures[1] Used for Hospital Care

	Personal Health Expenditures	Hospital Expenditures	Percentage Share
1980	217.2	100.5	46.3%
1990	616.8	250.4	40.6%
2000	1,165.4	415.5	35.7%
2005	1,697.1	609.4	35.9%
2010	2,190.0	815.9	37.3%
2014	2,563.6	971.8	37.9%

[1] Expenditures are in billions of dollars.

Data from National Center for Health Statistics. 2014. *Health, United States, 2013*. Hyattsville, MD: U.S. Department of Health and Human Services. p. 331; National Center for Health Statistics. 2016. *Health, United States, 2015*. Hyattsville, MD: U.S. Department of Health and Human Services. p. 295.

in 2013 (Figure 8-1). Notably, since 1998, the U.S. hospital capacity per 1,000 resident population has remained less than the level in 1946, when the Hill-Burton Act was passed. In those days, the additional hospital bed capacity may have been necessary because the settings for postdischarge continuity of care were not developed. Technological advances enabled the development of these alternative delivery settings. Hence, technology has played a major role in the tremendous advances in efficiency of the health care system.

Impact of Managed Care

In the 1990s, managed care became a growing force that transformed the delivery of health services in the United States. Managed care has emphasized cost-containment and the efficient delivery of services by stressing the use of alternative delivery settings whenever appropriate. Notably, greater market penetration by health maintenance organizations (HMOs) played a significant role in lowering hospital utilization and profitability (Clement and Grazier, 2001).

Hospital Closures

Between 1990 and 2000, more than 200 rural hospitals (8% of all rural hospitals) and nearly 300 urban hospitals (11% of all urban hospitals) closed for economic reasons (Office of Inspector General, 2003). Declining utilization was the main factor underlying this trend. Overall, the total number of community hospitals declined by 9% during the 1990s; the total number of beds in community hospitals declined by 11% (National Center for Health Statistics, 2013). Hospitals of all sizes throughout the United States either closed entire wings or converted those beds to alternative uses, such as outpatient care, long-term care, or rehabilitation services.

Since 2000, many government-run hospitals, at both the federal and local levels, have closed. For example, the number of hospitals operated by state and local governments declined from 1,163 in 2000 to 1,010 in 2013 (National Center for Health Statistics, 2016) because they could not complete with privately owned community hospitals.

▶ Some Key Utilization Measures and Operational Concepts

Discharges

The total number of patient discharges per 1,000 population (hospitalization rate) is one indicator of access to hospital inpatient services and of the extent of utilization. Because babies born in the hospital are not included in admissions, discharges provide a more accurate count of inpatients served by a hospital. **Discharge** data for a hospital indicate the total number of patients discharged from the hospital's acute care beds during a given period. Deaths in hospitals are counted as discharges.

In general, hospitalization rates and lengths of stay increase with age (**TABLE 8-2**). Females have a higher rate of hospitalization compared to males, but incur shorter lengths of stay. This holds true even when data are adjusted to account for pregnancy-related hospitalizations.

In 2012, Medicare paid for the largest number of hospitalizations, followed by private insurance and Medicaid. Approximately 2 million discharges were attributed to patients without insurance.

People living in low-income communities have higher hospitalization rates and greater lengths of stay compared to those living in higher-income communities. Poorer population groups are generally

TABLE 8-2 Discharges, Average Length of Stay, and Average Cost per Stay in U.S. Community Hospitals, 2012

Characteristics	Total Discharges (in Thousands)	Discharges per 1,000 Population (Hospitalization Rates)	Average Length of Stay (Days)	Average Cost per Stay ($)
Total	36,500	116.2	4.5	10,400
Age				
< 1 year	4,300	1070.9[1]	3.8	5,000
1–17 years	1,500	21.1	3.9	9,900
18–44 years	9,000	78.9	3.6	7,600

(continues)

TABLE 8-2 Discharges, Average Length of Stay, and Average Cost per Stay in U.S. Community Hospitals, 2012 (*continued*)

Characteristics	Total Discharges (in Thousands)	Discharges per 1,000 Population (Hospitalization Rates)	Average Length of Stay (Days)	Average Cost per Stay ($)
45–64 years	9,000	108.8	4.9	12,900
65–84 years	9,700	260.9	5.2	13,000
≥ 85 years	3,000	502.0	5.2	10,200
Gender				
Male	15,400	99.9	4.8	11,700
Female	21,000	132.0	4.3	9,400
Primary Payer				
Medicare	14,300	—	5.2	12,200
Medicaid	7,600	—	4.3	8,100
Private insurance	11,200	—	3.8	9,700
Uninsured	2,000	—	4.0	8,800
Community Income				
Low	10,900	136.8	4.6	9,700
Not low	24,700	106.1	4.4	10,600
Geographic Region				
Northeast	7,000	125.2	4.9	10,800
Midwest	8,200	122.4	4.3	10,200
South	14,100	120.4	4.5	9,300
West	7,200	97.2	4.2	12,300

[1] Includes hospital births.

Modified from Weiss, A. J., and A. Elixhauser. 2014. *Overview of hospital stays in the United States, 2012 (Statistical Brief #180)*. Rockville, MD: Agency for Healthcare Research and Quality. Available at: http://www.hcup-us.ahrq.gov/reports/statbriefs/sb180-Hospitalizations-United-States-2012.pdf. Accessed May 2017.

in poorer health and have less access to routine primary care. These patients also have higher levels of trust in the technical quality of hospital services compared to primary care (Kangovi et al., 2013).

The West, compared to other geographic regions in the United States, has lower hospitalization rates and lengths of stay. A high rate of managed care penetration is believed to be primarily responsible for this lower hospital utilization.

Inpatient Days

An **inpatient day** (also called a patient day) is a night spent in the hospital by a patient. The cumulative number of patient days over a certain period is known as **days of care**. Days of care per 1,000 population over the course of 1 year reflect utilization of inpatient services.

Average Length of Stay

Average length of stay (ALOS) is calculated by dividing the total days of care by the total number of discharges. Note that the ALOS is overstated when using admissions rather than discharges as the divisor. ALOS measures the number of days a patient, on average, spends in the hospital. Hence, this measure, when applied to individuals or specific groups of patients, is an indicator of severity of illness and resource use. In addition, ALOS has cost implications. Other things being equal, short hospital stays reduce the cost per discharge. **FIGURE 8-4** illustrates ALOS trends in community hospitals.

FIGURE 8-5 shows trends in ALOS by type of hospital ownership. Government-owned hospitals have higher lengths of stay, compared to private hospitals. Federal

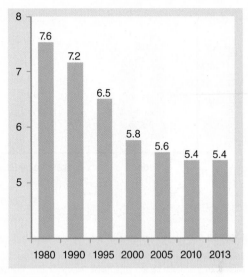

FIGURE 8-4 Trends in average length of stay in nonfederal short-stay hospitals, selected years.

Note: Lengths of stay have been somewhat overstated because they are calculated by dividing total inpatient days by admissions, instead of discharges.

Data from National Center for Health Statistics. 2016. *Health, United States, 2015.* Hyattsville, MD: Department of Health and Human Services. p. 281.

hospitals mainly include those in the Veterans Health Administration system, which serve an aging population. State and local government hospitals disproportionately serve the poor and uninsured.

Hospital Access and Utilization: Comparative Data

There has been increasing interest in comparing the U.S. health system to the health systems of other countries. For this purpose, the Organization for Economic Cooperation and Development (OECD) is a reliable source of comparative health care data. **TABLE 8-3** provides hospital utilization data for selected OECD members. Note that the data for the United States include all hospitals, whereas the data in Table 8-2 are confined to community hospitals.

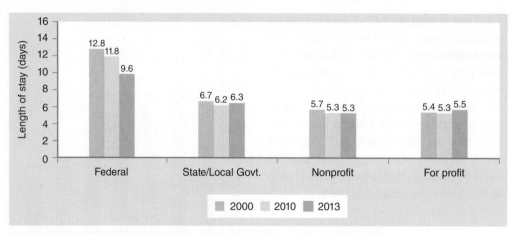

FIGURE 8-5 Average lengths of stay by U.S. hospital ownership, selected years.

Data from National Center for Health Statistics. 2013. *Health, United States, 2012.* Hyattsville, MD: U.S. Department of Health and Human Services. p. 307; National Center for Health Statistics. 2016. *Health, United States, 2015.* Hyattsville, MD: U.S. Department of Health and Human Services. p. 281.

TABLE 8-3 Inpatient Hospital Utilization: Comparative Data for Selected OECD Countries, 2012 (or Nearest Year)

	Acute Care Beds per 1,000 Population	Discharges per 1,000 Population	Average Length of Stay (Days)
Australia	3.4	159.5	5.0
Canada	1.7	82.5	7.7
France	3.4	168.5	5.6
Germany	5.3	244.2	9.3
United Kingdom	2.4	136.4	7.3
United States	2.6	125.5	4.8

Data from Organization for Economic Cooperation and Development (OECD). 2017. Health care utilization. *OECD Health Statistics [Database].* doi: http://dx.doi.org/10.1787/data-00542-en. Accessed May 2017.

Canada has the lowest number of hospital beds available and the lowest hospitalization rates. Germany has the highest utilization of hospital inpatient services. Hospital access and utilization in the United States fall somewhere in the middle of these extremes, except that it has the lowest ALOS.

Capacity

The number of beds set up and staffed for inpatient use determines the size or capacity of a hospital. Among all community hospitals in the United States, 84% have fewer than 300 beds (**FIGURE 8-6**).

Total number of community hospitals = 4,974
Total number of beds = 795,603

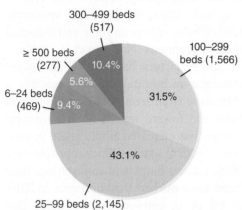

The average size of a community hospital was approximately 160 beds in 2013. The number of hospitals with fewer than 50 beds increased by 38% (from 1,198 to 1,655) between 2000 and 2013 (National Center for Health Statistics, 2016), primarily because of a dramatic rise in the number of physician-owned specialty hospitals (discussed later in the section "Specialty Hospitals").

Average Daily Census

The average number of inpatients receiving care each day in a hospital is called the **average daily census**. This measure is often used to define occupancy of inpatient beds in hospitals and other inpatient facilities. The total inpatient days during a given period (days of care) is divided by the number of days in that period to arrive at the average daily census. For example, if the number of total inpatient days for July is 3,131, then the average daily census for July is 101 (3,131/31).

Occupancy Rate

The **occupancy rate** for a given period is derived by dividing the average daily census for that period by the average number of beds (capacity). The resulting fraction is then expressed as a percentage (percent of beds occupied); it indicates the proportion of a hospital's total inpatient capacity actually utilized. Occupancy rates are also calculated for other types of inpatient facilities, such as nursing homes, and often used as a measure of performance.

FIGURE 8-7 shows the change in aggregate occupancy rates for U.S. community hospitals

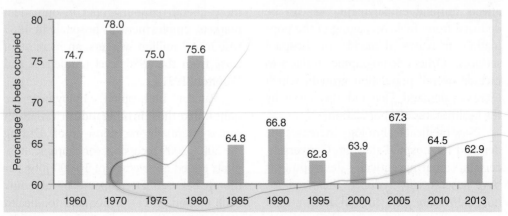

FIGURE 8-7 Change in occupancy rates in U.S. community hospitals, 1960–2013 (selected years).

from 1960 to 2013. Individual hospitals can compare their own occupancy rates against industry benchmarks. In a competitive environment, facilities with higher occupancy rates are considered more successful than those with lower occupancy rates.

▶ Factors That Affect Hospital Employment

In 2013, hospitals accounted for the largest number of jobs in the health care industry, and their workforce represented roughly 39% of total health care employment. More than 6 million people were employed by U.S. hospitals in 2013. The future also bodes well for health care jobs. Between 2012 and 2022, the hospital sector is projected to add 826,000 new jobs, although the largest growth in jobs will occur in the outpatient services sector (Torpey, 2014).

Demand for services is the most important factor that affects hospital employment. Demand is driven by changes in the size and nature of the U.S. population, advances in medical technology, and changes in health insurance (Goodman, 2006). Demand for services is the most important factor that affects hospital employment. As can be deduced from Table 8-2, aging of the population increases demand for hospital services. Other demographic influences include overall population growth, which increases demand. Demand also varies by the health status of a population.

New medical technology increases the demand for hospital staffing. Conversely, certain pharmaceutical developments have substantially reduced the need for hospitalization. The mental health field is especially noted for new pharmaceutical products that shorten hospital stays (Goodman, 2006). Hospital utilization is also significantly reduced for patients with human immunodeficiency virus (HIV)/acquired immunodeficiency syndrome (AIDS) who adhere to their antiretroviral therapy regimens (Nachega et al., 2010).

Other factors have had a downward influence on hospital jobs. For example, a shift away from treatment on an inpatient basis and toward treatment in outpatient settings has increased employment in various outpatient settings. Since approximately 1995, various outpatient care settings have hired more workers than hospitals. In 2010, 36.4% of all employment in health care and social assistance was in outpatient care settings; 28.5% of the employment was in hospitals (U.S. Census Bureau, 2012). This trend is likely to continue in the future.

Changes in reimbursement policy can also affect employment. Hospital employment declined by 2.3%, to approximately 4 million workers, over the 1983 to 1986 period when the hospital downsizing trend started with DRG-based PPS. Staff cuts, hiring freezes, and increased use of contract services were part of an economic belt-tightening effort initiated in response to declining inpatient admissions (Kahl and Clark, 1986). Later, as hospitals chased more liberal reimbursement in outpatient markets, employment in hospitals in 1989 rose to 4.3 million workers, an increase of 6.9% from the 1986 level (Anderson and Wootton, 1991).

Patterns in hospital employment are quite unlike those in other industries. Health care is essentially "recession-proof." During the 2007–2009 recession, for example, hospitals added an average of 10,000 jobs per month between December 2007 and July 2008 (Wood, 2011). If demand for health care services continues to rise because of the various factors discussed earlier, jobs will be added regardless of the overall economic conditions. Also, because health care jobs generally require personal interaction, they often cannot be outsourced or replaced with automation, as happens in some other industries (Torpey, 2014).

▶ Hospital Costs

Inpatient hospital services constitute the largest share of total health care expenditures in the United States, accounting for roughly one-third of the total expenditures (almost 38% of personal health expenditures). Pertinent cost data are presented in Table 8-1. The aggregate cost for inpatient hospital stays amounted to $381.4 billion in 2013, with 46% of these revenues being attributable to Medicare payments, 17% to Medicaid payments, 28% to private insurance payments, and 4% to other sources. Approximately 5% of the costs were attributed to uninsured persons (Torio and Moore, 2016).

Rise in Bad Debts

For hospitals, the Affordable Care Act (ACA) has been both a boon and a bane in regard to their finances. The sizable surge in the number of newly insured Medicaid recipients, who often continued to obtain care at hospital emergency rooms (Finkelstein et al., 2016), brought some new revenues into hospital coffers. Conversely, for patients with privately purchased insurance plans, rising deductibles created hardships for the insured when they had to pay for high-cost care in hospitals. Inability to pay increased the size of hospitals' bad debt loads—that is, revenues that cannot be collected (Murphy, 2016).

International Cost Comparisons

The International Federation of Health Plans has published comparative data on hospital costs for selected countries (**TABLE 8-4**).

TABLE 8-4 Cost per Inpatient Day in Selected Countries, 2012		
	Average Length of Stay (Days)	**Cost per Day ($)**
Australia	4.9	1,472
France	5.1	853
Netherlands	6.4	731
New Zealand	5.6	979
Spain	6.1	476
United States	5.4	4,287

Data from International Federation of Health Plans. 2012. *Comparative price report: Variation in medical and hospital prices by country*. Available at: http://www.vermontforsinglepayer.org/images/userfiles/file/2012iFHPPriceReportFINALApril3.pdf. Accessed May 2017; Organization for Economic Cooperation and Development (OECD). 2014. Average length of stay: Acute care. *Health: Key Tables from OECD*, no. 52. doi: http://dx.doi.org/10.1787/l-o-s-acutecare-table-2014-1-en.

According to these data, the cost per day in a U.S. hospital is 3 to 9 times the comparable cost in other developed nations. This difference persists despite the shorter lengths of stay in the United States compared to most countries. Clearly, hospitals in the United States charge far more than hospitals in other countries.

▶ Types of Hospitals

The U.S. hospital market includes a variety of institutional forms, including both private and government-owned hospitals. Most hospitals are private, nonprofit, short-stay, general hospitals (**FIGURE 8-8**). Private, for-profit (investor-owned) hospitals are next in predominance; then come the state and local government-owned hospitals and, finally, federal hospitals.

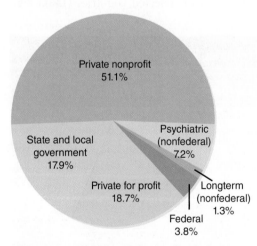

All hospitals = 5,617 (hospital units of institutions-prisons, college campuses, etc.-have been excluded)

FIGURE 8-8 Proportion of total U.S. hospitals by type of hospital, 2014.

Data from Health Forum. 2016. *Fast facts on U.S. hospitals*. Available at: http://www.aha.org/research/rc/stat-studies/fast-facts.shtml. Accessed October 30, 2016.

The endless variations in hospital characteristics defy any simple classification. The classification arrangements described in this section have been commonly used to differentiate among the various types of hospitals. Keep in mind, however, that these classifications are not mutually exclusive.

Classification by Ownership
Public Hospitals

Public hospitals are owned by agencies of federal, state, or local governments. Note that the word "public" does not have its ordinary meaning in this context. A public hospital, for instance, is not necessarily a hospital that is open to the general public.

Federal hospitals serve special groups of federal beneficiaries, such as Native Americans, military personnel, and veterans, rather than the general population. Veterans Affairs (VA) hospitals constitute the largest group among federal hospitals.

Local governments, such as counties and cities, operate hospitals to serve the general population. Many of these hospitals are located in large urban areas, where they function as an important safety net for the inner-city indigent and disadvantaged populations. Hence, Medicare, Medicaid, and state and local tax dollars pay for a large portion of the services these hospitals provide. Because of increasing financial pressures, many public hospitals have had to privatize or close in recent years. Out of the 1,444 state and local government-owned hospitals operating in the United States in 1990, 1,003 remained in operation in 2014 (Health Forum, 2016). Most hospitals operated by city and county governments are small to moderate size. Some large public hospitals are affiliated with medical schools; they play a significant role in training physicians and other health care professionals.

Compared to private hospitals, public hospitals incur higher utilization, at least in terms of ALOS (see Figure 8-5). ALOS is the highest in federal hospitals (9.6 days in 2013), and veterans are the biggest users of these hospitals. The number of discharges in VA hospitals increased from 579,000 in 2000 to 619,000 in 2014; the latter number actually represents a decrease from the 656,000 discharges that occurred in 2010, as the number of outpatient visits have increased substantially in recent years (National Center for Health Statistics, 2016).

Private Nonprofit Hospitals

Nonprofit hospitals are owned and operated by community associations or other nongovernment organizations. Their primary mission is to benefit the community in which they are located. Patient fees, third-party reimbursement, donations, and endowments cover their operating expenses. The private nonprofit sector constitutes the largest group of hospitals (Figure 8-8), accounting for 51% of all U.S. hospitals.

Private For-Profit Hospitals

For-profit **proprietary hospitals**—also referred to as **investor-owned hospitals** —are owned by individuals, partnerships, or corporations. They are operated for the financial benefit of the entity that owns the institution; in other words, they are accountable to their stockholders.

At the beginning of the 20th century, more than one-half of all U.S. hospitals were proprietary. Most of these hospitals were small and were established by physicians who wanted to hospitalize their own patients (Stewart, 1973). Later, most of these institutions were closed or acquired by community organizations or hospital corporations, due to population shifts, increased costs,

and the necessities of modern clinical practice (Raffel and Raffel, 1994).

Even though the nonprofit hospital sector has maintained its overall dominance of the U.S. hospital market, the numbers of for-profit hospitals and beds have increased quite substantially (**TABLE 8-5**). The greater increase in the number of hospitals compared to the number of beds and the significant reduction in the average size of U.S. hospitals reflect the growth of physician-owned specialty hospitals (discussed later in the section "Specialty Hospitals"), which are smaller in size than other community hospitals. However, private nonprofit hospitals continue to boast greater occupancy rates than for-profit hospitals.

Classification by Public Access

More than 87% of all U.S. hospitals are classified as community hospitals (National Center for Health Statistics, 2016). A **community hospital** is a nonfederal, short-stay hospital whose primary mission is to serve the general community. It may be a private for-profit facility, be a private nonprofit facility, or be owned by the state or local government, but not by the federal government (**FIGURE 8-9**). A community hospital can also be a general hospital or a specialty hospital. Noncommunity hospitals include hospitals operated by the federal government, such as VA hospitals to serve veterans; hospital units of institutions, such as prisons and infirmaries in colleges and universities; and long-stay hospitals.

Classification by Multiunit Affiliation

Hospitals are considered to be part of a multihospital chain—also referred to as a **multihospital system (MHS)**—when

TABLE 8-5 Changes in Number of U.S. Hospitals, Beds, Average Size, and Occupancy Rates

	2000	2013	Change
Private Nonprofit			
Number of hospitals	3,003	2,904	−3.3%
Number of beds	582,988	543,929	−6.7%
Average size	194	187	−3.6%
Occupancy rate	65.5%	64.5%	−1.5%
Private For-Profit			
Number of hospitals	749	1,060	41.5%
Number of beds	109,883	134,643	22.5%
Average size	147	127	−13.6%
Occupancy rate	55.9%	56.2%	0.5%

Data from National Center for Health Statistics. 2016. *Health, United States, 2015*. Hyattsville, MD: U.S. Department of Health and Human Services. p. 288.

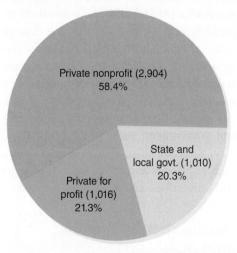

FIGURE 8-9 Breakdown of U.S. community hospitals by type of ownership, 2013.

Data from National Center for Health Statistics. 2016. *Health, United States, 2015*. Hyattsville, MD: U.S. Department of Health and Human Services. p. 288.

two or more hospitals are owned, leased, sponsored, or contractually managed by a central organization (Health Forum, 2016). MHSs exist in all three ownership types discussed earlier.

The number of hospitals in MHSs has grown annually since 2004, and the pace of consolidation that contributes to their formation has accelerated and is likely to continue. In 2014, more than 65% of U.S. hospitals were affiliated with MHSs, up from 52% in 2005 (Sanofi-Aventis, 2013, 2016). Most MHSs are operated by nonprofit corporations, but the three largest MHSs in the United States are actually for-profit corporations (**TABLE 8-6**). Not only

TABLE 8-6 The Largest U.S. Multihospital Chains,[1] 2014

Name of Hospital System (Location)	Number of Owned Hospitals	Number of Staffed Beds
Nonprofit Chains		
Ascension Health (St. Louis, MO)	55	11,079
Dignity Health (San Francisco, CA)	39	9,109
Kaiser Permanente (Oakland, CA)	38	8,591
Catholic Health Initiatives (Englewood, CO)	62	7,860
Trinity Health (Livonia, MI)	41	7,377
Adventist Health System (Altamonte Springs, FL)	37	6,698
North Shore-Long Island Jewish Health System (Great Neck, NY)	15	5,975
Providence Health and Services (Renton, WA)	26	5,768
CHRISTUS Health (Irving, TX)	23	5,084
Mercy (Chesterfield, MO)	30	4820
For-Profit Chains		
HCA (Nashville, TN)	156	33,415
Community Health Systems	208	26,289
Tenet Health System (Dallas, TX)	76	17,846
LifePoint Hospitals (Brentwood, TN)	55	5,237
Universal Health Services (King of Prussia, PA)	24	5,190
State and Local Government–Owned Chains		
New York City Health and Hospitals Corporation (New York, NY)	11	6,681

[1] Ranked by staffed beds in each category.

Data from Sanofi-Aventis. 2016. *Managed care digest series: Hospital/systems digest, 2016*. Bridgewater, NJ: Author.

are more hospitals joining MHSs, but the systems themselves are merging to form even larger systems (Burns et al., 2015).

Some of the advantages of multihospital chain affiliation include economies of scale, the ability to provide a wide spectrum of services, the ability to reach a variety of markets, increased access to capital, greater participation in managed care contracting, and access to management resources and expertise. Hospitals not affiliated with an MHS incur higher costs of operation ($5,709 per patient day versus $5,188 for all hospitals; Sanofi-Aventis, 2013). Even so, not all systems achieve a lower cost of operations (Burns et al., 2015).

The Veterans Health Administration (VHA) operates the single largest MHS in the United States, with more than 150 medical centers being owned by the federal government. In 2014, VHA hospitals had a total of 707,400 inpatient hospital discharges (Department of Veterans Affairs, 2016).

Classification by Type of Service

General Hospitals

A **general hospital** provides a variety of services, including general and specialized medicine, general and specialized surgery, and obstetrics, to meet almost all medical needs of the community it serves. It provides diagnostic, treatment, and surgical services for patients with a variety of medical conditions. Most hospitals in the United States are general hospitals.

The term "general hospital" does not imply that these hospitals are less specialized or that their care is inferior to that of specialty hospitals. The difference lies in the nature of services, not their quality. General hospitals provide a broader range of services for a larger variety of conditions, whereas specialty hospitals provide a narrow range of services for specific medical conditions or patient populations.

Specialty Hospitals

According to the North American Industry Classification System developed by the U.S. Census Bureau, **specialty hospitals** are establishments that primarily engage in providing diagnostic and medical treatment to inpatients with a specific type of disease or medical condition (but not services for psychiatric care or substance abuse). Specialty hospitals forge their own distinct service niches. Traditionally, the two most common types of specialty hospitals have been rehabilitation hospitals and children's hospitals. With increasing competition, however, other types of specialty hospitals have emerged to provide treatments that are also available in many general hospitals. Examples include orthopedic hospitals, cardiac hospitals, cancer (oncology) hospitals, and women's hospitals.

Physicians find such specialized hospitals more efficient, and in many instances, physicians are full or part owners of these hospitals. Affiliation with such hospitals gives physicians control over hospital operations, flexibility with their time, and opportunity to enhance their incomes.

Physician-Owned Specialty Hospitals. In the past, critics of physician-owned hospitals (POHs) have argued that physicians' ownership stakes in hospitals create a conflict of interest that could lead to increased utilization and health care costs (Hollingsworth et al., 2010). In a report to Congress, the Medicare Payment Advisory Commission (MedPAC, 2006) pointed out that POHs (1) have lower proportions of Medicaid-covered patients (2% to 3% of discharges) than community general hospitals (13% of discharges) in the same markets; (2) admit less severe, more profitable cases; (3) draw patients from community general hospitals, although general hospitals are typically able to compensate for the revenue loss; and (4) do not have lower costs per severity-adjusted discharge than competing general hospitals in the same markets. In addition, administrators of general hospitals have argued that specialty hospitals engage in "cream-skimming" insured patients, thereby leaving costly emergency and uncompensated cases to general hospitals (Snyder, 2003).

More recent research has concluded that POHs offer better patient satisfaction, albeit with higher total costs compared to other community hospitals. In spite of these higher costs, POHs operate at efficiency levels that are comparable to other hospitals (Lundgren et al., 2016). Although this research sheds new light on the controversy surrounding POHs, the results are preliminary and do not settle the debate over POHs.

The ACA closed the door on future physician-owned hospitals effective January 1, 2011, by mandating that hospitals could not be owned by physicians if those facilities wanted to receive Medicare payments. New or existing hospitals had to be certified by December 31, 2010, failing which they would be barred from participating in the Medicare program (Weaver, 2010). Existing physician-owned facilities also faced immediate restrictions on expansion. Payment by the government for health care is often accompanied by regulatory interventions in the delivery of health care by private providers. To skirt the new law, POHs expanded their operating hours, added room for magnetic resonance imaging (MRI) units and other imaging modalities, and launched same-day surgery units to perform procedures that do not require an inpatient stay (Mundy, 2013).

Psychiatric Hospitals

The primary function of a psychiatric inpatient facility is to provide diagnostic and treatment services for a variety of severe mental conditions, such as bipolar disorder, schizophrenia, severe depression, dual diagnosis (mental illness compounded by chemical dependency), and serious emotional disturbances in children and adolescents. The main services include psychiatric, psychological, and social work programs. A psychiatric hospital must also have a written agreement with a general hospital for the transfer of patients who may require medical, obstetric, or surgical services (Health Forum, 2001). Inpatient psychiatric facilities can be either freestanding hospitals or specialized psychiatric units in a general hospital.

State Mental Health Institutions. At one time, mental health institutions operated by state governments played a primary role in treating people with mental health conditions. Over time, various policy efforts focused on deinstitutionalizing people whose needs could be adequately met in community-based settings. Consequently, many of these institutions were either closed or some of their beds were taken out of service. Despite the reduction in number of beds, in 2014, more than 200 state-operated psychiatric hospitals nationwide served approximately

40,600 people on any given day. Many of those persons who are confined to state mental institutions fall into the forensic or sex offender categories, and others have complex psychiatric conditions (Parks and Radke, 2014). Psychiatric units in general hospitals, private psychiatric facilities, and outpatient mental health/behavioral health clinics treat the largest number of the patients with mental health disorders.

Rehabilitation Hospitals

Rehabilitation hospitals specialize in therapeutic services to restore the maximum level of functioning in patients who have suffered recent disability due to an episode of illness or an accident. According to Medicare rules, to be classified as a rehabilitation hospital, 75% of a hospital's inpatients must require intensive rehabilitation for conditions such as stroke, spinal cord injury, major multiple trauma, and brain injury (Grimaldi, 2002). Intensive rehabilitation refers to at least 3 hours of therapy per day. Rehabilitation hospitals also serve amputees, victims of accident or sports injuries, and individuals needing intensive cardiac rehabilitation. Facilities and staff are available to provide physical therapy, occupational therapy, and speech-language pathology. Most rehabilitation hospitals have special arrangements for psychological, social work, and vocational services and are required to have written arrangements with a general hospital for the transfer of patients who need medical, obstetric, or surgical care not available at the institution (Health Forum, 2001).

Inpatient rehabilitation facilities (IRFs) can be either freestanding hospitals or specialized rehab units in a general hospital.

Approximately 80% of these facilities are hospital based (MedPAC, 2016a). In 2014, approximately 1,180 IRFs were Medicare certified, and Medicare-covered patients accounted for approximately 60% of the caseload in these facilities (MedPAC, 2016a).

Children's Hospitals

Children's hospitals are community hospitals that typically have specialized facilities to deal mainly with complex, severe, or chronic illnesses among children. Nearly all children's hospitals provide neonatal intensive care units, pediatric intensive care units, trauma centers, and transplant services. Thus, these hospitals provide a wide range of high-intensity services for children, such as pediatric surgery, cardiology, orthopedic surgery, cancer treatment, HIV/AIDS treatment, and rehabilitation services (DelliFraine, 2006). Some specialize in services such as orthopedics or cancer treatment.

Children's hospitals can be freestanding or they can be pediatric centers located in major hospitals. Specialized pediatric departments of major medical centers have their own staffs, operating rooms, laboratories, and other facilities and are run as if they were a separate hospital within a hospital (Leonard, 2013). In most communities, no specialty children's hospitals exist; hence, general acute care hospitals serve as de facto children's hospitals (DelliFraine, 2006).

Classification by Length of Stay
Short-Stay Hospitals

A **short-stay hospital** is one in which the average length of stay is 25 days or less. Most hospitals fall in this category. Patients admitted to these hospitals suffer from acute conditions. Hospitals with average stays of more than 25 days are considered long-stay hospitals. These include state-run, as well as private, psychiatric hospitals; long-term care hospitals providing sub-acute care; and chronic disease hospitals.

Long-Term Care Hospitals

The majority of long-stay hospitals in the United States are **long-term care hospitals (LTCHs)**. A long-term care hospital is a special type of long-stay hospital described in section 1886(d)(1)(B)(iv) of the Social Security Act. LTCHs must meet Medicare's conditions of participation for acute care hospitals and must have an ALOS greater than 25 days. LTCHs serve patients who need postacute care, but have complex medical needs and may have multiple chronic problems requiring long-term hospitalization. Many patients are admitted directly to LTCHs from short-stay hospital intensive care units with respiratory/ventilator-dependent or other complex medical conditions.

The number of LTCHs in the United States grew rapidly—from 105 to 318 facilities between 1993 and 2003 (MedPAC, 2004), and then to 420 facilities in 2012 (MedPAC, 2014). Medicare accounted for approximately two-thirds of the revenues for these hospitals (MedPAC, 2014). Since April 2014, a moratorium has been in effect on the building of new LTCHs and the expansion of existing facilities; this moratorium will remain in effect through September 30, 2017 (Coons, 2014).

Classification by Location

Hospitals can be classified based on their location—that is, they can be either urban or rural. **Urban hospitals** are located in a county that is part of a metropolitan statistical area (MSA). The U.S. Census Bureau has defined an MSA as a geographic area that includes at least (1) one city with a population of 50,000 or more or (2) an urbanized area of at least 50,000 inhabitants and a total MSA population of at least 100,000. **Rural hospitals** are located in a county that is not part of an MSA. In 2014, 38% of all U.S. community hospitals were located in rural areas (Health Forum, 2016).

Rural hospitals provide care to nearly 51 million people (AHA, 2016), but face several challenges. They disproportionately rely on government payments because they serve a higher proportion of elderly and poor patients compared to urban hospitals. These government payments often do not cover the full cost of services. The financial viability of these hospitals is further put at risk because of their communities' low population density, which tends to keep hospital size small and patient volume low (AHA, 2011). Rural hospitals also face a sustained workforce shortage. The average age of hospital facilities begs for improvements and the demand for expensive new information systems climbs, yet these hospitals have only very limited access to capital financing (AHA, 2016).

Conversion to a facility that provides nonacute health care services, such as a primary care clinic, a long-term care facility, or a specialty hospital, is sometimes a viable alternative when closure threatens rural hospitals. For example, adoption of long-term care strategies has demonstrated to improve profitability of rural hospitals (Stuart et al., 2006).

Swing-Bed Hospitals

Subsequent to demonstration projects during the 1970s, the swing bed program for rural hospitals was authorized under the Omnibus Reconciliation Act of 1980. A hospital **swing bed** can be used for acute care or skilled nursing care as needed. The swing bed program enabled many rural hospitals to survive during a period of declining occupancy rates. It also enabled rural residents to access post-acute nursing care services, which were not otherwise available in many rural communities.

Because the swing bed program operates under two distinct payment systems, for acute hospital stays and skilled nursing facility (SNF) stays, Medicare rules require discharge of a patient from acute care in accordance with the rules that apply to SNFs—that is, a 3-day inpatient acute care stay is necessary to qualify for an SNF stay. In July 2002, the Centers for Medicare and Medicaid Services (CMS) brought hospital swing beds under the existing SNF PPS reimbursement, which has created financial pressures for rural hospitals. To overcome this drawback, many rural hospitals have switched to critical access hospital status.

Critical Access Hospitals

In an attempt to save some of the very small rural hospitals, the Balanced Budget Act of 1997 created the Medicare Rural Hospital Flexibility Program (MRHFP). Under this program, a rural hospital, upon meeting certain conditions, can file an application with Medicare to be classified as a **critical access hospital (CAH)**. To qualify as a CAH, the hospital should have no more than 25 acute care and/or swing beds and must provide 24-hour emergency medical services. It must also meet a distance test in relation to other hospitals. A CAH is allowed to have a 10-bed psychiatric unit, a 10-bed rehabilitation unit, and a distinct SNF.

CAHs are not subject to the prospective payment systems applicable to other health care providers; they receive cost-plus reimbursement for inpatient, outpatient, laboratory, therapy, and most postacute services in swing beds. Total payment to the hospital is fixed at 101% of reasonable costs. Because of their many financial advantages, the number of CAHs has jumped from 850 in 2003 (Mantone, 2005) to more than 1,300 today, representing 61% of all rural hospitals (MedPAC, 2015).

Other Rural Designations

To improve access in some remote locations, Congress created two additional rural hospital designations: sole community hospital and Medicare-dependent hospital.

Sole Community Hospitals. Hospitals can qualify for sole community hospital (SCH) status if, because of their remote locations, they are the sole source of hospital services in a wide geographic area. In some geographic locations, SCHs are important safety net providers. Approximately 17% of rural hospitals are classified as SCHs (MedPAC, 2015). These hospitals benefit from certain payment adjustments from Medicare.

Medicare-Dependent Hospitals. Small rural hospitals that may not qualify for the SCH designation may be classified as Medicare-dependent hospitals (MDHs) if at least 60% of their discharges are Medicare beneficiaries. In addition to PPS reimbursement, these hospitals receive payments that are partially based on their costs. Approximately 8% of rural hospitals are classified as MDHs (MedPAC, 2015).

Classification by Size

There is no standard way to classify hospitals by size. According to one classification scheme, hospitals with fewer than 100 beds would be classified as small, those with 100 to 500 beds as medium, and those with 500-plus beds as large. Others may classify by size a little differently. Fewer than half (47.5%) of all community hospitals in the United States have 100 beds or more (Figure 8-6).

Experience in the manufacturing and retail sectors of the economy suggests that large enterprises can often realize economies of scale. This benefit arises because certain overhead costs are fixed or semifixed—they do not increase proportionately as the size of the enterprise increases. Examples are administrative costs and plant maintenance costs.

In the hospital industry, the reverse may be happening. Coyne and colleagues (2009) showed that cost per adjusted patient-day was significantly higher in hospitals with more than 150 beds compared to hospitals with 40 to 150 beds, regardless of ownership type. The relatively higher costs in larger hospitals are likely attributable to the more extensive array of specialized and resource-intensive services that these hospitals must be equipped to provide. Such services require sophisticated technology and personnel with advanced training. Large teaching hospitals incur the additional costs of residency training and medical research. Higher costs in much smaller CAHs are likely attributable

to cost-based reimbursement, which does not provide any incentives to enforce cost controls.

Other Types of Hospitals

Teaching Hospitals

To be designated as a **teaching hospital**, a hospital must have one or more graduate residency programs approved by the AMA. The mere presence of nursing programs or training affiliations for other health professionals, such as therapists and dietitians, does not make an institution a teaching hospital.

The term **academic medical center** is commonly used when one or more hospitals, with or without affiliated outpatient clinics, are organized around a medical school. Apart from the training of physicians, research activities and clinical investigations become an important undertaking in such a center.

Among the largest and most prestigious teaching hospitals are the members of the Council of Teaching Hospitals and Health Systems (COTH), which has more than 400 members in the United States (including 64 VA medical centers) and Canada. They usually have substantial teaching and research programs and are affiliated with medical schools of large universities. The COTH member institutions train more than 100,000 new physicians each year (Association of American Medical Colleges [AAMC], 2013).

Three main traits separate teaching and nonteaching hospitals. First, teaching hospitals provide medical training to physicians, research opportunities to health services researchers, and specialized care to patients. These hospitals receive separate payments from Medicare (up to 140% of the national average) for the direct costs incurred in operating training programs for medical, dental, or podiatric residents. As part of the prospective DRG rates, these hospitals receive add-on payments to reflect the additional indirect costs of patient care associated with the training of medical residents (MedPAC, 2016b).

Second, teaching hospitals have a broader and more complex scope of services than nonteaching hospitals. These hospitals often operate several intensive care units, possess the latest medical technologies, and attract a diverse group of physicians representing most specialties and many subspecialties. Major teaching hospitals also offer many unique tertiary care services not generally found in other institutions, such as burn care, trauma care, and organ transplantation. Hence, teaching hospitals attract patients who frequently have more complicated diagnoses or need more complex procedures. Because of the greater case-mix complexity of teaching hospitals, greater resources are required for treatment.

Third, many of the major teaching hospitals are located in economically depressed, older inner-city areas and are owned by state or local governments. Consequently, these hospitals often provide disproportional amounts of uncompensated care to uninsured patients. For example, COTH member institutions provide nearly half of all hospital charity care in the United States (AAMC, 2013).

Church-Affiliated Hospitals

Various churches established hospitals mainly during the latter half of the 19th century and the early 20th century. For example, Catholic sisterhoods established the first church-sponsored hospitals in the United States. Later, Protestant denominations organized hospitals in accord with their missions of service, and Jewish philanthropic organizations opened hospitals so that Jewish patients could observe their dietary laws more faithfully and Jewish physicians could more easily find sites for training and work opportunities (Raffel, 1980).

Church-affiliated hospitals are often community general hospitals. They may be large or small, teaching or nonteaching. Affiliation with a medical school may also vary. Church-affiliated hospitals do not discriminate in rendering care; however, they are generally sensitive to the sponsoring denomination's special spiritual and/or dietary emphasis (Raffel and Raffel, 1994).

Osteopathic Hospitals

For all practical purposes, osteopathic hospitals are community general hospitals. In 1970, osteopathic hospitals became eligible to apply for registration with the AHA (1994). For many years after osteopathy was established as a separate branch of medicine in 1874, osteopaths had to develop their own hospitals because of antagonism from the established allopathic medical practitioners. Since then, both groups have inspected each other's medical schools and satisfied themselves that each is worth associating with and that each could serve on the other's faculties and practice side by side in the same hospitals (Raffel and Raffel, 1994).

Many osteopathic hospitals today are part of hospital systems and maintain their osteopathic identity within the context of these larger systems. An independent osteopathic hospital is no longer a necessity and seems to be economically out of place in today's market (Hilsenrath, 2006). Also, the operation of osteopathic hospitals has been found to be more costly and less productive in comparison to their counterparts (Sinay, 2005). Consequently, a number of these hospitals have closed.

▶ Expectations for Nonprofit Hospitals

Lay people often assume that nonprofit (sometimes called not-for-profit) health care corporations do not make a profit. In fact, every corporation—regardless of whether it is for profit or nonprofit—must make a profit (surplus of revenues over expenses) if it is to survive over the long term. No business can survive for long if it continually spends more than it takes in. That rule of economics holds true for both the nonprofit and for-profit sectors (Nudelman and Andrews, 1996).

The Internal Revenue Code, Section 501(c)(3), grants tax-exempt status to nonprofit organizations. As such, these institutions are exempt from federal, state, and local taxes, such as income taxes, sales taxes, and property taxes. In general, nonprofit organizations must (1) provide some defined public good, such as service, education, or community welfare; and (2) not distribute any profits to any individuals. In contrast, a major goal for a for-profit corporation is to provide its shareholders with a return on their investment, although it achieves this goal primarily by excelling at

its basic mission. For any health services provider, the basic mission is to deliver the highest-quality care at the most reasonable price possible.

Since 1969, a community-benefit standard has been applied to nonprofit hospitals. It broadly refers to services that the government would otherwise have to undertake (Owens, 2005). The standard was modified in 1983 to include specific criteria that hospitals must meet to qualify for tax exemption: a 24-hour emergency department, policy guidelines for treating the uninsured, and health promotion in the community (Alexander et al., 2009).

Section 4958 of the IRS code prohibits executive compensation that may be deemed unreasonable for tax-exempt organizations. Nonprofit hospitals must be prepared to demonstrate not only that they are paying salaries within some reasonable range of industry standards, but also that executives are bringing measurable value in key areas of operations, including community benefits (Appleby, 2004). Hence, it is recommended that some portion of hospital chief executive officers' salaries directly hinge on their performance in two critical areas (Newman et al., 2001): (1) organizational effectiveness, including financial performance, market share, quality, daily operations, and achievement of strategic objectives; and (2) community health, including charitable care, health promotion and education, and overall state of the community's health.

In many communities, nonprofit hospitals compete head-to-head with for-profit hospitals. For example, nonprofit hospitals frequently engage in the same kinds of aggressive marketplace behaviors that for-profit hospitals pursue. Generally, nonprofit hospitals operate in locations with higher average incomes, lower poverty rates, and lower rates of uninsurance than for-profit hospitals (Congressional Budget Office [CBO], 2006). Seven of the 10 most profitable hospitals in the United States in 2013 were nonprofit organizations (Ge and Anderson, 2016).

Institutional theory actually predicts such behavior. When for-profit and nonprofit organizations face similar regulatory, legal, and professional constraints, they often imitate each other (O'Connell and Brown, 2003). In the hospital industry, competition commonly occurs in the same communities for the same patients, with revenues coming from the same public and private third-party sources, and often involving the same physician providers who have admitting privileges at more than one hospital.

Empirical evidence has indicated that for-profit and nonprofit hospitals provide similar levels of charity and uncompensated care (Thorpe et al., 2000), but a later report by the CBO (2006) showed mixed results on this front. Nevertheless, lingering concerns over the issue of tax exemption in exchange for community benefits prompted the Internal Revenue Service (IRS) to require detailed financial documentation from nonprofit hospitals on their community benefit expenditures starting in 2009.

A study based on the initial IRS tax returns found that the scale of community benefits delivered by tax-exempt hospitals varied widely, from as little as 1% of operating expenses used for community benefits to as much as 20% (Young et al., 2013). Another recent study confirmed the existence of significant gaps in the delivery of community benefit services by nonprofit hospitals (Worthy et al., 2016).

In 2010, the Illinois Supreme Court, in *Provena v. Department of Revenue*, ruled that the plaintiff medical center was not entitled to charitable exemption for property taxes because it did not provide sufficient community benefits (Supreme Court of the State of Illinois, 2010). However, the debate over this issue continues, particularly over what is and what is not a community benefit, and whether giving tax-exempt status to certain hospitals has created an unequal and unfair system.

Nonprofit institutions face new demands to deliver community benefits under the ACA. The law requires nonprofit hospitals to (1) establish written financial assistance and emergency care policies, (2) limit charges for individuals who are eligible for assistance under the hospital's financial assistance policy, (3) limit certain billing and collection actions against those who fall within the guidelines of financial assistance, and (4) conduct a Community Health Needs Assessment and adopt an implementation strategy at least once every 3 years. Hospitals that fail to comply with the community health assessment mandate are subject to an excise tax (Betbeze, 2011; IRS, 2016).

▶ Some Management Concepts

From a management standpoint, hospitals are complex organizations. Compared to other business enterprises of similar size, both the external and internal environments of hospitals are more complex. A hospital is responsible to numerous stakeholders in its external environment, including the community, the government, insurers, managed care organizations (MCOs), and accreditation agencies. A hospital's organizational structure also differs substantially from that of other large organizations in the business world.

Hospital Governance

Hospital governance has traditionally assumed a tripartite structure, in which the three major sources of authority are the chief executive officer (CEO), the board of trustees, and the chief of staff (**FIGURE 8-10**). In earlier periods, when physicians operated their own hospitals, trustees dominated the hospitals. Trustees were often the source of capital investment, and their influence in the community brought prestige to the hospital. Later, as voluntary hospitals increased in number, the balance of power shifted

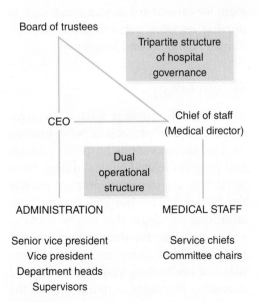

Board of trustees

Tripartite structure of hospital governance

CEO — Chief of staff (Medical director)

Dual operational structure

ADMINISTRATION — MEDICAL STAFF

Senior vice president
Vice president
Department heads
Supervisors

Service chiefs
Committee chairs

FIGURE 8-10 Hospital governance and operational structures.

into the hands of physicians because they played a critical role in bringing patients to the hospitals. As changes in the health care environment made the management of hospitals more complex, considerable power shifted from physicians to senior managers.

The medical staff constitute a separate organizational structure that operates in parallel to the administrative structure. Such a dual structure is rarely seen in other businesses and presents numerous opportunities for conflict between the CEO and the medical staff. Matters are further complicated when the lines of authority cross between the two structures. For example, nursing service, pharmacists, diagnostic technicians, and dietitians are administratively accountable to the CEO (via the vertical chain of command) but professionally accountable to the medical staff (Raffel and Raffel, 1994). Although most of the medical staff are not paid employees of the hospital, physicians' interest in employment has been growing as they seek ways to stabilize their incomes and achieve a better work-life balance in a changing health care landscape (Shoger, 2011).

Regardless of whether the physicians are independent practitioners or contracted employees of the hospital, they play a significant role in the hospital's success. It requires special skills on the part of the CEO to manage the dual structure to achieve the organization's overall objectives.

Board of Trustees

The **board of trustees** (also referred to as the governing body or board of directors) consists of influential business and community leaders. The board is legally responsible for the operations of the hospital. It has specific responsibilities for defining the hospital's mission and long-range direction; evaluating, from a strategic standpoint, major decisions such as incurring capital expenditures for building and equipment; approving annual budgets; and monitoring performance against plans and budgets. The CEO is a member of the board, and one or more physicians also sit on the board as voting members.

One of the most important responsibilities of the board is to appoint and evaluate the performance of the CEO, who is charged with providing the board with timely reports on the institution's progress toward achieving its mission and objectives. The board has the power to remove the CEO. In most hospitals, the board also approves the appointment of physicians and other professionals to the hospital's medical staff.

Boards often function through committees. Standing committees usually include executive, medical staff, human resources, finance, planning, quality improvement, and ethics. Special, or ad hoc, committees are established as needed. The two most important committees, from a governance standpoint, are the executive committee and the medical staff committee. The **executive committee** has continuing monitoring responsibility and authority over the hospital. Usually, it receives reports from other committees, monitors policy implementation, and makes recommendations. The **medical staff committee** is charged with managing medical staff relations. For example, this committee reviews admitting privileges and the

performance of the medical staff. There is also increased emphasis on the legal and ethical obligations of the hospital regarding patient safety, quality improvement, and patient satisfaction.

Chief Executive Officer

Formerly, the titles of "superintendent" and later "administrator" were commonly used for a hospital's chief executive. Now, "chief executive officer" and "president" are the titles typically used. The CEO's job is to accomplish the organization's mission and objectives by exhibiting leadership within the organization. The CEO has the ultimate responsibility for the hospital's day-to-day operations.

The CEO receives delegated authority from the board and is responsible for managing the organization with the help of senior managers. In large hospitals, these senior managers often carry the title of senior vice president or vice president for various key service areas, such as nursing services, rehabilitation services, human resources, and finance.

Medical Staff

The hospital's medical staff is an organized body of physicians who provide medical services to the hospital's patients and perform related clinical duties. Most physicians are in private practice outside the hospital. The hospital grants them admitting privileges that enable them to admit and care for their patients in the hospital. Other clinicians, such as dentists and podiatrists, may also be granted admitting privileges. Appointment to the medical staff is a formal process outlined in the hospital's medical staff bylaws. The medical staff use a framework of self-governance, which upholds the strong tradition of physician independence, but are formally accountable to the board. Lines of communication to the CEO and the board of trustees are established through various committee representations.

A medical director, or **chief of staff**, heads the medical staff. In all but the smallest hospitals, the medical staff are organizationally divided by major specialties into departments, such as anesthesiology, internal medicine, obstetrics and gynecology, orthopedic surgery, pathology, cardiology, and radiology. A **chief of service**, such as chief of cardiology, heads each specialty.

The medical staff generally have their own executive committee that sets general policies and is the main decision-making body in medical matters. Most hospitals have additional committees. The **credentials committee** grants and reviews admitting privileges for those already credentialed and for new doctors whose skills are yet untested. The **medical records committee** ensures that accurate documentation is maintained on the entire regimen of care given to each patient. This committee also oversees confidentiality issues related to medical records. The **utilization review committee** performs routine checks to ensure that inpatient placements, as well as the lengths of stay, are clinically appropriate. The **infection control committee** reviews policies and procedures for minimizing infections in the hospital. The **quality improvement committee** oversees the program for continual quality improvement.

▶ Licensure, Certification, and Accreditation

A license to operate a certain number of hospital beds is a basic regulatory requirement. State governments oversee the **licensure** of health care facilities, and each state sets its own standards for licensure. A state's department of health carries out licensure functions. State licensure standards strongly emphasize the physical plant's compliance with building codes, fire safety, climate control, space allocations, and sanitation. Minimum standards are also established for equipment and personnel. State licensure is not directly tied to the quality of care that a health care facility actually delivers.

All facilities must be licensed to operate, but they do not have to be certified or accredited. **Certification** gives a hospital the authority to participate in the Medicare and Medicaid programs. The U.S. Department of Health and Human Services (DHHS) has developed health, safety, and quality standards referred to as **conditions of participation**, and has the authority to enforce those standards for hospitals that participate in Medicare or Medicaid. The currently defined conditions focus primarily on the actual quality of care furnished to patients and the outcomes of that care. Each state's department of health verifies the actual compliance with the standards through periodic inspections.

In contrast to licensure and certification, which are government regulatory mechanisms, **accreditation** is a private undertaking designed to assure that accredited health care facilities meet certain basic standards. Seeking accreditation is voluntary, but the passage of Medicare in 1965 specified that accredited facilities were eligible for purposes of Medicare reimbursement. Accreditation of a hospital by the Joint Commission confers **deemed status** on the hospital, meaning the hospital is deemed to have met Medicare and Medicaid certification standards. Thus, an accredited hospital does not need to go through the certification process. Private organizations that have been approved by the CMS to confer deemed status are said to have "deeming authority." In addition to the Joint Commission, the American Osteopathic Association has deeming authority to accredit hospitals.

The Joint Commission also sets standards for and accredits long-term care facilities, psychiatric hospitals, substance abuse programs, outpatient surgery centers, urgent care clinics, group practices, community health centers, hospices, and home health agencies. Different sets of standards apply to each category of health care organization. Some facilities, such as nursing homes, do not receive deemed status as a result of accreditation and must also be certified by DHHS to receive Medicare and Medicaid reimbursement.

Over the years, the Joint Commission has refined its accreditation standards and process of verifying compliance. Since 2006, the Joint Commission has moved from scheduled to unannounced inspections, with the intention that hospitals should attempt to comply with all the standards all the time.

▶ The Magnet Recognition Program[1]

Magnet hospital is a special designation conferred by the American Nurses Credentialing Center, an affiliate of the American Nurses Association, that recognizes quality patient care, nursing excellence, and innovations in professional nursing practice in hospitals. This designation was created after a study of 163 hospitals was undertaken in 1983 by the American Academy of Nursing's Task Force on Nursing Practice in Hospitals. The study found that 41 of these hospitals had an environment that attracted and retained well-qualified nurses and promoted quality patient care. These hospitals were labeled "Magnet hospitals" because of their ability to attract and retain professional nurses. The characteristics that seemed to distinguish "Magnet" organizations from others became known as the Forces of Magnetism. The Forces of Magnetism have since been incorporated into quality indicators and standards of nursing practice as defined in the *ANA Nursing Administration: Scope & Standards of Practice*. The Magnet designation is granted after a thorough and lengthy process that includes review of data on quality indicators.

Studies show that visionary leadership, empowerment, and collaboration have an impact on development and maintenance of healthy work environments, and that the quality of patient care is related to the quality of the nurses' work environment (Kramer et al., 2011). Recent studies have pointed to better patient outcomes

---

[1] The Magnet Recognition Program is a registered trademark of the American Nurses Credentialing Center.

in Magnet hospitals compared to non-Magnet hospitals. For example, over a 13-year study period, better postsurgical outcomes were achieved in Magnet hospitals than in non-Magnet facilities (Friese et al., 2015). Admission to a Magnet hospital has also been associated with a 20% reduction in mortality among trauma patients (Evans et al., 2014).

▶ Ethical and Legal Issues in Patient Care

Ethical issues arise in all types of health services organizations, but the most significant ones occur in acute care hospitals. Increasing levels of technology create situations requiring decision making under complex circumstances. For example, life-sustaining therapies in intensive care and dealing with life and death issues commonly raise ethical concerns. Likewise, ethical issues arise in health care research and in experimental medicine. The Joint Commission requires accredited institutions to have mechanisms that allow patients, families, and employees to obtain resolution of ethical issues or issues that may present a conflict of interest (Hamric and Wocial, 2016).

Principles of Ethics

Ethics requires judgment. Because clear-cut rules are often not available in the health care environment, medical practitioners and managers must rely on certain well-established principles as guides to ethical decision making. Four important principles of ethics are respect for others, beneficence, nonmaleficence, and justice.

The principle of *respect for others* has four elements: autonomy, truth-telling, confidentiality, and fidelity. Autonomy allows people to govern themselves by choosing and pursuing a course of action without external coercion. In health care delivery, it refers to patient empowerment, which is ensured by obtaining consent for treatment, explaining the various treatment alternatives, allowing patients and their families to participate in decision making and selection of treatment options, and treating patients with respect and dignity. Constant tension exists between autonomy and paternalism, the view that someone else must decide what the patient will undergo without the patient's involvement. Truth-telling requires a caregiver to be honest. This principle often needs to be balanced with nonmaleficence because a tension is created when truth-telling would result in harm to the patient. The principle of confidentiality sometimes becomes a source of conflict when the legal system requires disclosure of patient information. Fidelity means performing one's duty, keeping one's word, and keeping promises.

The principle of *beneficence* means that hospitals and caregivers have a moral obligation to benefit others. A health services organization is ethically obligated to do all it can to alleviate suffering caused by ill health and injury. This obligation includes providing a certain amount of charity care to the financially needy.

The principle of *nonmaleficence* means that medical professionals have a moral obligation not to harm others. Of course, many health care interventions, including certain preventive measures such as immunization, carry risks. Hence, in health care, nonmaleficence requires that the potential benefits from medical treatment sufficiently outweigh the potential harm.

The principle of *justice* encompasses fairness and equality. It denounces discrimination in the delivery of health care.

Legal Rights

Legal issues arise in areas of patient competency and the patient's right to refuse treatment. Although the right of mentally competent patients to refuse medical care is well established, the desires of incompetent or comatose patients present ethical challenges. Unless such patients have expressed their wishes in advance, family members or legal guardians may end up making decisions regarding sustained medical treatment, or state laws may govern such decisions. Medical and legal experts and family members may differ, often bitterly, on the controversial issue of withdrawing nutrition and other life support means for dying patients. The battle over this decision for Theresa Schiavo, a Florida patient, made national news in 2004 and demonstrated how vociferous these debates can be. However, certain legal mechanisms have been established to deal with the issues of patients' rights.

Bill of Rights and Informed Consent

The Patient Self-Determination Act of 1990 applies to all health care facilities participating in Medicare or Medicaid. This law requires hospitals and other facilities to provide all patients, upon admission, with information on patients' rights. Most hospitals and other inpatient institutions have developed what is referred to as a **patient's bill of rights**. This document reflects the law concerning issues such as confidentiality and consent. Other patient rights include the right to make decisions regarding medical care, be informed about diagnosis and treatment, refuse treatment, and formulate advance directives.

Based on the principle of autonomy, **informed consent** refers to the patient's right to make an informed choice regarding medical treatment. The current climate in medical ethics supports honest and complete disclosure of medical information. In 1972, the Board of Trustees of the AHA affirmed the document known as the Patient's Bill of Rights, which states that patients have the right to obtain from their physicians complete current information concerning their diagnosis, treatment, and prognosis, in terms the patients can be reasonably expected to understand (Rosner, 2004). Informed consent is customarily obtained via a signature on preprinted forms and becomes part of the patient's medical record.

Certain principles governing patients' rights are being incorporated into provider mindsets and organizational culture within the **patient-centered care** model. Involving patients in their own treatment, grounding treatment decisions in patients' preferences, and creating a caregiving environment in which staff solicit patients' input and meet their needs for information and education collectively promote patient-centered care (Cross, 2004).

Advance Directives

Advance directives specify the patient's wishes regarding continuation or withdrawal of treatment when the patient lacks decision-making capacity. Advance directives are intended to ensure that the patient's end-of-life wishes are carried out.

Three types of advance directives are in common use: do-not-resuscitate orders, living wills, and durable powers of attorney.

- A **do-not-resuscitate order** directs medical caregivers not to administer any artificial means to resuscitate the person when his or her heart or breathing stops. It is based on the theory that a patient may prefer to die rather than live when strong odds are against a good quality of life after cardiopulmonary resuscitation, because severe disabilities would likely remain.

- A **living will** communicates a patient's wishes regarding medical treatment when he or she is unable to make decisions due to terminal illness or incapacitation. The main drawback of a living will is that it is general in nature and does not cover all possible situations.

- A **durable power of attorney** for health care is a written legal document in which the patient appoints another individual to act as the patient's agent for purposes of health care decision making in the event that the patient is unable or unwilling to make such decisions. Although a durable power of attorney can cover most circumstances, its main drawback is that the appointed person may not act in the same manner in which the patient would have acted had he or she remained competent.

Mechanisms for Ethical Decision Making

Many health care organizations, especially large acute care hospitals, have **ethics committees** charged with developing guidelines and standards for ethical decision making in the delivery of health care (Paris, 1995). Ethics committees are also responsible for resolving issues related to medical ethics. Such committees are multidisciplinary, including physicians, nurses, clergy, social workers, legal experts, ethicists, and administrators.

Although physicians and other caregivers have moral responsibilities on the clinical side, the health care executive who leads the health services organization must also assume the role of a moral agent. As a **moral agent**, the manager morally affects and is morally affected by actions taken. Although executives are entrusted with the fiduciary responsibility to act prudently in managing the affairs of the organization, their responsibilities to patients must take precedence.

In governing the affairs of an organization, health care executives must recognize that ethics is much more than obeying the law. The law represents only the minimum standard of morality established by society. Similarly, health care professionals must recognize that, even though they are bound by the law, they also have a higher calling—one that includes numerous positive duties to patients, society, and each other (Darr, 1991).

▶ Summary

Hospitals are institutions engaged primarily in the delivery of inpatient acute care services, although many have branched out to provide postacute and outpatient services. In the United States, almshouses and pesthouses first evolved into public hospitals to serve the poor. Subsequently, voluntary hospitals were established to serve all classes of people. Advances in medical science, improvements in hygiene, and evolution of nursing care transformed hospitals into institutions of medical practice, many of which then became important centers of medical training and research. Since the 1980s, economic pressures have led many hospitals to consolidate. Health systems that offer a full continuum of health care services now exist in many locations.

Hospitals in the United States went through an expansion phase in the mid-20th century that lasted until the mid-1980s. The Hill-Burton Act of 1946 was the greatest single factor contributing to this increase in the nation's bed supply. The government later played an equally important role in reducing inpatient utilization by establishing the prospective payment system. Some of the key measures of inpatient utilization are discharges, inpatient days, average length of stay, capacity, average daily census, and occupancy rates. The growth of managed care has also been significant in reducing inpatient utilization. Despite these accomplishments, hospital costs have not abated, and U.S. hospitals remain the most expensive in the world.

Hospitals can be classified in numerous ways, and the various classification schemes help differentiate one hospital from another. Performance statistics by hospital type can help executives compare their hospital to others in the same category. Although most U.S. hospitals are general community hospitals, various specialty hospitals treat specific types of patients or conditions. Roughly half of all U.S. community hospitals are nonprofit organizations, but physician-owned specialty hospitals have proliferated in recent years.

Most public and voluntary hospitals are nonprofit and, as such, these institutions enjoy some tax advantages. They are expected to provide community benefits that are equivalent in value to the tax subsidies received; however, many nonprofit hospitals emulate the behavior of their for-profit counterparts. Ongoing concerns about nonprofit hospitals' compliance with the expectations attached to their tax-exempt status have invited greater scrutiny and reporting requirements from the Internal Revenue Service.

The ACA put restrictions on opening of new physician-owned specialty hospitals and expansion of existing ones as a condition for participating in Medicare. This law also placed new demands on nonprofit hospitals to provide community benefits.

Hospitals are among the most complex organizations to manage; they must satisfy numerous external stakeholders and manage a complex internal governance structure. A hospital cannot legally operate unless it is licensed by the state in which it is located. To participate in the Medicare and Medicaid programs, a hospital can voluntarily apply for accreditation by the Joint Commission. Magnet hospitals are recognized for their ability to recruit and retain qualified nurses and to deliver high-quality patient care.

Ethical decision making has been a special area of concern for hospitals. From a medical standpoint, ethical issues often pertain to patient privacy, confidentiality, informed consent, and end-of-life treatment. Bills of rights and advance directives are two of the legal means to address these issues. Active ethics committees develop policies and standards, and deal with ethical issues as they arise.

▶ **Test Your Understanding**

Terminology

academic medical center
accreditation
advance directives
average daily census
average length of stay
　(ALOS)
board of trustees
certification
chief of service
chief of staff
community hospital
conditions of participation
credentials committee
critical access hospital
　(CAH)
days of care
deemed status
discharge
do-not-resuscitate order
durable power of attorney

ethics committees
executive committee
general hospital
hospital
infection control
　committee
informed consent
inpatient
inpatient day
investor-owned hospitals
licensure
living will
long-term care hospitals
　(LTCHs)
Magnet hospital
medical records
　committee
medical staff committee
moral agent

multihospital system
　(MHS)
occupancy rate
patient-centered care
patient's bill of rights
proprietary hospitals
public hospitals
quality improvement
　committee
rehabilitation hospitals
rural hospitals
short-stay hospital
specialty hospitals
swing bed
teaching hospital
urban hospitals
utilization review
　committee
voluntary hospitals

Review Questions

1. What is the difference between inpatient and outpatient services?
2. As hospitals evolved from rudimentary custodial and quarantine facilities to their current state, how did their purpose and function change?
3. What were the main factors responsible for the growth of hospitals until the latter part of the 20th century?
4. Name the three main forces that were responsible for hospital downsizing. How did each of these forces affect the decline in inpatient hospital utilization?
5. What is a voluntary hospital? How did voluntary hospitals evolve in the United States?
6. Discuss the role of government in the growth, as well as the decline, of hospitals in the United States.
7. What are inpatient days? What is the significance of this measure?
8. How does hospital utilization vary according to a person's age, gender, and socioeconomic status?
9. Explain the factors that affect hospital employment.
10. Discuss the different types of public hospitals and the roles they play in

the delivery of health care services in the United States.

11. What are some of the differences between private nonprofit and for-profit hospitals?

12. What is a long-term care hospital (LTCH)? What role does it play in health care delivery in the United States?

13. The table gives some operational statistics for two hospitals located in the same community. Use the table to answer the following questions.

    a. Calculate the following measures for each hospital (wherever appropriate, calculate the measure for each pay type). Discuss the meaning and significance of each measure, and point out the differences between the two hospitals.
       (i) Hospital capacity
       (ii) ALOS
       (iii) Occupancy rate
    b. Operationally, which hospital is performing better? Why?
    c. Do you think the nonprofit hospital is meeting its community benefit obligations in exchange for its tax-exempt status? Explain.
    d. Do you think the hospitals have a problem with excess capacity? If so, what would you recommend?

14. Why have physicians developed their own specialty hospitals? What main criticisms have these hospitals faced?

Calendar Year 2016	Nonprofit Community Hospital (A)	Proprietary Community Hospital (B)
Number of beds in operation	320	240
Total discharges	12,051	9,230
Medicare	5,130	3,876
Medicaid	3,565	2,118
Private insurance	3,356	3,236
Total hospital days	72,421	51,684
Medicare	36,935	26,359
Medicaid	23,175	12,921
Private insurance	12,311	12,404
Total inpatient revenues	$45,755,000	$35,800,000
Dollar value of community benefits	$5,000,000	$3,500,000

15. What criteria does Medicare use to classify a hospital as a rehabilitation hospital?

16. How do you differentiate between a community hospital and a noncommunity hospital?

17. What is a critical access hospital (CAH)? Why was this designation created?

18. What are some of the main differences between teaching and non-teaching hospitals?

19. Discuss some of the issues relative to the tax-exempt status of nonprofit hospitals. What does the Internal Revenue Service require from these hospitals in terms of documentation?

20. Discuss the governance of a modern hospital.

21. In the context of hospitals, what are the differences between licensure, certification, and accreditation?

22. What can a hospital do to address some of the difficult ethical problems relative to end-of-life treatment?

▶ References

Alexander, J. A., et al. 2009. How do system-affiliated hospitals fare in providing community benefit? *Inquiry* 46, no. 1: 72–91.

American Hospital Association (AHA). 1990. *Hospital statistics 1990–1991 edition*. Chicago, IL: Author.

American Hospital Association (AHA). 1994. *AHA guide to the health care field 1994 edition*. Chicago, IL: Author.

American Hospital Association (AHA). 2011. *The opportunities and challenges for rural hospitals in an era of health reform*. Washington, DC: AHA and Avalere Health.

American Hospital Association (AHA). 2016. *Rural health care*. Available at: http://www.aha.org/advocacy-issues/rural/index.shtml. Accessed October 2016.

Anderson, K., and B. Wootton. 1991. Changes in hospital staffing patterns. *Monthly Labor Review* 114, no. 3: 3–9.

Appleby, J. 2004, September 30. IRS looking closely at what non-profits pay. *USA Today*, p. 02b.

Arndt, M., and B. Bigelow. 2006. Toward the creation of an institutional logic for the management of hospitals: Efficiency in the early nineteen hundreds. *Medical Care Research and Review* 63, no. 3: 369–394.

Association of American Medical Colleges (AAMC). 2013. *Teaching hospitals*. Available at: https://www.aamc.org/about/teachinghospitals. Accessed August 2013.

Balotsky, E. R. 2005. Is it resources, habit or both: Interpreting twenty years of hospital strategic response to prospective payment. *Health Care Management Review* 30, no. 4: 337–346.

Betbeze, P. 2011. Reassessing community benefit. *Health Leaders Magazine* 14, no. 1: 50.

Burns, L. R., et al. 2015. Is the system really the solution? Operating costs in hospital systems. *Medical Care Research and Review* 72, no. 3: 247–272.

Clement, J. P., and K. L. Grazier. 2001. HMO penetration: Has it hurt public hospitals? *Journal of Health Care Finance* 28, no. 1: 25–38.

Congressional Budget Office (CBO). 2006. *Non-profit hospitals and the provision of community benefits*. Available at: http://www.cbo.gov/sites/default/files/cbofiles/ftpdocs/76xx/doc7695/12-06-nonprofit.pdf. Accessed August 2013.

Coons, T. W. 2014. *Medicare's LTCH moratorium: CMS issues instructions and proposed regulation*. Available at: https://www.bakerdonelson.com/medicares-ltch-moratorium-cms-issues-instructions-and-proposed-regulation. Accessed May 2017.

Coyne, J. S., et al. 2009. Hospital cost and efficiency: So hospital size and ownership type really matter? *Journal of Healthcare Management* 54, no. 3: 163–174.

Cross, G. M. 2004, November. What does patient-centered care mean for the VA? *Forum*, Academy Health. pp. 1–2, 8.

Darr, K. 1991. *Ethics in health services management.* 2nd ed. Baltimore, MD: Health Professions Press.

DelliFraine, J. L. 2006. Communities with and without children's hospitals: Where do the sickest children receive care? *Hospital Topics* 84, no. 3: 19–28.

Department of Veterans Affairs. 2016. *Selected Veterans Health Administration characteristics: FY 2002 to FY 2014.* Available at: http://www.va.gov/vetdata/Utilization.asp. Accessed October 2016.

Evans, T., et al. 2014. Magnet hospitals are a magnet for higher survival rates at adult trauma centers. *Journal of Trauma and Acute Care Surgery* 77, no. 1: 89–94.

Feldstein, M. 1971. *The rising cost of hospital care.* Washington, DC: Information Resource Press.

Feldstein, P. J. 1993. *Health care economics.* 4th ed. Albany, NY: Delmar Publishers.

Finkelstein, A. N., et al. 2016. Effect of Medicaid coverage on ED use: Further evidence from Oregon's experiment. *New England Journal of Medicine* 375, no. 16: 1505–1507.

Friese, C. R., et al. 2015. Hospitals in "Magnet" program show better patient outcomes on mortality measures compared to non-"Magnet" hospitals. *Health Affairs* 34, no. 6: 986–992.

Ge, B., and G. F. Anderson. 2016. A more detailed understanding of factors associated with hospital profitability. *Health Affairs* 35, no. 5: 889–897.

Goodman, W. C. 2006, June. Employment in hospitals: Unconventional patterns over time. *Monthly Labor Review.* Washington, DC: Bureau of Labor Statistics.

Grimaldi, P. L. 2002. Inpatient rehabilitation facilities are now paid prospective rates. *Journal of Health Care Finance* 28, no. 3: 32–48.

Haglund, C. L., and W. L. Dowling. 1993. The hospital. In: *Introduction to health services.* 4th ed. S. J. Williams and P. R. Torrens, eds. Albany, NY: Delmar Publishers. pp. 135–176.

Hamric, A. B., and L. D. Wocial. 2016. Institutional ethics resources: Creating moral spaces. *Hastings Center Report* 46 (suppl): S22–S27.

Health Forum. 2001. *AHA guide to the health care field: 2001–2002 edition.* Chicago, IL: Author.

Health Forum. 2016. *Fast facts on U.S. hospitals.* Available at: http://www.aha.org/research/rc/stat-studies/fast-facts.shtml. Accessed October 30, 2016.

Hilsenrath, P. E. 2006. Osteopathic medicine in transition: Postmortem of the Osteopathic Medical Center of Texas. *Journal of the American Osteopathic Association* 106, no. 9: 558–561.

Hollingsworth, J. M., et al. 2010. Physician ownership of ambulatory surgery centers linked to higher volume of surgeries. *Health Affairs* 29, no. 4: 683.

Internal Revenue Service (IRS). 2016. *New requirements for 501(c)(3) hospitals under the Affordable Care Act.* Available at: http://www.irs.gov/Charities-Non-Profits/Charitable-Organizations/New-Requirements-for-501c3-Hospitals-Under-the-Affordable-Care-Act. Accessed May 2017.

International Federation of Health Plans. 2012. *Comparative price report: Variation in medical and hospital prices by country.* Available at: http://www.vermontforsinglepayer.org/images/userfiles/file/2012iFHPPriceReportFINAL April3.pdf. Accessed May 2017.

Kahl, A., and D. E. Clark. 1986. Employment in health services: Long-term trends and projections. *Monthly Labor Review* 109, no. 8: 17–36.

Kangovi, S., et al. 2013. Understanding why patients of low socioeconomic status prefer hospitals over ambulatory care. *Health Affairs* 32, no. 7: 1196–1203.

Kramer, M., et al. 2011. Clinical nurses in Magnet hospitals confirm productive, healthy unit work environments. *Journal of Nursing Management* 19, no. 1: 5–17.

Leonard, K. 2013. Best children's hospitals 2013-14: Overview and honor roll. *U.S. News & World Report.* Available at: http://health.usnews.com/health-news/best-childrens-hospitals/articles/2013/06/11/best-childrens-hospitals-2013-14-overview-of-the-rankings-and-honor-roll. Accessed July 2013.

Lundgren, D. K., et al. 2016. Are the Affordable Care Act restrictions warranted? A contemporary statewide analysis of physician-owned hospitals. *Journal of Arthroplasty* 31, no. 9: 1857–1861.

Mantone, J. 2005. Critical time at rural hospitals. *Modern Healthcare* 35, no. 10: 22.

Medicare Payment Advisory Commission (MedPAC). 2004. *New approaches in Medicare: Report to the Congress.* Washington, DC: Author.

Medicare Payment Advisory Commission (MedPAC). 2006. *Report to the Congress: Physician-owned* specialty hospitals revisited. Washington, DC: Author.

Medicare Payment Advisory Commission (MedPAC). 2014. Long-term care hospital services. In: *Report to Congress: Medicare payment policy.* Washington, DC: Author. pp. 263–295.

Medicare Payment Advisory Commission (MedPAC). 2015. *Critical access hospital payment system.* Washington, DC: Author.

Medicare Payment Advisory Commission (MedPAC). 2016a. *Inpatient rehabilitation facilities payment system.* Washington, DC: Author.

Medicare Payment Advisory Commission (MedPAC). 2016b. *Hospital acute inpatient services payment system.* Washington, DC: Author.

Mundy, A. 2013, May 14. Doc-owned hospitals prep to fight. *Wall Street Journal U.S. Edition*, p. B1.

Murphy, B. 2016. Bad debt on the rise for hospitals nationally: 4 takeaways. *Becker's Hospital CFO.* Available at: http://www.beckershospitalreview.com/finance/bad-debt-on-the-rise-for-hospitals-nationally-4-takeaways.html. Accessed February 2017.

Nachega, J. B., et al. 2010. Association of antiretroviral therapy adherence and health care costs. *Annals of Internal Medicine* 152, no. 1: 18–25.

National Center for Health Statistics. 2002. *Health, United States, 2002.* Hyattsville, MD: Department of Health and Human Services.

National Center for Health Statistics. 2013. *Health, United States, 2012.* Hyattsville, MD: Department of Health and Human Services.

National Center for Health Statistics. 2014. *Health, United States, 2013.* Hyattsville, MD: U.S. Department of Health and Human Services.

National Center for Health Statistics. 2016. *Health, United States, 2015.* Hyattsville, MD: Department of Health and Human Services.

Newman, J. F., et al. 2001. CEO performance appraisal: Review and recommendations. *Journal of Healthcare Management* 46, no. 1: 21–37.

Nudelman, P. M., and L. M. Andrews. 1996. The "value added" of not-for-profit health plans. *New England Journal of Medicine* 334, no. 16: 1057–1059.

O'Connell, L., and S. L. Brown. 2003. Do nonprofit HMOs eliminate racial disparities in cardiac care? *Journal of Healthcare Finance* 30, no. 2: 84–94.

Office of Inspector General. 2003. *Trends in urban hospital closure: 1990–2000.* Available at: http://oig.hhs.gov/oei/reports/oei-04-02-00611.pdf. Accessed August 2013.

Organization for Economic Cooperation and Development (OECD). 2014. Average length of stay: Acute care. *Health: Key Tables from OECD*, no. 52. doi: http://dx.doi.org/10.1787/l-o-s-acutecare-table-2014-1-en.

Organization for Economic Cooperation and Development (OECD). 2017. Health care utilization. *OECD Health Statistics [Database].* doi: http://dx.doi.org/10.1787/data-00542-en. Accessed May 2017.

Owens, B. 2005. The plight of the not-for-profit. *Journal of Healthcare Management* 50, no. 4: 237–250.

Paris, M. 1995. The medical staff. In: *Health care administration: Principles, practices, structure, and delivery.* 2nd ed. L. F. Wolper, ed. Gaithersburg, MD: Aspen Publishers. pp. 32–46.

Parks, J., and A. Q. Radke. 2014. *The vital role of state psychiatric hospitals.* Alexandria, VA: National Association of State Mental Health Program Directors.

Raffel, M. W. 1980. *The US health system: Origins and functions.* New York, NY: John Wiley and Sons.

Raffel, M. W., and N. K. Raffel. 1994. *The US health system: Origins and functions.* 4th ed. Albany, NY: Delmar Publishers.

Roemer, M. I. 1961. Bed supply and hospital utilization: A natural experiment. *Hospitals* 35, no. 21: 36–42.

Rosner, F. 2004. Informing the patient about a fatal disease: From paternalism to autonomy: The Jewish view. *Cancer Investigation* 22, no. 6: 949–953.

Sanofi-Aventis. 2013. *Managed care digest series: Hospital/systems digest, 2013.* Bridgewater, NJ: Author.

Sanofi-Aventis. 2016. *Managed care digest series: Hospital/systems digest, 2016.* Bridgewater, NJ: Author.

Shoger, T. R. 2011. Commonsense contracts. *Trustees* 64, no. 1: 6–7.

Sinay, T. 2005. Cost structure of osteopathic hospitals and their local counterparts in the USA: Are they any different? *Social Science and Medicine* 60, no. 8: 1805–1814.

Snyder, J. 2003, February 23. Specialty hospitals on rise: Facilities source of controversy. *The Arizona Republic.*

Stewart, D. A. 1973. The history and status of proprietary hospitals. *Blue Cross Reports—Research Series 9*. Chicago, IL: Blue Cross Association.

Stuart, B., et al. 2006. Financial consequences of rural hospital long-term care strategies. *Health Care Management Review* 31, no. 2: 145–155.

Supreme Court of the State of Illinois. 2010. *Provena Covenant Medical Center et al. v. the Department of Revenue et al.* Docket no. 107328. Opinion filed March 18, 2010. Available at: http://www.state.il.us/court/Opinions/SupremeCourt/2010/March/107328.pdf. Accessed February 2011.

Teisberg, E. D., et al. 1991. *The hospital sector in 1992*. Boston, MA: Harvard Business School.

Thorpe, K. E., et al. 2000. Hospital conversions, margins, and the provision of uncompensated care. *Health Affairs* 19, no. 6: 187–194.

Torio, C. M., and B. J. Moore. 2016. *National inpatient hospital costs: The most expensive conditions by payer, 2013 (Statistical Brief #204)*. Available at: https://www.hcup-us.ahrq.gov/reports/statbriefs/sb204-Most-Expensive-Hospital-Conditions.pdf. Accessed February 2017.

Torpey, E. 2014, Spring. Healthcare: Millions of jobs now and in the future. *Occupational Outlook Quarterly*. Bureau of Labor Statistics.

U.S. Census Bureau. 2012. *Statistical abstract of the United States, 2012*. Washington, DC: Author.

Vogt, W. B., and R. Town. 2006. *How has hospital consolidation affected the price and quality of hospital care?* Princeton, NJ: Robert Wood Johnson Foundation.

Weaver, C. 2010. Physician-owned hospitals racing to meet health law deadline. *Kaiser Health News*. Available at: http://www.kaiserhealthnews.org/Stories/2010/October/28/physician-owned-hospitals.aspx. Accessed February 2011.

Weiss, A. J., and A. Elixhauser. 2014. *Overview of hospital stays in the United States, 2012 (Statistical Brief #180)*. Rockville, MD: Agency for Healthcare Research and Quality. Available at: http://www.hcup-us.ahrq.gov/reports/statbriefs/sb180-Hospitalizations-United-States-2012.pdf. Accessed May 2017.

Wolfson, J., and S. L. Hopes. 1994. What makes tax-exempt hospitals special? *Healthcare Financial Management* 4, no. 7: 56–60.

Wood, C. A. 2011. Employment in health care: A crutch for the ailing economy during the 2007–09 recession. *Monthly Labor Review*. Washington, DC: Bureau of Labor Statistics.

Worthy, J. C., et al. 2016. Analysis of the community benefit standard in Texas hospitals. *Journal of Healthcare Management* 61, no. 2: 94–102.

Young, G. J., et al. 2013. Provision of community benefits by tax-exempt U.S. hospitals. *New England Journal of Medicine* 368, no. 16: 1519–1527.

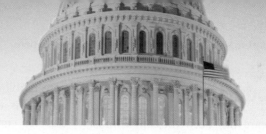

CHAPTER 9

Managed Care and Integrated Organizations

LEARNING OBJECTIVES

- Review the link between the development of managed care and earlier organizational forms in the U.S. health care delivery system.
- Grasp the basic concepts of managed care and how managed care organizations achieve cost savings.
- Distinguish between the main types of managed care organizations.
- Examine the different models under which health maintenance organizations are organized and explain the advantages and disadvantages of each model.
- Describe why managed care did not achieve its cost-control objectives.
- Discuss the driving forces behind organizational integration and strategies commonly used to achieve integration.
- Describe highly integrated health care systems—namely, integrated delivery systems and accountable care organizations.

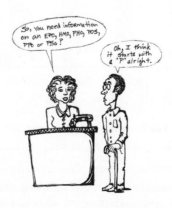

▶ Introduction

Managed care has been the single most dominant force that has fundamentally transformed the delivery of health care in the United States since the 1990s. It is noteworthy that even the Affordable Care Act (ACA) of 2010, the most sweeping health care reform initiative in recent memory, did not attempt to obliterate managed care and had to work within its parameters. Managed care is firmly entrenched in the U.S. health care system and shows no signs of disappearing in the future.

In 2016, employer-sponsored health insurance enrolled fewer than 1% of employees in traditional fee-for-service plans (**FIGURE 9-1**), which have reached a point of near extinction. In recent years, high-deductible health plans (HDHPs) have gained popularity and the share of managed care enrollment has declined proportionately; this trend is likely to continue. In HDHPs, consumers control the use of a savings feature to pay out-of-pocket expenses up to a certain limit, and subsequently fall back on health insurance to cover additional expenses.

Although managed care originated in the United States, its tools have spread internationally. For instance, general practitioners in several European countries regulate access to specialists and have responsibility over a per-capita annual budget (Deom et al., 2010).

In the United States, the transition to managed care became necessary as employers grappled with the unaffordable excesses associated with unrestrained delivery of services, which had led to spiraling health insurance premiums. In the traditional insurance system (also referred to

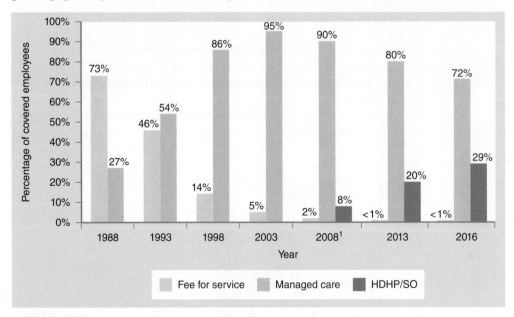

FIGURE 9-1 Percentage of worker enrollment in health plans, selected years.

[1] In 2008, the survey started to include High Deductible Health Plans paired with a savings option (HDHP/SO).

Data from Kaiser Family Foundation and Health Research and Educational Trust (Kaiser/HRET). 2003. *Employer health benefits: 2003 annual survey.* Menlo Park, CA: Author; Kaiser Family Foundation and Health Research and Educational Trust (Kaiser/HRET). 2016. *Employer health benefits: 2016 annual survey.* Menlo Park, CA: Author.

as fee-for-service or indemnity insurance) that prevailed prior to managed care, insurance companies had no incentive to manage how services were delivered and how the providers were paid. With no controls over delivery and payment, costs got out of hand. The only way to control the runaway costs was to integrate delivery and payment with the functions of financing and insurance. This integration of functions was accomplished through managed care.

As employers increasingly abandoned traditional insurance and switched to managed care as a defense against rising insurance costs, managed care started wielding enormous buying power over physicians and hospitals. Providers saw this dominance as a threat to their independence and earnings. For their part, insureds who had previously been able to seek any provider of their choice now had some restrictions placed on that freedom. Subsequently, there ensued the "managed care backlash": As a result of opposition from physicians and consumers and increased regulation from policymakers in the 1990s, managed care organizations (MCOs) were forced to relax tight controls over health care utilization and payments to providers. Some diversification within the industry also occurred, as more than one type of managed care plan became available. Consequently, managed care evolved into something quite different from what it was originally intended to be and, eventually, had limited success in controlling health care costs.

The balancing of power on the demand and supply sides of the market led to organizational integration. To counter the erosion of their marketplace power, providers began forming integrated organizations led by hospitals. On the other side of the equation, the managed care industry itself has consolidated by absorbing weaker competitors and, more recently, joining providers in organizational integration. As a result, the U.S. health care delivery landscape has been radically transformed. Managed care faces ongoing challenges of how to further manage cost escalations in hospital care, prescription drugs, and other areas of health care delivery.

▶ What Is Managed Care?

Managed care is an organized approach to delivering a comprehensive array of health care services to a group of enrolled members through efficient management of services needed by the members and negotiation of prices or payment arrangements with providers. Managed care is generally discussed in two different contexts. First, and more commonly, it refers to an approach for providing health care services that has two main features: (1) integration of the financing, insurance, delivery, and payment functions within one organizational setting (**FIGURE 9-2**) and (2) formal control over utilization. Second, the term "managed care" can refer to an MCO, which can take a variety of forms discussed in this chapter. In this context, managed care is an organization that delivers health care services using the approach just discussed.

Financing

In a managed care system, premiums are based on negotiated contracts between employers and the MCO. A fixed premium per enrollee includes all health care services provided for in the contract, and premiums cannot be raised during the term of the contract.

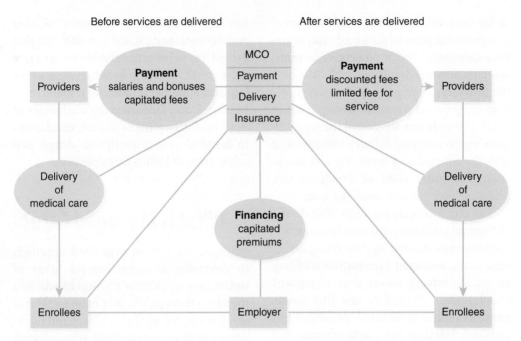

Before services are delivered   After services are delivered

FIGURE 9-2 Integration of health care delivery functions through managed care.

Insurance

The MCO functions like an insurance company by assuming all risk. In other words, it takes the financial responsibility if the total cost of services provided exceeds the revenue from fixed premiums.

Delivery

In an ideal scenario, an MCO would operate its own hospitals and outpatient clinics and employ its own physicians. Some large MCOs actually do employ their own physicians on salary. Others have concluded mergers with hospitals and/or group practices. Most MCOs, however, arrange the delivery of medical services through contracts with physicians, clinics, and hospitals operating independently.

Payment

MCOs use three main types of payment arrangements with providers: capitation, discounted fees, and salaries. The three methods allow risk sharing in varying degrees between the MCO and the providers. Risk sharing puts the burden on the providers to be cost-conscious and to curtail unnecessary utilization. Sometimes, a limited amount of fee-for-service reimbursement is used for specialized services.

Capitation refers to the payment of a fixed monthly fee per member to a health care provider. All health care services are included in the one set fee, so that risk shifts from the MCO to the provider.

Discounted fee arrangements can be regarded as a modified form of fee for service. After the delivery of services, the provider can bill the MCO for each service separately but is paid according to a prenegotiated schedule called a **fee schedule**. In this case, risk is borne by the MCO, but the MCO can lower its costs by paying discounted rates. Providers agree to discount their regular fees in exchange for the volume of business the MCO brings them.

A third method of payment is salaries, often coupled with bonuses or withholdings. In this case, the provider is an employee of the MCO. Physicians get paid fixed salaries. At the end of the year, a pool of money is distributed among the physicians in the form of bonuses based on various performance measures. Hence, under this method of payment, some risk shifts from the MCO to the physicians. Research demonstrates that financial incentives for providers result in higher performance on care effectiveness measures (Borenstein et al., 2004). Financial incentives have also been shown to have a modest positive effect on quality, particularly in staff- and group model HMOs (Tisnado et al., 2008).

Cost containment is not the only objective managed care seeks to achieve, although the potential for cost containment has been the driving force behind the phenomenal growth of managed care. MCOs are also involved in initiatives that improve health and wellness, disease management, enrollee satisfaction, quality of care, and overall organizational performance.

▶ Evolution of Managed Care

The concept of managed care is not new, even though the widespread application of the concept is a more recent phenomenon. The principles on which managed care is based have been around for nearly a century. For example, the first private health insurance arrangement for hospital services (known as the Baylor Plan) in the United States was based on capitation (**EXHIBIT 9-1**). In 1929, this plan started enrolling teachers for a fixed monthly fee per enrollee that was paid to Baylor Hospital; no insurance company was involved in the arrangement.

The idea of managed care evolved from what the medical establishment pejoratively referred to as the corporate practice of medicine. Even before private health insurance became widespread, these practices were used sporadically as cost-effective means of providing health care services to certain groups of people. Contract practice takes the idea of capitation a step further by incorporating a defined group of enrollees. Here, an employer is the financier that contracts with one or more providers to furnish health care to a group of enrollees—the employees—at a predetermined fee per enrollee.

Prepaid group practice goes another step further. First, it preserves the principles of capitation, bearing of risk by the provider, and a defined group of enrollees whose health care contract is financed by their employer. It then adds the delivery of comprehensive services. Prepaid practice, which gave rise to health maintenance organizations (HMOs) in the mid-1970s, was well established in the form of plans such as the Kaiser Foundation Health Plan (Oakland, California, 1942), the Group Health Cooperative of Puget Sound (Seattle, Washington, 1947), and the Health Insurance Plan of Greater New York (1947).

Managed care has incorporated certain cost-control features such as utilization management to control inefficient use of health care services, discounted fees

EXHIBIT 9-1 The Evolution of Managed Care

Health insurance	Capitation Bearing of risk by providers

Initially, health insurance combined the insurance, delivery, and payment functions of health care, as seen in the Baylor Plan, but further evolution of this initial concept was thwarted by organized medicine. Contract practice moved toward the integration of these functions, bypassing the insurance companies.

Contract practice	Defined group of enrollees Capitation or salary Bearing of risk by providers

↓

Prepaid group practice	Comprehensive services Defined group of enrollees Capitation Bearing of risk by providers

↓

Managed care	Utilization controls Comprehensive services Defined group of enrollees Capitation, discounted fees, or salary Limited fee for service Limits on choice of providers Sharing of risk with providers Financial incentives to providers Accountability for plan performance

and salaries as alternative methods of payment to providers, limits on the choice of providers from whom enrollees can obtain services, and accountability to the stakeholders by evaluating performance on certain quantifiable measures. The objectives are to limit inefficient utilization of services, to contract with providers who agree to certain policies and standards in the delivery of care, and to measure the MCO's overall performance.

Accreditation of Managed Care Organizations

The National Committee for Quality Assurance (NCQA), a private nonprofit organization, began accrediting MCOs in

1991. Accreditation emerged in response to the demand for standardized, objective information about the quality of MCOs. Participation in the accreditation program is voluntary, but nearly half of MCOs in the United States are accredited. To be accredited, MCOs must comply with NCQA standards. Compliance is determined by a review process and evaluation by physicians and managed care experts. A national oversight committee of physicians supervises the process. Accreditation is combined with a rating system that has six status categories: excellent, commendable, accredited, provisional, interim, and denied.

Quality Assessment in Managed Care

Developed by the NCQA, Healthcare Effectiveness Data and Information Set (HEDIS) performance measures date back to 1989. Originally designed for private employers' needs as purchasers of health insurance, HEDIS has been adapted for use by the general public, public insurers, and regulators. More than 90% of all U.S. health plans use HEDIS measures to evaluate performance on important dimensions of clinical care and service. These measures have also been used quite extensively to compare the quality of care in health plans.

HEDIS 2017 contains more than 80 measures across seven domains (NCQA, 2017):

- Effectiveness of care (e.g., immunizations, screenings, management of chronic conditions)
- Access and availability of care (e.g., access to preventive services, treatment for alcohol and drug dependency, prenatal and postpartum care)
- Experience of care (e.g., the adult and child versions of CAHPS Health Plan Survey 5.0H)
- Utilization (e.g., appropriate frequency of visits, inpatient utilization, mental health utilization)
- Relative resource use (resource use for conditions such as diabetes, heart diseases, hypertension, and asthma)
- Health plan descriptive information, which includes board certification of physicians, enrollments, and race/ethnic diversity of the enrolled population, among other details
- Measures collected using electronic clinical data systems (e.g., use of electronic health records [EHRs])

The HEDIS program has been criticized because disclosure is voluntary. Despite this concern, the overall quality of care has consistently improved among all plans reporting to the NCQA (DoBias, 2008).

▶ Growth of Managed Care

As previously mentioned, the main impetus for managed care's growth was rapid cost escalations during the 1970s and 1980s under the dominant fee-for-service system. Employers, who in many instances paid the entire cost of health insurance premiums on their employees' behalf, began switching to managed care only after they experienced notable escalations in premium costs. The Health Maintenance Organization Act of 1973 provided some federal support for the creation of HMOs and created widespread awareness of an alternative to fee-for-service medicine.

Flaws in the Fee-for-Service Model

Traditional fee-for-service health insurance is also referred to as **indemnity insurance**. An indemnity plan allows the insured to obtain health care services anywhere and from any physician or hospital. Indemnity insurance and fee-for-service reimbursement to providers are closely intertwined.

Uncontrolled Utilization

In fee-for-service practice of medicine, moral hazard prevailed. In a system dominated by specialists and an absence of primary care gatekeeping, patients were free to go to any provider. Care received from specialists and utilization of sophisticated technology gave patients the impression of high quality. Competition was driven by such impressions rather than by cost or assessed quality. Physicians and hospitals competed for patients by offering the most up-to-date technologies and the most attractive practice settings (Wilkerson et al., 1997).

Despite research conducted to study this issue over the years, both in the United States and elsewhere, the notion of provider-induced demand has been controversial. Nevertheless, ample evidence exists that providers had an incentive to promote higher utilization in pursuit of higher revenues when controls over utilization were inadequate (Nguyen and Derrick, 1997; Rice and Labelle, 1989; Yip, 1998). Hence, a 10% reduction in fees, for example, would not necessarily translate into a 10% reduction in total expenditures on physician services because physicians generated demand in response to real fee reductions (Rice and Labelle, 1989).

Uncontrolled Prices and Payment

In traditional indemnity insurance, the insurance company exercised little control over providers' charges or patients' utilization of services. Providers set charges at an artificially high level and billed insurance an item-by-item claim. The insurance company was merely a passive payer of claims—it paid what the providers billed, limited only by what the insurer deemed as usual, customary, and reasonable. The insurance company had little incentive to control costs because it could simply increase the premiums the following year based on utilization during the previous year.

Focus on Illness Rather Than Wellness

Indemnity insurance paid for services only when a specific medical diagnosis was reported on the insurance claim; thus, visits for preventive checkups were not covered. The fee-for-service system also presented a second, even bigger problem: Indemnity insurance provided more thorough coverage when a person was hospitalized, and the physician was paid for daily hospital visits when the patient was being treated in the hospital. Thus, costly hospitalization of patients was lucrative for both the physicians and hospitals.

Employers' Response to Rise in Premiums

When it first appeared, the concept of managed care was designed to compete against fee-for-service medicine. Until the 1980s, HMOs were the predominant form of managed care. The price-based competition from HMOs was often referred to as "shadow pricing," because HMOs typically offered more benefits and somewhat lower premiums than indemnity plans (Zelman, 1996). At this stage, however, managed care plans had limited appeal. Individuals covered by indemnity insurance saw little benefit in joining a plan that would restrict their choice of providers. Most providers also saw little benefit in contracting with HMOs that might restrict their potential income or alter their style of practice (Wilkerson et al., 1997). For the most part, employers remained passive.

Between 1980 and 1990, the total cost of private health insurance increased at an average annual rate of more than 12% (**FIGURE 9-3**). Economic realities forced employers to make the transition from indemnity plans to managed care. Among the U.S. population with employer-based health insurance, the proportion of those enrolled in various managed care plans jumped from 27% in 1988 to 86% in 1998, and then to 95% in 2003 (see Figure 9-1).

Weakened Economic Position of Providers

Indirectly, excess capacity in the health care delivery system may have contributed to the growth of managed care (McGuire,

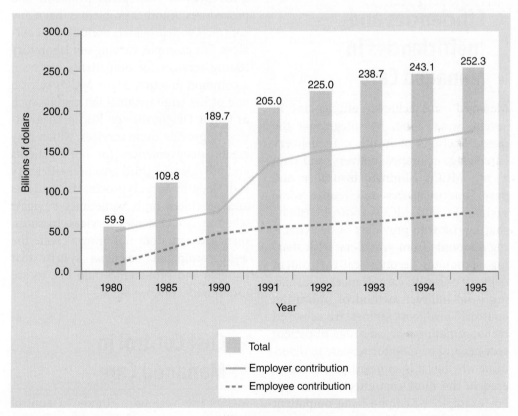

FIGURE 9-3 Growth in the cost of U.S. health insurance (private employers), 1980–1995.

Data from National Center for Health Statistics. 1998. *Health, United States, 1998.* Hyattsville, MD: U.S. Department of Health and Human Services. p. 348.

1994). This relationship perhaps initially arose because the Medicare prospective payment system, introduced in the mid-1980s, had a marked impact on hospital economics. Left with significant unused capacity in the form of empty beds, hospitals had substantially weakened bargaining power. Physicians initially showed great resistance to managed care but, as the financing of health care quickly shifted toward managed care, found they could not resist the growing momentum. In most cases, physicians were left with the stark choice of participating or being left out.

▶ ## Efficiencies and Inefficiencies in Managed Care

Managed care achieves efficiencies in several ways. First, by integrating the quad functions of health care delivery (financing, insurance, delivery, and payment), MCOs eliminate insurance and payer intermediaries and realize some savings. Second, MCOs control costs by sharing risk with providers or by extracting discounts from providers. Risk sharing promotes economically prudent delivery of health care. Hence, risk sharing is an indirect method of utilization control. Third, cost savings are achieved by coordinating a broad range of patient services and by monitoring care to determine whether it is appropriate and delivered in the most cost-effective settings. For example, by emphasizing outpatient services, MCOs achieve lower rates of hospital utilization. Some evidence also suggests that HMO plans incur lower

utilization of costly procedures, compared to non-HMO plans (Miller and Luft, 1997). Fourth, gatekeeping reduces moral hazard. Finally, a focus on wellness and preventive services saves money through illness prevention, as well as through early detection and treatment of more serious illnesses.

Although many of the cost-control measures adopted by managed care have been applauded, other results have not been so commendable. The complexity of having to deal with numerous plans does not add value to the delivery of health care. Administrative inefficiencies are created for providers, who must deal with differences in each plan's protocols and procedures. Another problem is that many contracts with providers exclude some services. For example, carving out laboratory testing services for outpatients has been a common practice. Many MCOs rely on one of the large national lab chains, such as Quest Diagnostics or Roche Diagnostics, to provide these services, which may create inconveniences for both patients and providers. A third area of inefficiency is the lengthy appeals process that patients and providers must sometimes navigate when an MCO denies services. In short, managed care does not always create the well-coordinated, seamless system that patients and providers would like to see (Southwick, 1997).

▶ ## Cost Control in Managed Care

MCOs use various methods to control utilization and to deliver cost-effective care. The need for utilization management emanates from the fact that, in the United

States, approximately 10% of patients—typically those with chronic or complex medical conditions—account for 70% of overall health care spending (Berk and Monheit, 2001). Moreover, recent estimates suggest that nearly one-third of health care spending in the United States is a result of unnecessary care (Levine and Mulligan, 2015).

Utilization management requires (1) an expert evaluation of which services are medically necessary in a given case and steps to ensure that unnecessary services are minimized, (2) a determination of how the medically necessary services can be provided most inexpensively while maintaining acceptable quality standards, and (3) a review of the process of care and changes in the patient's condition to revise the course of medical treatment if necessary. Utilization management of institutional inpatient services takes priority because the cost of hospital care represents nearly 50% of the total costs that health plans pay for medical services (Melnick et al., 2011).

Earlier concerns raised about the potential for negative effects of managed care's cost-containment strategies on the physician–patient relationship proved unfounded. Physicians seem to have managed the relationships with their patients without letting external factors compromise patient satisfaction and trust (Keating et al., 2007).

The following methods are often used for utilization monitoring and control:

- Choice restriction
- Care coordination
- Disease management
- Pharmaceutical management
- Utilization review
- Practice profiling

Not all MCOs use all of these mechanisms. Traditionally, HMOs have employed tighter utilization controls than other managed care plans.

Choice Restriction

Traditional indemnity insurance gave the insured open access to any provider, whether generalist or specialist. Such indiscretion led to overutilization of services. Most managed care plans impose some restrictions on where and from whom the patient can obtain medical care. Patients still have a choice of physicians, but the choice is limited to physicians who are either employees of the MCO or have established contracts with the MCO. A physician who has formal affiliations with an MCO is said to be on the **panel** of the MCO. In a **closed-panel** (or closed-access or in-network) plan, services obtained from providers outside the panel are not covered by the plan. By contrast, an **open-panel** (or open-access or out-of-network option) plan allows access to providers outside the panel, but enrollees almost always have to pay higher out-of-pocket costs.

Because the MCO has greater control over providers who are on its panel, utilization is better managed under closed-panel plans, compared to those that allow access outside the panel. From the enrollees' standpoint, the restricted choice of providers is a trade-off for lower out-of-pocket costs. Earlier, during the growth phase of managed care, choice restriction had caused dissatisfaction among enrollees. Since then, an increasing number of both low-income and higher-income Americans have indicated their willingness to limit their choice of providers to save on out-of-pocket medical costs (Tu, 2005).

Care Coordination

Physicians control the utilization of most health care services. But their practice patterns sometimes come with a caveat: More expensive health care services do not always equate to better health. Except in primary care, most of the increase in health care spending has not produced improved clinical outcomes (Kravitz, 2008). Yet, driven by consumer demand, the U.S. health care system favors specialty care over primary care. In addition, U.S. consumers, who are bombarded by advertisements for expensive new pharmaceuticals, often expect their physicians to prescribe the latest drugs even when an older and cheaper drug may be quite satisfactory in obtaining expected results.

To address such paradoxes, certain MCOs have required that their enrollees must have a primary care physician (PCP) who coordinates all health care services. This mechanism is referred to as "gatekeeping." It emphasizes preventive care, routine physical examinations, and other primary care services. When gatekeeping is used, secondary-level services (**FIGURE 9-4**) are obtained only on referral from the primary care physician. Gatekeeping strategies have been shown to result in modest cost savings (Pati et al., 2005), although one Swiss study showed savings of 15% to 19% per person for individuals enrolled in a gatekeeping plan compared to those enrolled in a fee-for-service plan (Schwenkglenks et al., 2006).

Another care coordination model used by some MCOs is **case management**. This model relies on a client-centered approach for evaluating and coordinating care, particularly for patients who have complex, potentially costly problems that

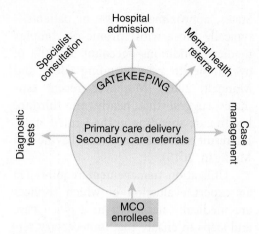

FIGURE 9-4 Care coordination and utilization control through gatekeeping.

require a variety of services from multiple providers over an extended period. Examples of conditions managed through this model include acquired immunodeficiency syndrome (AIDS), spinal cord injury, bone marrow transplant, lupus, cystic fibrosis, and severe workplace injuries. Patients with these conditions need expensive secondary and tertiary care services more often than primary care. Comorbidities require care coordination of multiple health issues comprehensively. In such circumstances, a primary care gatekeeper cannot adequately coordinate all of the patient's needs, as these needs may frequently change.

In case management, an experienced health care professional, such as a nurse practitioner, with knowledge of available health care resources coordinates an individual's total health care in consultation with primary and secondary care providers. Based on the patient's needs, which change over time, services are arranged so that they are delivered in the most appropriate and cost-effective settings (**FIGURE 9-5**).

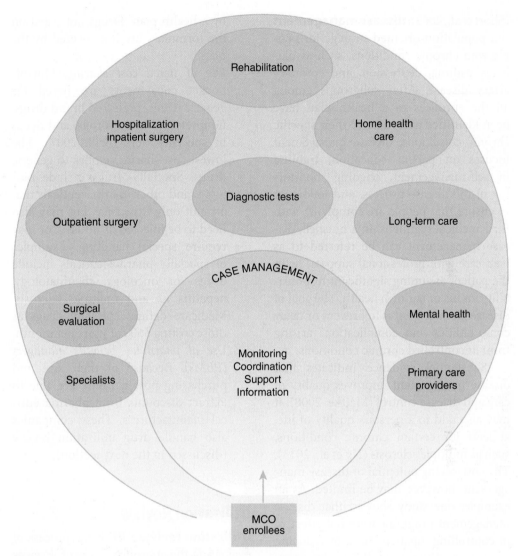

FIGURE 9-5 Case management function in care coordination.

In one study, advanced case management strategies used for high-risk populations in five states resulted in reduced costs for health care while improving the delivery of services (Lattimer, 2005). Medicare Coordinated Care Demonstration Programs have also shown reductions in hospital admissions, ranging from 8% to 33%, for high-risk patients enrolled in case management programs (Brown et al., 2012).

Disease Management

Whereas case management is typically highly individualized and focuses on coordinating the care of high-risk patients with multiple or complex medical conditions

(Short et al., 2003), **disease management** is a population-oriented strategy for people with chronic conditions, such as diabetes, asthma, depression, and coronary artery disease. After subgroups among all the enrollees in a health plan have been identified according to their specific chronic conditions, disease management focuses on patient education, training in self-management, ongoing monitoring of the disease process, and follow-up to ensure that people are complying with their medical regimens. In a nutshell, disease management can be referred to as "self-care with professional support," with the patient assuming significant responsibility for his or her own health. The goal of disease management is to prevent or delay comorbidities and complications arising from uncontrolled chronic conditions.

Substantial evidence indicates that disease management improves quality of care and disease control (Mattke, 2008). It may also add to a person's quality of life, at least for certain chronic conditions, such as multiple sclerosis (Ng et al., 2013). The cost-saving potential of disease management, however, may be limited. As an example, one study showed that disease management programs were not effective in controlling inpatient costs or reducing emergency department (ED) admissions for patients with diabetes (Conti, 2013).

Pharmaceutical Management

In the decade of 2000–2010, expenditures on prescription drugs increased more rapidly than total personal health care expenditures. To manage these rising costs, health plans use three main strategies:

- *Use of drug formularies.* A **formulary** is a list of prescription drugs approved by a health plan. Drugs not listed on the formulary are not covered by the plan.

- *Use of tiered cost sharing.* Out-of-pocket copayments are tiered for generic drugs, preferred brand drugs, nonpreferred brand drugs, and drugs in specialty tiers (Brill, 2007). The lowest cost sharing applies to generic drugs. Specialty drugs include biologics and other pharmaceuticals that are not only expensive, but may also need to be injected or infused, or may require special handling. Examples of specialty pharmaceuticals include drugs for oncology, rheumatology, hepatitis C, and multiple sclerosis. Medicare defines specialty drugs as those costing $600 or more per month.

- *Use of pharmacy benefits managers (PBMs).* Because of their size and purchasing power, PBMs are able to extract discounts from pharmaceutical manufacturers. These companies also handle drug utilization review (discussed in the next section).

Utilization Review

Utilization review (UR) is the process of evaluating the appropriateness of services provided. It is sometimes misunderstood as a mechanism for denying services, but its main objective is to ensure that appropriate levels of services are delivered, care is cost-efficient, and subsequent care is planned. Hence, quality of care has become an important component of UR. Drug UR practices have also become common because of ongoing increases in the utilization and cost of prescription drugs. Misuse of certain drugs can not only waste resources, but also harm patients.

Three main types of UR are distinguished based on when the review is undertaken: prospective, concurrent, and retrospective. All three also apply to pharmaceutical management.

Prospective Utilization Review

Prospective utilization review determines the appropriateness of utilization before the care is actually delivered. An example of prospective UR is the decision by a primary care gatekeeper to refer or not refer a patient to a specialist. However, not all managed care plans use gatekeepers. Some plans require the enrollee or the provider to call the plan administrators for preauthorization (also called precertification) of services for hospital admissions and surgical procedures. In case of an emergency admission to an inpatient facility, plans generally require notification within 24 hours. Plans use preestablished clinical guidelines to authorize hospitalization and assign an initial length of stay.

In drug UR, formularies are the first step in prospective review. Subsequently, the PBM can require preauthorization for certain drugs and biologics.

In inpatient care, one objective of prospective UR is to prevent unnecessary or inappropriate institutionalization; however, it also serves other functions. The prospective review system notifies the concurrent review system of a new case so that length of stay can be monitored and additional days of care be authorized when necessary.

Concurrent Utilization Review

Concurrent utilization review determines, on a daily basis, the length of stay necessary in a hospital. It also monitors the use of ancillary services and ensures that the selected medical treatment is appropriate and necessary. Concurrent UR is a critical undertaking when hospitals receive prospective reimbursement because the length of stay determines the profitability, or lack thereof, in a given case. Optimal drug therapy and management have been shown to reduce length of stay in hospitals in addition to reducing drug utilization and cost (Chen et al., 2009).

Concurrent UR is closely linked to **discharge planning**, which focuses on ensuring postdischarge continuity of care. For example, if a patient is admitted with a hip fracture, it is important to determine whether a rehabilitation hospital or a skilled nursing facility would be more appropriate for convalescent care. If the patient requires care in a skilled nursing facility, discharge planning must find out whether the appropriate level of rehabilitation services would be available and how long the plan will pay for rehabilitation therapies in a long-term care setting. For a patient who will be discharged home, subsequent home health services and durable medical equipment (DME) may be necessary. The objective of discharge planning is "to get all the ducks in a row" to provide seamless services at the lowest cost and in the best interest of the patient.

Retrospective Utilization Review

Retrospective utilization review refers to the review of utilization after services have been delivered. A close examination of medical records is undertaken to assess the appropriateness of care. Retrospective review may also involve an analysis of utilization data to determine patterns of overutilization or underutilization. It allows monitoring of billing accuracy and compilation of provider-specific practice patterns, with feedback then being given to physicians. Such statistical data can be helpful for taking corrective action and for monitoring subsequent progress.

Retrospective drug review can help reduce inappropriate use of controlled substances, among other things (Daubresse et al., 2013). It enables clinical pharmacists to intervene with the prescribing physician to emphasize therapeutic appropriateness and drug interactions that can affect future prescribing habits (Angalakuditi and Gomes, 2011; Starner et al., 2009).

Practice Profiling

Practice profiling refers to the monitoring of physician-specific practice patterns and the comparison of individual practice patterns to some norm. It may incorporate results of patient satisfaction surveys and compliance with clinical practice guidelines. Profiling can be used to decide which providers have the right fit with the plan's managed care philosophy and goals. The profile reports are also used to give feedback to physicians so they can modify their own behavior of medical practice. Profiling may be combined with financial incentives to boost compliance with standard practice patterns. To date, research has produced inconsistent results about the effectiveness of physician feedback and financial incentives on improving quality of care.

▶ Types of Managed Care Organizations

HMOs were the most common type of MCO until, in the late 1970s, commercial insurance companies developed preferred provider organizations (PPOs) to compete with HMOs. Today, many health insurance companies in the United States offer different types of managed care plans. For example, the largest health insurers in the United States, such as United Healthcare, Blue Cross/Blue Shield, Humana, and Aetna, operate both HMOs and PPOs. Moreover, many HMOs offer what is referred to as **triple-option plans**. These plans combine the features of indemnity insurance, HMO, and PPO; the insured has the flexibility to choose which feature to use when seeking out health care services. The three main types of managed care arrangements discussed in this section are HMOs, PPOs, and point-of-service (POS) plans.

Health Maintenance Organization

A **health maintenance organization (HMO)** is distinguished from other types of plans by the following main characteristics:

- Traditionally, indemnity insurance paid for medical care only when a person was ill, whereas an HMO not only provided medical care during illness but also offered a variety of services to help people maintain their health. The ACA removed this distinction, as almost all health plans are required to provide preventive services.
- The enrollee is generally required to choose a PCP from the panel of physicians. The PCP delivers services in accordance with a gatekeeping model.
- The provider receives a capitated fee regardless of whether the enrollee uses health care services and regardless of the quantity of services used.
- All health care must be obtained from in-network hospitals, physicians, and other health care providers. Hybrid

plans that have an HMO component, such as POS and triple-option plans, allow out-of-network use at a higher out-of-pocket cost.

- Specialty services, such as mental health and substance abuse treatment, are frequently carved out. A **carve-out** is a special contract outside regular capitation that an HMO funds separately—for example, a contract with a managed behavioral health care organization (MBHO) for mental health services.
- The HMO is responsible for ensuring that services comply with certain established standards of quality.

In the employer-based health insurance market, HMO enrollment grew rapidly in the first half of the 1990s, peaking in 1996 (**FIGURE 9-6**). Subsequently, PPO and POS plans became more popular. HMOs fell into disfavor with enrollees because these plans were the most restrictive regarding choice of providers and utilization controls. Since 2013, however, HMO enrollment has been stable. Conversely, the majority of Medicaid beneficiaries have been enrolled in HMO plans (discussed in the section "Medicaid Enrollment").

Four HMO models are commonly used: staff, group, network, and independent practice association (IPA). These models differ primarily in their arrangements with participating physicians. Some HMOs cannot be categorized neatly into any one of the four models because they may use a hybrid arrangement, referred to as a **mixed model**. An example of a mixed model is an HMO that is partially organized as a staff model, employing its own physicians, and partially relies on the group model by contracting with a group practice.

Staff Model

A **staff model** HMO employs its own salaried physicians. Based on the physician's productivity and the HMO's performance, bonuses may be added to the salary. Physicians work only for their employer HMO and provide services to that HMO's enrollees (Rakich et al., 1992). Staff model HMOs must employ physicians in all the common specialties to provide for the health care needs of their members. Contracts with selected subspecialties are established for infrequently needed services. The HMO operates one or more ambulatory care facilities that contain physicians' offices; employs support staff; and may have ancillary support facilities, such as laboratory and radiology departments. In most instances, the HMO contracts with area hospitals for inpatient services (Wagner, 1995).

Compared to other HMO models, staff model HMOs can exercise a greater degree of control over the practice patterns of their physicians. These HMOs also offer

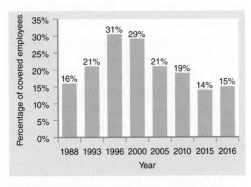

FIGURE 9-6 Percentage of covered employees enrolled in HMO plans, selected years.

Data from Kaiser Family Foundation and Health Research and Educational Trust (Kaiser/HRET). 2016. *Employer health benefits: 2016 annual survey.* Menlo Park, CA: Author.

the convenience of "one-stop shopping" for their enrollees because most routinely needed services are located in the same clinic (Wagner, 1995).

Staff model HMOs also present several disadvantages. The fixed-salary expense can be high, requiring these HMOs to have a large number of enrollees to cover their operating expenses. Enrollees also have a limited choice of physicians. When expanding into new markets, a staff model HMO requires heavy capital outlays (Wagner, 1995). Because of such disadvantages, the staff model has been the least popular.

Group Model

A **group model** HMO contracts with a single multispecialty group practice and contracts separately with one or more hospitals to provide comprehensive services to its members. The group practice employs the physicians, not the HMO. The HMO pays an all-inclusive capitation fee to the group practice to provide physician services to its members. The group practice may have contracts with other MCOs as well.

Large groups are usually attractive to HMOs because they deliver a large block of physicians with one contract. However, a large group contract can also be a downside for the HMO. If the contract is lost, the HMO will have difficulty meeting its service obligations to the enrollees.

As for other advantages, the group model HMO is able to avoid large expenditures in fixed salaries and facilities. Affiliation with a reputable multispecialty group practice lends the HMO prestige and creates a perception of quality among its enrollees. On the down side, enrollees may find the choice of physicians limited.

Network Model

Under the **network model**, the HMO contracts with more than one medical group practice. This model is especially adaptable to large metropolitan areas and widespread geographic regions where group practices are located. A common arrangement in the network model is to have contracts only with primary care group (PCG) practices. Enrollees may select PCPs from any of these groups. Each group is paid a capitation fee based on the number of enrollees, and is responsible for providing all physician services. The group can make referrals to specialists but is financially responsible for reimbursing them for any referrals made. In some cases, the HMO may contract with a panel of specialists, in which case referrals can be made only to physicians serving on the panel (Wagner, 1995).

The network model can offer a wider choice of physicians than the staff or group model. The main disadvantage is the dilution of utilization control.

Independent Practice Association Model

In 1954, a variant of the prepaid group practice plan was established by the San Joaquin County Foundation for Medical Care in Stockton, California. This plan, which was a prototype of the **IPA model**, was initiated by the San Joaquin County Medical Society (MacColl, 1966). As a result of political pressures from organized medicine, this form of HMO was specifically included in the HMO Act of 1973 (Mackie and Decker, 1981).

An **independent practice association (IPA)** is a legal entity separate from the HMO. The IPA contracts with both independent solo practitioners and group practices. The HMO then contracts with the IPA instead of contracting with individual physicians or group practices (**FIGURE 9-7**). Hence, the IPA is an intermediary representing a large number of physicians. The HMO pays a capitation amount to the IPA, but the IPA retains administrative control over how it pays its physicians. For example, it may reimburse physicians through capitation, or it may use some other means, such as a modified fee for service. The IPA often shares risk with the physicians and assumes the responsibility for utilization management and quality assessment. The IPA also carries stop-loss reinsurance, or the HMO may provide stop-loss coverage to prevent the IPA from going bankrupt (Kongstvedt and Plocher, 1995).

Under the IPA model, the HMO is still responsible for providing health care services to its enrollees, but the logistics of arranging physician services shifts to the IPA. This approach relieves the HMO of the administrative burden of establishing contracts with numerous providers and managing utilization. Financial risk also transfers to the IPA. The IPA model provides an expanded choice of providers to enrollees. It also allows small groups and individual physicians the opportunity to participate in managed care and get a slice of the revenues.

Community physicians may independently establish IPAs, or the HMO may create an IPA and invite community physicians to participate in it. An IPA may also be hospital based and structured so that only physicians from one or two hospitals are eligible to participate in the IPA (Wagner, 1995). One major disadvantage of the IPA model is that, if a contract is lost, the HMO loses a large number of participating physicians.

The IPA acts as a buffer between the HMO and physicians. Hence, the IPA does not have as much leverage in changing physician behavior as a staff or a group model HMO would have. In addition, many IPAs have a surplus of specialists, which creates some pressure to use their services (Kongstvedt and Plocher, 1995).

Of the four HMO models, the IPA model has been the most successful in terms of share of all enrollments over time. Its success likely reflects the wider choice of physicians that the enrollees have and the buffer an IPA creates between the HMO and its practicing physicians.

Preferred Provider Organization

A **preferred provider organization (PPO)** is distinguished from other types of managed care plans by the following main characteristics:

- The PPO establishes contracts with a select group of physicians and hospitals. These providers on the PPO's panel are referred to as "preferred providers."
- Generally, the PPO allows an open-panel option in which the enrollee can use out-of-network providers, but incurs higher cost sharing. The additional out-of-pocket expenses act largely as a deterrent to going outside the panel. If a PPO

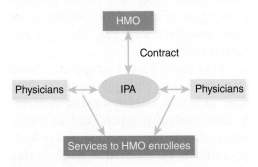

FIGURE 9-7 The IPA-HMO model.

does not provide an out-of-network option, it is referred to as an **exclusive provider plan**.

- Instead of using capitation as a method of payment, PPOs make discounted fee arrangements with providers. The discounts can range between 25% and 35% of the providers' established charges. Negotiated payment arrangements with hospitals can be based on diagnosis-related groups (DRGs), bundled charges for certain services, or discounts. Hence, no direct risk sharing with providers is involved.

- PPOs apply fewer restrictions to the care-seeking behavior of enrollees. In most instances, primary care gatekeeping is not employed. Prior authorization (retrospective UR) is generally employed only for hospitalization and high-cost outpatient procedures (Robinson, 2002).

Insurance companies (including Blue Cross and Blue Shield), independent investors, and hospital alliances own most PPOs. Other PPOs are owned by HMOs, and some are jointly sponsored by a hospital and physicians. As a less stringent choice of managed care for both enrollees and providers, PPOs have enjoyed remarkable success. After reaching their peak enrollment of 61% of covered employees in 2005 (**FIGURE 9-8**), enrollment in PPOs has declined as high-deductible health plans have gained popularity in recent years.

Point-of-Service Plans

A **point-of-service (POS) plan** combines features of classic HMOs with some of the characteristics of patient choice found in PPOs. Hence, these plans are a type of hybrid plan, also referred to as open-ended HMOs. When first brought on the market,

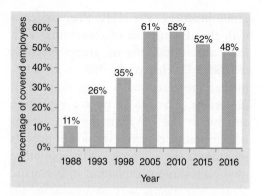

FIGURE 9-8 Percentage of covered employees enrolled in PPO plans, selected years.

Data from Kaiser Family Foundation and Health Research and Educational Trust (Kaiser/HRET). 2002. *Employer health benefits: 2002 annual survey.* Menlo Park, CA: Author; Kaiser Family Foundation and Health Research and Educational Trust (Kaiser/HRET). 2016. *Employer health benefits: 2016 annual survey.* Menlo Park, CA: Author.

these plans had a two-pronged objective: (1) retain the benefits of tight utilization management found in HMOs but (2) offer an alternative to their unpopular feature of restricted provider choice. The features borrowed from HMOs were capitation or other risk-sharing payment arrangements with providers and the gatekeeping method of utilization control. The feature borrowed from PPOs was the patient's ability to choose between an in-network or out-of-network provider at the point (time) of receiving services—hence, the name "point of service." Of course, the enrollee had to pay extra for the privilege of using out-of-network providers because these providers were paid their fee-for-service charges.

POS plans grew in popularity soon after they first emerged in 1988. Over time, as HMOs relaxed some of their utilization control practices and as PPOs, which already offered a choice of providers, proliferated, the need for a hybrid plan became less important to consumers. After reaching a peak in popularity in 1998 and

1999, employee enrollment in POS plans declined sharply, although enrollments have stabilized in recent years (**FIGURE 9-9**).

▶ Trends in Managed Care

Managed care has become a mature industry in the United States. In the employment-based health insurance market, indemnity insurance has almost entirely disappeared. In the government sector, states have increasingly enrolled Medicaid beneficiaries in managed care plans. Medicare beneficiaries have also found value for their premium dollars by enrolling in Medicare Advantage (MA) plans.

Employment-Based Health Insurance Enrollment

PPOs continue to dominate employment-based health insurance enrollments (**FIGURE 9-10**). HDHPs continue to gain momentum, and are particularly attractive for young, healthy individuals and families. Their growth has cut into the share of managed care (Figure 9-1).

Medicaid Enrollment

Waivers under the Social Security Act, particularly sections 1115 and 1915(b), first allowed states to enroll their Medicaid recipients in managed care plans. Subsequently, the Balanced Budget Act of 1997 gave states the authority to implement mandatory managed care programs without requiring federal waivers (Moscovice et al., 1998). As a result, enrollment of Medicaid beneficiaries in HMOs has grown rapidly, from 56% of all Medicaid beneficiaries in 2000 to almost 85% in 2015 (Sanofi-Aventis, 2013, 2016). The influx of new Medicaid-insured individuals into

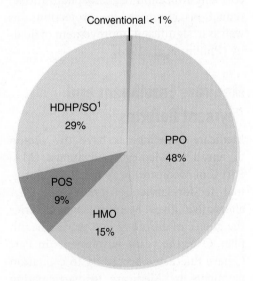

FIGURE 9-10 Share of managed care enrollments in employer-based health plans, 2016.

[1] High-deductible health plan with a savings option.

Note: Numbers may not add to 100 because of rounding.

Data from Kaiser Family Foundation and Health Research and Educational Trust (Kaiser/HRET). 2016. *Employer health benefits: 2016 annual survey.* Menlo Park, CA: Author.

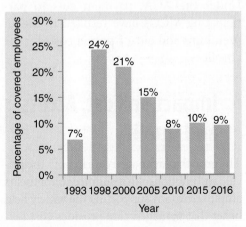

FIGURE 9-9 Percentage of covered employees enrolled in POS plans, selected years.

Data from Kaiser Family Foundation and Health Research and Educational Trust (Kaiser/HRET). 2002. *Employer health benefits: 2002 annual survey.* Menlo Park, CA: Author; Kaiser Family Foundation and Health Research and Educational Trust (Kaiser/HRET). 2016. *Employer health benefits: 2016 annual survey.* Menlo Park, CA: Author.

the U.S. health care market under the ACA is at least partially responsible for the increase: The managed care penetration rate for Medicaid was 77% in 2010 and 2011, before the ACA became effective (Sanofi-Aventis, 2016).

Some states have developed a different model of managing health care delivery, particularly in rural areas where managed care has not flourished. Medicaid **primary care case management (PCCM)** is a model that requires a Medicaid enrollee to choose a PCP; the PCP is then responsible for coordinating the enrollee's care and is paid a monthly fee for doing so, on top of the payment for providing medical services. In general, all medical services are reimbursed on a fee-for-service basis. Most states now use the PCCM model. In a research study, the PCCM program in Illinois was found to result in substantial cost and utilization (e.g., hospitalizations) reductions compared to projections, as well as in significant improvement of quality (Phillips et al., 2014).

Medicare Enrollment and Payment Reforms

Medicare beneficiaries have the option to enroll in Medicare Advantage (MA; Part C of Medicare) or remain in the original fee-for-service program. The MA alternative gives Medicare beneficiaries the choice of enrolling in a private health plan. Over the years, enrollments in Part C have fluctuated according to capitation payments by Medicare to participating MCOs. For example, a 10% increase in payments increased enrollment by 9.6% (Morrisey et al., 2013). Conversely, cuts in Medicare's capitation rates have decreased enrollments, as fewer MCOs are willing

to participate in Part C under that condition. For example, the Balanced Budget Act of 1997 reduced payments to HMOs. As HMOs withdrew from the Medicare program, 800,000 beneficiaries lost their HMO coverage between 2000 and 2001 (Aventis Pharmaceuticals and SMG Marketing-Verispan, 2002).

Between 2003 and 2007, the Centers for Medicare and Medicaid Services (CMS) rolled out a new payment plan that included risk adjustments based on hierarchical condition categories, which represent major medical conditions that are ranked on the basis of disease severity and cost. The resulting risk-adjusted payments accounted for the health status of each beneficiary. Between 2009 and 2013, enrollment in MA plans grew by 10% annually, exceeding 14 million enrollees across the United States in 2013, or 28% of the total Medicare population (Gold et al., 2013). More recently, the rate of growth in MA enrollment has slowed, and reached 31.7% in 2015 (Sanofi-Aventis, 2016). Under the ACA, payment cuts to participating MCOs have resulted in higher premiums and out-of-pocket costs for the enrollees.

▶ Impact on Cost, Access, and Quality

The growth of managed care in both the private and public health insurance sectors bears ample testimony supporting the widely held belief that managed care provides cost savings and better value for money than traditional indemnity insurance. Widespread use of managed care may also be a testament to a few problematic issues related to health care access and quality. Even as managed care has become the primary vehicle for providing health insurance through employers and to a large extent through Medicaid, Medicare has remained an open field for studying differences between managed care and indemnity insurance.

Influence on Cost Containment

Managed care has been widely credited with slowing the rate of growth in health care expenditures during the 1990s. In the insurance sector, growth rates for premiums slowed during the first half of the 1990s, and by 1996 they had fallen below the rate of inflation (Morrisey and Ohsfeldt, 2003). In the provider sector, between 1990 and 1998, hospitals in areas experiencing high growth in managed care enrollments saw revenue and cost growth rates that were 18 percentage points less than those for hospitals in areas with low managed care enrollments, although this cost-containment effect plateaued after 1998 (Shen, 2005). Cost reductions were also noted in the outpatient sector.

Eventually, a backlash from both enrollees and providers prompted MCOs to back away from aggressive cost-control measures. Hence, the full cost-containment potential of managed care was never realized. For example, the "any willing provider" laws and "freedom of choice" laws (discussed later in the section "Regulation of Managed Care") passed by many states caused premiums to rise and reversed any gains in cost containment made by MCOs (Dugan, 2015). Unfortunately, alternatives for reducing the spiraling costs in the U.S. health care delivery system have not emerged since then. Future cost reductions are not likely to be realized without some mechanism to rationally control utilization, particularly the use of expensive technology.

Impact on Access

Managed care enrollees have good access to primary and preventive care. Baker and colleagues (2004) found that timely breast cancer and cervical cancer screening was twice as likely for women receiving services in geographic areas with greater HMO market share, compared to women in areas with low managed care penetration. More recent studies have reported similar findings on health screenings and diabetes care (Ayanian et al., 2013; Hung et al., 2016). In MA plans, better access to primary care may have been responsible for lowering the risk of preventable hospitalizations. This effect has been particularly beneficial for ethnic/minority groups (Basu, 2012). For some minority groups, disparities in diabetes care are also found to be smaller in MA plans compared to fee-for-service Medicare (Mahmoudi et al., 2016).

In the ACA era, the influx of new Medicaid-insured patients into the managed care market has resulted in limited access to certain health care services for those enrolled in the Medicaid program. Among this population, ED use has increased as well as unmet prescription drug needs. This population also often experiences difficulty seeing a specialist. A major factor in these experiences is the low reimbursement rates in Medicaid programs, which do not encourage providers to take on Medicaid-covered clients (Caswell and Long, 2015). Collectively, these factors may mean that Medicaid-insured patients will have difficulty accessing medical care services.

Influence on Quality of Care

It is not surprising that quality varies across health care plans; however, the overall quality of care in managed care plans has been found to be at least equivalent to that in traditional fee-for-service plans. Despite anecdotes, individual perceptions, and isolated stories propagated by the news media during the 1990s, no comprehensive research to date has clearly demonstrated that managed care's growth has come at the expense of quality in health care. In fact, the available evidence points mostly in the opposite direction. A comprehensive review of the literature by Miller and Luft (2002) concluded that HMO and non-HMO plans provided roughly equal quality of care, as measured by a wide range of conditions, diseases, and interventions. At the same time, HMOs were found to decrease the use of hospitals and other expensive resources. Hence, managed care plans have been cost-effective while delivering levels of quality that are either comparable to or better than those with traditional indemnity plans.

Higher managed care penetration has been associated with increased quality in hospitals based on indicators such as inappropriate utilization, wound infections, and iatrogenic complications (Sari, 2002). More recent studies comparing quality of care in Medicare fee-for-service and MA plans showed that the level of quality, as evaluated by breast cancer screening, quality of diabetes care, cholesterol testing, testing for cardiovascular disease, and various HEDIS measures, was significantly higher in MA plans (Ayanian et al., 2013; Brennan and Shepard, 2010). MA plans are also associated with a reduction in preventable hospitalizations—for example, with urinary tract infections that can be detected early and treated with medications (Nicholas, 2013).

Evidence also suggests that financial pressures do not lead to significant changes in physician behavior because, under capitation, a physician takes full responsibility for the patient's overall care (Eikel, 2002). This is particularly true for life-saving treatment decisions, such as treatment of patients with cancer (Bourjolly et al., 2004). Concerns about disparities in quality of care, based on race and socioeconomic status, are also largely unfounded (DeFrancesco, 2002).

On the flip side, some evidence suggests that quality of care may be lower in for-profit health plans, compared to nonprofit plans (Himmelstein et al., 1999; Schneider et al., 2005). In addition, some evidence indicates that, in MCOs serving Medicaid-insured patients under a capitation scheme, the enrollees may not receive certain services for which the PCPs do not get additional compensation, which may have some impact on quality of care (Quast et al., 2008). After adjusting data for differences in risk, enrollees in MA plans have been found to have a substantially higher likelihood of hospital readmission within 30 days of discharge compared to beneficiaries in original Medicare plan (Friedman et al., 2012). In Medicare Advantage Special Needs Plans (MA-SNPs), the HEDIS measure for osteoporosis testing was found to be worse than in the original Medicare program, although performance on fall risk management was better (Grace et al., 2013).

In the delivery of mental health, earlier reports had suggested that poorer patient outcomes occurred in managed care plans (Rogers et al., 1993; Wells et al., 1989), although later investigations reached the opposite conclusion. In an examination of qualitative and quantitative aspects of specialty managed outpatient mental health treatment, managed care plans were found to achieve cost savings but not at the expense of quality of care (Goldman et al., 2003).

Managed Care Backlash, Regulation, and the Aftermath

The large-scale transition of health care delivery to managed care in the 1990s was met with widespread criticism, which turned into a backlash from consumers, physicians, and legislators across the United States. Three main reasons were behind the discontentment, and widespread media frenzy further shaped unsympathetic public opinion toward managed care.

First, to restrain the spiraling costs of health insurance premiums, employers around the country switched to managed care by dropping, in many instances, traditional indemnity plans that had allowed enrollees to choose any physician or hospital. A large number of employees experienced at least some loss of freedom and, to some extent, faced barriers to free access.

Second, insureds did not see a reduction in their own share of the premium costs or a drop in their out-of-pocket expenses under managed care.

Third, when faced with tight utilization management from MCOs, physicians became openly hostile toward managed care. In national surveys, managed care penetration was found to be negatively correlated with physicians' satisfaction (Landon et al., 2003). Much

of this discontent stemmed from pressure to change the way physicians had traditionally practiced medicine, which had not included any accountability for appropriateness of utilization and costs. Physicians' vocal discontent no doubt also influenced patients' views about managed care. Both physicians and patients perceived that managed care would drive a wedge between the patient–physician relationship.

Ultimately, as the momentum continued to shift toward enrollment in managed care, physicians had little choice except to contract with managed care or face the prospect of losing patients. Employees had little choice except to enroll in managed care plans, or personally bear significantly higher premium costs, or go without health insurance altogether. As this drama unfolded, employers largely remained passive, as their main objective of reducing their own premium costs had been attained.

Regulation of Managed Care

In response to widespread complaints and negative publicity about managed care, many state legislators were prompted to take action because the state governments are primarily responsible for overseeing issues pertaining to health insurance. To address the complaints, states passed an extensive array of anti-managed care legislation: Between 1990 and 1999, states adopted more than 1,000 distinct regulatory provisions against managed care (Kronebusch et al., 2009). At the federal level, the U.S. Congress passed the Newborns' and Mothers' Health Protection Act of 1996, although numerous states already had laws against "drive-through deliveries." The federal law prohibits a health plan from providing less than a 48-hour inpatient maternity coverage for a mother and her child following a normal vaginal delivery and less than a 96-hour coverage following a cesarean section.

Two types of state-legislated statutes are noteworthy:

- *Any willing provider laws* require admission of any provider into a network as long as that provider can abide by the terms and conditions of network membership. A little more than half of all states have such statutes (Noble, 2014). Proponents of such laws argue that they broaden the choice of providers for consumers; opponents contend they raise costs and eliminate price competition. The latter charge arises because the laws weaken MCOs' ability to select providers on the basis of obtaining reduced prices in exchange for the volume of business the MCOs would bring to the providers.
- *Freedom of choice laws* require MCOs to allow their enrollees to seek care from providers outside the panel, and not be penalized for it. Again, the argument in favor of these laws is expansion of choice. Those opposing the laws argue that they increase costs and dilute MCOs' ability to control quality.

Other regulations adopted by many states addressed financial incentives to physicians for curtailing utilization, the right of patients to have an expeditious appeal in case of denial of services, and mandates to include certain benefits in health plans (e.g., chiropractic services, women's health screening, diabetic supplies, obesity care). Some states' legislation included provisions giving enrollees the right to seek civil remedy in the courts for negligent actions of health plans, including denial of services. While anti-managed care legislation may have provided both consumers and providers with certain protections, it also had negative effects by increasing costs (Hurley and Draper, 2002).

The Aftermath

The backlash and anti-managed care laws produced their intended effects, as MCOs scaled back tight controls on utilization and took significant steps to develop better relationships with physicians and other providers. Physicians and hospitals found bargaining power shifting in their direction, mainly through organizational integration, and the providers were able to push back on MCOs by terminating contracts or negotiating more favorable payment arrangements (Short et al., 2001; Strunk et al., 2001).

The balance achieved between the bargaining powers of MCOs on the one hand and providers on the other hand has left consumers in the middle. Employers have been forced to absorb the lion's share of rising premiums and they, in turn, have passed some of those costs on to their employees through higher cost sharing.

▶ Organizational Integration

The term **integration** refers to various strategies that health care organizations employ to achieve economies of operation, diversify existing operations by offering new products or services, or gain market share. In the United States, the integration movement began with hospital mergers and acquisitions during the 1990s and early 2000s—a phenomenon that was national in scope. Numerous reasons can drive hospital consolidation, such as technology, effects of reimbursement, and growth of services in alternative delivery settings, but the role of managed care cannot be underestimated. For instance, some evidence indicates that hospitals gained increased pricing power over MCOs subsequent to consolidations (Capps and Dranove, 2004). Ginsburg (2005) reached the same conclusion: "Hospitals correctly perceived that by merging with others in the same community, they would increase their leverage with health plans" (p. 1514).

Subsequent to the hospital consolidations, physician groups sought to align themselves with hospitals to maintain their autonomy and find refuge from the growing influence of managed care. Hospitals saw such arrangements as mutually beneficial, as increasingly more health care services were moving to the outpatient sector. Large hospital systems were particularly attracted to group practices because group practices could offer a large slice of the patient market to the participating hospitals.

Later, the formation of integrated delivery systems sought to achieve **diversification**—that is, addition of new services that the organization had not offered before. For example, a hospital engaging in diversification may enter into the market for postacute long-term care services by converting an unused acute care wing into a long-term care facility or by acquiring an existing nursing home. In sprawling urban areas, integrated organizations saw the opportunity to more efficiently provide services to the growing populations in these communities.

The highly integrated Kaiser Permanente model, which has been in use in California since the 1940s, has long been known for its cost-effective care with high-quality services to its enrollees. This model has even influenced the mindsets and policy development within many European health care systems (Strandberg-Larsen et al., 2007).

Integration Strategies

Various integration strategies are illustrated in **FIGURE 9-11**. Three strategies are especially popular: (1) outright ownership, such as through a merger or acquisition; (2) joining hands with another organization in the common ownership of an entity; or (3) having a stake in an organization without owning it.

Mergers and Acquisitions

Mergers and acquisitions involve integration of existing assets. **Acquisition** refers to the purchase of one organization by another. The acquired company ceases to exist as a separate entity and is absorbed into the purchasing corporation. A **merger** involves a mutual agreement to unify two or more organizations into a single entity. The separate assets of two organizations are consolidated, typically under a new name. Both entities cease to exist, and a new corporation forms. A merger requires the willingness of all parties, after they have assessed the advantages and disadvantages of merging their organizations.

Small hospitals may merge to gain efficiencies by eliminating duplication of services. A large hospital may acquire smaller hospitals to serve as satellites in a major

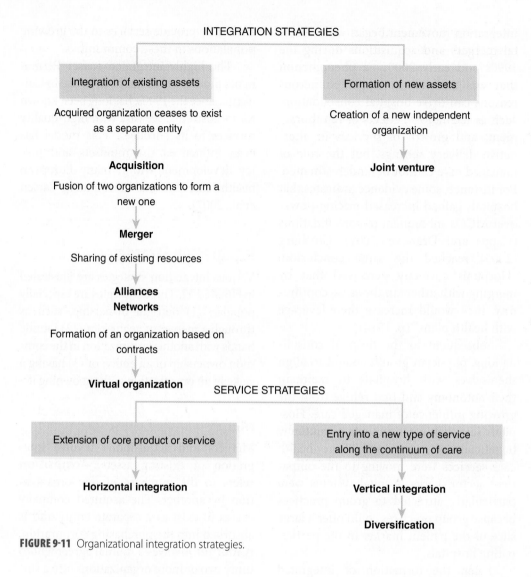

FIGURE 9-11 Organizational integration strategies.

metropolitan area with sprawling suburbs. A regional health system may form after a large hospital has acquired smaller hospitals and certain providers of long-term care, outpatient care, and rehabilitation to diversify its services. Multifacility nursing home chains and home health firms often acquire other facilities as a means to enter new geographic markets.

Joint Ventures

A **joint venture** is formed when two or more institutions share resources to create a new organization to pursue a common purpose (Pelfrey and Theisen, 1989). Each partner in a joint venture continues to conduct business independently. The new company created by the partners also remains independent.

Joint ventures are often used as a diversification strategy when the new service can benefit all the partners and when competing against each other for that service would be undesirable. For example, hospitals in a given region may engage in a joint venture to form a home health agency that benefits all partners. An acute care hospital, a multispecialty physician group practice, a skilled nursing facility, and an insurer may join to offer a managed care plan (Carson et al., 1995). Each of these participants would continue to operate its own business, but they would all have a common stake in the new MCO.

Alliances

In one respect, the health care industry is unique in that organizations often develop cooperative arrangements with rival providers. Cooperation instead of competition, in some situations, eliminates duplication of services while ensuring that all the health needs of the community are fulfilled (Carson et al., 1995). An **alliance** is an agreement between two organizations to share their existing resources without joint ownership of assets.

The main advantages of alliances are threefold:

- Alliances are relatively simple to form.
- Alliances provide the opportunity to evaluate the financial and legal ramifications of the arrangement before a potential "marriage" takes place. Forming an alliance gives organizations the opportunity to evaluate the advantages of an eventual merger.
- Alliances require little financial commitment and can be easily dissolved, similar to an engagement prior to a marriage.

Even when a merger is not contemplated, alliance members can reap the benefits of consolidation while maintaining their independence (Butcher, 2016).

Networks. A network is formed through alliances with numerous providers. It is built around a core organization, such as an MCO, a hospital, or a large group practice. An IPA is also a type of network in which physicians are brought under the umbrella of a nonphysician organization.

Virtual Organizations. Alliances and networks often involve resource-sharing arrangements between organizations. However, when contractual arrangements between organizations form a new organization, the result is referred to as a virtual organization or an organization without walls. The formation of networks based on contractual arrangements is called **virtual integration**. IPAs are a prime example of virtual organizations. The main advantage of virtual organizations is that they require less capital to enter new geographic or service markets (Gabel, 1997). They also bring together scattered entities under one mutually cooperative arrangement. For example, solo practitioners and small group practices can be brought under the umbrella of an IPA.

Service Strategies
Horizontal Integration

Horizontal integration is a growth strategy in which a health care delivery organization extends its core product or service. Commonly, the services are similar to or are substitutes for existing services. Horizontal integration may be achieved through internal development, acquisition, or merger. Horizontally linked organizations may be closely coupled through ownership or loosely coupled through alliances. The main objective of horizontal integration is to control the geographic distribution of a certain type of health care service. Multi-hospital chains, nursing facility chains, or a chain of drugstores, all under the same management, with member facilities offering the same core services or products, are horizontally integrated. Diversification into new products and/or services is not achieved through horizontal integration.

Vertical Integration

Vertical integration links services at different stages in the production process of health care—for example, organization of primary care, acute care, postacute services, and a hospital. The main objective of vertical integration is to increase the comprehensiveness and continuity of care across a continuum of health care services. Hence, vertical integration is a diversification strategy.

Vertical integration may be achieved through acquisitions, mergers, joint ventures, or alliances. Formation of networks and virtual organizations can also involve vertical integration. Vertically integrated regional health systems may be the best-positioned organizations to become the providers of choice for managed care or for direct contracting with self-insured employers (Brown, 1996).

▶ Basic Forms of Integration

The major participants in organizational integration have been physicians and hospitals. Other clinical and nonclinical entities may also be involved, as described in some of the previous examples. In the past, several different types of configurations emerged; however, success of these models was spotty. Lack of experience, misplaced administrative controls, misaligned financial incentives, and unfavorable economic trends were some of the reasons why many of these models failed to gain momentum. A few—namely, management services organizations and physician–hospital organizations—have survived. By comparison, the number of provider-sponsored organizations has greatly declined.

Management Services Organizations

During the dominant phase of MCOs in the 1980s and early 1990s, physicians recognized that they needed management expertise if their practices were to survive in the complex health care environment. In recognition of this need, the **management services organization (MSO)** emerged to supply management expertise, administrative tools, and information technology to physician group practices. Today, MSO services are needed mainly by smaller group practices because they find it uneconomical to employ full-time managers. Dental service organizations have also emerged in recent years to provide management and support services to dental clinics.

Physician–Hospital Organizations

A **physician–hospital organization (PHO)** is a legal entity that forms an alliance between a hospital and local physicians. In addition to contracting with MCOs, if a PHO is large enough, it can contract its services directly to employers, while engaging a third-party administrator to process claims.

Between 1998 and 2000, the number of hospitals associated with PHOs more than doubled. Subsequently, many PHOs failed because of poor management, undercapitalization, and federal antitrust scrutiny. Physician and hospital integration subsequently gained momentum in a health care system that continues to evolve in complex ways. For example, PHOs are often in a prime position to function as accountable care organizations (discussed in the section "Accountable Care Organizations").

Today, hospitals seem to be in the driver's seat, as physicians are increasingly turning to hospitals for financial support. There has been a growing trend of physicians leaving their private practices to seek hospital employment. Among the factors underlying this trend are declines in reimbursement, increases in practice expenses, complexities associated with newer demands such as EHRs, and desire of younger physicians to be employees rather than owners (Jessee, 2011; Minich-Pourshadi, 2013). Hence, some PHOs are becoming more tightly integrated.

Provider-Sponsored Organizations

A risk-bearing entity that incorporated the insurance function into integrated clinical delivery—referred to as a **provider-sponsored organization (PSO)**—emerged in the 1990s. PSOs are sponsored by physicians, by hospitals, or jointly by physicians and hospitals; they compete with regular MCOs by agreeing to provide health care to a defined group of enrollees under capitation. The PSO bypasses the insurance "middleman" by contracting directly with employers and public insurers.

PSOs attracted national attention in 1996 when Congress proposed that PSOs could legitimately participate in Medicare risk contracts. Later, the Balanced Budget Act of 1997 opened up the Medicare market to PSOs as an option to HMOs under the Medicare+Choice program (the precursor to MA). The Balanced Budget Act also required these entities to carry adequate coverage for risk protection.

The initial appeal of PSOs was their promise to deal with patients directly rather than through contracted arrangements, as an HMO would. However, after they suffered financial losses, PSOs failed in large numbers. In many instances, larger HMOs acquired PSOs. One major reason for PSO failures has been their lack of experience with risk management (the insurance function).

More recently, provider organizations have again begun seeking to sponsor their own health plans. Approximately 13% of health systems in the United States already offer health plans in one or more markets (*Trustee*, 2015).

▶ Highly Integrated Health Care Systems

Highly integrated systems are vertically integrated systems that generally include a hospital, a physician component, and at least one systemwide contract with a payer, such as Medicare or MCO. The payers may stipulate some responsibility for quality and cost.

The pace of integration in the U.S. health care system has continued to intensify. Perhaps the primary reason for the drive toward integration is the ongoing evolution of the overall system toward value-based payment models and accountability for population health. In this changing landscape, many organizations have realized that forming partnerships with other providers allows them to share best practices, combine resources, coordinate information technology, strengthen supply chain purchasing power, and reduce the overall cost of providing care to their patient population (Letourneau, 2014).

Some evidence indicates that organizational integration does not negatively affect the quality of care. In addition, the appropriate use of services, such as ED use, may be better aligned in an integrated system (Carlin et al., 2015).

Integrated Delivery Systems

An **integrated delivery system (IDS)**, also called an "integrated delivery network," is a network of organizations that provides or arranges to provide a coordinated continuum of services to a defined population and is willing to be held clinically and fiscally accountable for the outcomes and health status of the population serviced (Shortell et al., 1993). An IDS encompasses various forms of ownership and other strategic linkages among hospitals, physicians, and insurers. One of its objectives is to achieve greater integration of health care services along the continuum of care (Shortell and Hull, 1996). In 2015, more than 54% of all U.S. health care providers were affiliated with IDSs (*Drug Store News*, 2016).

Managed care market domination prompted providers to integrate for three main reasons. First, for MCOs, it is more cost-effective to contract with organizations that offer comprehensive services to ensure a full spectrum of services to the MCO's enrollees—and providers have a vested interest in making their organizations attractive to MCOs. Second, MCOs seek providers who can render services in a cost-efficient manner and who will take responsibility for the quality of those services; in turn, providers seek greater efficiencies by joining with other organizations or by diversifying into providing new services. Large organizations are in a better position to acquire up-to-date management and information systems to monitor their operations and successfully address inefficiencies. Third, hospitals, physicians, and other providers have been concerned with protecting their autonomy. By forging linkages, these providers can strengthen their bargaining power when dealing with MCOs.

Satisfaction of members enrolled in health plans that are integrated with IDSs—such as the Health Alliance Plan and the Kaiser Foundation Health Plan—is considerably higher than member satisfaction with plans in which the provider and the payer are not part of the same organization. In addition, members enrolled in integrated plans have a better understanding of their coverage and the processes necessary to receive services (J. D. Power and Associates, 2011).

A recent comprehensive review of the literature concluded that IDSs may reduce utilization without affecting quality negatively. In some cases, IDSs have lowered health care utilization, but cost savings have not materialized (Hwang et al., 2013). In other cases, IDSs may actually increase costs without any gains in quality (Kralewski et al., 2014).

Accountable Care Organizations

In a general sense, an **accountable care organization (ACO)** is an integrated group of providers who are willing and able to take responsibility for improving the overall health status, care efficiency, and satisfaction with care for a defined population (DeVore and Champion, 2011). ACOs are motivated to eliminate unnecessary care because their contract payments from insurers cover the entire continuum of care (Song and Fisher, 2016).

In an attempt to realize the threefold expectation of cost, quality, and improvement in population health, ACOs use mechanisms already prevalent in managed care and IDSs—disease management, care coordination, sharing of cost savings with providers, use of information technology, and so forth (Burns and Pauly, 2012). Consequently, the operational strategies available to ACOs are not much different from what their predecessors have used. Because ACOs are organizationally based on the IDS model, they may not achieve cost efficiencies, as these outcomes are often lacking in IDSs.

The formation of ACOs in the Medicare program has been closely tied to the ACA of 2010. Within the more-regulated environment under the ACA, payment reforms hold both "carrots and sticks." The general evolution of payment reform is guided by value-based payments (as opposed to volume-based payments), in which incentives are aligned with the goal of achieving better health outcomes for the dollars spent. For example, a shared savings program, implemented in 2013, authorized Medicare to pay additional funds to providers if an ACO achieved targeted cost savings while meeting defined quality objectives. Spending reductions under this program actually exceeded bonus payments to ACOs in 2014. Hence, shared savings may be a fiscally viable alternative payment model for Medicare (McWilliams, 2016).

As might be expected, ACOs have diverse contracting arrangements with payers and demonstrate wide variations in their performance. Some evidence suggests that ACOs with commercial payer contracts in the private market produce better value. They have higher quality scores at lower benchmark expenditures, compared with ACOs that have only public contracts with Medicare and Medicaid (Peiris et al., 2016). It is too early to speculate how such differences might affect the future of ACOs. Of particular interest would be the continuity of the shared savings program, and its ongoing success, given the disparities in efficiencies achieved by ACOs. On the supply side, however, many ACOs have sustained financial losses because the shared savings bonuses have not covered the cost of delivering population health (Chen et al., 2016).

Today, ACOs remain in their infancy. Their eventual success or failure will depend on their ability to consistently deliver value and reduce the cost of health care. The main barrier to such an achievement is a U.S. health care delivery system and U.S. consumer expectations that put a premium on specialty care and use of the latest technology (including new drugs), without taking into account any concerns about value. Indeed, early results suggest that, in the short term, ACOs may focus largely on primary care-related strategies to achieve cost reductions while doing little to coordinate specialty care, acute care, and postacute care—steps that will certainly be necessary in the longer term (Lewis et al., 2016).

Lack of clarity also exists on three main issues related to ACOs:

- While hospitals and larger clinics are joining hands to form ACOs, smaller physician practices may get left out of the picture, preventing them from reaping any benefits that the ACOs may provide.

- It remains to be seen how safety-net providers, including community health centers and public hospitals—which have long experience in caring for vulnerable populations—will be included in ACOs (Witgert and Hess, 2012).
- Under certain conditions, ACOs could dominate a geographic market, reduce competition, and harm consumers through higher prices or lower quality of care.

The last concern can be addressed through existing antitrust laws. **Antitrust** policy consists of federal and state laws that prohibit or regulate certain types of business practices—namely, price fixing, price discrimination, exclusive contracting arrangements, and acquisitions and mergers that may stifle competition. Bacher and colleagues (2013) argued that antitrust policy faces a trade-off in regard to ACOs. On the one hand, pursuit of market competitiveness would limit ACOs' size and geographic reach. On the other hand, antitrust policies may make it more difficult for ACOs to effectively integrate their operations to achieve economies of scale and care coordination.

Payer–Provider Integration

In a radically changing health care system, payer–provider integration is on the rise. For example, insurance companies have started to acquire large physician practice groups and health systems as a strategy to gain more control over the delivery of health care (Berarducci et al., 2012).

It is early in the game, but collaboration between managed care and providers as risk-bearing entities could become the next major trend. Because most MCOs already have expertise in managing financial risk, these organizations would stand a much better chance to succeed than the earlier PSOs. If this trend does take off, the same provider entities that had rebelled against the growing power of managed care not too long ago would now join hands with it out of a mutual fear of the encroachment of a much more powerful adversary—the government.

▶ Summary

Managed care evolved through the integration of the insurance function with the concepts of contract practice and prepaid group practice of the late 19th and early 20th centuries. Even though managed care has since become the dominant medium through which the vast majority of Americans obtain health care services, its full potential to achieve cost-effectiveness has been thwarted by opposition from providers, consumers, and policymakers. Participation in the HEDIS program, however, has improved the quality of services provided by MCOs.

The growing power of managed care was one main factor that triggered integration among health care providers. The pace of integration between physicians, hospitals, and other providers has continued to accelerate in recent years. Highly integrated organizations are held accountable for achieving specific objectives related to costs, quality, and consumer satisfaction. Cost containment, however, remains an elusive goal, perhaps because the U.S. health care delivery system continues to be plagued by an overemphasis on specialization and overuse of costly technology.

▶ Test Your Understanding

Terminology

accountable care
  organization (ACO)
acquisition
alliance
antitrust
carve-out
case management
closed-panel
concurrent utilization
  review
discharge planning
disease management
diversification
exclusive provider plan
fee schedule
formulary
group model
health maintenance
  organization (HMO)

horizontal integration
indemnity insurance
independent practice
  association (IPA)
integrated delivery system
  (IDS)
integration
IPA model
joint venture
management services
  organization (MSO)
merger
mixed model
network model
open-panel
panel
physician–hospital
  organization (PHO)

point-of-service
  (POS) plan
practice profiling
preferred provider
  organization (PPO)
primary care case
  management (PCCM)
prospective utilization
  review
provider-sponsored
  organization (PSO)
retrospective utilization
  review
staff model
triple-option plans
utilization review (UR)
vertical integration
virtual integration

Review Questions

1. What are some of the key differences between traditional indemnity insurance and managed care?
2. What are the three main payment mechanisms used in managed care? With each mechanism, who bears the risk?
3. Explain how the fee-for-service practice of medicine led to uncontrolled utilization.
4. How do MCOs achieve cost-efficiencies by integrating the quad functions, risk sharing with providers, and care coordination? What are some of the inefficiencies created by managed care?

5. Discuss the concept of utilization monitoring and control.
6. How does case management achieve efficiencies in the delivery of health care? How does case management differ from disease management?
7. Explain how MCOs engage in pharmaceutical management. How does utilization review apply to drug management?
8. Describe the three utilization review methods, giving appropriate examples. Discuss the benefits of each type of utilization review.
9. What is an HMO? How does it differ from a PPO?

10. Briefly explain the four main models for organizing an HMO. Discuss the advantages and disadvantages of each model.

11. What is a point-of-service plan? Why did it initially grow in popularity? What caused its subsequent decline?

12. To what extent has managed care been successful in containing health care costs?

13. Has the quality of health care declined as a result of managed care? Explain.

14. What is organizational integration? What is its ultimate aim? Why did health care organizations integrate?

15. What is the difference between a merger and an acquisition? What is the purpose of these organizational consolidations? Give examples.

16. When would a joint venture be considered a preferable integration strategy?

17. What is the main advantage of two organizations forming an alliance?

18. State the main strategic objectives of horizontal and vertical integration.

19. What is an accountable care organization (ACO)? Describe its current status in U.S. health care delivery.

▶ **References**

Angalakuditi, M., and J. Gomes. 2011. Retrospective drug utilization review: Impact of pharmacist interventions on physician prescribing. *Clinicoeconomics and Outcomes Research* 3: 105–108.

Aventis Pharmaceuticals and SMG Marketing-Verispan. 2002. *Managed care digest series: HMO-PPO/Medicare–Medicaid digest*. Bridgewater, NJ: Aventis Pharmaceuticals.

Ayanian, J. Z., et al. 2013. Medicare beneficiaries more likely to receive appropriate ambulatory services in HMOs than in traditional Medicare. *Health Affairs* 32, no. 7: 1228–1235.

Bacher, G. E., et al. 2013. Regulatory neutrality is essential to establishing a level playing field for accountable care organizations. *Health Affairs* 32, no. 8: 1426–1432.

Baker, L., et al. 2004. The effect of area HMO market share on cancer screening. *Health Services Research* 39, no. 6: 1751–1772.

Basu, J. 2012. Medicare managed care and primary care quality: Examining racial/ethnic effects across states. *Health Care Management Science* 15, no. 1: 15–28.

Berarducci, J., et al. 2012. New partnership opportunities for payers and providers. *Healthcare Financial Management* 66, no. 10: 58–61.

Berk, M. L., and A. C. Monheit. 2001. The concentration of health expenditures revisited. *Health Affairs* 20, no. 2: 9–18.

Borenstein, J., et al. 2004. The association between quality improvement activities performed by managed care organizations and quality of care. *American Journal of Medicine* 117, no. 5: 297–304.

Bourjolly, J. N., et al. 2004. The impact of managed health care in the United States on women with breast cancer and the providers who treat them. *Cancer Nursing* 27, no. 1: 45–54.

Brennan, N., and M. Shepard. 2010. Comparing quality of care in the Medicare program. *American Journal of Managed Care* 16, no. 11: 841–848.

Brill, J. V. 2007. Trends in prescription drug plans delivering the Medicare Part D prescription drug benefit. *American Journal of Health-System Pharmacy* 64 (suppl 10): S3–S6.

Brown, M. 1996. Mergers, networking, and vertical integration: Managed care and investor-owned hospitals. *Health Care Management Review* 21, no. 1: 29–37.

Brown, R. S., et al. 2012. Six features of Medicare Coordinated Care Demonstration Programs that cut hospital admission of high-risk patients. *Health Affairs* 31, no. 6: 1156–1166.

Burns, L. R., and M. V. Pauly. 2012. Accountable care organization may have difficulty avoiding the failures of integrated delivery networks of the 1990s. *Health Affairs* 31, no. 11: 2407–2416.

Butcher, L. 2016. Building alliances to stay independent. *Hospitals & Health Networks* 90, no. 7: 46–52.

Capps, C., and D. Dranove. 2004. Hospital consolidation and negotiated PPO prices. *Health Affairs* 23, no. 2: 175–181.

Carlin, C. S., et al. 2015. Changes in quality of health care delivery after vertical integration. *Health Services Research* 50, no. 4: 1043–1068.

Carson, K. D., et al. 1995. *Management of healthcare organizations.* Cincinnati, OH: South-Western College Publishing.

Caswell, K. J., and S. K. Long. 2015. The expanding role of managed care in the Medicaid program: Implications for health care access, use, and expenditures for nonelderly adults. *Inquiry* 52. doi: 10.1177/0046958015575524.

Chen, C., et al. 2009. Evaluation of a nurse practitioner–led care management model in reducing inpatient drug utilization and cost. *Nursing Economics* 27, no. 3: 160–168.

Chen, C. T., et al. 2016. Transforming healthcare delivery: Why and how accountable care organizations must evolve. *Journal of Hospital Medicine* 11, no. 9: 658–661.

Conti, M. S. 2013. Effect of Medicaid disease management programs on emergency admissions and inpatient costs. *Health Services Research* 48, no. 4: 1359–1374.

Daubresse, M., et al. 2013. Impact of a drug utilization review program on high-risk use of prescription controlled substances. *Pharmacoepidemiology and Drug Safety* 23, no. 4: 419–427.

DeFrancesco, L. B. 2002. HMO enrollees experience fewer disparities than older insured populations. *Findings Brief: Health Care Financing & Organization* 5, no. 2: 1–2.

Deom, M., et al. 2010. What doctors think about the impact of managed care tools on quality of care, costs, autonomy, and relations with patients. *BMC Health Services Research* 10, no. 331: 2–8.

DeVore, S., and R. W. Champion. 2011. Driving population health through accountable care organizations. *Health Affairs* 30, no. 1: 41–50.

DoBias, M. 2008. Uneven results. *Modern Healthcare* 38, no. 40: 12.

Drug Store News. 2016. Healthcare delivery changes. *Drug Store News* 38, no. 8 (special section): 31–35.

Dugan, J. 2015. Trends in managed care cost containment: An analysis of the managed care backlash. *Health Economics* 24, no. 12: 1604–1618.

Eikel, C. V. 2002. Fewer patient visits under capitation offset by improved quality of care: Study brings evidence to debate over physician payment methods. *Findings Brief: Health Care Financing & Organization* 5, no. 3: 1–2.

Friedman, B., et al. 2012. Likelihood of hospital readmission after first discharge: Medicare Advantage vs. fee-for-service patients. *Inquiry* 49, no. 3: 202–213.

Gabel, J. 1997. Ten ways HMOs have changed during the 1990s. *Health Affairs* 16, no. 3: 134–145.

Ginsburg, P. B. 2005. Competition in health care: Its evolution over the past decade. *Health Affairs* 24, no. 6: 1512–1522.

Gold, M., et al. 2013. *Medicare Advantage 2013 spotlight: Enrollment market update.* Menlo Park, CA: Kaiser Family Foundation.

Goldman, W., et al. 2003. A four-year study of enhancing outpatient psychotherapy in managed care. *Psychiatric Services* 54, no. 1: 41–49.

Grace, S. C., et al. 2013. Health-related quality of life and quality of care in specialized Medicare managed care plans. *Journal of Ambulatory Care Management* 36, no. 1: 72–84.

Himmelstein, D., et al. 1999. Quality of care in investor-owned vs not-for-profit HMOs. *Journal of the American Medical Association* 282, no. 2: 159–163.

Hung, A., et al. 2016. The effect of Medicare Advantage enrollment on mammographic screening. *American Journal of Managed Care* 22, no. 2: e53–e59.

Hurley, R. E., and D. A. Draper. 2002. Health plan responses to managed care regulation. *Managed Care Quarterly* 10, no. 4: 30–42.

Hwang, W., et al. 2013. Effects of integrated delivery system on cost and quality. *American Journal of Managed Care* 19, no. 5: e175–e184.

J. D. Power and Associates. 2011. *Press release: J.D. Power and Associates reports: Members of health plans with integrated delivery models are more satisfied than members without integrated plans.*

Available at: http://content2.businesscenter.jd
power.com/JDPAContent/CorpComm/News
/content/Releases/pdf/2011028-natl.pdf.
Accessed September 2013.

Jessee, W. F. 2011. Is there an ACO in your future? *MGMA Connexion* 11, no. 1: 5–6.

Kaiser Family Foundation and Health Research and Educational Trust (Kaiser/HRET). 2002. *Employer health benefits: 2002 annual survey*. Menlo Park, CA: Author.

Kaiser Family Foundation and Health Research and Educational Trust (Kaiser/HRET). 2003. *Employer health benefits: 2003 annual survey*. Menlo Park, CA: Author.

Kaiser Family Foundation and Health Research and Educational Trust (Kaiser/HRET). 2016. *Employer health benefits: 2016 annual survey*. Menlo Park, CA: Author.

Keating, N. L., et al. 2007. The influence of cost containment strategies and physicians' financial arrangements on patients' trust and satisfaction. *Journal of Ambulatory Care Management* 30, no. 2: 92–104.

Kongstvedt, P. R., and D. W. Plocher. 1995. Integrated health care delivery systems. In: *Essentials of managed health care*. P. R. Kongstvedt, ed. Gaithersburg, MD: Aspen Publishers. pp. 35–49.

Kralewski, J., et al. 2014. Do integrated health care systems provide lower-cost, higher-quality care? *Physician Executive* 40, no. 2: 14–18.

Kravitz, R. 2008. Beyond gatekeeping: Enlisting patients as agents for quality and cost-containment. *Journal of General Internal Medicine* 23, no. 10: 1722–1723.

Kronebusch, K., et al. 2009. Managed care regulation in the states: The impact on physicians' practices and clinical autonomy. *Journal of Health Politics, Policy, and Law* 34, no. 2: 219–259.

Landon, B. E., et al. 2003. Changes in career satisfaction among primary care and specialist physicians, 1997–2001. *Journal of the American Medical Association* 289, no. 4: 442–449.

Lattimer, C. 2005. Advanced care management strategies reduce costs and improve patient health in high-risk insurance pools. *Lippincott's Case Management* 10, no. 5: 261–263.

Letourneau, R. 2014. Partnering for better population health management. *Health Leaders Magazine* 17, no. 4: 48–51.

Levine, D., and J. Mulligan. 2015. Overutilization, overutilized. *Journal of Health Politics, Policy & Law* 40, no. 2: 421–437.

Lewis, V. A., et al. 2016. Clinical coordination in accountable care organizations: A qualitative study. *Health Care Management Review*. [Epub ahead of print]. doi: 10.1097/HMR.0000000000000141.

MacColl, W. A. 1966. *Group practice and prepayment of medical care*. Washington, DC: Public Affairs Press.

Mackie, D. L., and D. K. Decker. 1981. *Group and IPA HMOs*. Gaithersburg, MD: Aspen Publishers.

Mahmoudi, E., et al. 2016. Does Medicare managed care reduce racial/ethnic disparities in diabetes prevention care and healthcare expenditure? *American Journal of Managed Care* 22, no. 10: e360–e367.

Mattke, S. 2008. Is there disease management backlash? *American Journal of Managed Care* 14, no. 6: 349–350.

McGuire, J. P. 1994. The growth of managed care. *Health Care Financial Management* 48, no. 8: 10.

McWilliams, J. M. 2016. Changes in Medicare shared savings program savings from 2013 to 2014. *Journal of the American Medical Association* 316, no. 16: 1711–1713.

Melnick, G. A., et al. 2011. The increased concentration of health plan markets can benefit consumers through lower hospital prices. *Health Affairs* 30, no. 9: 1728–1733.

Miller, R. H., and H. S. Luft. 1997. Does managed care lead to better or worse quality of care? *Health Affairs* 16, no. 5: 7–26.

Miller, R. H., and H. S. Luft. 2002. HMO plan performance update: An analysis of the literature, 1997–2001. *Health Affairs* 21, no. 4: 63–86.

Minich-Pourshadi, K. 2013. The drive to hire docs. *Health Leaders Magazine* 16, no. 2: 46–51.

Morrisey, M. A., et al. 2013. Favorable selection, risk adjustment, and the Medicare Advantage program. *Health Services Research* 48, no. 3: 1039–1056.

Morrisey, M. A., and R. L. Ohsfeldt. 2003. Do "any willing provider" and "freedom of choice" laws affect HMO market share? *Inquiry* 40, no. 4: 362–374.

Moscovice, I., et al. 1998. Expanding rural managed care: Enrollment patterns and prospects. *Health Affairs* 17, no. 1: 172–179.

National Center for Health Statistics. 1998. *Health, United States, 1998*. Hyattsville, MD: U.S. Department of Health and Human Services.

National Committee for Quality Assurance (NCQA). 2017. *HEDIS 2017 measures*. Available at: http://www.ncqa.org/Portals/0/HEDISQM/HEDIS2017/HEDIS%202017%20Volume%202%20List%20of%20Measures.pdf?ver=2016-06-27-135433-350. Accessed January 3, 2017.

Ng, A., et al. 2013. Self-efficacy and health status improve after a wellness program in persons with multiple sclerosis. *Disability & Rehabilitation* 35, no. 12: 1039–1044.

Nguyen, N. X., and F. W. Derrick. 1997. Physician behavioral response to a Medicare price reduction. *Health Services Research* 32, no. 3: 283–298.

Nicholas, L. H. 2013. Better quality of care or healthier patients? Hospital utilization by Medicare Advantage and fee-for-service enrollees. *Forum for Health Economics & Policy* 16, no. 1: 137–161.

Noble, A. 2014. *Any willing or authorized providers.* National Conference of State Legislatures. Available at: http://www.ncsl.org/research/health/any-willing-or-authorized-providers.aspx. Accessed January 11, 2017.

Pati, S., et al. 2005. Health expenditures for privately insured adults enrolled in managed care gatekeeping vs indemnity plans. *American Journal of Public Health* 95, no. 2: 286–291.

Peiris, D., et al. 2016. ACOs holding commercial contracts are larger and more efficient than noncommercial ACOs. *Health Affairs* 35, no. 10: 1849–1856.

Pelfrey, S., and B. A. Theisen. 1989. Joint venture in health care. *Journal of Nursing Administration* 19, no. 4: 39–42.

Phillips, R. L., et al. 2014. Cost, utilization, and quality of care: An evaluation of Illinois' Medicaid primary care case management program. *Annals of Family Medicine* 12, no. 5: 408–417.

Quast, T., et al. 2008. Does the quality of care in Medicaid MCOs vary with the form of physician compensation? *Health Economics* 17, no. 4: 545–550.

Rakich, J. S., et al. 1992. *Managing health services organizations*. 3rd ed. Baltimore, MD: Health Professions Press.

Rice, T. H., and R. J. Labelle. 1989. Do physicians induce demand for medical services? *Journal of Health Politics, Policy and Law* 14, no. 3: 587–600.

Robinson, J. C. 2002. Renewed emphasis on consumer cost sharing in health insurance benefit design. *Health Affairs Web Exclusives* 2002: W139–W154.

Rogers, W. H., et al. 1993. Outcomes for adult outpatients with depression under prepaid or fee-for-service care: Results from the Medical Outcomes Study. *Archives of General Psychiatry* 50, no. 7: 517–525.

Sanofi-Aventis. 2013. *Managed care digest series, 2013: Public payer digest*. Bridgewater, NJ: Author.

Sanofi-Aventis. 2016. *Managed care digest series, 2016: Public payer digest*. Bridgewater, NJ: Author.

Sari, N. 2002. Do competition and managed care improve quality? *Health Economics* 11, no. 7: 571–584.

Schneider, E. C., et al. 2005. Quality of care in for-profit and not-for-profit health plans enrolling Medicare beneficiaries. *American Journal of Medicine* 118, no. 12: 1392–1400.

Schwenkglenks, M., et al. 2006. Economic efficiency of gatekeeping compared with fee for service plans: A Swiss example. *Journal of Epidemiology and Community Health* 60, no. 1: 24–30.

Shen, Y. 2005. *Is managed care still an effective cost containment device?* Freeman Spogli Institute for International Studies at Stanford University. Available at: http://fsi.stanford.edu/events/is_managed_care_still_an_effective_cost_containment_device. Accessed May 2011.

Short, A. C., et al. 2001. *Provider network instability: Implications for choice, costs, and continuity of care.* Community Tracking Study Issue Brief No. 39. Washington, DC: Center for Studying Health System Change.

Short, A. C., et al. 2003, October. *Disease management: A leap of faith to lower-cost, higher-quality health care.* Issue Brief No. 69. Washington, DC: Center for Studying Health System Change.

Shortell, S. M., and K. E. Hull. 1996. The new organization of the health care delivery system.

In: *Strategic choices for a changing health care system*. S. H. Altman and U. E. Reinhardt, eds. Chicago, IL: Health Administration Press.

Shortell, S. M., et al. 1993. Creating organized delivery systems: The barriers and facilitators. *Hospital and Health Services Administration* 38, no. 4: 447–466.

Song, Z., and E. S. Fisher. 2016. The ACO experiment in infancy: Looking back and looking forward. *Journal of the American Medical Association* 316, no. 7: 705–706.

Southwick, K. 1997. Case study: How United Health-Care and two contracting hospitals address cost and quality in era of hyper-competition. *Strategies for Healthcare Excellence* (COR Healthcare Resources) 10, no. 8: 1–9.

Starner, C. I., et al. 2009. Effect of retrospective drug utilization review on potentially inappropriate prescribing in the elderly. *American Journal of Geriatric Pharmacotherapy* 7, no. 1: 11–19.

Strandberg-Larsen, M., et al. 2007. Kaiser Permanente revisited: Can European health care systems learn? *Eurohealth* 13, no. 4: 24–26.

Strunk, B. C., et al. 2001. Tracking health care costs. *Health Affairs Suppl. Web Exclusives* W39–W50.

Tisnado, D. M., et al. 2008. Financial incentives for quality in breast cancer care. *American Journal of Managed Care* 14, no. 7: 457–466.

Trustee. 2015. Considering a provider-backed health plan? Strategic considerations for executives & boards. *Trustee* 68, no. 10: 23–24.

Tu, H. T. 2005. *More Americans willing to limit physician–hospital choice for lower medical costs.*

Issue Brief No. 94. Washington, DC: Center for Studying Health System Change.

Wagner, E. R. 1995. Types of managed care organizations. In: *Essentials of managed health care*. P. R. Kongstvedt, ed. Gaithersburg, MD: Aspen Publishers. pp. 24–34.

Wells, K. B., et al. 1989. Detection of depressive disorder for patients receiving prepaid or fee-for-service care: Results from the Medical Outcomes Study. *Journal of the American Medical Association* 262, no. 23: 3298–3302.

Wilkerson, J. D., et al. 1997. The emerging competitive managed care marketplace. In: *Competitive managed care: The emerging health care system*. J. D. Wilkerson et al., eds. San Francisco, CA: Jossey-Bass Publishers.

Witgert, K., and C. Hess. 2012. Including safety-net providers in integrated delivery systems: Issues and options for policymakers. *Issue Brief: Commonwealth Fund pub. 1617*, 20: 1–18. Available at: http://www.nashp.org/sites /default/files/Including.SN_.Providers.in _.IDS_.pdf. Accessed May 2017.

Yip, W. C. 1998. Physician response to Medicare fee reductions: Changes in the volume of coronary artery bypass graft (CABG) surgeries in the Medicare and private sectors. *Journal of Health Economics* 17, no. 6: 675–699.

Zelman, W. A. 1996. *The changing health care marketplace*. San Francisco, CA: Jossey-Bass Publishers.

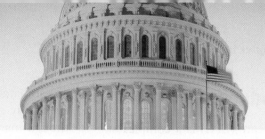

CHAPTER 10
Long-Term Care

LEARNING OBJECTIVES

- Describe the concept of long-term care (LTC) and its main features.
- Discuss the various types of LTC services.
- Describe who needs LTC and why.
- Identify the large variety of home- and community-based LTC services, and who pays for these services.
- Describe LTC institutions and the levels of services they provide.
- Discuss specialized LTC facilities and continuing care retirement communities.
- Explore institutional trends, utilization, and costs.
- Explore the various aspects of private LTC insurance.

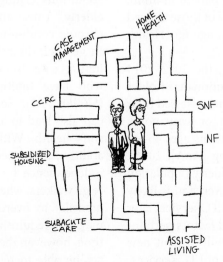

"Now, honey, where are we supposed to go from here?"

▶ Introduction

Long-term care (LTC) is a complex subsystem within the larger, even more complex U.S. health care delivery system. It escapes a simple definition. It encompasses numerous services. Several different sources of financing are associated with the different services. The sources of public financing have their own eligibility criteria, so not everyone qualifies. Regular health insurance does not cover LTC; if it does, the coverage is limited. Private insurance just for LTC has made limited headway. Even many people using LTC services do not realize that they are receiving LTC because often the recipients of those services are not in a nursing home.

An estimated 9 million Americans of all ages use paid LTC services annually (Harris-Kojetin et al., 2016). Although LTC services are not restricted to the elderly (people age 65 and older), the elderly are the predominant users of this care and most LTC services have been designed with the elderly patient in mind. Even so, an estimated 37% of those in need of LTC are younger than age 65 (Health Policy Institute, 2003).

In a survey covering the 2012–2014 period, 44% of noninstitutionalized older persons in the United States assessed their own health as excellent or very good, compared to 55% for persons ages 45–64 (Administration on Aging [AoA], 2016). The growing nonwhite elderly population is in poorer health, however, and is likely to face a greater need for LTC services later in life. Social and cultural factors pertaining to minority groups will present new challenges in the delivery of LTC services.

According to the U.S. Department of Health and Human Services (DHHS; 2017), an estimated 70% of older Americans will eventually need some type of LTC, even though many may never leave their own homes. Surveys over time have shown that the vast majority of older Americans wish to stay in their own homes indefinitely. Community-based services are not only preferred by most older people, but are also more economical. Hence, these services have grown more rapidly than LTC institutions. To reflect this shift, the term "long-term services and supports" (LTSS), has been suggested to refer to a broad spectrum of LTC options (Reinhard et al., 2011).

The clients of LTC need a variety of health care services over time. Hence, LTC cannot be an isolated component of the health care delivery system. Ideally, the LTC system will interface with the rest of the system to provide an easy transition among the various types of health care settings and services, both LTC and non-LTC.

Many individuals require LTC because of functional deficits arising from chronic conditions (Hung et al., 2012). Among elderly Americans, 80% have multiple chronic conditions (Gerteis et al., 2014). In general, disability and functional limitations rise dramatically among persons who have multiple chronic conditions (**FIGURE 10-1**). Serious illness or injury can also lead to a rapid decline in a person's health. With certain types of disabilities, many people can maintain their independence by using adaptive devices (e.g., walkers, wheelchairs, adaptive eating utensils) to overcome their deficits and may not require any LTC services. Over time, however, the individual may no longer be able to perform certain common tasks of daily living because of functional decline; LTC services are then needed.

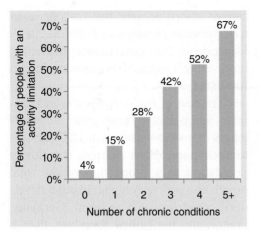

FIGURE 10-1 People with multiple chronic conditions are more likely to have activity limitations.

Reproduced from Partnership for Solutions and Johns Hopkins University. 2002. *Chronic conditions: Making the case for ongoing care.* Baltimore, MD: Johns Hopkins University. p. 12.

Cognitive impairment may also lead to functional decline. **Cognitive impairment** is a mental disorder that is indicated by a person having difficulty remembering, learning new things, concentrating, or making decisions that affect the individual's everyday life. Cognitive impairment ranges from mild to severe, and may lead to disturbing behaviors. Cognitive impairment with or without dementia contributes to neuropsychiatric symptoms and increased disability (Tabert et al., 2002).

Two common indicators used to assess functional limitations are the activities of daily living (ADLs) scale and instrumental activities of daily living (IADLs). As examples, ADLs include a person's ability to bathe, dress, and eat; IADLs include a person's ability to prepare meals, do housework, and manage medication use. Limitations in ADLs indicate a more severe decline in a person's functional status than limitations in IADLs do. People receiving care in nursing homes have a greater degree of ADL decline compared

to people who can live at home or in community housing that offers some support services (**FIGURE 10-2**).

In 2014, a person who attained the age of 65 could expect to live for another 19 years (National Center for Health Statistics, 2016). As the elderly population in the United States continues to grow, issues related to chronic conditions, accompanying disability, and the need for LTC services will intensify. By 2030, 20% of

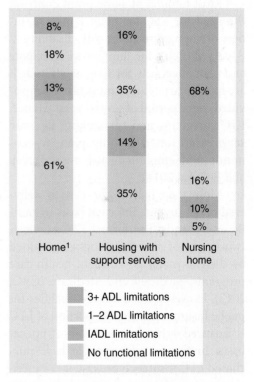

FIGURE 10-2 Medicare enrollees age 65 and older with functional limitations according to where they live, 2009.

[1] Living at home does not mean living at home alone. Housing with support services may offer meals, housekeeping, laundry, or help with medications.

Note: Numbers may not add to 100 because of rounding.

Reproduced from Federal Interagency Forum on Aging-Related Statistics. 2012. *Older Americans 2012: Key indicators of well-being.* Washington, DC: US Government Printing Office. p. 61.

the total U.S. population is projected to be elderly, up from 14.5% in 2014. The population consisting of people age 85 or older is expected to grow the fastest of all age groups in the country over this span of time. That growth in the elderly population will bring a corresponding surge in the number of elderly people with functional and cognitive limitations. Hence, the need for assistance is expected to increase sharply in the coming decades (Congressional Budget Office [CBO], 2013).

Most families at some point confront the need for LTC for older family members or younger relatives with disability. It is very difficult for families to anticipate and plan effectively for LTC needs, which are highly variable and must often be provided over a period of several years. Hence, LTC caregiving and careseeking for paid services are often accompanied by economic and emotional challenges (Kwak and Polivka, 2014).

More than half of the care is delivered on an unpaid, informal basis by family and friends. For formal LTC services, two-thirds of the financing is provided by the two major government health care programs, Medicaid and Medicare (CBO, 2013). However, not everyone qualifies for public insurance. A smaller portion of LTC is financed privately on an out-of-pocket basis. In the past, few people have purchased LTC insurance because it is expensive. As costs rise, even fewer people may be able to afford LTC insurance in the future.

Paying for LTC is one of the great financial burdens for individuals and the United States as a nation. Even as the number of people needing LTC services grows inexorably, the capacity of people to pay for services will likely decline. Even now, Americans with the median income cannot afford to pay the cost of most LTC services (Kwak and Polivka, 2014). Dependence on government financing, however, will put an enormous burden on future taxpayers.

The rest of the developed world also faces aging-related problems and challenges in providing adequate LTC services to their populations. Indeed, the elderly population as a proportion of the total population is already higher in other developed countries, such as Japan, Germany, France, and the United Kingdom, than it is in the United States. Clearly, the U.S. health care system is not alone in facing tough challenges in regard to LTC.

This chapter provides an overview of LTC, its main clients, various types of community-based and institutional services, and financing of these services. LTC services form a continuum, from basic help to more advanced care, to address the varied needs of a heterogeneous population. Even the elderly, who are the predominant users of LTC services, are not a homogeneous group; thus, they need a diverse group of services to meet their LTC needs.

▶ The Nature of Long-Term Care

Long-term care (LTC) can be defined as a variety of individualized, well-coordinated services that promote the maximum possible independence for people with functional limitations and are provided over an extended period of time in accordance with a holistic approach, while maximizing the care recipients' quality of life. To the extent possible, the delivery of LTC should employ appropriate current technology and available evidence-based practices. LTC is unique in health care delivery, and is multidimensional.

Variety of Services

A variety of LTC services are necessary because individual needs, as determined by health status, finances, and other factors, vary greatly among people who require these services. Hence, services should (1) fit the needs of different individuals, (2) address their changing needs over time, and (3) suit their personal preferences.

Individualized Services

LTC services are tailored to the needs of the individual patient. Those needs are determined by an assessment of the individual's current physical, mental, and emotional condition. Other factors used for making the assessment include a history of the patient's medical and psychosocial conditions; a social history of family relationships, former occupation, and leisure activities; and cultural factors, such as racial and ethnic background, language, and religious practices. The information obtained from a comprehensive assessment is used to develop an individualized plan of care that addresses each type of need through customized interventions.

Well-Coordinated Total Care

LTC providers are responsible for managing the total health care needs of an individual client. **Total care** requires that any health care need is recognized, evaluated, and addressed by appropriate clinical professionals (Singh, 2016). Hence, LTC must interface with non-LTC services (**FIGURE 10-3**). The main non-LTC services include primary care, mental health services, acute care hospitals, and various outpatient services, such as those provided by specialist physicians, dentists, optometrists, podiatrists, diagnostic labs, and imaging centers.

Patients needing LTC often require coordination among many different health care services as different needs arise over time. For most people, managing the myriad of health care services, eligibility requirements, and financing is an overwhelming challenge. Hence, case management (discussed later under "Case Management") becomes an important service for many people. One key role of case management is to match client needs with available services that are likely to best address those needs, regardless of whether they are obtained within the LTC sector or from the non-LTC sector.

Maintenance of Residual Function

As a person ages, chronic ailments, comorbidity, disability, and dependency tend to follow each other in a roughly linear sequence. Serious physical or mental illness, accidents, severe birth defects, and cognitive impairment may also lead to functional decline and create dependency. In some cases, the dependency is short term; in other cases, it lasts longer, perhaps even for the rest of the person's life.

Dependency, because of a loss of ability to independently perform certain IADL and/or ADL functions, creates the need for LTC. Caregiver assistance becomes necessary when a person is either unable or unwilling to perform daily living tasks. In that case, LTC has two main goals: (1) to

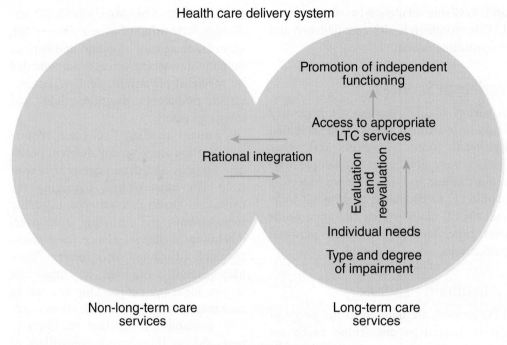

Health care delivery system

Promotion of independent functioning

Access to appropriate LTC services

Rational integration

Evaluation and reevaluation

Individual needs

Type and degree of impairment

Non-long-term care services

Long-term care services

KEY CHARACTERISTICS

1. The LTC system is rationally integrated with the rest of the health care delivery system. This rational integration facilitates easy access to services between the two components of the health care delivery system.
2. Appropriate placement of the patient within the LTC system is based on an assessment of individual needs. For example, individual needs determine whether and when institutionalization may be necessary.
3. The LTC system accommodates changes in individual needs by providing access to appropriate LTC services as determined by a reevaluation of needs.
4. LTC services are designed to compensate for existing impairment and have the objective of promoting independence to the extent possible.

FIGURE 10-3 Key characteristics of a well-designed long-term care system.

maintain residual function—that is, whatever ability to function a person still has; and (2) to prevent further decline. These goals are accomplished by letting the person do as much as possible for himself or herself. Some patients—such as a comatose patient in a persistent vegetative state, for example—may be totally dependent on a caregiver.

Extended Period of Care

For most LTC clients, the delivery of various services extends over a relatively long period because the underlying causes of functional decline are often irreversible. In other cases, rehabilitation therapies or postacute convalescence may be needed for a relatively short duration, generally less than 90 days, with the patient subsequently returning to independent living. People receiving community-based LTC services generally need them for a long duration to prevent institutionalization. A smaller number of LTC recipients need institutional care for an extended period, or even indefinitely. Examples include people with severe dementia, incontinence of bowel and bladder, severe psychiatric or behavioral issues, or unstable postacute conditions, and those in a comatose/vegetative state.

Holistic Care

The holistic approach to health care delivery focuses on every aspect of what makes a person whole and complete. A person's needs and preferences are incorporated into medical care delivery and all aspects of daily living. Physical aspects of care include medical exams, nursing care, medications, and rehabilitation treatments. The individual's mental and emotional well-being are addressed, for example, by minimizing stress and anxiety. Opportunities are created for socializing with family, friends, and volunteers. Pursuit of spirituality and religious faith is encouraged.

Quality of Life

A sense of satisfaction, fulfillment, and self-worth are regarded as critical patient outcomes in any health care delivery setting. They take on added significance in LTC because (1) a loss of self-worth often accompanies disability and (2) patients remain in LTC settings for relatively long periods, with little hope of full recovery in most instances.

Quality of life is a multifaceted concept that recognizes at least five factors: lifestyle pursuits, living environment, clinical palliation, human factors, and personal choices.

- Lifestyle factors are associated with personal enrichment and making one's life meaningful through activities one enjoys. Many older people still enjoy pursuing their former leisure activities, such as woodworking, crocheting, knitting, gardening, and fishing. Even those whose function has declined to a vegetative or comatose state must be engaged in something that promotes sensory awakening through visual, auditory, olfactory, and tactile stimulation.
- The living environment must be comfortable, safe, and appealing to the senses. Cleanliness, décor, furnishings, and other aesthetic features are important.
- Clinical **palliation** should be available for relief from unpleasant symptoms, such as pain or nausea, for instance, when a patient is undergoing chemotherapy.
- Human factors refer to caregiver attitudes and practices that emphasize caring, compassion, respect, and preservation of human dignity for the patient. Institutionalized patients find it disconcerting to have lost their autonomy and independence. Quality of life is enhanced when patients residing in a LTC facility, who are often referred to as residents, have some latitude to govern their own lives, and have adequate privacy.
- Being able to make personal choices is important to most people. In nursing facilities, for example, food is often the primary area of discontentment, which can be addressed by offering a selection of menu choices. Also, the ability

to set one's own schedule is important to most people. Many elderly resent being awakened early in the morning when caregivers begin their responsibilities to care for patients' hygiene, bathing, and grooming.

Use of Current Technology

Technology offers one avenue for at least mitigating the impending challenges of the growing need for LTC. In addition, technology can improve overall safety and quality of care. For example, a **personal emergency response system (PERS)** enables an at-risk elderly person living alone at home to summon help in an emergency at any time during the day or night. A fall detector can be used at home or in an institution. Electronic medication dispensers are programmed to dispense pills and sound an alarm as reminders for a person to take prescribed medications. Technology also enables remote monitoring of patients who live independently. Examples of technology used in institutional settings include global positioning systems (GPS) to monitor a patient who may wander away, sensor technology to prevent and heal pressure ulcers by detecting moisture levels and length of time spent in one position, use of robotic pets, and pedometers to measure daily activity levels (Morley, 2012).

Use of Evidence-Based Practices

Evidence-based care incorporates the use of best practices that have been evaluated for effectiveness and safety through clinical research. Best practices are often found in clinical practice guidelines, which provide directions and protocols for treatment interventions for specific health conditions. The American Medical Directors Association (AMDA), for example, publishes clinical practice guidelines on important topics related to the treatment of common clinical conditions in long-term care. Evidence-based protocols are meant to be used for staff training and in caregiving routines to improve quality of care. Studies show that the use of evidence-based practices in nursing homes can reduce falls (Teresi et al., 2013), prevent pressure ulcers (Niederhauser et al., 2012; Riordan and Voegeli, 2009), and increase satisfaction among nurses (Barba et al., 2012).

▶ Long-Term Care Services

The large array of LTC services can include a combination of different types of services depending on an individual's assessed needs at a given point in time, as new needs arise, and as needs change over time. Such services include the following:

- Medical care, nursing, and rehabilitation
- Mental health services and dementia care
- Social support
- Preventive and therapeutic long-term care
- Informal and formal care
- Respite care
- Community-based and institutional services
- Housing
- End-of-life care

Medical Care, Nursing, and Rehabilitation

Medical care, nursing, and rehabilitation services focus on three main areas: (1) postacute continuity of care, (2) clinical management of chronic illness and comorbidity, and (3) restoration or maintenance of physical function. LTC often becomes necessary after the treatment of an acute episode in a hospital. However, patients in LTC settings may also experience acute episodes, such as pneumonia, bone fracture, or stroke, and require admission to a general hospital. The elderly are more prone to hospitalization compared to younger age groups; that is, younger patients are more likely to be treated as outpatients, whereas older patients may be admitted as inpatients for the same medical conditions.

Nurses, rehabilitation therapists, nutritionists, and other professionals typically provide medical care in LTC settings under the direction of a physician. Preventing complications from chronic conditions (tertiary prevention) is an important aspect of LTC.

Mental Health Services and Dementia Care

It is erroneous to believe that mental disorders are a normal part of aging. Nevertheless, an estimated 25% of older adults have depression, anxiety disorders, or other significant psychiatric conditions, and mental health disorders are frequently comorbid in older adults, occurring in conjunction with common chronic illnesses such as diabetes, cardiac disease, and arthritis (Robinson, 2010). Psychiatric symptoms and cognitive decline are particularly common among nursing home residents (Scocco et al., 2006). Mental disorders range in severity from problematic to disabling to fatal.

Major barriers must be overcome in the delivery of mental health care. In general, assessing psychiatric illness in geriatric patients can be difficult, especially

since comorbidity may obscure the diagnosis. For example, patients with multiple chronic illnesses may display symptoms of either dementia or depression that are attributed to their primary medical condition rather than to an underlying psychiatric illness (Tune, 2001). Hence, elderly people with mental disorders are less likely than younger adults to receive correct diagnoses and needed mental health care.

With the growing prevalence of dementia in the United States and around the world, caring for patients with dementia has become a major focus in LTC. **Dementia** is a general term for progressive and irreversible decline in cognition, thinking, and memory. The risk of dementia increases with age. Approximately 15% of people older than 70 years of age have dementia (Hurd et al., 2013), the majority of whom have **Alzheimer's disease**—a progressive degenerative disease of the brain that produces memory loss, confusion, irritability, and severe functional decline. Alzheimer's disease affects approximately 5 million older Americans in the United States (Alzheimer's Association, 2013).

Although people with mild dementia may receive home-based care, almost 40% of people with dementia receive institutional LTC. Among institutionalized patients, almost 72% have a diagnosis of dementia, according to one study (Helmer et al., 2006).

Social Support

LTC clients need social and emotional support to help them cope with changing life events that may cause stress, frustration, anger, fear, grief, or other emotional imbalances. Adaptation to new surroundings and new people becomes necessary when a patient leaves his or her own home and moves to supportive housing or a nursing home. Social support is also needed when problems and issues arise in the interactions among people within social systems. For example, conflicts may arise between what a patient wants for himself or herself and what the family thinks is best for the patient. Conflicts may also arise between patients and caregivers.

Social services are also necessary to facilitate the coordination of total care needs. Examples include transportation services, information, counseling, recreation, and spiritual support. For people residing in LTC facilities, remaining connected with the community and the outside world is an important aspect of social support.

Preventive and Therapeutic Long-Term Care

In the context of LTC, prevention generally refers to preventing or delaying institutionalization. Various community-based LTC services perform a preventive function by providing good nutrition and access to services, such as vaccinations, flu shots, and routine medical care. Therapeutic services, such as nursing care, rehabilitation, and therapeutic diets, are specified in a plan of care and administered as directed by a physician.

Informal and Formal Care

Among the elderly who receive LTC services in the United States, 80% live in private homes (CBO, 2013). Contrary to popular belief, most LTC services in the United States are provided informally by family, friends, and surrogates such as neighbors and members from church or other community organizations. An estimated 92% of community-dwelling residents receive unpaid help (Kaye et al., 2010), and there are approximately 40 to 50 million informal caregivers in the United States (O'Shaughnessy, 2013). Family members also play an important role in managing the often critical transitions between settings of care delivery, such as between the hospital and the nursing home, and between the hospital and the home (Levine et al., 2010). They also play an important role in monitoring adequacy of services when the patient is placed in an institution (O'Shaughnessy, 2013).

Informal care reduces the use of formal home health care and delays nursing home entry (Van Houtven and Norton, 2004). In a population of disabled elderly people, insufficient informal care is associated with overall discontinuation of living at home, all-cause mortality, hospitalization, and institutionalization (Kuzuya et al., 2011).

Given their enormous, though often underappreciated role in LTC, unpaid caregivers are the largest source of financing of these services (Holtz-Eakin, 2005). The economic value of informal caregiving could be as high as $470 billion per year in the United States (Reinhard et al., 2015).

The pool of informal caregivers in the United States, in relation to the growing elderly population needing LTC, is expected to shrink rather dramatically in the future. Various reports suggest that the number of older people who are divorced, unmarried, or without children has been on the rise. Such people may have to depend on paid services, although it remains unclear how the services will be financed. If the government ends up filling the financing gaps, the burden will fall on future taxpayers.

Respite Care

Family caregivers often experience a range of physical, emotional, social, and financial problems. Negative feelings, such as anger, dissatisfaction, guilt, frustration, tension, and family conflict, are some common issues faced by these caregivers. Under such pressures, caregivers may experience stress and burnout. **Respite care** is the most frequently suggested intervention to address family caregivers' feelings of stress and burnout. Its objective is to provide relief or assistance to caregivers for limited periods, thereby allowing them some free time without subjecting the patient to neglect. Respite care can include any kind of LTC service, such as adult day care, which allows people to work during the day, or temporary institutionalization, which allows families to take some time off.

Community-Based and Institutional Services

For many people who need LTC, the availability of community-based services provided by formal agencies becomes an important factor in living independently. Such services are brought to the patient's home or delivered in a community-based location; hence, these services are collectively referred to as home- and community-based services (HCBS). HCBS have a fourfold objective: (1) to deliver LTC in the most economical and least restrictive setting whenever appropriate, (2) to supplement informal caregiving when advanced services are needed or to substitute informal services when a person lacks a social network to receive informal care, (3) to provide temporary respite to informal caregivers, and (4) to delay or prevent institutionalization.

Institutionalization can be for a long-term or short-term duration. As can be inferred from Figure 10-2, functional deficits in three or more ADLs dramatically raise the probability that an individual will need institutional care. The main goals for institutional care are (1) to deliver therapeutic services in accordance with the plan of care, (2) to provide professional help for ADL functions that the patient cannot perform, (3) to implement measures to prevent further loss of remaining function, and (4) to coordinate services with non-LTC providers to address the patient's total care needs.

FIGURE 10-4 illustrates various types of HCBS and institutional LTC settings. For many patients, there are complex interlinkages between services that are brought to the patients and services that they obtain by being physically transferred to receive them.

Housing

In the LTC context, housing refers to noninstitutional housing other than a person's own home. It includes independent living facilities and retirement living centers/communities—both private and public—that may or may not provide support services, such as meals, housekeeping, transportation, and scheduled recreational activities. Residents have their self-contained apartments or individual cottages that allow maximum privacy, and they can come and go as they please. Occasional needs for LTC services are met by obtaining home health care through an outside agency. Institutions, in contrast, are distinguished by services that go beyond basic support services to include therapeutic services delivered in accordance with a plan of care.

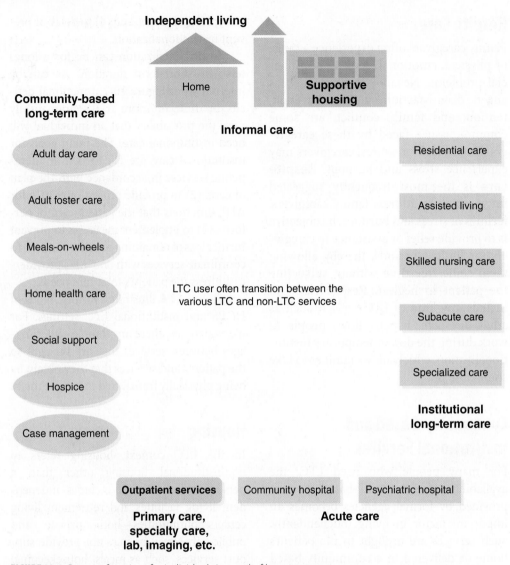

FIGURE 10-4 Range of services for individuals in need of long-term care.

Modified with permission from Taylor & Francis from Singh, D. A. 1997. *Nursing home administrators: Their influence on quality of care.* New York: Garland Publishing, Inc. p. 15.

Housing that supports independent living for the elderly and for disabled persons must take into account physical function and safety issues. Examples of supportive features include safety pull-cords to summon help in an emergency, grab bars in bathrooms to prevent falls, kitchenettes that allow the preparation of meals or snacks,

railings in hallways to assist in mobility, and easy means of access to the outdoors.

Private Housing

Upscale retirement centers abound in which the residents can expect to pay a fairly substantial entrance fee plus a monthly rental or maintenance fee. These complexes have various types of recreational facilities and social programs. The fees often include the evening meal. Housekeeping services and transportation may also be included.

Public Housing

More modest housing complexes provide government-assisted, subsidized housing for low-income people. The U.S. Department of Housing and Urban Development (HUD) administers three main kinds of rent subsidy programs: (1) federal aid to local housing agencies, which allows them to offer reduced rent to low-income tenants; (2) vouchers that a tenant can apply toward renting housing of his or her choice; and (3) public housing operated by the government (less commonly available). HUD also provides federal funds to nonprofit sponsors to help them construct rental housing that includes support services.

End-of-Life Care

Dealing with death and dying is very much a part of LTC. End-of-life care focuses on preventing needless pain and distress for terminally ill patients and their families, and places a high emphasis on maintaining patient dignity and comfort.

Roughly three-fourths of all deaths in the United States occur in people who are 65 years or older. Among the elderly, 28% of all deaths are related to heart disease and 22% are attributable to cancer (National Center for Health Statistics, 2010). Other diseases that often prove fatal to elderly persons include stroke, chronic lower respiratory disease, Alzheimer's disease, diabetes, pneumonia, and influenza.

Care professionals seem to be well positioned to provide end-of-life care in some LTC settings. In others, terminal patients are referred to hospice services; patients are either transferred to a freestanding hospice or the services are brought to the patient wherever the patient resides.

▶ Users of Long-Term Care

As mentioned previously, the elderly are the main consumers of LTC services. Nevertheless, approximately 50% of LTC users are younger than age 65, including some children and young adults (**FIGURE 10-5**).

Some children have functional impairments because of congenital disorders, such as cerebral palsy, autism, spina bifida, and epilepsy. These children grow up with physical disability and need help with ADLs. The term **developmental disability (DD)** describes the general physical incapacity that such children may face at a very early age. Those who acquire such dysfunctions are referred to as developmentally disabled. **Intellectual disability (ID)**—that is, below-average intellectual capacity, which can be caused by a disorder

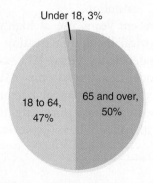

FIGURE 10-5 Users of long-term care by age group.

Data from Iglehart, J. K. 2016. Future of long-term care and the expanding role of Medicaid managed care. *New England Journal of Medicine* 374: 182–187.

such as Down syndrome—also leads to DD status in most cases. The close association between the two is reflected in the term intellectual/developmental disability (IDD). Approximately 14% of children in the 3–17 age group are developmentally disabled; boys are almost twice as likely as girls to have this kind of disability (Boyle et al., 2011). Those with severe ID and/or DD are also likely to have disturbing behavioral issues and usually require institutional care in specialized facilities.

IDD is also prevalent among young adults, but some persons with IDD live into their 70s or beyond (Robinson, 2012). These individuals present special challenges because of their combined low intellectual and physical function.

Other young adults have permanent disabilities stemming from neurologic malfunctions, degenerative conditions, traumatic injury, or surgical complications. For example, multiple sclerosis is the most common cause of neurologic disability in young adults (Compston and Coles, 2002). Severe injury to the head, spinal cord, or limbs can occur in victims of vehicle crashes, sports mishaps, or industrial accidents. Subsequent to receiving acute care, they often must spend years in a LTC institution.

In recent years, use of highly active antiretroviral therapy in treating human immunodeficiency virus (HIV)/acquired immunodeficiency syndrome (AIDS) has increased the life span of persons with this disease.[1] Those surviving to older ages with HIV/AIDS, however, often face an accelerated aging accompanied by increased comorbidity and decline in health and function, leading to premature disablement—both physical and cognitive (Leveille and Thapa, 2017). Patients with HIV/AIDS are at a high risk of developing heart disease, certain cancers, and kidney disease (Karpiak and Havlik, 2017). In LTC settings, people with HIV/AIDS are often younger than other populations, male, and unmarried (Foebel et al., 2015). They may be disconnected from traditional informal support networks, and rely heavily on formal care providers (Shippy and Karpiak, 2005).

Patients with HIV/AIDS have a variety of medical and social needs that evolve over time. Those changing needs may require transitions between community-based services, nursing homes, and hospitals. Care coordination for these patients results in fewer unmet needs for supportive services and often better utilization of services (Vargas and Cunningham, 2006). Discrimination in providing services to people with HIV/AIDS is a violation of federal law.

▶ Level of Care Continuum

The importance of providing different levels of services to a heterogeneous population has given rise to a continuum of clinical categories, ranging from basic personal care to subacute care and specialized services.

---

[1] An HIV/AIDS diagnosis prior to the mid-1990s often meant a miserable death because of the total collapse of the patient's immune system (Karpiak and Havlik, 2017).

Personal Care

Personal care refers to light assistance with basic ADLs. Delivery of these services is largely the domain of **paraprofessionals**—personnel who provide basic ADL services, such as personal care attendants, certified nursing assistants (CNAs), and therapy aides. Personal care can be provided by informal caregivers, home health agencies, adult day care, adult foster care, and residential and assisted living facilities. Other levels of care often include a component of personal care.

Custodial Care

Custodial care is nonmedical care provided to support and maintain the patient's condition. It requires no active medical or nursing treatments. Services provided are designed to maintain rather than restore functioning, with an emphasis on preventing further deterioration. Examples are personal care with basic ADLs, range-of-motion exercises, bowel and bladder training, and assisted walking. Custodial services are rendered by paraprofessionals, such as aides, rather than by licensed nurses or therapists. The settings in which custodial care is provided resemble those in which personal care is offered.

Restorative Care

Restorative care or rehabilitation involves short-term therapy treatments to help a person regain or improve physical function. It is provided immediately after the onset of a disability. Examples of cases requiring short-term restorative therapy include orthopedic surgery, stroke, limb amputation, and prolonged illness. Treatments are rendered by physical therapists, occupational therapists, and speech–language pathologists. Restorative care can be provided by home health agencies, rehabilitation hospitals, outpatient rehabilitation clinics, adult day care centers, and assisted living and skilled nursing facilities.

Skilled Nursing Care

Skilled nursing care is medically oriented care provided mainly by a licensed nurse under the overall direction of a physician in accordance with a plan of care. Delivery of care includes assessment and reassessment to determine the patient's care needs, monitoring of acute and unstable chronic conditions, and a variety of treatments that may include wound care, tube care management, intravenous (IV) therapy, oncology care, HIV/AIDS care, and management of neurological conditions. Rehabilitation therapies often form an important component of skilled nursing care. Home health agencies and skilled nursing facilities provide skilled nursing care.

Subacute Care

The term **subacute care** applies to postacute services for people who remain critically ill during the postacute phase of illness or injury or who have complex conditions that require ongoing monitoring and treatment or intensive rehabilitation. Micheletti and Shlala (1995) suggested four categories of subacute care services exist: (1) extensive care (e.g., parenteral feeding, tracheostomy), (2) special care (e.g., postburn care, pressure ulcers, IV therapy, tube feedings), (3) clinically complex care (e.g., wound care, postsurgical care), and (4) intensive rehabilitation.

▶ # Home- and Community-Based Services

Financing for formal HCBS comes from a variety of sources: private out-of-pocket payments, private long-term care insurance, Medicaid, Medicare, and other public sources. Under the Older Americans Act of 1965, federal funds are granted to states for a variety of community-based services, such as nutrition programs for the elderly, case management, homemaker services, and transportation services (Kowlessar et al., 2015). These services are available to Americans age 60 years and older, particularly those with social or economic need. The federal AoA oversees the program. LTC programs across the United States are carried out primarily through an administrative network of state agencies on aging, area agencies on aging, and Native American tribal organizations.

In 1981, the HCBS waiver program was enacted under Section 1915(c) of the Social Security Act. Because nursing home services are mandated under Medicaid, the 1915(c) waivers allow states to expand community-based LTC services under the Medicaid program. Services are available to those Medicaid beneficiaries who would otherwise require institutional care.

Some federal funding available to the states under Title XX Social Services Block Grants from DHHS may also be used for community-based LTC services when such services prevent or reduce inappropriate institutionalization. Some states also provide limited assistance with ADLs in a person's home under the Medicaid Personal Care Services program. Although nearly all states provide HCBS

to Medicaid beneficiaries, the eligibility requirements, available services, and the scope and extent of these services differ considerably across states and between geographical areas within states (National Health Policy Forum, 2013).

Even though national LTC policy has taken unprecedented steps to shift services from institutions to HBCS, researchers have identified several needs that continue to go unmet. For example, some acute health problems and mental health issues are inadequately accommodated in HCBS. Additional unmet needs relate to the inadequate HCBS workforce, transportation barriers, and limited supportive housing options for care recipients (Robison et al., 2012).

A 1999 decision by the U.S. Supreme Court (*Olmstead v. L.C.*) directed states to provide community-based services for persons with disabilities—including persons with IDD, physical disabilities, and mental illness—when such services are determined to be appropriate by health care professionals. Also, states must develop a comprehensive working plan to place qualified people with IDD in less restrictive settings. Most adults with IDD now live in community housing with support services.

Even though Medicaid recipients have been the main beneficiaries of policies that promote HCBS, approximately one-fifth of community-dwelling Medicare recipients have serious physical or cognitive limitations, and three-fourths have three or more chronic conditions. Only one-fourth of these Medicare recipients qualify for Medicaid (Davis et al., 2016). Hence, there are serious gaps in their ability to receive LTC services on a continuous basis. Medicare pays for HCBS, but for home health care only when eligibility criteria are met. The patients must be homebound, have a plan of treatment and periodic review by a physician, and require intermittent or part-time skilled nursing care and/or rehabilitation therapies.

Home Health Care

The organizational setup for home health care commonly involves a community- or hospital-based home health agency that sends health care professionals and paraprofessionals to patients' homes to deliver services approved by a physician. Skilled nursing care is the service most often received by home health patients (**FIGURE 10-6**).

Of the 12,400 home health agencies in the United States, the majority are private for-profit organizations, and almost all are certified by Medicare (Harris-Kojetin et al., 2016). Medicare is the single largest payer for home health services in

the country, though Medicaid is not far behind (**FIGURE 10-7**).

Preliminary evidence indicates that a properly structured home care program may actually reduce disability among older adults, thereby leading to a strong preventive effect. In a demonstration project funded by the Centers for Medicare and Medicaid Services (CMS), 75% of the elderly participants in the project showed improved performance of ADLs after receiving 5 months of home-based services from an interprofessional team. The average number of ADLs in which the participants had difficulty declined from 3.9 to 2.0 after the 5-month program (Szanton et al., 2016).

Adult Day Care

Adult day care (ADC), also referred to as "adult day service," is a daytime group program designed to meet the needs of functionally and/or cognitively impaired

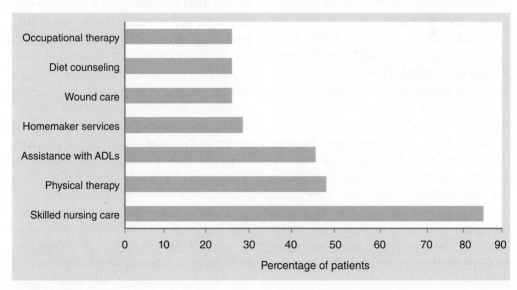

FIGURE 10-6 Most frequently provided services to home health patients.

Data from Jones, A. L., et al. 2012. *Characteristics and use of home health care by men and women aged 65 and over. National health statistics reports, No. 52.* Hyattsville, MD: National Center for Health Statistics.

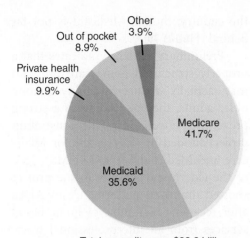

Total expenditures = $83.2 billion

FIGURE 10-7 Sources of payment for home health care, 2014.

Data from National Center for Health Statistics. 2016. *Health, United States, 2015.* Hyattsville, MD: U.S. Department of Health and Human Services. p. 298.

adults and to provide partial respite to family caregivers so they can work during the day or pursue other responsibilities of life. ADC is designed for people who live with their families, but cannot remain alone during the day because of physical or mental conditions.

There are an estimated 4,800 ADC centers across the United States (Harris-Kojetin et al., 2016). These centers operate programs during normal business hours 5 days per week, although some offer evening and weekend services as well.

Most ADC services are highly focused on prevention and health maintenance, with the objective of preventing or delaying institutionalization, but they also incorporate nursing care, psychosocial therapies, and rehabilitation. As such, ADC services, in many instances, have become alternatives to home health care and assisted living and/or a transitional step before placement in a long-term care institution.

Not all ADC centers provide the same level of services. Almost 70% of these programs provide nursing care, 50% offer rehabilitation services, 50% provide social services, one-third offer mental health services, one-third offer podiatry services, and one-fourth have pharmacy services available (Harris-Kojetin et al., 2016). Most provide transportation services. Group socialization, therapeutic recreational activities, and meals are included. Nearly half of the participants in ADC programs have dementia, and 50% of ADC centers offer specialized programs for these patients (MetLife Mature Market Institute, 2010).

Medicaid provides some funding for ADC services under Section 1915(c) waivers. Medicare does not pay for ADC services but may cover rehabilitation services under Part B.

Adult Foster Care

Adult foster care (AFC) is a service characterized by small, family-run homes providing room, board, and varying levels of supervision, oversight, and personal care to nonrelated adults who are unable to care for themselves ("AARP studies adult foster care for the elderly," 1996). Foster care provides services in a community-based dwelling in an environment that promotes the feeling of being part of a family unit (Stahl, 1997). Participants in the program are elderly or disabled individuals who have a medical diagnosis, a psychiatric diagnosis, or a need for personal care. Typically, the caregiving family resides in part of the home. To maintain the family environment, most states license fewer than 10 beds per family unit.

This type of program differs widely from state to state and goes by several names, including adult family care, community residential care, and domiciliary care. Each state has established its own standards for the licensing of AFCs. Funding for AFCs may come from Medicaid, private insurance, or personal sources. Medicare does not pay for AFC services but may cover rehabilitation services under Part B.

Senior Centers

Senior centers are local community centers for older adults where seniors can congregate and socialize. Many centers offer one or more meals daily. Others sponsor wellness programs, health education, counseling services, recreational activities, information and referrals, and limited health care services, including health screening, especially for glaucoma and hypertension. Nearly all senior centers receive some public funding. Other common funding sources are United Way and private donations.

Home-Delivered and Congregate Meals

The Elderly Nutrition Program (ENP) is the nation's oldest framework for providing community- and home-based preventive nutrition in the United States. This program has been in operation since 1972 for congregate meals, and since 1978 for home-delivered meals. The ENP program was authorized under the Older Americans Act, which also provides the majority of its funding. Additional funds are provided through Title XX block grants, 1915(c) waivers, and private donations.

The ENP provides a hot noon meal 5 days per week to Americans 60 years and older (and their spouses) who cannot prepare a nutritionally balanced noon meal for themselves. Home-delivered meals for homebound persons are commonly referred to as **meals-on-wheels**. Ambulatory clients are encouraged to get their meals at senior centers or other congregate settings, where they also have the opportunity to socialize. Roughly 60% of the meals are home delivered; the other 40% are served in congregate settings (Kowlessar et al., 2015).

ENP services successfully meet the needs of the community-dwelling vulnerable elderly people. For example, participants in the meals-on-wheels program are more than twice as likely as the general population to be in poor or fair health, more than half live alone, more than one-third are age 85 or older, and more than one-third have difficulty with three or more ADLs (Kowlessar et al., 2015).

It is a common practice for local-area Agencies on Aging to contract out the preparation and delivery of ENP meals to local nursing homes, hospitals, or religious organizations. In the meals-on-wheels program, volunteers carry the meals to homebound participants. Congregate meals may be served on the premises of participating facilities, such as hospitals and nursing homes, or at local senior centers or religious establishments.

Homemaker Services

Depending on availability of funds, states may provide limited housekeeping and chore services—such as essential shopping, light cleaning, meal preparation, and minor home repairs—to low-income people. Homemaker programs may be staffed largely or entirely by volunteers. The Medicaid program may pay for some homemaker services, or these services may be funded through the local seniors programs under Title XX Social Services Block Grants or the Older Americans Act. Besides the limited public funding options that help a relatively small number of people, private homemaker service agencies have sprung up across the nation.

Continuing Care at Home

Continuing care at home (CCAH) is a new model of home-based care that has only recently emerged. Its growth has been slow because of regulatory issues at the state government level. CCAH programs are an extension of the continuing care retirement center (CCRC) model that has been in existence for a number of years. As discussed later in this chapter, CCRCs provide a continuum of housing and institutional LTC services on one campus. Thus, CCRCs are also at the forefront of developing these home-based programs.

To participate in the CCAH program, clients are required to pay an initial lump-sum fee and a monthly fee under a contract that guarantees a person's future LTC care. To qualify, a person must be in good health and not need LTC services at the time of enrollment. CCAH services typically include care coordination, routine home maintenance, home health care, transportation, meals, and social and wellness programs (Spellman and Brod, 2014). Most services are provided at the client's home with the objective of delaying institutionalization. When institutional services are needed, the client receives them at the CCRC's assisted living and/or skilled nursing care facilities or at subcontracted local facilities.

Case Management

Case management involves evaluating a patient's physical, medical, and psychosocial needs; preparing a plan to address those needs and identifying services that would be most appropriate, including LTC; determining eligibility for services and how those services would be financed; making referrals to those services; coordinating the delivery of services; and reevaluating needs as circumstances change over time. Two main case management models are prominent today.

Brokerage Model

In the **brokerage model**, once needs have been independently assessed, case managers arrange services through other providers. The case manager is usually a freestanding agent who is mainly responsible for linking the client with other organizations, agencies, and service providers, but has no formal administrative or financial relationship with these entities. Needs assessment, development of a service plan, and making referrals are the main functions of case management in this model. There is minimal coordination and monitoring of services.

In the public domain, most states have implemented preadmission screening rules through a brokerage model. The purpose of this screening is to determine whether a Medicaid beneficiary's needs can be better met in a nursing facility or through HCBS. In addition, federal regulations require an evaluation of a patient for mental illness and/or ID before such a patient can be admitted to a Medicaid-certified nursing facility (see the discussion of nursing facility certification under "Skilled Nursing Facilities"); this process is called

Preadmission Screening and Resident Review (PASRR). The purpose of this requirement is to determine whether a nursing facility is the best alternative for individuals with serious mental illness or ID or whether their needs can be adequately met in community-based settings.

Managed Care/Integrated Model

The managed care/integrated model of case management has two main features: (1) capitation as a method of payment and (2) all-inclusive services within the fixed capitation fee. Several states contract with health maintenance organizations (HMOs) to provide integrated services that include care coordination, various community-based services, and nursing home placement when indicated to primarily Medicaid recipients. In 2012, an estimated 389,000 people received Medicaid-covered LTC services through managed care contracts, up from 105,000 in 2004 (Burwell and Saucier, 2013), and the program is expected to continue to grow.

A slightly different model, but one that is also based on capitation payments, is the **Program of All-Inclusive Care for the Elderly (PACE).** This program is available in most states to people 55 years and older. It focuses on frail elderly who have already been certified for nursing home placement under Medicare and/or Medicaid. PACE's purpose is to prevent the progression of disability, and to keep the participants out of nursing homes. At the core of the program is ADC, augmented by home care and meals-on-wheels (Gross et al., 2004).

PACE was authorized under the Balanced Budget Act of 1997 after the On Lok project in San Francisco demonstrated that, in many instances, LTC institutionalization could be prevented through appropriate case management. Under this program, all medical care and social services are coordinated by a PACE team. PACE has no deductibles and copayments, which is an incentive for qualified individuals to participate. The program has been shown to result in reduced numbers of hospitalizations and rehospitalizations (Meret-Hanke, 2011), and substantial cost savings over alternative models of LTC delivery (Wieland et al., 2013).

Recent Policies Related to Community-Based Services

The two main policies discussed here simply continue the patchwork of options that benefit mainly Medicaid recipients while leaving many of the Medicare recipients with unmet LTC needs.

Money Follows the Person

The **Money Follows the Person (MFP)** demonstration program was codified in the Deficit Reduction Act (DRA) of 2005 to provide adequate federal funding to states for the sole purpose of moving qualified people whose care is funded by Medicaid from nursing homes back into community-based settings. The precursors to the MFP program were demonstration projects in most states, launched between 1998 and 2002 through federal grants, that showed successful transitioning of many nursing home residents back to their communities. Under the MFP program, funds that had previously been used by the state to pay for nursing home care are applied toward HCBS. The Affordable Care Act (ACA) amended the DRA by extending the MFP program through 2016 but allows the states to use the funds through 2020 (Reinhard, 2012).

The MFP program continues to show slow but steady success in transitioning people out of nursing homes. Between 2008 and 2014, almost 52,000 people made this transition. Research shows an overall decline in the rates of re-institutionalization within 12 months of an individual's transition to the community. In addition, declines in Medicaid and Medicare expenditures after transition of all target populations have been noted (Irvin et al., 2015). Critics point to the exclusion of assisted living facilities and AFC homes (if they house more than four people) from the program. Another drawback has been a shortage of skillful, trained coordinators to work with nursing home clients to ensure they make a successful transition to the community (Reinhard, 2012).

Community First Choice

The ACA created financial incentives for states to establish "attendant services and supports" to deliver personal care to individuals with disabilities. To qualify for the Community First Choice program, which supplies such care, the individual must be eligible for Medicaid and have an income that does not exceed 150% of the federal poverty level (Mann, 2011). To date, only a few states have implemented this program.

▶ Institutional Long-Term Care Continuum

Institutional LTC is appropriate for patients whose needs cannot be adequately met in a community-based setting. Apart from a patient's clinical condition, factors such as inability to live alone or lack of social support may suggest a need for the individual to be in an institution. The institutional sector of LTC offers a continuum of services (Figure 10-4), from institutions that offer only basic personal and custodial care to those that provide skilled nursing, subacute care, or specialized services. Some sources lump residential and personal care facilities together with community-based care. In terms of care delivery, some overlap exists between assisted living and skilled nursing care. Hence, the distinction between some of the institutional categories is not always clear-cut.

For institutions at the lower end of the continuum, and even in independent living and supportive housing, the concept of **aging-in-place** has become important, particularly from the viewpoint of consumer choice. This concept refers to older people's preference and expectation to stay in one place for as long as possible and to delay or avoid transfer to an institution where the acuity level of patients is higher. In independent and supportive housing, management often faces the dilemma of how to continue to house residents who have escalating needs for care—for example, when patients develop incontinence of bladder or bowel.

Most care in LTC institutions is provided by nonphysician staff, such as nurses, CNAs, dietitians, social workers, and therapists. Residents have the right to be treated by a physician of their choice, who makes periodic rounds to monitor the care being delivered. Between rounds, the professional nursing staff communicate with the physician, especially when changes in a patient's condition are observed or treatment orders are not producing the desired results. By law, a transfer agreement with a local hospital must be in place to facilitate transition between the acute care and LTC facilities. At the onset of an acute episode, such as pneumonia or injury from a fall, the patient is transferred to a hospital.

Residential and Personal Care Facilities

Residential and personal care facilities are also known as "domiciliary care facilities," "board-and-care homes," or "sheltered care facilities." Sometimes AFC homes are included in this category. These facilities provide physically supportive dwelling units, monitoring and/or assistance with medications, oversight, and personal or custodial care. No nursing or medical services are provided. To maintain a residential rather than an institutional environment, many such facilities limit the admission of residents with severe disabilities, but some may take patients with mild levels of mental dysfunction. Services are provided by paraprofessionals rather than by licensed personnel. Minimal staffing is provided 24 hours a day for supervision and assistive purposes. More advanced services can be arranged through an external home health agency when needed.

In terms of the level of comfort, these kinds of facilities can range from spartan to deluxe. The latter are often private-pay facilities. For people who have limited incomes, Supplemental Security Income (SSI) can be used along with other types of government assistance funds to pay for residence. Services include meals, housekeeping and laundry services, and social and recreational activities.

Assisted Living Facilities

An **assisted living facility (ALF)** provides personal care, 24-hour supervision, social services, recreational activities, and some nursing and rehabilitation services. These facilities are appropriate for people who cannot function independently but do not require skilled nursing care. Some ALFs, however, now offer Alzheimer's/dementia care (Hoban, 2013). ALFs operate predominantly on a private-pay basis; the vast majority of the residents use their own financial resources to pay for the care in these facilities. To maintain the desired residential environment, ALFs generally have private accommodations, rather than the semi-private accommodations that are common in skilled nursing facilities.

All states now require ALFs to be licensed. In the absence of federal standards, regulations vary from state to state. These regulations continue to evolve in response to the rising acuity levels of residents. More than half of the residents in ALFs have considerable health care needs, such as nursing care, and assistance with transfers, medications, eating, and dressing. Yet, in one research study, fewer than half of the facilities were found to have registered nurses or licensed practical nurses (Han et al., 2016). Because of the lack of regulatory oversight over ALFs, evaluations of their quality are practically nonexistent.

Skilled Nursing Facilities

A **skilled nursing facility (SNF)** is a typical nursing home at the higher end of the institutional continuum. Patients are generally transferred from a hospital to the SNF after an acute episode, and the care needs of these patients have become increasingly more complex, requiring much higher levels of staffing for SNFs compared to ALFs. Although many nursing home residents stay for a long period of time (sometimes for years), short-term stays for convalescence and rehabilitation under Medicare coverage have become common.

Patients in nursing homes most often suffer from bladder incontinence, depression, Alzheimer's-type dementia, and bowel incontinence. Changes in the main chronic conditions noted in these patients between 2005 and 2015 point to an increase in the acuity level of nursing home residents (**FIGURE 10-8**)—an outgrowth of the HCBS policies discussed previously, as lower-need residents have been moved out to community-based settings.

The nursing home environment is generally more institutional and clinical than the residential environment emphasized in ALFs. In recent years, a movement, loosely referred to as "culture change," has sought to transform the existing facilities into more homelike and vibrant living environments. Newer facilities are being built with innovative designs that offer a sense of community living, a greater degree of privacy, and enriched environments that promote physical and psychological well-being and reduce boredom and stress (see Singh, 2016, Chapter 7).

SNFs are heavily regulated through licensure and certification requirements. All facilities in a particular state must be licensed, and licensing regulations differ considerably from state to state. Most licensing regulations establish minimum qualifications required for administrators and other staff, prescribe minimum staffing levels, establish standards for building construction, and require compliance with the national fire and safety codes. To admit patients covered under the Medicaid and/or Medicare programs, nursing homes must also be certified and must demonstrate compliance with the federal certification standards enforced by the CMS.

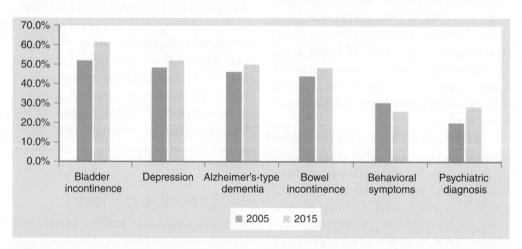

FIGURE 10-8 Changes in the percentages of nursing home residents with various conditions between 2005 and 2015.

Data from Sanofi-Aventis. 2007. *Managed care digest series: Senior care digest, 2007.* Bridgewater, NJ: Author. p. 12; Sanofi-Aventis. 2016. *Managed care digest series: Public payer digest, 2016.* Bridgewater, NJ: Author. p. 43.

The Nursing Home Reform Act, passed in 1987, created two categories for certification purposes. A nursing home certified to admit Medicare patients is called an SNF. This facility can be freestanding or a **distinct part**—that is, a section of a nursing home that is distinctly separate and distinguishable from the rest of the facility. When SNF certification applies to a distinct part, Medicare patients can be admitted only to that section. A nursing home certified for Medicaid only (but not for Medicare) is called a **nursing facility (NF)**. A facility may be dually certified as an SNF and an NF. Facilities having **dual certification** can admit Medicare- and/or Medicaid-insured patients to any part of the facility. Hence, most nursing homes have opted for dual certification. The federal certification standards governing SNFs and NFs are essentially the same. Medicare- and Medicaid-insured patients do not receive two different levels of services; rather, the SNF and NF categories have been created to account for the two distinct sources of public financing.

The term "facility" does not necessarily refer to a separate physical structure in this context. The term can be used for the facility as a whole, or, within the context of licensure and certification, it may apply more specifically to different sections or units of a building (distinct parts) with different certifications or no certification (**FIGURE 10-9**).

A small proportion of facilities have elected not to participate in the Medicaid and/or Medicare programs. They can admit only patients who can pay privately, either out of pocket or through private LTC insurance. These facilities are described as **noncertified**; however, they must be licensed under the state licensure regulations. **Private-pay patients**—those not covered by either Medicare or Medicaid for nursing home care—are not restricted

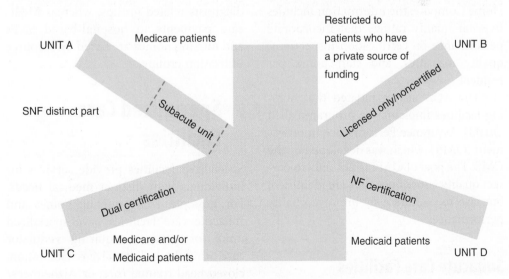

FIGURE 10-9 Distinctly certified units in a nursing home.

to noncertified facilities. These patients also may be admitted to SNF- or NF-certified beds. Thus, the restriction applies only to Medicare- and Medicaid-insured patients, who cannot be admitted to non-certified facilities.

The ACA requires that in case of an LTC facility closure, administrators of an SNF or NF must provide written notice to residents, their legal representatives, and other stakeholders at least 60 days prior to closure. The administrators are also required to furnish a plan for relocating residents. To participate in Medicare and/or Medicaid, nursing facilities must also institute effective compliance and ethics programs (Farhat, 2013).

Licensure and certification standards define minimum standards of quality with which nursing homes must comply, and such compliance is verified through periodic inspections. The CMS provides Web-accessible information on nursing homes' compliance and quality for consumers through a program called Nursing Home Compare; the information includes five-star quality ratings that incorporate performance on certification inspections, quality measures, and staff hours per resident.

The ACA also mandated that nursing facilities implement a program called Quality Assurance Performance Improvement (QAPI), which was developed by the CMS. The goal of QAPI is not only to correct quality issues once they are identified, but also to continuously improve quality performance.

Subacute Care Facilities

The three main institutional locations for subacute care—long-term care hospitals (LTCHs), hospital transitional care units/ extended care units (HTCUs/ECUs) certified as SNFs, and freestanding nursing homes—vary in terms of availability, cost, and quality. Selection of the most appropriate setting for a specific patient is governed by numerous factors, both clinical and nonclinical. The main nonclinical factor is the availability of subacute care services in a given location (Buntin et al., 2005).

In terms of costs, LTCHs are the most expensive. In some cases, nursing homes are a more cost-effective alternative to LTCHs. Because of their high cost, LTCHs are appropriate for medically stable, post-intensive care unit patients (Medicare Payment Advisory Commission [MedPAC], 2016).

Postacute needs can vary widely among patients, but there is no uniform system of clinical assessment and payment for subacute care. Medicare uses different payment methodologies for the different settings. For example, LTCHs are paid according to severity-based diagnosis-related groups, whereas Medicare payments to hospital-based SNFs and nursing homes are based on resource utilization groups.

▶ Specialized Care Facilities

Specialized facilities provide services for individuals with distinct medical needs. For example, some nursing homes and subacute care facilities have specialized units for patients requiring ventilator care, wound care, intensive rehabilitation, closed head trauma care, or Alzheimer's/dementia care. Specialized facilities also exist for IDD patients who require active treatment.

Intermediate Care Facilities for Individuals with Intellectual Disabilities

In 1971, Section 1905(d) of the Social Security Act authorized Medicaid coverage for the care of IDD patients in specialized facilities. Most of these patients have other disabilities in addition to ID. For example, many (1) are nonambulatory; (2) have seizure disorders, behavioral problems, mental illness, or visual or hearing impairments; or (3) have a combination of these conditions. For the care of these patients, federal regulations have provided a separate certification category for LTC facilities classified as intermediate care facilities for individuals with intellectual disabilities (ICF/IIDs; formerly known as intermediate care facilities for the mentally retarded [ICF/MRs]). The primary purpose of ICF/IIDs is to furnish nursing and rehabilitative services that involve "active treatment." Active treatment entails aggressive and consistent specialized programs that include skill training to help the patients function as independently as possible. More than 6,000 ICF/IDD facilities serve more than 100,000 individuals in all 50 states (CMS, 2013).

Alzheimer's Facilities

Informal caregivers, ADC centers, and ALFs can all play a role in the care of patients with dementia, but specialized Alzheimer's facilities are often needed for those who have severe dementia or when comorbid conditions are present. Modern Alzheimer's facilities have small-group living arrangements, copious use of natural lighting, pastel colors, pleasant surroundings, protected pathways for wandering, and special programming. All these features are integrated to minimize agitation, anxiety, disruptiveness, and combativeness among patients with severe dementia.

▶ Continuing Care Retirement Communities

A **continuing care retirement community (CCRC)** integrates and coordinates independent living and institutional components of the LTC continuum. As a convenience factor, different levels of services are all located on one campus. CCRCs also guarantee delivery of higher-level services when future needs arise. Services include independent living in cottages or apartments with or without support services, and medical and nursing care, rehabilitation, and social services in an ALF or SNF. Residents enter these communities when they are still relatively healthy.

CCRCs, for the most part, require private financing, with the exception of services delivered in a Medicare-certified SNF. Three types of CCRC contracts are common in the industry:

- A life care or extended contract comprises a complete package of services that includes a commitment to provide unlimited future LTC services without an increase in the monthly fee.
- A modified contract provides for support services in independent living and includes a limited number of days of care in assisted living and SNF without an increase in the monthly fee.
- A fee-for-service contract includes only support services in independent living; higher levels of services must be paid for out of pocket at the prevailing rates.

There is a wide variation in entrance and monthly fees for CCRCs based on amenities and the type of contract. In the state of New York, for example, entrance fees begin at approximately $115,000 for a single-person independent living unit; monthly fees begin at approximately $2,100 (New York Department of Health, 2016). There are currently more than 2,000 CCRCs in the United States.

▶ # Institutional Trends, Utilization, and Costs

With the emphasis in government policy placed on community-based care, the institutional LTC sector has undergone significant changes over time. For example, the number of nursing home beds per 1,000 population age 65 and older has steadily declined, decreasing from 49.7 in 2000 to an all-time low of 35.1 in 2015 (Sanofi-Aventis, 2016). The number of assisted living facility beds, in contrast, increased from 779,700 in 2011 to 789,800 in 2015 (Sanofi-Aventis, 2016). Over time, community-based services and assisted living have absorbed much of the care that was previously delivered by nursing homes. Consequently, nursing homes have experienced a gradual decline in occupancy rates, from 86.0% in 1992 (National Center for Health Statistics, 1997) to 82.4% in 2000, and then to 80.8% in 2014 (National Center for Health Statistics, 2016). **TABLE 10-1** presents available data on the trends, capacity, utilization, and prices for nursing homes, hospital-based SNFs, and assisted living facilities.

The hospital industry has drastically cut back on the number of SNFs it operates. The number of hospital-based SNFs declined from 1,233 in 2005 to 681 in 2014 (Sanofi-Aventis, 2007, 2016). In 2005, 17.8% of hospitals operated SNFs; in 2014, only 9.5% of hospitals operated such facilities (Sanofi-Aventis, 2007, 2016). Medicare regulations and changes in reimbursement are the likely causes of this decline. Some of the hospital-based SNFs may have been converted to LTCHs, which saw an increase in their numbers over time.

For some time, ALFs were the fastest-growing segment of the institutional continuum, with their numbers steadily rising from 13,544 facilities in 2005 to 15,781 in 2010. Since then, the growth has moderated substantially, with 15,836 facilities being in operation in 2015 (Sanofi-Aventis, 2007, 2016).

Another notable aspect of the LTC market is the rising cost of institutional care, as shown in Table 10-1. Aggregate national nursing home expenditures, however, decreased from 6.2% of total U.S. health care spending in 2000 to 5.1% in 2014 (National Center for Health Statistics, 2016, p. 295), as other health care sectors, such as prescription drugs and hospital services, consumed a greater share of the national health care expenditures.

Five nursing home chains operate a little more than 9% of all U.S. nursing homes: Genesis Healthcare (419 facilities), Golden Living (297 facilities), HCR Manor Care (280 facilities), Life Care Centers of America (215 facilities), and Consulate Health Care (190 facilities) (Sanofi-Aventis, 2016). According to Sanofi-Aventis (2016), more than 10% of the nation's ALFs are operated by the five largest ALF chains: Brookdale Senior Living (993 ALFs), Sunrise Senior Living (238 ALFs), Enlivant (184 ALFs), Five Star Quality Care (159 ALFs), and Atria Senior Living (135 ALFs).

TABLE 10-1 Trends in Number of Long-Term Care Facilities, Beds/Resident Capacity, and Prices, Selected Years

Type of Facility	Number of Facilities	Total Bed Capacity	Beds per 1,000 Population	Occupancy Rate	Average Length of Stay (Days)	Average Price (Annual)
Nursing homes						
2010	15,004	1,667,900	41.4	83.3%	188	$67,525[1]
2015	15,219	1,678,200	35.1	81.5%	180	$80,300[1]
Hospital-based skilled nursing facilities						
2009	930 (13.2% of hospitals)			74.5%	145.0	
2014	681 (9.5% of hospitals)			71.8%	160.4	
Assisted living facilities						
2010	15,781	779,700 (2011)				$38,220[2]
2015	15,836	789,800				$43,200[2]

[1] Annual national median price for a semi-private room (private-pay).
[2] Annual national median price for a private one-bedroom unit (private-pay).

Data from Genworth Financial, Inc. 2010. *Genworth 2010 cost of care survey*. Richmond, VA: Author; Genworth Financial, Inc. 2015. *Genworth 2015 cost of care survey*. Richmond, VA: Author; Sanofi-Aventis. 2016. *Managed care digest series: Public payer digest, 2016*. Bridgewater, NJ: Author.

Most nursing home care is financed by Medicaid (**FIGURE 10-10**). Government policies pushing for HCBS options for Medicaid recipients have been successful in shifting funds away nursing home care. Consequently, the share of total Medicaid spending used for nursing home care declined from 45.5% in 2000 to 35.0% in 2014 (National Center for Health Statistics, 2016, pp. 297, 298). The payment per Medicaid beneficiary receiving care in a nursing home was $28,060 in 2012 (National Center for Health Statistics, 2016, p. 334), compared to $73,000 for a private-pay patient (Genworth Financial, 2012). Private sources (mainly, a combination of out-of-pocket payments and private insurance) also cover a sizable portion of nursing home expenses (Figure 10-10). Total private financing, however, has been declining for a number of years.

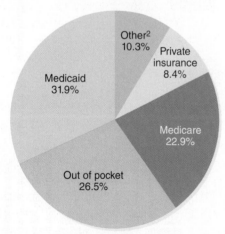

Total nursing home and CCRC
expenditures = 155.6 billion (5.1%
of national health expenditures)

FIGURE 10-10 Sources of financing nursing home care, 2014.[1]

[1] Nonhospital-based facilities; data include CCRCs.
[2] Mainly includes Department of Veterans Affairs, other federal programs, workers' compensation, and other private funds.
Data from National Center for Health Statistics. 2016. *Health, United States, 2015.* Hyattsville, MD: U.S. Department of Health and Human Services. p. 298.

▶ Insurance for Long-Term Care

Private LTC insurance is separate from regular health insurance, as the latter does not cover LTC costs. Medicare, which is the major health insurance program for elderly Americans, also does not cover most LTC services. Medicaid requires spending down most of one's assets to poverty levels to qualify for LTC coverage. As the cost of LTC continues to rise, most people are likely to have few options for paying for such care. Moreover, most are unprepared to cope with the high risk of needing LTC in their retirement years, a period when incomes for most people also dwindle. LTC expenditures may potentially eat into the income and savings of a large portion of middle-class retirees, jeopardizing their standard of living (Ameriks et al., 2016).

After experiencing rapid growth until 2006, the number of people carrying LTC insurance has leveled off. One area of growth comprises combination or hybrid products that combine LTC benefits with either life insurance or an annuity. These products can pay out if LTC is needed, but if not needed, they provide a death benefit or annuity payout (Ameriks et al., 2016).

As the elderly continue to live longer, claims paid by LTC insurers have risen sharply. Consequently, premiums have become unaffordable for most middle-income people. Also, a large number of LTC insurers have left the market altogether. Insurers have faced challenges in anticipating future costs and the ability to spread the risk over a large number of people because of leveling sales of LTC policies. For several years, the ratio of actual to expected losses from claim payments has exceeded 100%.

In fact, between 2010 and 2014, the LTC insurance industry experienced deterioration in its financial performance because the underlying morbidity assumptions used in the initial pricing of premiums were too low (Ameriks et al., 2016).

Public policy has created few incentives to spur the growth of LTC insurance. The DRA of 2005 created the Long-Term Care Insurance Partnership Program, which allowed individuals who purchase private LTC insurance to shield part of their financial assets when they became eligible to receive Medicaid benefits for LTC. This policy seems to have had some effect in spurring the purchase of LTC insurance. By 2015, slightly more than two out of every five new LTC policies sold were Partnership policies (Ameriks et al., 2016). More than half the states provide tax incentives for the purchase of LTC insurance, but there is little evidence that such incentives have played a noticeable role in persuading consumers to purchase LTC insurance (Ameriks et al., 2016).

The ACA did little to address the impending dilemma of how to provide LTC—a dilemma that many people will face as they age. The impending burden on Medicaid and Medicare will be unsustainable. Hence, LTC financing is at a critical juncture.

▶ Summary

The need for long-term care arises when an individual is no longer able to perform ADL and/or IADL functions because of a severe chronic condition, multiple illnesses, or cognitive impairment. Such individuals need both LTC and non-LTC services on an ongoing basis. LTC is unique within health care delivery, and is multidimensional.

LTC includes medical care, nursing, rehabilitation, social support, mental health care, housing alternatives, and end-of-life care. LTC services often complement what people with impaired functioning can do for themselves. Informal caregivers provide the bulk of LTC services in the United States. Respite care can provide family members with temporary relief from the burden of caregiving. When the required intensity of care exceeds the capabilities of informal caregivers, alternatives include professional community-based services to supplement informal care.

Institutional services vary from basic personal assistance to more complex skilled nursing care and subacute care. Institutional care can be of long or short duration. People with severe dementia, incontinence, severe psychiatric or behavioral issues, or unstable postacute conditions, and those in a comatose/vegetative state may need nursing home care for a long time. Other patients may require short-term postacute convalescence and restorative care. A continuing care retirement community offers independent living and institution-based LTC services. Specialized institutions exist for people with Alzheimer's disease or severe intellectual or developmental disability.

Nursing homes require federal SNF certification to admit Medicare patients and NF certification to admit Medicaid patients. Most facility beds in the United States are dually certified as both SNFs and NFs. Medicaid is the most common source of funding for nursing home care.

The LTC industry has become more competitive as services offered by community-based and institutional options have started to overlap. Within the institutional sector, the number of nursing homes and beds has been declining; this trend is more pronounced in hospital-based SNFs. Conversely, ALFs have experienced remarkable growth, which is moderating.

Although costs for LTC provided in the public sector continue to rise, few people have purchased private LTC insurance. Better government policies are needed to spur growth in private insurance, as Medicaid and Medicare expenditures for LTC will be unsustainable in the long term.

▶ Test Your Understanding

Terminology

adult day care (ADC)
adult foster care (AFC)
aging-in-place
Alzheimer's disease
assisted living facility (ALF)
brokerage model
case management
cognitive impairment
continuing care retirement community (CCRC)
custodial care
dementia
developmental disability (DD)
distinct part

dual certification
evidence-based care
intellectual disability (ID)
long-term care (LTC)
meals-on-wheels
Money Follows the Person (MFP)
noncertified
nursing facility (NF)
palliation
paraprofessionals
personal care
personal emergency response system (PERS)

Preadmission Screening and Resident Review (PASRR)
private-pay patients
Program of All-Inclusive Care for the Elderly (PACE)
quality of life
respite care
restorative care
senior centers
skilled nursing care
skilled nursing facility (SNF)
subacute care
total care

Review Questions

1. Long-term care services must be individualized, integrated, and coordinated. Elaborate on this statement, pointing out why these elements are essential in the delivery of LTC.

2. Age is not the primary determinant for long-term care. Comment on this statement, explaining why this is or is not true.

3. What is meant by "quality of life"? Briefly discuss the five main features of this multifaceted concept.

4. What are some of the challenges in the delivery of mental health services for the elderly?

5. Discuss the preventive and therapeutic aspects of long-term care.

6. How do formal and informal long-term care differ? What is the importance of informal care in LTC delivery?

7. What are the main goals of community-based and institution-based LTC services?

8. What is respite care? Why is it needed?

9. Distinguish between supportive housing and institutional long-term care.

10. Why do some children and adolescents need long-term care?

11. Why has long-term care become an important service for people with HIV/AIDS?

12. Briefly discuss the brokerage model of case management and the PACE program.

13. What is meant by the continuum of institutional long-term care? Discuss the clinical services delivered by residential/personal care facilities, assisted living facilities, and skilled nursing facilities.

14. What is the difference between licensure and certification? What are the two types of certifications? What purpose does each serve from (a) a clinical standpoint and (b) a financial standpoint?

15. Describe a continuing care retirement community. Include in your response the financing and contractual arrangements.

16. Discuss the main issues with private long-term care insurance. Briefly explain the Long-Term Care Insurance Partnership Program.

▶ References

AARP studies adult foster care for the elderly. 1996. *Public Health Reports* 111, no. 4: 295.

Administration on Aging (AoA). 2016. *Profile of older Americans: 2015*. Available at: http://www.aoa.acl.gov/Aging_Statistics/Profile/2015/14.aspx. Accessed December 2016.

Alzheimer's Association. 2013. *Alzheimer's facts and figures*. Available at: http://www.alz.org/alzheimers_disease_facts_and_figures.asp#prevalence. Accessed August 2013.

Ameriks, J., et al. 2016. *The state of long-term care insurance: The market, challenges, and future innovations*. Kansas City, MO: National Association of Insurance Commissioners.

Barba, B. E., et al. 2012. Quality geriatric care as perceived by nurses in long-term and acute care settings. *Journal of Clinical Nursing* 21, no. 5/6: 833–840.

Boyle, C. A., et al. 2011. Trends in the prevalence of developmental disabilities in US children, 1997–2008. *Pediatrics* 127, no. 6: 1034–1042.

Buntin, M. B., et al. 2005. How much is postacute care use affected by its availability? *Health Services Research* 40, no. 2: 413–434.

Burwell, B., and P. Saucier. 2013. Managed long-term services and supports programs are a cornerstone for fully integrated care. *Generations* 37, no. 2: 33–38.

Centers for Medicare and Medicaid Services (CMS). 2013. *Intermediate care facilities for individuals with intellectual disabilities (ICFs/IID)*. Available at: http://www.cms.gov/Medicare/Provider-Enrollment-and-Certification/CertificationandComplianc/ICFMRs.html. Accessed August 2013.

Compston, A., and A. Coles. 2002. Multiple sclerosis. *Lancet* 359, no. 9313: 1221–1231.

Congressional Budget Office (CBO). 2013. *Rising demand for long-term services and supports for elderly people*. Available at: https://www.cbo.gov/sites/default/files/cbofiles/attachments/44363-LTC.pdf. Accessed December 2016.

Davis, K., et al. 2016. Medicare help at home. *Health Affairs Blog*. Available at: http://healthaffairs.org/blog/2016/04/13/medicare-help-at-home. Accessed December 2016.

Department of Health and Human Services (DHHS). 2017. *Long-term care: Find your path forward*. Available at: https://longtermcare.acl.gov/. Accessed May 2017.

Farhat, T. 2013. Compliance clock ticks. *McKnight's Long-Term Care News* 34, no. 2: 30–31.

Federal Interagency Forum on Aging-Related Statistics. 2012. *Older Americans 2012: Key indicators of well-being.* Washington, DC: US Government Printing Office.

Foebel, A. D., et al. 2015. Comparing the characteristics of people living with and without HIV in long-term care and home care in Ontario, Canada. *AIDS Care* 27, no. 10: 1343–1353.

Genworth Financial, Inc. 2010. *Genworth 2010 cost of care survey.* Richmond, VA: Author.

Genworth Financial, Inc. 2015. *Genworth 2015 cost of care survey.* Richmond, VA: Author.

Gerteis, J., et al. 2014. *Multiple chronic conditions chartbook: 2010 medical expenditure panel survey data.* Rockville, MD: Agency for Healthcare Research and Quality.

Gross, D. L., et al. 2004. The growing pains of integrated health care for the elderly: Lessons from the expansion of PACE. *Milbank Quarterly* 82, no. 2: 257–282.

Han, K., et al. 2016. Variations across U.S. assisted living facilities: Admissions, resident care needs, and staffing. *Journal of Nursing Scholarship* 49: 24–32.

Harris-Kojetin, L., et al. 2016. *Long-term care providers and services users in the United States: Data from the National Study of Long-Term Care Providers, 2013–2014.* Hyattsville, MD: National Center for Health Statistics.

Health Policy Institute. 2003. *Who needs long-term care? Long-Term Care Financing Project.* Georgetown University. Available at: http://ltc.georgetown.edu/pdfs/whois.pdf. Accessed August 2013.

Helmer, C., et al. 2006. Dementia in subjects aged 75 years or over within the PAQUID cohort: Prevalence and burden by severity. *Dementia and Geriatric Cognitive Disorders* 22, no. 1: 87–94.

Hoban, S. 2013. Assisted living 2013: On the upswing. *Long-Term Living: For the Continuing Care Professional* 62, no. 3: 28–30.

Holtz-Eakin, D. 2005, April 27. *CBO testimony: The cost of financing of long-term care services.* Before the Subcommittee on Health Committee on Energy and Commerce, U.S. House of Representatives.

Hung, W. W., et al. 2012. Association of chronic diseases and impairments with disability in older adults: A decade of change? *Medical Care* 50, no. 6: 501–507.

Hurd, M. D., et al. 2013. Monetary costs of dementia in the United States. *New England Journal of Medicine* 368, no. 14: 1326–1334.

Iglehart, J. K. 2016. Future of long-term care and the expanding role of Medicaid managed care. *New England Journal of Medicine* 374: 182–187.

Irvin, C. V. 2015. *Money Follows the Person 2014 annual evaluation report.* Cambridge, MA: Mathematica Policy Research.

Jones, A. L., et al. 2012. *Characteristics and use of home health care by men and women aged 65 and over. National health statistics reports, No. 52.* Hyattsville, MD: National Center for Health Statistics.

Karpiak, S. E., and R. Havlik. 2017. Are HIV-infected older adults aging differently? *Interdisciplinary Topics in Gerontology and Geriatrics* 42: 11–27.

Kaye, H. S., et al. 2010. Long-term care: Who gets it, who provides it, who pays, and how much? *Health Affairs* 29, no. 1: 11–21.

Kowlessar, N., et al. 2015. *Older Americans Act Nutrition Programs.* Research Brief Number 8. Administration on Aging. Available at: https://aoa.acl.gov/Program_Results/docs/2015/AoA-Research-Brief-8-2015.pdf. Accessed December 2016.

Kuzuya, M., et al. 2011. Impact of informal care levels on discontinuation of living at home in community-dwelling dependent elderly using various community-based services. *Archives of Gerontology & Geriatrics* 52, no. 2: 127–132.

Kwak, J., and L. J. Polivka. 2014. *The future of long-term care and the aging network.* American Society on Aging. Available at: http://www.asaging.org/blog/future-long-term-care-and-aging-network. Accessed December 2016.

Leveille, S. G., and S. Thapa. 2017. Disability among persons aging with HIV/AIDS. *Interdisciplinary Topics in Gerontology and Geriatrics* 42: 101–118.

Levine, C., et al. 2010. Bridging troubled waters: Family caregivers, transitions, and long-term care. *Health Affairs* 29, no. 1: 116–124.

Mann, C. 2011. *CMCS informational bulletin.* Available at: https://www.medicaid.gov/federal-policy-guidance/downloads/2-28-11-recent-developments-in-medicaid.pdf. Accessed December 2016.

Medicare Payment Advisory Commission (MedPAC). 2016. *Long-term care hospital services: Assessing payment adequacy and updating payments.*

Report to Congress. Washington, DC: Medicare Payment Advisory Commission.

Meret-Hanke, L. A. 2011. Effects of the Program of All-inclusive Care for the Elderly on hospital use. *Gerontologist* 51, no. 6: 774–785.

MetLife Mature Market Institute. 2010. *The MetLife national study of adult day services.* Westport, CT: Metropolitan Life Insurance Company.

Micheletti, J. A., and T. J. Shlala. 1995. Understanding and operationalizing subacute services. *Nursing Management* 26, no. 6: 49–56.

Morley, J. E. 2012. High technology coming to a nursing home near you. *Journal of the American Medical Directors Association* 13, no. 5: 409–412.

National Center for Health Statistics. 1997. *Health, United States, 1996–97.* Hyattsville, MD: U.S. Department of Health and Human Services.

National Center for Health Statistics. 2010. *Health, United States, 2010.* Hyattsville, MD: U.S. Department of Health and Human Services.

National Center for Health Statistics. 2016. *Health, United States, 2015.* Hyattsville, MD: U.S. Department of Health and Human Services.

National Health Policy Forum. 2013. *State variation in long-term services and supports: Location, location, location. Forum Session, July 19, 2013.* Washington, DC: George Washington University.

New York Department of Health. 2016. *Continuing care retirement communities & fee-for-service continuing care retirement communities.* Available at: https://www.health.ny.gov/facilities/long_term _care/retirement_communities/continuing _care/. Accessed December 2016.

Niederhauser, A., et al. 2012. Comprehensive programs for preventing pressure ulcers: A review of the literature. *Advances in Skin & Wound Care* 25, no. 4: 167–188.

O'Shaughnessy, C. V. 2013. *Family caregivers: The primary providers of assistance to people with functional limitations and chronic impairments.* National Health Policy Forum, Background Paper No. 84. Available at: https:// www.nhpf.org/library/background-papers /BP84_FamilyCaregiving_01-11-13.pdf. Accessed December 2016.

Partnership for Solutions and Johns Hopkins University. 2002. *Chronic conditions: Making the case for ongoing care.* Baltimore, MD: Johns Hopkins University.

Reinhard, S. C. 2012. Money Follows the Person: Un-burning bridges and facilitating a return to the community. *Generations* 36, no. 1: 52–58.

Reinhard, S. C., et al. 2011. How the Affordable Care Act can help move states toward a high-performing system of long-term services and supports. *Health Affairs* 30, no. 3: 447–453.

Reinhard, S. C., et al. 2015. *Valuing the invaluable: 2015 update undeniable progress, but big gaps remain.* AARP. Available at: http://www.aarp .org/content/dam/aarp/ppi/2015/valuing -the-invaluable-2015-update-new.pdf. Accessed December 2016.

Riordan, J., and D. Voegeli. 2009. Prevention and treatment of pressure ulcers. *British Journal of Nursing* 18, no. 20: S20–S27.

Robinson, K. M. 2010. Policy issues in mental health among the elderly. *Nursing Clinics of North America* 45, no. 4: 627–634.

Robinson, L. M. 2012. Growing health disparities for persons who are aging with intellectual and developmental disabilities: The social work linchpin. *Journal of Gerontological Social Work* 55, no. 2: 175–190.

Robison, J., et al. 2012. Transition from home care to nursing home: Unmet needs in a home- and community-based program for older adults. *Journal of Aging and Social Policy* 24, no. 3: 251–270.

Sanofi-Aventis. 2007. *Managed care digest series: Senior care digest, 2007.* Bridgewater, NJ: Author.

Sanofi-Aventis. 2016. *Managed care digest series: Public payer digest, 2016.* Bridgewater, NJ: Author.

Scocco, P., et al. 2006. Nursing home institutionalization: A source of *eustress* or *distress* for the elderly. *International Journal of Geriatric Psychiatry* 21, no. 3: 281–287.

Shippy, R. A., and S. E. Karpiak. 2005. Perceptions of support among older adults with HIV. *Research on Aging* 27, no. 3: 290–306.

Singh, D. A. 1997. *Nursing home administrators: Their influence on quality of care.* New York: Garland Publishing, Inc.

Singh, D. A. 2016. *Effective management of long-term care facilities.* 3rd ed. Burlington, MA: Jones & Bartlett Learning.

Spellman, S., and K. Brod. 2014. Continuing care at home. *Senior Housing & Care Journal* 22, no. 1: 112–118.

Stahl, C. 1997, September. Adult foster care: An alternative to SNFs? *ADVANCE for Occupational Therapists*, p. 18.

Szanton, S. L., et al. 2016. Home-based care program reduces disability and promotes aging in place. *Health Affairs* 35, no. 9: 1558–1563.

Tabert, M. H., et al. 2002. Functional deficits in patients with mild cognitive impairments: Prediction of AD. *Neurology* 58: 758–764.

Teresi, J. A., et al. 2013. Comparative effectiveness of implementing evidence-based education and best practices in nursing homes: Effects on falls, quality-of-life and societal costs. *International Journal of Nursing Studies* 50, no. 4: 448–463.

Tune, L. 2001. Assessing psychiatric illness in geriatric patients. *Clinical Cornerstone* 3, no. 3: 23–36.

Van Houtven, C. H., and E. Norton. 2004. Informal care and health care use of older adults. *Journal of Health Economics* 23, no. 6: 1159–1180.

Vargas, R. B., and W. E. Cunningham. 2006. Evolving trends in medical care-coordination for patients with HIV and AIDS. *Current HIV /AIDS Reports* 3, no. 4: 149–153.

Wieland, D., et al. 2013. Does Medicaid pay more to a Program of All-Inclusive Care for the Elderly (PACE) than for fee-for-service long-term care? *Journal of Gerontology. Series A, Biological Sciences and Medical Sciences* 68, no. 1: 47–55.

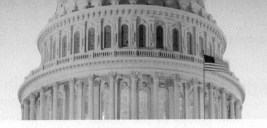

CHAPTER 11

Health Services for Special Populations

LEARNING OBJECTIVES

- Describe population groups facing greater challenges and barriers in accessing health care services.
- Identify racial and ethnic disparities in health status.
- Discuss the health concerns of U.S. children and the health services available to them.
- Discuss the health concerns of U.S. women and the health services available to them.
- Describe rural health challenges and measures taken to improve access to care in rural populations.
- Describe the characteristics and health concerns of homeless populations and migrant workers.
- Describe the U.S. mental health system.
- Summarize the AIDS epidemic in the United States, the population groups affected by it, and the services available to patients with HIV/AIDS.
- Identify the benefits of the Affordable Care Act for certain vulnerable groups.

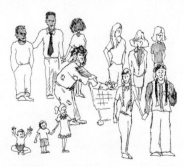

They all have something in common.

▶ Introduction

Certain population groups in the United States face greater challenges than the general population in accessing timely and needed health care services (Shortell et al., 1996). As a consequence, members of these groups are at greater risk of poor physical, psychological, and/or social health (Aday, 1993). Various terms are used to describe these populations, such as "underserved populations," "medically underserved," "medically disadvantaged," "underprivileged," and "American underclasses." The causes of their vulnerability are largely attributable to unequal social, economic, health, and geographic conditions. These population groups consist of racial and ethnic minorities, uninsured children, women, persons living in rural areas, homeless individuals and families, mentally ill individuals, chronically ill and disabled individuals, and persons with **human immunodeficiency**

virus (HIV)/acquired immunodeficiency syndrome (AIDS). These population groups are more vulnerable than the general population and experience greater barriers in access to care, financing of care, and racial or cultural acceptance.

After presenting a conceptual framework to study vulnerable populations, this chapter defines these special population groups, describes their health needs, and summarizes the major challenges they face. The potential impact of the Affordable Care Act (ACA) on vulnerable populations is also discussed.

▶ Framework to Study Vulnerable Populations

The vulnerability framework (**EXHIBIT 11-1**) is an integrated approach to studying vulnerability (Shi and Stevens, 2010). From a health perspective, *vulnerability* refers to

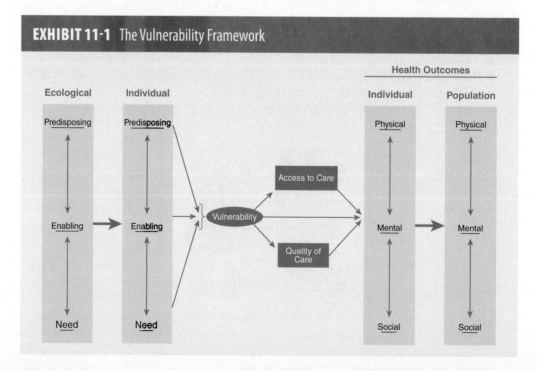

EXHIBIT 11-1 The Vulnerability Framework

the likelihood of experiencing poor health or illness. Poor health can be manifested physically, psychologically, and socially. Because poor health along one dimension is likely to be compounded by poor health along others, the health needs are greater for those persons with problems along multiple dimensions compared to those persons with problems along a single dimension.

According to the framework, vulnerability is determined by a convergence of (1) predisposing, (2) enabling, and (3) need characteristics at both individual and ecological (contextual) levels (**EXHIBIT 11-2**). Not only do these predisposing, enabling, and need characteristics converge and determine individuals' access to health care, but they also ultimately influence individuals' risk of contracting illness or, for those already sick, recovering from illness. Individuals with multiple risks (i.e., a combination of two or more vulnerability traits) typically experience worse access to care, care of lesser quality, and inferior health status than do those with fewer vulnerability traits.

Understanding vulnerability as a combination or convergence of disparate factors is preferred over studying individual factors separately because vulnerability, when defined as a convergence of risks, best captures reality. This approach not only reflects the co-occurrence of risk factors, but also underscores the belief that it is difficult to address disparities related to one risk factor without addressing others.

This vulnerability model has a number of distinctive characteristics. First, it is a comprehensive model, including both individual and ecological attributes of risk. Second, it is a general model, focusing on the attributes of vulnerability for the total population rather than vulnerable traits of subpopulations. Although we recognize individual differences in exposure to risks, we also think that some common, cross-cutting traits affect all vulnerable populations. Third, a major distinction of our model is its emphasis on the convergence of vulnerability. In other words, the effects of experiencing multiple vulnerable traits may lead to cumulative vulnerability that is additive or even multiplicative.

EXHIBIT 11-2 Predisposing, Enabling, and Need Characteristics of Vulnerability

Predisposing characteristics:
- Racial/ethnic characteristics
- Gender and age (women and children)
- Geographic location (rural health)

Enabling characteristics:
- Insurance status (uninsured)
- Homelessness

Need characteristics:
- Mental health
- Chronic illness/disability
- HIV/AIDS

▶ Racial/Ethnic Minorities

The 2010 U.S. census questionnaire listed 15 racial categories, as well as places to write in specific races not listed on the form (U.S. Census Bureau, 2009). These racial categories were White, Black, American Indian or Alaska Native, Asian Indian, Chinese, Filipino, Japanese, Korean, Vietnamese, Other Asian, Native Hawaiian, Guamanian or Chamorro, Samoan, Other Pacific Islander, or some other race. Respondents could choose more than one race.

The U.S. Census Bureau (2015) estimated that, in 2015, more than 38% of the U.S. population was made up of minorities: black or African Americans (13.3%), Hispanics or Latinos (17.6%), Asians (5.6%), Native Hawaiian and Other Pacific Islanders (0.2%), and American Indian and Alaska Natives (1.2%). In addition, 2.6% of all Americans self-identified as being two or more races (U.S. Census Bureau, 2010a).

Significant differences exist across the various racial/ethnic groups on health-related lifestyles and health status. For example, in 2014, the percentage of live births in which the neonate weighed less than 2,500 grams (low birth weight) was greatest among blacks, followed by Asians or Pacific Islanders, American Indians or Native Americans, Hispanics, and whites (**FIGURE 11-1**). Asians and Pacific Islanders were most likely to begin prenatal care during their first trimester,

followed by whites, Hispanics, blacks, and American Indians or Alaska Natives (**TABLE 11-1**). Mothers of whites and individuals of Asian and Pacific Islander origin were least likely to smoke cigarettes during pregnancy, followed by Hispanics, blacks, and American Indians or Alaska Natives; mothers in the last group had a smoking rate more than double that of any other group (18%) (**FIGURE 11-2**). The white adult population is more likely to consume alcohol than other races (**FIGURE 11-3**). Among women 40 years of age and older, utilization of mammography is the highest among whites and lowest among Hispanics (**FIGURE 11-4**).

Black Americans

Black Americans are more likely to be economically disadvantaged than whites. They also fall behind in health status, despite progress made during the past few

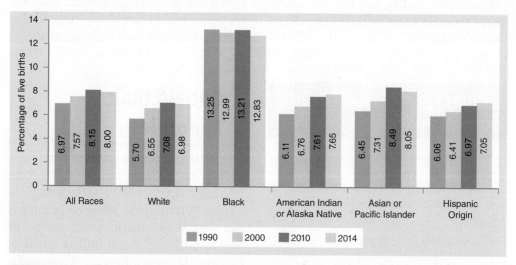

FIGURE 11-1 Percentage of U.S. live births weighing less than 2,500 grams by mother's detailed race.

Data from National Center for Health Statistics (NCHS). 2016b. *Health, United States, 2015.* Hyattsville, MD: U.S. Department of Health and Human Services. p. 74.

TABLE 11-1 Characteristics of U.S. Mothers by Race/Ethnicity

Item	1970	1980	1990	2000	2010	2014
Prenatal Care Began During First Trimester						
All mothers	68.0	76.3	75.8	83.2	83.2	84.8
White	72.3	79.2	79.2	85.0	84.7	86.6
Black	44.2	62.4	60.6	74.3	76.0	80.8
American Indian or Alaskan Native	38.2	55.8	57.9	69.3	69.5	76.7
Asian or Pacific Islander	—	73.7	75.1	84.0	84.8	86.4
Hispanic origin	—	60.2	60.2	74.4	77.3	83.3
Education of Mother 16 Years or More						
All mothers	8.6	14.0	17.5	24.7	26.6[1]	20.2
White	9.6	15.5	19.3	26.3	27.9[1]	25.0
Black	2.8	6.2	7.2	11.7	13.4[1]	12.5
American Indian or Alaska Native	2.7	3.5	4.4	7.8	8.5[1]	12.2
Asian or Pacific Islander	—	30.8	31.0	42.8	47.1[1]	35.1
Hispanic origin	—	4.2	5.1	7.6	8.7[1]	8.4

(continues)

TABLE 11-1 Characteristics of U.S. Mothers by Race/Ethnicity (*continued*)						
Item	**1970**	**1980**	**1990**	**2000**	**2010**	**2014**
Low Birth Weight (Less Than 2,500 Grams)						
All mothers	7.93	6.84	6.97	7.57	8.15	8.00
White	6.85	5.72	5.70	6.55	7.08	6.98
Black	13.90	12.69	13.25	12.99	13.21	12.83
American Indian or Alaska Native	7.97	6.44	6.11	6.76	7.61	7.65
Asian or Pacific Islander	—	6.68	6.45	7.31	8.49	8.05
Hispanic origin (selected states)	—	6.12	6.06	6.41	6.97	7.05

[1] Data from 2008.
Note: Numbers are percentages.

Data from National Center for Health Statistics (NCHS). 2010. *Health, United States, 2009*. Hyattsville, MD: U.S. Department of Health and Human Services. pp. 159, 163; National Center for Health Statistics (NCHS). 2013. *Health, United States, 2012*. Hyattsville, MD: U.S. Department of Health and Human Services. p. 144; National Center for Health Statistics (NCHS). 2016b. *Health, United States, 2015*. Hyattsville, MD: U.S. Department of Health and Human Services. p. 74.

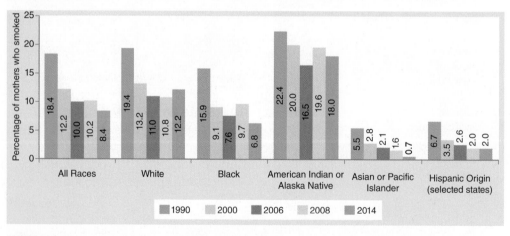

FIGURE 11-2 Percentage of U.S. mothers who smoked cigarettes during pregnancy according to mother's race.

Data from Centers for Disease Control and Prevention (CDC). 2016d. *Smoking prevalence and cessation before and during pregnancy: Data from the birth certificate*, 2014. National Vital Statistics Reports 65. Available at: https://www.cdc.gov/nchs/data/nvsr/nvsr65/nvsr65_01.pdf. Accessed July 2017.

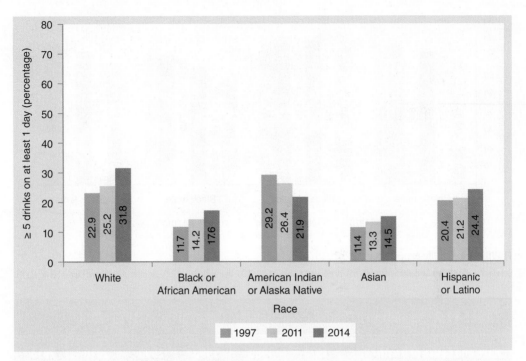

FIGURE 11-3 Alcohol consumption by persons 18 years of age and older.

Data from National Center for Health Statistics (NCHS). 2014a. *National Health Interview Survey.* Available at: https://www.cdc.gov/nchs/nhis/. Accessed March 2017.

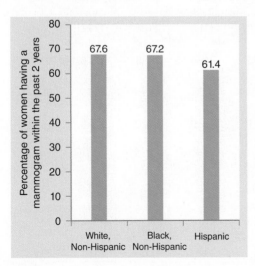

FIGURE 11-4 Use of mammography by women 40 years of age and older, 2013.

Data from National Center for Health Statistics (NCHS). 2016b. *Health, United States, 2015.* Hyattsville, MD: U.S. Department of Health and Human Services. p. 246.

decades. Blacks have shorter life expectancies than whites (**FIGURE 11-5**); higher age-adjusted death rates for a majority of leading causes of death (**TABLE 11-2**); higher age-adjusted maternal mortality rates (**FIGURE 11-6**); and higher infant, neonatal, and postneonatal mortality rates (**TABLE 11-3**). On self-reported measures of health status, blacks are more likely to report fair or poor health status compared to whites (**FIGURE 11-7**). In terms of behavioral risks, black males are slightly more likely to smoke cigarettes than white males (21.7% versus 18.8%), but white females are more likely to smoke than black females (16% versus 13.4%) (**FIGURE 11-8**), although smoking among black females has increased in recent years. Conversely, blacks have lower

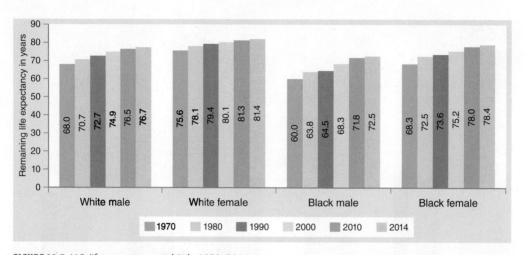

FIGURE 11-5 U.S. life expectancy at birth, 1970–2014.

Data from National Center for Health Statistics (NCHS). **2016b.** *Health, United States, 2015*. Hyattsville, MD: U.S. Department of Health and Human Services. p. 93.

TABLE 11-2 Age-Adjusted Death Rates for Selected Causes of Death, 1970–2014

Race and Cause of Death	1970	1980	1990	2000	2010	2014
All Persons: Deaths per 100,000 Standard Population						
All causes	1,222.6	1,039.1	938.7	869.0	747.0	724.6
Diseases of the heart	492.7	412.1	321.8	257.6	179.1	167.0
Ischemic heart disease	—	345.2	249.6	186.8	113.6	98.8
Cerebrovascular diseases	147.7	96.2	65.3	60.9	39.1	36.5
Malignant neoplasms	198.6	207.9	216.0	199.6	172.8	161.2
Chronic lower respiratory diseases	21.3	28.3	37.2	44.2	42.2	40.5
Influenza and pneumonia	41.7	31.4	36.8	23.7	15.1	15.1
Chronic liver disease and cirrhosis	17.8	15.1	11.1	9.5	9.4	10.4
Diabetes mellitus	24.3	18.1	20.7	25.0	20.8	20.9
Human immunodeficiency virus (HIV) disease	—	—	10.2	5.2	2.6	2.0

Unintentional injuries	60.1	46.4	36.3	34.9	38.0	40.5
Motor vehicle-related injuries	27.6	22.3	18.5	15.4	11.3	10.8
Suicide	13.1	12.2	12.5	10.4	12.1	13.0
Homicide	8.8	10.4	9.4	5.9	5.3	5.1
White						
All causes	1,193.3	1,012.7	909.8	849.8	741.8	725.4
Diseases of the heart	492.2	409.4	317.0	253.4	176.9	165.9
Ischemic heart disease	—	347.6	249.7	185.6	113.5	99.3
Cerebrovascular diseases	143.5	93.2	62.8	58.8	37.7	35.2
Malignant neoplasms	196.7	204.2	211.6	197.2	172.4	161.9
Chronic lower respiratory diseases	21.8	29.3	38.3	46.0	44.6	43.1
Influenza and pneumonia	39.8	30.9	36.4	23.5	14.9	15.1
Chronic liver disease and cirrhosis	16.6	13.9	10.5	9.6	9.9	11.2
Diabetes mellitus	22.9	16.7	18.8	22.8	19.0	19.3
Human immunodeficiency virus (HIV) disease	—	—	8.3	2.8	1.4	1.1
Unintentional injuries	57.8	45.3	35.5	35.1	40.3	43.1
Motor vehicle-related injuries	27.1	22.6	18.5	15.6	11.7	11.1
Suicide	13.8	13.0	13.4	11.3	13.6	14.7
Homicide	4.7	6.7	5.5	3.6	3.3	3.0
Black						
All causes	1,518.1	1,314.8	1,250.3	1,121.4	898.2	849.3

(continues)

TABLE 11-2 Age-Adjusted Death Rates for Selected Causes of Death, 1970–2014 (*continued*)

Race and Cause of Death	1970	1980	1990	2000	2010	2014
Diseases of the heart	512.0	455.3	391.5	324.8	224.9	206.3
Ischemic heart disease	—	334.5	267.0	218.3	131.2	112.8
Cerebrovascular diseases	197.1	129.1	91.6	81.9	53.0	49.7
Malignant neoplasms	225.3	256.4	279.5	248.5	203.8	185.6
Chronic lower respiratory diseases	16.2	19.2	28.1	31.6	29.0	28.4
Influenza and pneumonia	57.2	34.4	39.4	25.6	16.8	16.1
Chronic liver disease and cirrhosis	28.1	25.0	16.5	9.4	6.7	7.2
Diabetes mellitus	38.8	32.7	40.5	49.5	38.7	37.3
Human immunodeficiency virus (HIV) disease	—	—	26.7	23.3	11.6	8.3
Unintentional injuries	78.3	57.6	43.8	37.7	31.3	33.8
Motor vehicle-related injuries	31.1	20.2	18.8	15.7	10.9	11.1
Suicide	6.2	6.5	7.1	5.5	5.2	5.5
Homicide	44.0	39.0	36.3	20.5	17.7	17.2

Data from National Center for Health Statistics (NCHS). 2016b. *Health, United States, 2015*. Hyattsville, MD: U.S. Department of Health and Human Services. pp. 99–101.

levels of serum cholesterol than whites (**TABLE 11-4**). Rates of heart disease and stroke deaths are highest among non-Hispanic blacks, and rates of hypertension are highest among this racial group as well. Non-Hispanic black women are more likely to lose more expected years of life due to breast cancer than non-Hispanic whites (Hung et al., 2016). The prevalence of diabetes is highest among Hispanics and non-Hispanic blacks compared to non-Hispanic whites (National Center for Health Statistics [NCHS], 2016b).

Hispanic Americans

The Hispanic segment of the U.S. population is growing at a significantly faster rate than other population segments. Between 2000 and 2010, the Hispanic

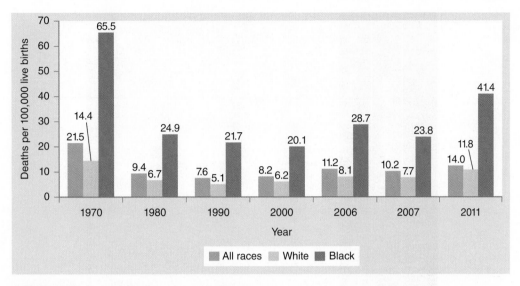

FIGURE 11-6 Age-adjusted maternal mortality rates.

Data from National Center for Health Statistics (NCHS). 2011. *Health, United States, 2010*. Hyattsville, MD: U.S. Department of Health and Human Services. p. 231; Centers for Disease Control and Prevention (CDC). 2016e. *Pregnancy Mortality Surveillance System*. Available at: https://www.cdc.gov/reproductivehealth /maternalinfanthealth/pmss.html. Accessed July 2017.

segment increased by 43%, compared to a 10% increase for the total U.S. population (U.S. Census Bureau, 2011a, 2011b). In 2014, the U.S. Hispanic population numbered nearly 55 million; it is projected to reach 119 million by 2060.

Hispanic Americans are also one of the youngest groups in the United States. In 2014, the median age for Hispanic Americans was 28.4 years, compared to 43.1 years for non-Hispanic whites. In 2013, 9.7% of Hispanics were younger than age 5, compared to 5.1% of non-Hispanic whites (U.S. Census Bureau, 2013). In 2012, 25.6% of Hispanic persons lived below the federal poverty level (FPL), compared to 9.7% of non-Hispanic white persons (U.S. Census Bureau, 2013).

Many Hispanic Americans experience significant barriers in accessing medical care. This represents a greater problem for those from Central America (39% foreign born) than those from South America (25.6% foreign born) and Mexico (32.6%

foreign born). Place of birth also contributes to some Hispanic people's inability to speak English, which is another factor associated with reduced access to medical services (Solis et al., 1990).

Because of their relatively low education levels, Hispanic Americans have higher unemployment rates than non-Hispanic whites (5.6% versus 4.0% in 2016; U.S. Bureau of Labor Statistics, 2016) and are more likely to be employed in semiskilled, nonprofessional occupations (U.S. Census Bureau, 2011a). Consequently, Hispanic Americans are more likely to be uninsured or underinsured than non-Hispanic whites. In 2014, 25.5% of Hispanic persons were uninsured, compared to 13.3% of non-Hispanic whites and 13.7% of non-Hispanic blacks or African Americans (NCHS, 2016b). Among Hispanics, 27.2% of Mexican Americans were uninsured, followed by 19.4% of Cubans, 13.0% of Puerto Ricans, and 26.2% of other Hispanics (NCHS, 2016b).

TABLE 11-3 Infant, Neonatal, and Postneonatal Mortality Rates by Mother's Race (per 1,000 Live Births)

Race of Mother	Infant Deaths						Neonatal Deaths						Postneonatal Deaths					
	1983	1990	2000	2008	2013		1983	1990	2000	2008	2013		1983	1990	2000	2008	2013	
All mothers	10.9	8.9	6.9	6.6	6.0		7.1	5.7	4.6	4.3	4.0		3.8	3.2	2.3	2.3	1.9	
White	9.3	7.3	5.7	5.6	5.1		6.1	4.6	3.8	3.6	3.4		3.2	2.7	1.9	2.0	1.6	
Black	19.2	16.9	13.5	12.4	10.8		12.5	11.1	9.1	8.1	7.3		6.7	5.9	4.3	4.3	3.5	
American Indian or Alaska Native	15.2	13.1	8.3	8.4	7.6		7.5	6.1	4.4	4.2	4.1		7.7	7.0	3.9	4.2	3.5	
Asian or Pacific Islander	8.3	6.6	4.9	4.5	4.1		5.2	3.9	3.4	3.1	3.0		3.1	2.7	1.4	1.4	1.1	
Hispanic origin (selected states)	9.5	7.5	5.6	5.6	5.0		6.2	4.8	3.8	3.9	3.6		3.3	2.9	1.8	1.8	1.5	

Data from National Center for Health Statistics (NCHS). 2013. *Health, United States, 2012.* Hyattsville, MD: U.S. Department of Health and Human Services. p. 66; National Center for Health Statistics (NCHS). 2016b. *Health, United States, 2015.* Hyattsville, MD: U.S. Department of Health and Human Services. p. 86.

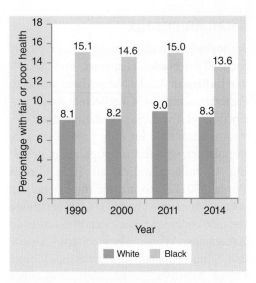

FIGURE 11-7 Respondent-assessed health status.

Data from *Health, United States, 1995*. p. 172; *Health, United States, 2012*. p. 168; *Health, United States, 2015*. p. 182.

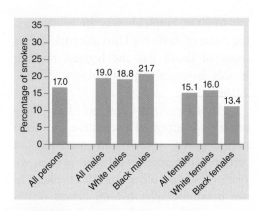

FIGURE 11-8 Current cigarette smoking by persons 18 years of age and older, age adjusted, 2014.

Data from National Center for Health Statistics (NCHS). 2016b. *Health, United States, 2015*. Hyattsville, MD: U.S. Department of Health and Human Services. p. 186.

TABLE 11-4 Selected Health Risks Among Persons 20 Years and Older, 2011–2014

Sex and Race[1]	% with Hypertension	% with Cholesterol Level $\geq$ 240 mg/dL	% That Is Overweight
Both sexes	30.4	27.8	69.5
White			
Male	30.2	29.4	73.7
Female	28.0	28.0	63.5
Black			
Male	42.4	24.5	69.6
Female	44.0	25.7	82.0

[1] 20–74 years, age adjusted.

Data from National Center for Health Statistics (NCHS). 2016b. *Health, United States, 2015*. Hyattsville, MD: U.S. Department of Health and Human Services. pp. 202, 204, 216.

In 2006, homicide was the ninth leading cause of death for Hispanic males. This cause of death has the highest ranking in this group, along with blacks (NCHS, 2016b).

Hispanic Americans are less likely to take advantage of preventive care than non-Hispanic whites and members of certain other races. Hispanic women 40 years of age or older were least likely to use mammography (61.4% versus 66.8% for non-Hispanic whites and 67.1% for non-Hispanic blacks; see Figure 11-4). In 2014, fewer Hispanic mothers began their prenatal care during the first trimester than the U.S. average (83.3% of Hispanic mothers versus 84.8% as the U.S. average; see Table 11-1). Among Hispanics 2 years of age and older in 2014, 59.7% had at least one dental visit during a year, compared to 67.7% for non-Hispanic whites (NCHS, 2016b).

People of Hispanic origin also experience greater behavioral risks than whites and members of certain other racial/ethnic groups. For example, among individuals 18 years and older in 2014, a higher proportion of Hispanics drank five or more alcoholic drinks per day than people of other ethnic origins (24.4% for Hispanics versus 17.6% for blacks and 14.5% for Asians; see Figure 11-3). In contrast, fewer Hispanics smoked compared to people from other ethnic groups. In 2014, 15.7% of Hispanic males 18 years and older identified themselves as "current smokers," compared to 20.0% of non-Hispanic white males and 21.8% of non-Hispanic black males (NCHS, 2016b). Among female adults, 7.3% of Hispanics smoked in 2014, compared to 16.4% of non-Hispanic whites and 14.2% of non-Hispanic blacks (NCHS, 2016b).

Asian Americans

Minority health epidemiology has typically focused on blacks, Hispanics, and American Indians or Alaska Natives because Asian Americans represent a relatively small proportion of the U.S. population. In 2015, Asians accounted for only 5.6% of the U.S. population, with this subpopulation including 19 million individuals (U.S. Census Bureau, 2012a). To include the diversity of Asian Americans, the NCHS has expanded the race codes into nine categories for Asian Americans: White, Black, Native American, Chinese, Japanese, Hawaiian, Filipino, Other Asian/Pacific Islanders, and other races. Nevertheless, even the category of "Other Asian/Pacific Islander" is extremely heterogeneous, encompassing 21 subgroups with different health profiles.

Asian Americans constitute one of the fastest-growing population segments in the United States. The growth rate for this population was 43% between 2000 and 2010, compared to 10% for the U.S. population as a whole (U.S. Census Bureau, 2012a). The U.S. Census Bureau (2010b) projected that the Asian American population would reach 16.5 million by 2015.

In education, income, and health, Asian Americans and Pacific Islanders (AA/PIs) are very diverse. In 2013, 86.2% of AA/PIs 25 years of age or older had at least graduated from high school, compared with 87.6% of non-Hispanic whites; in addition, the percentage of AA/PIs with a bachelor's degree or higher was 51.3%, compared to 30.3% for non-Hispanic whites (U.S. Census Bureau, 2012a). Educational attainment varies greatly among the subgroups, however. For example, between 2007 and 2009, 94% of adults of Japanese descent had graduated from high school, whereas that rate was 72% for adults of Vietnamese descent and only 61% for Hmong adults (U.S. Census Bureau, 2010a).

In 2013, the median income for Asian males (aged 15 years and older) was $72,472, compared to $40,963 for non-Hispanic white males (U.S. Census Bureau, 2010a). In addition, a smaller percentage of Asians (12.7%) lived below the FPL, compared to blacks (27.4%), and Hispanics (23.5%) (U.S. Census Bureau, 2011c).

One study found that Chinese, Asian Indian, Filipino, and other AA/PI children were more likely to be without contact with a health professional, compared to non-Hispanic white children. Citizenship/nativity status, maternal education attainment, and poverty status were all significant independent risk factors for health care access and utilization (Yu et al., 2004). In addition, cultural practices and attitudes may prevent AA/PI women from receiving adequate preventive care, such as Pap smears and breast cancer screening. Overall, the AA/PI population reported lower Pap smear test utilization; in 2013, 65.3% of AA/PI women aged 18 and older had a Pap smear test, compared with 68.7% of non-Hispanic whites, 75.3% of non-Hispanic blacks, and 70.5% of Hispanics (NCHS, 2016b).

Failure to recognize the heterogeneity of this minority population sometimes contributes to the myth that the entire AA/PI population is both healthy and economically successful. In fact, the heterogeneity of the AA/PI population is reflected in the various indicators of health status. For instance, people of Vietnamese descent are more likely to assess their own health status as fair or poor, compared to people of Korean, Chinese, Filipino, Asian Indian, and Japanese descent (NCHS, 2014a). The

incidence of overweight and obesity varies greatly, with Filipino adults being 70% more likely to be obese than the rest of the AA/PI population. In terms of the total U.S. population, overall smoking rates are the lowest among AA/PIs. Nevertheless, 22% of Koreans are current smokers—a rate higher than that for black (17%) and Hispanic adults (10%). Compared with whites, Asian Indians are more than twice as likely to have diabetes (Centers for Disease Control and Prevention [CDC], 2015a).

American Indians and Alaska Natives

More than three-fourths of the American Indian and Alaska Native (AIAN) population resides in rural and urban areas outside of reservations or off-reservation trust lands (U.S. Census Bureau, 2011d). According to the Census Bureau (2011d), the AIAN population is growing at a rate of 26.7% per year. Concomitantly, demand for expanded health care services within this population has been increasing for several decades and is becoming more acute. The incidence and prevalence of certain diseases and conditions—such as diabetes, hypertension, infant mortality and morbidity, chemical dependency, and AIDS- and HIV-related morbidity—in the AIAN population are all high enough to be matters of prime concern. Compared to the general U.S. population, Native Americans also have much higher death rates from alcoholism, tuberculosis, diabetes, injuries, suicide, and homicide (Indian Health Service [IHS], 2010a).

It is also no secret that Native Americans continue to occupy the bottom of the socioeconomic strata in the United States. AIANs are approximately twice as likely to be poor and unemployed as other Americans (U.S. Census Bureau, 2011d). Nevertheless, the health status of American Indians appears to be improving. For example, the mortality rate among Native American expectant mothers dropped from 28.5 deaths per 100,000 live births in 1972–1974 to 8.3 deaths per 100,000 live births in 2007–2009 (IHS, 2014); infant mortality declined from 8.3 deaths per 1,000 births in 2000 to 7.6 deaths per 1,000 births in 2013 (NCHS, 2016b). Even with these gains, Native Americans continue to experience significant health disparities compared to the general U.S. population. The life expectancy of Native Americans is 4.6 years less than that for the U.S. population as a whole (IHS, 2010a). Native Americans die at higher rates than other Americans from alcohol abuse (519% higher), tuberculosis (500% higher), diabetes (195% higher), unintentional injuries (149% higher), homicide (92% higher), and suicide (72% higher) (IHS, 2010a).

The provision of health services to American Indians by the federal government was first negotiated in 1832, as partial compensation for land cessions. Subsequent laws have expanded the scope of services and allowed American Indians greater autonomy in planning, developing, and administering their own health care programs. These laws explicitly permit the practice of traditional as well as Western medicine.

Indian Health Care Improvement Act

The Indian Health Care Improvement Act of 1976 (IHCIA), which was amended in 1980, outlined a 7-year effort to help bring American Indian health to a level of parity with the general population. Although this goal of health parity remains unmet, the IHCIA has at least been successful in minimizing prejudice, building trust, and putting responsibility back into the hands of American Indians. The Affordable Care Act included the permanent reauthorization of the IHCIA.

Indian Health Service

The goal of the federal program administered by the Indian Health Service (IHS) is to ensure that comprehensive and culturally acceptable health services are available to AIANs (IHS, 2013). The IHS (2010b) serves the members and descendants of more than 560 federally recognized AIAN tribes. The health care needs of a rapidly expanding American Indian population have grown faster than medical care resources, however, and most American Indian communities continue to be medically underserved.

IHS is divided into 12 area offices, each responsible for program operations in a particular geographic area. Each area office is composed of branches dealing with various administrative and health-related services. Delivery of health services is the responsibility of 161 tribally managed service units operating at the local level (IHS, 2010b). The IHS mandate has been made particularly difficult because the locations of Indian reservation communities are among the least geographically accessible in the United States (Burks, 1992).

Besides rendering primary and preventive care, special initiatives focus on areas such as injury control, alcoholism, diabetes, mental health, maternal and child health, Indian youth and children, elder care, and HIV/AIDS (IHS, 1999a). Additional areas of focus include domestic violence and child abuse, oral health, and sanitation (IHS, 1999b). Even with the limitations in the IHS's scope of service, many American Indians do not avail themselves of the system's services. More than half of low-income uninsured Indians do not have access to IHS. Among the low-income population, Indians with HIS access fared better than uninsured Indians (Zuckerman et al., 2004).

▶ The Uninsured

The *Health Services Financing* chapter discussed the number of uninsured people in the United States and the reasons why so many Americans have been without health insurance. Although the rate of uninsurance among adults has increased, lack of health insurance coverage among children declined from 8.9% in 2008 to 4.5% in 2015 (NCHS, 2016a), mainly because of the success of the Children's Health Insurance Program (CHIP).

Ethnic minorities are more likely than whites to lack health insurance. The U.S. Census Bureau (2014) estimated that, in 2014, 19.9% of Hispanic residents were uninsured, compared with 11.8% of blacks, 9.3% of Asian Americans, and 7.6% of whites. Most of the uninsured population comprises young workers (O'Neill and O'Neill, 2009). Lack of coverage is also more prevalent in the southern and western regions of the United States, and among individuals who lack a college degree.

Generally, uninsured persons are in poorer health than the general population (NCHS, 2016a). Studies have also shown that the uninsured use fewer health services than the insured (CDC, 2010a). In 2015, 54% of uninsured people reported having no regular source of health care (Kaiser Family Foundation, 2016d).

Decreased utilization of lower-cost preventive services—a characteristic of the uninsured population—can ultimately result in an increased need for more expensive emergency health care. Even when the uninsured can access health care, they often have serious problems paying their medical bills. In 2015, 20% of uninsured people postponed obtaining needed prescription drugs because of cost concerns, compared to 12% of those with public insurance and 6% of privately insured people (Kaiser Family Foundation, 2016d).

The plight of the uninsured affects those who have insurance as well. Medical expenditures for uncompensated care to the uninsured were estimated to total $85 billion in 2013 (Kaiser Family Foundation, 2014a). Much of this cost was absorbed by Medicaid, federal grants to nonprofit hospitals, and charitable organizations.

The ACA did make sizable progress in reducing the number of uninsured in the United States. It is not clear how the new reform proposal in the form of the American Health Care Act (AHCA) will address the ongoing problem of uninsurance.

▶ Children

There were approximately 74 million children younger than 18 years living in the United States in 2015, representing 23% of the total population. Approximately 15.5 million children (21%) lived in households with incomes below the U.S. Census Bureau's poverty threshold. The racial and ethnic diversity of U.S. children continues to increase; notably, Hispanic children represented more than 25% of all U.S. children in 2015, up from 8.8% in 1980. Nearly 20% of U.S. children younger than 18 years have a special health care need, defined as having a chronic medical, behavioral, or developmental condition lasting 12 months or longer and experiencing a service-related or functional consequence (Federal Interagency Forum on Child and Family Statistics, 2016).

Excess body weight in children is associated with excess morbidity during childhood and excess body weight in adulthood. From 1988–1994 to 2011–2014, the percentage of children age 6–17 years with obesity increased by 8 percentage points, from 11% to 19%. During the same time period, the percentage of children with obesity increased by 7 percentage points for white, non-Hispanic children; by 9 percentage points for black, non-Hispanic children; and by 10 percentage points for Mexican American children (NCHS, 2014b). Children living in rural areas were more likely to be overweight or obese than their urban counterparts. In addition, children with lower household incomes were significantly more likely to be overweight or obese than those living in households with higher incomes. The rate of overweight and obesity among children in households with incomes below 100% of the FPL was approximately twice that of children with household incomes of 400% or more of the FPL (Health Resources and Services Administration [HRSA], 2015).

Health insurance is a major determinant of access to and utilization of health care. From 2000 to 2014, the percentage of children with public coverage increased and the percentage with no health insurance and with private health insurance declined (Federal Interagency Forum on Child and Family Statistics, 2016). The proportion of children younger than 18 years without health insurance was 4.5% in 2015 (CDC, 2016b), but the coverage rates

varied across races and ethnicities. Hispanic children were more likely to be uninsured (10%) than white, non-Hispanic and black, non-Hispanic children (4% each). White, non-Hispanic children were more likely to have private insurance (68%) compared to Hispanic children (31%) and black, non-Hispanic children (34%). In urban and large rural areas, children living in households with the lowest incomes were less likely to have health insurance than their peers living in households with the highest income categories. For instance, 95.3% of children in large rural areas with household incomes below 100% of the FPL had current health insurance, compared to 98.2% of those with household incomes of 400% or more of the FPL. Among children living in households with incomes below 100% of the FPL, children in small and large rural areas were significantly more likely to have health insurance than those in urban areas—94.7% and 95.3% versus 91.2%, respectively (HRSA, 2015).

Unintentional injuries are the leading cause of death for children and adolescents. In 2014, 35% of deaths among adolescents age 15–19 and 30% of deaths among children age 1–14 were due to unintentional injuries. For both age groups, motor vehicle–related (MVR) injury was the leading cause of unintentional injury death (NCHS, 2016b).

Asthma is one of the most common childhood chronic diseases. The prevalence of asthma among U.S. children doubled from 1980 to 1995, but then increased more slowly during the 2000s. More than 10 million U.S. children younger than age 18 (14%) have ever been diagnosed with asthma; 6.8 million children still have asthma (9%) (Federal Interagency Forum on Child and Family Statistics, 2016). In

2014, 13% of black, non-Hispanic children were reported to currently have asthma, compared with 8% of white, non-Hispanic children; 8% of Hispanic children; and 6% of Asian, non-Hispanic children.

Depression has a significant impact on adolescent development and well-being. In 2014, approximately 11% of youths ages 12–17 had a major depressive episode (MDE) during the past year—a higher prevalence than was reported in 2004 (9%). Among children ages 2-17 years who had an ongoing emotional, developmental, or behavioral problem, 61.0% had received mental health care or counseling in the previous year (Federal Interagency Forum on Child and Family Statistics, 2016; HRSA, 2015).

Vaccination rates for children for selected diseases differ by race, poverty status, and area of residence (**TABLE 11-5**). White children have greater vaccination rates for diphtheria/tetanus/pertussis (DTP), polio, measles, *Haemophilus influenzae* serotype b

TABLE 11-5 Vaccinations of Children 19–35 Months of Age for Selected Diseases According to Race, Poverty Status, and Residence in a Metropolitan Statistical Area (MSA), 2014 (%)

Vaccination	Total	Race		Poverty Status		Inside MSA	
		White	Black	Below Poverty	At or Above Poverty	Inner City	Remaining Areas
DTP[1]	84	86	80	79	87	84	85
Polio[2]	93	93	92	92	95	93	94
Measles-containing vaccines or measles/mumps/rubella[3]	92	91	90	90	93	92	91
HIB[4]	82	84	75	83	76	81	83
Combined series[5]	72	73	65	66	75	71	73

[1] Diphtheria/tetanus/pertussis, four doses or more.
[2] Three doses or more.
[3] Respondents were asked about measles-containing or measles/mumps/rubella (MMR) vaccines.
[4] *Haemophilus influenzae* type b, three doses or more.
[5] The combined series consists of four doses of DTP vaccine, three doses of polio vaccine, and one dose of measles-containing vaccine (4:3:1:3:3:1).

Data from National Center for Health Statistics (NCHS). 2016b. *Health, United States, 2015*. Hyattsville, MD: U.S. Department of Health and Human Services. p. 238.

(Hib), and combined series compared to blacks. Children who come from families with incomes below the FPL, or who live in inner-city areas, have lower vaccination rates than other children.

Children's health has certain unique aspects in terms of delivery of health care. Among these factors are children's developmental vulnerability, dependency, and differential patterns of morbidity and mortality. **Developmental vulnerability** refers to the rapid and cumulative physical and emotional changes that characterize childhood and the potential impact that illness, injury, or disruptive family and social circumstances can have on a child's life-course trajectory. **Dependency** refers to children's special circumstances that require adults—parents, school officials, caregivers, and sometimes neighbors—to recognize and respond to their health needs, seek health care services on their behalf, authorize treatment, and comply with recommended treatment regimens. These dependency relationships can be complex, change over time, and affect utilization of health services by children.

Children and the U.S. Health Care System

The various programs that serve children have distinct eligibility, administrative, and funding criteria that can present barriers to access. The patchwork of disconnected programs also makes it difficult to obtain health care in an integrated and coordinated fashion. These programs can be categorized into three broad sectors: the personal medical and preventive services sector, the population-based community health services sector, and the health-related support services sector.

Personal medical and preventive health services include primary and specialty medical services, which are delivered in private and public medical offices, health centers, and hospitals. Personal medical services are principally funded by private health insurance, Medicaid, and out-of-pocket payments.

Population-based community health services include community-wide health promotion and disease prevention services. Examples are immunization delivery and monitoring programs, lead screening and abatement programs, and child abuse and neglect prevention. Other health services include special child abuse treatment programs and rehabilitative services for children with complex congenital conditions or other chronic and debilitating diseases. Community-based programs also provide assurance and coordination functions, such as case management and referral programs, for children with chronic diseases and early interventions and monitoring for infants at risk for developmental disabilities. Funding for this sector comes from federal programs, such as Medicaid's Early Periodic Screening, Diagnosis, and Treatment (EPSDT) program; Title V (Maternal and Child Health) of the Social Security Act; and other categorical programs.

Health-related support services include nutrition education, early intervention, rehabilitation, and family support programs, among other services. An example of a rehabilitation service is education and psychotherapy for children with HIV. Family support services include parent education and skill building in families with infants at risk for developmental delay because of physiological or social conditions, such as low birth weight or very low income. Funding for these services comes from diverse agencies, such as the U.S. Department of Agriculture, which funds the Special Supplemental Nutrition Program for Women, Infants, and Children (WIC), and the U.S. Department of Education, which funds the Individuals with Disabilities Education Act (IDEA).

▶ Women

In 2015, the U.S. population was estimated to include more than 320 million individuals, with females accounting for 50.8% of the total population (U.S. Census Bureau, 2016). Women are playing an increasingly important role in the delivery of health care. Not only do women remain the leading providers of care in the nursing profession, but they are also well represented in various other health professions, including allopathic and osteopathic medicine, dentistry, podiatry, and optometry (**FIGURE 11-9**).

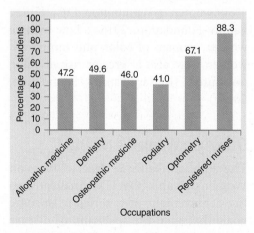

FIGURE 11-9 Percentage of female students of total enrollment in schools for selected health occupations, 2013–2014.

Data from Association of American Medical Colleges (AAMC). 2017. *The state of women in academic medicine: The pipeline and pathways to leadership, 2013-2014.* Available at: https://www.aamc.org/members /gwims/statistics/#bench.

Women in the United States can expect to live about 4.8 years longer than men (NCHS, 2013), but they suffer greater morbidity and poorer health outcomes. Morbidity is greater among women than among men, even after childbearing-related conditions are factored out. For instance, nearly 38% of women report having chronic conditions that require ongoing medical treatment, compared to 30% of men (Salganicoff et al., 2005). Women also have a higher prevalence of certain health problems than men over the course of their lifetimes (Sechzer et al., 1996). Heart disease and stroke account for a higher percentage of deaths among women than among men at all stages of life. Approximately 42% of women who have heart attacks die within a year, compared to 24% of men who have heart attacks (Misra, 2001). Research has also demonstrated that women are more likely to experience functional limitations due to health than men (35% and 26%, respectively; NCHS, 2013).

Among respondents to the 2014 National Health Interview Survey, 60.2% of women reported being in excellent or very good health, while 26.8% reported being in good health and 13% reported being in fair or poor health (NCHS, 2016a). Self-reported health status was similar among men and women but varied greatly with age and educational attainment (NCHS, 2016a). Overall, though, women reported more physically and mentally unhealthy days than men. Women reported an average of 4.2 days of poor physical health, compared to 3.5 days per month for men in 2014. Similarly, women reported an average of 4.2 mentally unhealthy days, while men reported an average of 3.1 such days per month (CDC, 2014a).

The CDC defines binge drinking as consuming four or more drinks on a single occasion for women and five or more drinks on a single occasion for men. In 2015, men were more likely than women to report both binge drinking (29.9% versus 17.4%, respectively) in 1 day at least once in the past year. However, among women, incidence of heavy drinking increased from 11.2% in 2004 to 17.4% in 2015 (NCHS, 2016a). An estimated 13.6% of women 18 years and older currently smoke cigarettes, with this rate having declined in recent years (NCHS, 2016a).

Overweight and obesity are associated with an increased risk of numerous diseases and conditions. In 2011–2014, 38.8% of U.S. women 20 years and older were obese, which was higher than the corresponding rate for men (34.5%). In addition, obesity has increased significantly over the past decade for non-Hispanic black and Mexican American women, contributing to widening health disparities. The rates of obesity among females in 2011–2014 were 36.2% in non-Hispanic white women, 56.9% in non-Hispanic black women, and 45.0% in Hispanic women (NCHS, 2016b).

In 2014, 1,298,177 women ages 18 and older died in the United States. Of these deaths, nearly half were attributable to heart disease and cancer—responsible for 22.3% and 21.6% of deaths, respectively. Compared to men, women also had a greater relative burden of mortality from chronic lower respiratory disease (6%), which was the third leading cause of death for women but the fourth leading cause for men. After stroke, Alzheimer's disease was the fifth leading cause of death for women; by comparison, it ranked eighth

as a cause of death for men (CDC, 2015b). Between 2000 and 2014, three causes of death increased in relative burden among women: chronic lower respiratory diseases (from 5.1% to 6.0% of deaths), Alzheimer's disease (from 2.9% to 5% of deaths), and unintentional injury (from 2.6% to 3.9% of deaths) (CDC, 2015b).

In terms of health insurance coverage, most of the 98 million women ages 19 to 64 residing in the United States had some form of coverage in 2015 (Kaiser Family Foundation, 2016c). However, gaps in private-sector and publicly funded programs left 11% of women uninsured. In addition, women were less likely than men to be insured through their own jobs (35% versus 44%, respectively) and more likely to be covered as a dependent (24% versus 16%, respectively) (Kaiser Family Foundation, 2016c). There was considerable state-level variation in uninsured rates across the United States, with these rates ranging from 21% of women in Texas to 4% of women in Washington, D.C. (Kaiser Family Foundation, 2016c). Low-income women, women of color, and immigrant women were also at greater risk of being uninsured (Kaiser Family Foundation, 2016c).

Office on Women's Health

The Public Health Service's Office on Women's Health (OWH) is dedicated to the achievement of a series of specific goals that span the spectrum of disease and disability. These goals range across the life cycle and address cultural and ethnic differences among women. OWH promotes, coordinates, and implements a comprehensive women's health agenda on research, service delivery, and education across various government agencies.

OWH was responsible for implementing the National Action Plan on Breast Cancer (NAPBC), a major public–private partnership dedicated to improving the diagnosis, treatment, and prevention of breast cancer through research, service delivery, and education. OWH also worked to implement measures to prevent physical and sexual abuse against women, as delineated in the Violence Against Women Act of 1994. This agency is currently active in projects promoting breastfeeding, women's health education and research, girl and adolescent health, and heart health.

Within the Substance Abuse and Mental Health Services Administration (SAMHSA), the Advisory Committee for Women's Services has targeted six areas for special attention: physical and sexual abuse of women; women as caregivers; women with mental and addictive disorders; women with HIV/AIDS, sexually transmitted diseases, and/or tuberculosis; older women; and women detained in the criminal justice system.

The Women's Health Initiative, supported by the National Institutes of Health (NIH), was the largest clinical trial conducted in U.S. history, involving more than 161,000 women (NIH, 2002). It focused on diseases that are the major causes of death and disability among women—heart disease, cancer, and osteoporosis. In 2002, the Women's Health Initiative published a groundbreaking study, finding detrimental effects of postmenopausal hormone therapy on women's development of invasive breast cancer, coronary heart disease, stroke, and pulmonary embolism (NIH, 2002).

Women and the U.S. Health Care System

Women face a distinct disadvantage in obtaining employer-based health insurance coverage because they are more likely than men to work part-time, receive lower wages, and have interruptions in their work histories. Hence, married women are more likely to be covered as dependents under their husbands' plans and are at a higher risk of being uninsured. Women also place greater reliance on Medicaid for their health care coverage. In 2014, 11.9% of women were uninsured compared to 14.7% of men, while 21.4% of women were covered by Medicaid compared to 17.8% of men (NCHS, 2016b).

Women are more likely than men to use contraceptives (**FIGURE 11-10**), but contraceptives have been among the most

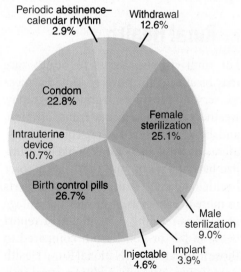

Percentage of woman using contraception is 62.2.

FIGURE 11-10 Contraceptive use in the past month among women 15–44 years old, 2011–2013.

Note: Numbers may not add to 100 because of rounding.

Data from National Center for Health Statistics (NCHS). 2016b. *Health, United States, 2015*. Hyattsville, MD: U.S. Department of Health and Human Services. pp. 81–82.

poorly covered reproductive health care service in the United States. As of September 2013, 28 states required private health insurance plans to cover prescription contraceptives if they covered other prescription drugs (Guttmacher Institute, 2013).

The ACA required private insurance to cover, with no cost sharing, a wide variety of preventive services and additional services for women, including Food and Drug Administration (FDA)-approved prescription contraceptives, domestic violence screening, breastfeeding supports, and human papillomavirus (HPV) testing. Although such services are not required under Medicaid, several states have started to cover all preventive services important for women with or without cost sharing (Kaiser Family Foundation, 2013). It remains to be seen how these services may be affected by the ACA replacement.

▶ Rural Health

For rural citizens, access to health care may be affected by poverty, long distances to service providers, rural topography, weather conditions, lack of transportation, and being uninsured. Consequently, residents of rural areas are less likely to utilize health services, and they have poorer health outcomes than their counterparts in more urban areas. A greater percentage of persons residing in a rural area report being in fair or poor health compared to those in urban areas (National Rural Health Association, 2016). In addition, rural residents are more likely to report health problems, such as headaches and back and neck pain, than urban residents—17.2% versus 14.7%, respectively (CDC, 2012a, 2012b).

People in rural areas are more likely than urban residents to forgo or delay care due to cost—15.6% versus 13.3%, respectively (Ziller et al., 2015). Across all races and ethnicities, rural residents have lower levels of insurance coverage. Among Hispanic rural residents, 45.3% do not have health insurance, compared to 40.9% of urban Hispanics. Among whites, 21.3% of rural residents were uninsured, compared to 13.1% of urban residents (U.S. Census Bureau, 2014; Ziller, 2014). The uninsured often do not have a usual source of care (Larson & Fleishman, 2003).

Geographic maldistribution that creates a shortage of health care professionals in rural settings results in barriers in access to care. As of January 2017, there were approximately 6,600 designated primary care health professional shortage areas (HPSAs), 5,500 dental HPSAs, and 4,600 mental health HPSAs in the United States (HRSA, 2017). Nearly 21% of the U.S. population resides in areas where primary care health professionals are in short supply (HRSA, Bureau of Health Professions, 2013a). More than 33 million Americans live in a nonmetropolitan federally designated health professional shortage area (HRSA, Bureau of Health Professions, 2013). The scarcity of health care providers encompasses a broad spectrum of professionals, including pediatricians, obstetricians, internists, dentists, nurses, and allied health professionals (Patton and Puskin, 1990). Rural hospitals are often under financial strain, which results in these facilities generally being smaller hospitals that provide fewer services than urban hospitals.

Various steps have been taken to improve access in rural America, including the promotion of the National Health

Service Corps (NHSC), the designation of HPSAs and medically underserved areas (MUAs), the development of community and migrant health centers (C/MHCs), and the enactment of the Rural Health Clinics Act. In 2015, there were 4,099 certified rural health clinics throughout the United States (Kaiser Family Foundation, 2015). In addition, the Office of Rural Health Policy, within the Health Resources and Services Administration of the U.S. Department of Health and Human Services (DHHS), was established in 1987 to promote better health care in rural America (HRSA, Office of Rural Health Policy, 2015). Several measures and enhanced funding have been initiated to improve rural emergency medical services, to bolster the rural health workforce, and to develop behavior health capacity in rural areas (National Conference of State Legislatures, 2013).

National Health Service Corps

NHSC was created in 1970, under the Emergency Health Personnel Act, with the intention being to recruit and retain physicians to provide needed services in areas with physician shortages. A 1972 amendment created a scholarship program targeting HPSAs. The scholarship and loan repayment program applies to doctors, dentists, nurse practitioners, midwives, and mental health professionals who serve a minimum of 2 years in underserved areas. Since 1972, more than 50,000 health professionals have been placed in medically underserved communities in hospitals and clinics (HRSA, Bureau of Health Professions, 2013). Currently, nearly 10,400 health professionals are providing services under NHSC (HRSA, NHSC, 2017).

Health Professional Shortage Areas

The Health Professions Educational Assistance Act of 1976 provided the designation criteria for health manpower shortage areas, later renamed health professional shortage areas (HRSA, Bureau of Health Professions, 2007). The act provided that three different types of HPSAs could be designated: geographic areas, population groups, and medical facilities.

A geographic area must meet the following three criteria for designation as a primary care HPSA:

1. The geographic area involved must be rational for the delivery of health services.
2. One of the following conditions must prevail in the area:
   - The area has a population to full-time equivalent primary care physician (PCP) ratio of at least 3,500:1.
   - The area has a population to full-time equivalent PCP ratio of less than 3,500:1 but greater than 3,000:1, and has unusually high needs for primary care services or insufficient capacity of existing primary care providers.
3. Primary care professionals in contiguous areas are overutilized, excessively distant, or inaccessible to the population of the area under consideration (HRSA, Bureau of Health Professions, 2007).

A population group can be designated as an HPSA for primary care if it can be demonstrated that access barriers prevent members of the group from using local providers. Medium- and maximum-security federal and state correctional institutions and public or nonprofit private residential facilities can be designated as facility-based HPSAs. HPSAs are classified on a scale of 1 to 4, with scores of 1 and 2 signifying areas of greatest need.

Medically Underserved Areas

The primary purpose of the MUA designation, which was established in the HMO Act of 1973, was to target the community health center and rural health clinic programs. The 1973 statute required that several factors be considered in designating MUAs, such as available health resources in relation to area size and population, health indices, and care and demographic factors affecting the need for care. To meet this mandate, the Index of Medical Underservice was developed, comprising four variables:

- Percentage of population below poverty income levels
- Percentage of population 65 years of age and older
- Infant mortality rates
- Number of primary care practitioners per 1,000 population

The index yields a single numerical value on a scale from 0 to 100; any area with a value less than 62 (the median of all counties) is designated as an MUA.

▶ Migrant Workers

Migrant workers are farm workers who travel long distances from their primary residence or lack a primary residence entirely, either due to seasonal crop changes or work availability. While their exact number is difficult to assess due to citizenship issues and the transient nature of this population, it is widely accepted that there are at least 3 million migrant workers in the United States (Larson and Plascencia, 1993; Migrant Health Promotion, 2013; National Center for Farmworker Health, 2012; Rust, 1990). The migrant population is largely composed of racial and ethnic minorities. As of 2009, 72% of migrant workers in the United States were born in Mexico or Central America (U.S. Department of Labor, 2011).

In 2009, the average annual income of a family in which at least one member is a migrant worker was between $17,500 and $19,999. Furthermore, only 43% of workers were currently receiving any public assistance (U.S. Department of Labor, 2011). As of 2013–2014, approximately 84% of migrant workers were uninsured (U.S. Department of Labor, 2016). Furthermore, approximately 30% of female migrant workers who become pregnant do not have their first prenatal visit until their second trimester, and approximately 14% do not have their first visit until their third trimester (Bircher, 2009). In addition to the occupational health risks to which this population is exposed, their lack of access to and utilization of health services translates into poor health outcomes.

The rate of obesity among migrant workers has risen to 81% of males and 76% of females (Villarejo et al., 2000). These rates are not found among migrant workers during their first year in the United States, so dietary changes in later years likely account for these high rates of obesity. In addition to higher rates of chronic conditions, migrant populations are at greater risk for developing infectious diseases. Notably, in part due to their living conditions, migrant workers are at greater risk of contracting tuberculosis (TB). In total, 388 agricultural worker patients were diagnosed with TB at migrant health centers in 2011, equating to a prevalence rate of 48.8 cases per 100,000 population. In comparison, non-agricultural worker patients at all health centers in 2011 had a prevalence rate of 33.1 TB cases per 100,000 population (National Center for Farmworker Health, 2015). The rate of HIV/AIDS is also considerably higher in the migrant worker population than in the general population, with observed rates between 5% and 26% (National Center for Farmworker Health, 2011).

To address the growing health needs of this population, services have been provided to migrant workers and their families through state programs and through HRSA's Migrant Health Program.

Community and Migrant Health Centers

Community and migrant health centers (C/MHCs) provide services to low-income populations on a sliding-fee scale, thereby addressing both geographic and financial barriers to access. Whereas community health centers must be located in areas designated as MUAs, migrant centers must be located in "high-impact" areas, defined as areas that serve at least 4,000 migrant and/or seasonal farm workers for at least 2 months per year. For more than 4 decades, C/MHCs have provided primary care and preventive health services to populations in designated MUAs. Because of a shortage of physicians, C/MHCs heavily rely on nonphysician providers (NPPs) to deliver care. In 2015, C/MHCs served

approximately 898,950 migrants and seasonal farm workers (HRSA, 2015).

Rural Health Clinics Act

The Rural Health Clinics Act was developed in 1977 to respond to the concern that isolated rural communities could not generate sufficient revenue to support the services of a physician. In many cases, the only sources of primary care or emergency services in these areas were NPPs, who were ineligible at that time for Medicare or Medicaid reimbursement. The Rural Health Clinics Act permitted physician assistants (PAs), nurse practitioners (NPs), and certified nurse-midwives (CNMs) associated with rural clinics to practice without the direct supervision of a physician; enabled rural health clinics (but not NPPs directly) to be reimbursed by Medicare and Medicaid for their services; and tied the level of Medicaid payment to the level established by Medicare.

To be designated as a rural health clinic, a public- or private-sector physician practice, clinic, or hospital must meet several criteria, including location in an MUA, geographic HPSA, or a population-based HPSA. More than 4,000 rural health clinics currently provide primary care services to more than 8 million people in 50 states (HRSA, 2015).

▶ The Homeless

Although their exact number is unknown, an estimated 3.5 million people (1.35 million of whom are children) are likely to experience homelessness in a given year (National Law Center on Homelessness and Poverty, 2015). Across the United States, approximately 1 in 200 people became homeless in 2011 (U.S. Department of Housing and Urban Development [HUD], 2012). Although most homeless persons live in major urban areas, a surprising 27.7% live in suburban and rural areas (HUD, 2012).

The adult homeless population is composed of 63% men and 37% women (HUD, 2012). An estimated 22.8% of all homeless people are children younger than the age of 18, 35.8% are families with children, and 14% are veterans (HUD, 2012).

Homeless women, in particular, face major difficulties: economic and housing needs and special gender-related issues that include pregnancy, childcare responsibilities, family violence, fragmented family support, job discrimination, and wage discrepancies. The economic standing of women is often more unstable than that of men, and women are more likely to live in poverty than men. In 2015, 17 million women were living in poverty in the United States, of whom 46% were in extreme poverty (National Women's Law Center, 2015). The low wages and extreme poverty faced by women increase their risk for becoming homeless. In addition, domestic violence is a factor that contributes to family homelessness, with 18% of families citing this issue as the main cause of their status (U.S. Conference of Mayors, 2011). Among all homeless women, 1 in 4 state that their homelessness was a direct result of violence committed against them (Jasinski, 2005). Homeless women, regardless of parenting status, should be linked with social services, family support, self-help, and housing resources. Mentally ill women caring for children need additional consideration, with an emphasis on parenting skills and special services for children. Thus, homelessness is a multifaceted problem related to personal, social, and economic factors.

The economic picture for homeless persons is dismal, and suggests that homeless persons are severely lacking in the financial and educational resources necessary to access health care. A majority (60%) of mothers living in poverty who have ever been homeless did not complete high school (Institute for Children, Poverty, and Homelessness, 2011). In addition, approximately 38% of the homeless population is unsheltered, living in the streets or outside (National Alliance to End Homelessness, 2012). Receipt of public benefits among the homeless is low. For example, a survey revealed that among more than 9,000 clients served by Maryland's Health Care for the Homeless, 75% were uninsured (Health Care for the Homeless, 2012). The number of homeless individuals who receive public benefits remains low because of federal restrictions that prohibit giving federal help to persons without a physical street address.

The shortage of adequate low-income housing is the major precipitating factor for homelessness. Unemployment, personal or family life crises, rent increases that are out of proportion to inflation, and reduction in public benefits can also directly result in the loss of a home. Illness, by comparison, tends to result in the loss of a home in a more indirect way. Another indirect cause of homelessness is deinstitutionalization of individuals from public mental hospitals, substance abuse programs, and overcrowded prisons and jails.

Community-based residential alternatives for mentally ill individuals vary from independent apartments to group homes staffed by paid caregivers. Independent living may involve either separate apartments or single-room occupancy units in large hotels, whereas group homes are staffed during at least a portion of the day and traditionally provide some on-site mental health services (Schutt and Goldfinger, 1996).

The homeless—both adults and children—have a high prevalence of untreated acute and chronic medical, mental health, and substance abuse problems. The reasons for this increased prevalence are debatable. Some argue that people may become homeless because of a physical or mental illness. Others argue that homelessness itself may lead to the development of physical and mental disability because homelessness is associated with specific risk factors such as excessive use of alcohol, illegal drugs, and cigarettes; sleeping in an upright position, which results in venous stasis and its consequences; extensive walking in poorly fitting shoes; and grossly inadequate nutrition. While the reasons for the generally poorer health of the homeless may not be agreed upon, the outcomes are easily seen. Homeless adults typically have eight to nine medical conditions or illnesses (Breakey et al., 1989). Homeless children have a risk of mortality nearly double that of housed children (Kerker et al., 2011).

Homeless persons are also at a greater risk of assault and victimization regardless of whether they live in a shelter or outdoors. Many are exposed to extreme heat, cold, and other weather conditions. They are also exposed to illness because of overcrowding in shelters and overexposure to weather.

Between 2015 and 2016, the number of people experiencing homelessness in the United States declined by 3%; these decreases occurred mostly because of people staying in sheltered locations, whereas homelessness increased among people staying in unsheltered locations (HUD, 2016). Chronic homelessness among individuals declined by 7% between 2015 and 2016 (HUD, 2016).

Barriers to Health Care

The homeless face barriers to obtaining ambulatory services but incur high rates of hospitalization. A high use of inpatient services in this manner amounts to the substitution of inpatient care for outpatient services. Both individual factors (competing needs, substance dependence, and mental illness) and system factors (availability, cost, convenience, and appropriateness of care) account for the barriers to adequate ambulatory services.

Other barriers to accessing health care include lack of accessible transportation to medical care providers and competing needs for basic food, shelter, and income, which often take precedence over obtaining health services or following through with a prescribed treatment plan. Homeless individuals who experience psychological distress and disabling mental illness may be in the greatest need of health services, yet may be the least able to obtain them. This inability to obtain health care may be attributable to such individual traits of mental illness as paranoia, disorientation, unconventional health beliefs, lack of social support, lack of organizational skills to gain access to needed services, and fear of authority figures and institutions resulting from previous institutionalization. The social conditions of street life also affect compliance with medical care, as unsheltered persons often lack proper sanitation and a stable place to store medications. In addition, they lack resources to obtain proper food for the medically indicated diets necessary for conditions such as diabetes or hypertension.

Federal efforts to provide medical services to the homeless population are delivered primarily through the Health Care for the Homeless (HCH) program. Community health centers supported by the 1985 Robert Wood Johnson Foundation/Pew Memorial Trust HCH program (subsequently covered by the 1987 McKinney Homeless Assistance Act) have addressed many of the access and quality-of-care issues faced by the homeless. In 2015, U.S. community health centers served approximately 1.2 million homeless patients (HRSA, 2015). A walk-in appointment system reduces access barriers at these medical facilities. Medical care, routine laboratory tests, substance abuse counseling, and some medications are provided free of charge to eliminate financial barriers.

The Mental Health Services for the Homeless Block Grant program sets aside funds for states to implement services for homeless persons with mental illness. These services include outreach services; community mental health services; rehabilitation; referrals to inpatient treatment, primary care, and substance abuse services; case management services; and supportive services in residential settings.

Services for homeless veterans are provided through the Department of Veterans Affairs (VA). The Homeless Chronically Mentally Ill Veterans Program provides outreach, case management

services, and psychiatric residential treatment for homeless mentally ill veterans in community-based facilities in 45 U.S. cities. Homelessness among veterans declined by 47% between 2009 and 2016 (HUD, 2016). The Domiciliary Care for Homeless Veterans Program addresses the health needs of veterans who have psychiatric illnesses or alcohol or drug abuse problems; it offers over 2,000 beds at 43 sites across the United States (U.S. Department of Veterans Affairs, 2012). This program had nearly 8,000 episodes of care in 2010 (U.S. Department of Veterans Affairs, 2012).

The Salvation Army also provides a variety of social, rehabilitation, and support services for homeless persons. Its centers include adult rehabilitation and food programs and permanent and transitional housing.

▶ Mental Health

Mental disorders are common psychiatric illnesses affecting adults and present a serious public health problem in the United States. Mental disorders are among the leading cause of disability for the U.S. population (CDC, 2014b). Mental illness is a risk factor for death from suicide, cardiovascular disease, and cancer. Suicide is currently the tenth leading cause of death in the United States and the fourth leading cause of death among persons age 22–44 (CDC, 2015b). Non-Hispanic white men 85 years or older have one of the highest rates of suicide—approximately 50 suicide deaths per 100,000 population (Population Reference Bureau, 2006). AIAN males are at higher risk for suicides as well; their mortality rate from this cause is approximately 16 suicide deaths per 100,000 population (CDC, 2015b).

Mental health disorders can be either psychological or biological in nature. Many mental health diseases—including mental retardation (MR), developmental disabilities (DD), and schizophrenia—are now known to be biological in origin. Other behaviors, including those related to personality disorders and neurotic behaviors, are still subject to interpretation and professional judgment.

National studies have concluded that the most common mental disorders are phobias; substance abuse, including alcohol and drug dependence; and affective disorders, including depression. Schizophrenia is considerably less common, affecting an estimated 0.6% of the U.S. population (Reeves et al., 2011).

Nearly one in five adults experiences a mental disorder every year (National Institute of Mental Health [NIMH], 2015). In 2015, 43.4 million adults (18 years or older) had a mental illness, including 9.8 million adults with severe mental illness (SMI) (NIMH, 2015). Among adults with any diagnosable mental disorder, 62.1% did not seek mental health treatment (SAMHSA, 2012a, 2012b). Prevalence of SMI was higher among Medicaid recipients, women, and individuals in the 18–25 age group (SAMHSA, 2012a, 2012b).

The mental health of children has drawn increasing attention in recent years. More than 1 in 5 children has a mental disorder—a higher rate than that for adults; approximately 4 million children or adolescents have SMIs (NIMH, 2015). Only half of those children diagnosed with mental health disorders receive mental health services

(U.S. Public Health Service, 2000). If left untreated, mental health problems in children can lead to more severe and/ or co-occurring mental illness (Kessler et al., 1997).

Most mental health services are provided in the general medical sector—a concept first described by Regier and colleagues (1988) as the de facto mental health service system—rather than through formal mental health specialist services. The de facto system combines specialty mental health services with general counseling services, such as those provided in primary care settings, nursing homes, and community health centers by ministers, counselors, self-help groups, families, and friends. Specifically, mental health services are provided through public and private resources in both inpatient and outpatient facilities. These facilities include state and county mental hospitals, private psychiatric hospitals, nonfederal general hospital psychiatric services, VA psychiatric services, residential treatment centers, and freestanding psychiatric outpatient clinics (**TABLE 11-6**).

Total expenditures for mental disorders have increased dramatically in the last few decades, from $31 billion in 1986 to $172 billion in 2009 (SAMHSA, 2014b). Nevertheless, only 37.9% of all individuals with mental illness received mental health services, and only 48.5% of individuals covered under Medicaid/CHIP received care in 2010 (SAMHSA, 2012a, 2012b). The U.S. **mental health system** essentially consists of two subsystems: one primarily for individuals with insurance coverage or private funds, and the other for those persons without private coverage.

TABLE 11-6 Mental Health Organizations, 2010

Service and Organization	Number of Mental Health Organizations
All organizations	10,374
Psychiatric hospitals	648
General hospitals	1,170
Outpatient clinics	6,305
Residential treatment centers for emotionally disturbed children	781
All other	1,470

Data from Substance Abuse and Mental Health Services Administration (SAMHSA). 2014a. *National Mental Health Services Survey (N-MHSS): 2010*. Data on Mental Health Treatment Facilities. BHSIS Series S-69, HHS Publication No. (SMA) 14–4837. Rockville, MD: Author.

Barriers to Mental Health Care

Two main barriers to access for mental health care are commonly experienced across the United States: prohibitive costs of services and shortage of available mental health professionals. In 2013, among young adults who delayed or did not seek needed mental health care, 50.1% stated that their failure to seek care was due to the prohibitive cost of treatment (SAMHSA, 2015). In addition to being unable to cover the high costs of care, many individuals currently reside in a mental health care health professional shortage area. A mental health HPSA is defined as an area in which the population to mental health professional ratio equals 30,000 people to 1 mental health professional and 30,000 people to 1 psychiatrist (Kaiser Family Foundation, 2017). As of 2017, there were more than 4,600 mental health HPSAs across the United States (Kaiser Family Foundation, 2017). This shortage translates to the available services being able to meet only 56% of the need for mental health services, leaving a large number of patients without needed care (Kaiser Family Foundation, 2017).

The Uninsured and Mental Health

Patients without insurance coverage or personal financial resources are treated in state and county mental health hospitals and in community mental health clinics. Care is also provided in short-term, acute care hospitals and emergency departments. Local governments are the providers of last resort, with the ultimate responsibility to provide somatic and mental health services for all citizens regardless of ability to pay.

The Insured and Mental Health

For patients who have insurance coverage or personal ability to pay, availability of both inpatient and ambulatory mental health care has expanded tremendously in recent decades. Inpatient mental health services for patients with insurance are usually provided through private psychiatric hospitals. These hospitals may operate on either a nonprofit or a for-profit basis. Notably, there has been substantial growth in national chains of for-profit mental health hospitals.

Patients with insurance coverage are also more likely to receive care through the offices of private psychiatrists, clinical psychologists, and licensed social workers. In addition, mental health services are provided by the VA and by the military health care system; however, access to these services is limited based on eligibility.

Managed Care and Mental Health

Managed care has expanded its services to include delivery of mental health care. Many state and local governments have also contracted with managed care organizations (MCOs) to manage their full health care benefits packages, which include mental health and substance abuse services for their Medicaid enrollees.

Many health maintenance organizations (HMOs) contract with specialized companies that provide managed behavioral health care, an arrangement called a carve-out; such carve-outs are implemented mainly because HMOs typically lack the in-house capacity to provide treatment. Using case managers and reviewers, most of whom are psychiatric nurses, social workers, and psychologists, these specialized companies oversee and authorize the use of mental health and substance abuse services. The case reviewers, using clinical protocols to guide them, assign patients to the least expensive appropriate treatment, emphasizing outpatient alternatives over inpatient care. Working with computerized databases, a reviewer studies a patient's particular problem and then authorizes an appointment with an appropriate provider in the company's selective network. On average, psychiatrists constitute approximately 4.5% of any given provider network, psychologists 18%, counselors 17%, and psychiatric social workers 65% (NIMH, 2015).

Mental Health Professionals

A variety of professionals provide mental health services (**TABLE 11-7**), including, but not limited, to psychiatrists, psychologists, social workers, nurses, counselors, and therapists.

Psychiatrists are physicians who specialize in the diagnosis and treatment of mental disorders. They receive postgraduate specialty training in mental health after completing medical school. Psychiatric residencies cover medical—as well as behavioral—diagnosis and treatments. A relatively small proportion of the total mental health workforce consists of psychiatrists, but they exercise disproportionate influence in the system by virtue of their authority to prescribe drugs and admit patients to hospitals.

Psychologists usually hold a doctoral degree, although some have master's degrees. These professionals are trained in interpreting and changing the behavior of people. Psychologists cannot prescribe drugs, but they provide a wide range of services to patients with neurotic and behavioral problems. Psychologists use such techniques as psychotherapy and counseling, which psychiatrists typically do not engage in. Psychoanalysis is a subspecialty in mental health that involves the use of intensive treatment by both psychiatrists and psychologists.

TABLE 11-7 Mental Health Providers by Discipline, Selected Years

Staff Discipline	Number	Year
Psychiatrists	33,727	2011
Child and adolescent psychiatrists	6,398	2009
Psychologists	95,545	2011
Clinical social workers	193,038	2008
Psychiatric nurses	13,701	2011
Substance abuse counselors	48,080	2011
Counselors	144,567	2011
Marriage and family therapists	62,316	2011

Data from Substance Abuse and Mental Health Services Administration (SAMHSA). 2013. *Behavioral health, United States, 2012.* Available at: http://archive .samhsa.gov/data/2012BehavioralHealthUS/2012-BHUS.pdf.

Social workers receive training in various aspects of mental health services, particularly counseling. These professionals are trained at the master's degree level. They also compete with psychologists for patients.

Nurses are involved in mental health care through the subspecialty of psychiatric nursing. Specialty training for nurses had its origins in the latter part of the 1800s. Nurses provide a wide range of mental health services.

Many other health care professionals contribute to the array of available services, including marriage and family counselors, recreational therapists, and vocational counselors. Numerous people work in related areas, such as adult day care (ADC) and alcohol/drug abuse counseling, and as psychiatric aides in institutional settings.

▶ The Chronically Ill

Chronic diseases are now the leading cause of death in the United States—heart disease, cancer, and stroke account for more than 50% of all U.S. deaths each year. Overall, 7 out of 10 deaths each year are from chronic diseases (CDC, 2016c). Heart disease is the number one cause of death in the United States, with a mortality rate of 167 deaths per 100,000 persons (NCHS, 2016b). The prevalence of heart disease from 2013 to 2014 was 10.7%, which is equal to 36.1 million Americans having some form of this disease (NCHS, 2016b). In 2010, more than 1 in 4 adults (80 million Americans) had more than one chronic illness (Ward and Schiller, 2013).

Chronic disease results in adverse consequences such as limitations on daily life activities. Among normal-weight adults with one or more chronic illnesses, the number of sick or unhealthy days they experience each month leads to loss of productivity that costs more than $15 billion per year (Witters and Agrawal, 2011). For overweight or obese adults with one or more chronic illnesses, this loss is more than double—an estimated $32 billion annually. Overall, the total loss of productivity due to overweight, obesity, or other chronic illnesses is estimated at more than $153 billion each year.

The loss in human potential and work days notwithstanding, chronic disease is expensive. Chronic disease places a huge economic demand on the United States. Treatment of people with chronic diseases accounts for 86% of total U.S. health care costs, which amounted to $2.9 trillion in 2013 (CDC, 2015c). In 2008, expenditures related to obesity were an estimated $147 billion (Finkelstein et al., 2009). The total estimated cost of diagnosed diabetes in 2012 was $245 billion, including $176 billion in direct medical costs and $69 billion in decreased productivity (CDC, 2016c). For the years 2009–2012, the economic cost due to smoking was estimated to exceed $289 billion per year (CDC, 2016c). In addition, costs related to heart disease totaled more than $475 billion in 2009 (Lloyd-Jones et al., 2009).

Much of the burden of chronic diseases results from four modifiable risk behaviors: physical activity, nutrition, smoking, and alcohol use (CDC, 2010b). In 2011, more than half (52%) of adults 18 years or older did not meet the CDC's recommendations for aerobic exercise or physical activity. In addition, 76% did not meet the recommendations for muscle-strengthening physical activity (CDC, 2016c). There has also been a decline in participation in physical education classes among high school students, from 42% in 1991 to 31% in 2011.

In addition, the U.S. population as a whole suffers from poor nutrition. In 2011, more than one-third (36%) of adolescents and 38% of adults said they ate fruits less than once a day, while 38% of adolescents and 23% of adults said they ate vegetables less than once a day (CDC, 2016c).

More detailed coverage on chronic diseases can be found in the *Beliefs, Values, and Health* chapter.

Disability

As of 2015, approximately 53 million people in the United States had a disability (CDC, 2015d). The prevalence of disability increases with age, with 70.5% of adults age 80 or older having a disability (U.S. Census Bureau, 2012b). The chronic conditions most responsible for disabilities are arthritis, heart disease, back problems, asthma, and diabetes (Kraus et al., 1996). Disabled individuals tend to be covered by public insurance (30% by Medicare and 10% by Medicaid), whereas those who have no disabilities are more likely to have private health insurance (U.S. Census Bureau, 2011e). In addition, Medicaid is the primary payer (40%) for long-term services and supports for disabled individuals, including nursing facility stays and home- and community-based services (Kaiser Family Foundation, 2014a).

Disability can be categorized as mental, physical, or social; tests of disability tend to be more sensitive to some categories than others. Physical disability usually relates to a person's mobility and other basic activities performed in daily life, mental disability involves both the cognitive and emotional states, and social disability is considered the most severe disability because management of social roles requires both physical and mental well-being (Ostir et al., 1999).

The two commonly used measures of disability—activities of daily living (ADLs) and instrumental activities of daily living (IADLs)—are covered in the *Beliefs, Values, and Health* chapter. Another tool for assessing disability is the Survey of Income and Program Participation (SIPP), which measures disability by asking participants about functional limitations (difficulty in performing activities such as seeing, hearing, walking, and having one's speech understood). The ADL and IADL scales are more widely used than the SIPP.

Despite the availability of community-based and institutional long-term care services for people with functional limitations, many people do not get the help they need with the basic tasks of personal care. It is estimated that approximately one in five individuals with an ADL limitation does not receive needed assistance (Newcomer et al., 2005). Furthermore, racial minorities are more likely to experience unmet personal assistance needs (Newcomer et al., 2005).

▶ **HIV/AIDS**

FIGURE 11-11 illustrates trends in AIDS reporting. The number of AIDS cases reported increased between 1987 and 1993, decreased between 1994 and 1999, increased between 2000 and 2004, and has decreased since 2005 (U.S. Census Bureau, 2010c).

In the United States, deaths from AIDS declined 19% between 2005 and 2014 (CDC, 2016a). Declines in reported AIDS cases are attributed to new treatments; decreasing death rates may reflect the fact that benefits from new treatments are being fully realized. Consequently, the number of people living with AIDS has continued to increase. In 2010, 487,692 people were living with AIDS; by comparison, that figure was 341,332 in 2001 (CDC, 2011).

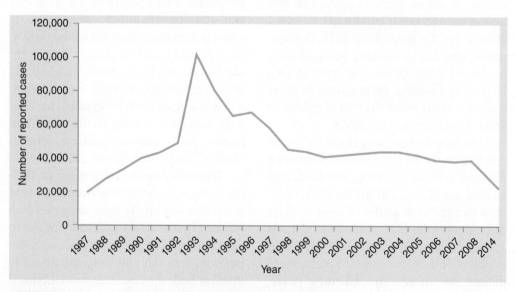

FIGURE 11-11 AIDS cases reported in the United States, 1987–2014.

Data from Centers for Disease Control and Prevention, Statistical Abstracts of the United States, 2001, p. 119; Statistical Abstracts of the United States, 2007, p. 120; Statistical Abstracts of the United States, 2008, p. 121; Statistical Abstracts of the United States, 2009, p. 120; Statistical Abstracts of the United States, 2010, p. 122.; Statistical Abstracts of the United States, 2012, p. 125; Centers for Disease Control and Prevention (CDC). 2016a. *HIV in the United States: At a glance.* Available at: https://www.cdc.gov/hiv/statistics/overview/ataglance.html. Accessed March 2017.

Among blacks, Hispanics, and minority women, AIDS/HIV is still a major public health concern. In 2014, males and blacks continued to have significantly higher rates of HIV/AIDS than females and whites (**TABLE 11-8**). Notably, only among black males is HIV a leading cause of death (CDC, 2012c). In 2011, rates of AIDS cases were 51.3 cases per 100,000 people in the black population, 16.2 cases per 100,000 people in the Hispanic population, and 4.9 cases per 100,000 people in the white population (CDC, 2012d). Blacks accounted for a rate of annual diagnoses that was 8 times greater than the rate for whites in 2009 (CDC, 2013c). Racial differences in HIV/AIDS infection probably reflect social, economic, behavioral, and other factors associated with HIV transmission risks.

TABLE 11-8 AIDS Cases Reported in the United States, 2010–2014 Cumulative and 2014

Characteristic	2010–2014 Cumulative		2014	
	Number	**Percentage**	**Number**	**Percentage**
Total	1,201,185	100.0	44,073	100.0
Sex				
Male (13 years and older)	947,580	78.9	35,571	80.7
Female (13 years and older)	244,044	20.3	8,328	18.9
Children younger than 13 years	9,561	0.8	174	0.4
Race/Ethnic Group				
White	436,952	38.1	12,025	27.3
Black	499,734	41.9	19,540	44.3
Hispanic	217,650	17.5	10,201	23.1
Asian	9,689	0.8	1,046	2.4
Native Hawaiian or other Pacific Islander	842	0.1	58	0.1
American Indian/Alaska Native	3,498	0.3	222	0.5

Data from National Center for Health Statistics (NCHS). 2016b. *Health, United States, 2015*. Hyattsville, MD: U.S. Department of Health and Human Services. p. 154.

HIV Infection in Rural Communities

In 2015, 39,513 people were diagnosed with HIV infection in the United States, and 18,303 people were diagnosed with AIDS. Since the HIV/AIDS epidemic began in the early 1980s, a total of 1,216,917 people have been diagnosed with AIDS in the United States (CDC, 2016a).

Rural persons with HIV and AIDS are more likely to be young, non-white, and female, and to have acquired their infection through heterosexual contact. Additionally, a growing number of these HIV-infected persons live in the rural South, a region historically characterized by a disproportionate number of poor and minority persons, strong religious beliefs and sanctions, and decreased access to comprehensive health services (CDC, 1995). Trends in new cases of HIV and AIDS in rural areas indicate that poor and non-white residents are disproportionately affected by these diseases (Aday, 1993; Lam and Liu, 1994).

HIV in Children

In the absence of specific therapy to interrupt transmission of HIV, an HIV-infected woman has a 20% chance of having a child born with HIV (Cooper et al., 2000). Building on previous success with zidovudine monotherapy in the 1990s, clinical studies established the efficacy of antiretroviral therapy in reducing the mother-to-child transmission rate when administered prenatally (Cooper et al., 2000). Use of antiretroviral therapy has resulted in a decrease of the rate of mother-to-child transmission to only 2% (Cooper et al., 2000). Guidelines on the use of antiretroviral drugs in pregnant HIV/AIDS-infected women have now been established (NIH, 2012; World Health Organization, 2004). The importance of preventing perinatal transmission is underscored by the fact that 68% of all AIDS cases among U.S. children are caused by mother-to-child transmission in pregnancy, labor, delivery, or breastfeeding (CDC, 2016a).

Children who are born with AIDS suffer from failure to thrive, which leaves them unable to grow and develop as healthy children. Without intervention, failure to thrive may lead to developmental delays that can have negative lifetime consequences for the child and his or her family.

HIV in Women

Women account for a rapidly growing proportion of the population with HIV/AIDS. In 2015, women represented 51% of HIV/AIDS cases worldwide (UN Women, 2015). For black U.S. women age 15 to 44 and Hispanic women age 25 to 44, HIV/AIDS was among the top 10 causes of death in 2010 (CDC, 2013a). For women in general, heterosexual sexual practices, followed by injection drug use (IDU), are the greatest causes of HIV exposure (CDC, 2017). Aside from the inherent risks of IDU, drug use contributes to a higher risk of contracting HIV if heterosexual sex with an IDU user occurs or when sex is traded for drugs or money (CDC, 2013b). Black and Hispanic minority women are at particular risk for these modes of exposure. Despite accounting for less than one-fourth of the total U.S. female population, black and Hispanic women represent more than three-fourths (76%) of all AIDS cases in women (CDC, 2017).

HIV/AIDS-Related Issues

Need for Research

HIV-related research is currently focusing on the development of a vaccine to prevent HIV-negative people from acquiring HIV. Researchers are also seeking to develop a therapeutic vaccine to prevent HIV-positive people from developing symptoms of AIDS.

People with HIV/AIDS cover a broad spectrum of social classes, races, ethnicities, sexual orientations, and genders. Therefore, behavioral intervention research should focus particularly on the subpopulations most vulnerable to HIV infection and are in urgent need of preventive interventions. These groups include gay youth and young adults, especially those who are black and Hispanic; disenfranchised and impoverished women; heterosexual men, especially those who are black and Hispanic; inner-city youth; and out-of-treatment substance abusers and their sexual partners. Research should focus on not only the individual, but also the impact of broader interventions (e.g., among drug users or those involved in sexual networks or community-wide groups) that change behavioral norms and consequently, affecting individual behavior (Merson, 1996).

Public Health Concerns

Trends related to AIDS underscore the synergy between poverty and intravenous drug use. Further, control of the HIV epidemic among the poor is hampered by this population's preoccupation with other problems related to survival, such as homelessness, crime, and lack of access to adequate health care.

Additionally, a relationship exists between the current tuberculosis epidemic and HIV. Indeed, tuberculosis, which is classified as an **opportunistic infection (OI)** in the HIV/AIDS setting, is the leading cause of death among HIV-infected people on a worldwide basis. Tuberculosis in HIV-infected persons is also a particular public health concern because HIV-infected persons are at greater risk of developing multidrug-resistant tuberculosis. Multidrug-resistant tuberculosis is understandably difficult to treat and can be fatal (CDC, 1999a, 1999b).

Reducing the spread of AIDS requires understanding and acceptance of a variety of sexual issues, ranging from the concept that even heterosexual men may engage in anonymous homosexual intercourse to the difficulty that adolescents may have controlling their sexual urges. Prejudice against gays and lesbians is manifested as **homophobia**, a fear and/or hatred of these individuals. Homophobia explains the initially slow policy-related response to the HIV epidemic.

Unfortunately, testing for HIV may not limit the virus's spread because many people who learn their HIV status do not change the behaviors that contribute to its spread. HIV infection has no cure, and current treatments do not affect the transmissibility of HIV.

In some cases, criminal law has been used to contain the spread of HIV and to protect public health. For example, some U.S. laws require that persons convicted of sex offenses be tested for HIV. Most of these laws, however, are disproportionately enforced against prostitutes. These laws suggest that persons who test positive for HIV may receive longer prison sentences; however, it is questionable whether this type of punishment actually reduces the spread of HIV.

Health promotion efforts, including those used to reduce the transmission of HIV, are often hamstrung by psychosocial and other factors. For example, humans generally have difficulty changing their behaviors. Further, much human behavior is associated with functional needs (e.g., unsafe sex might fulfill a need for intimacy). Social learning theory explains that behavior change first requires knowledge, followed by a change of attitude or perspective.

Discrimination

HIV-positive people may experience discrimination in access to health care. The policies of various government agencies intended to help have also had a discriminatory impact on people with HIV/AIDS. For example, the Social Security Administration has not historically considered many of the HIV-related symptoms of women and IV drug users in adjudicating disability claims. Although the Department of Defense provides adequate medical care to individuals who acquire HIV in the military, recruits who test positive for HIV cannot join the military.

Provider Training

Increased knowledge about HIV and personal contact with people who have HIV have improved the attitudes of health care providers toward individuals with HIV and contributed to their willingness to care for people with HIV. Training of health care professionals should encompass not only medical and treatment-related information, but also a range of competencies related to interpersonal skills.

In the area of psychosocial skills, the following characteristics are essential in an effectively trained provider: good communication skills (ability to establish rapport, ask questions, and listen), positive attitudes (respect, empowerment, trust), and an approach that incorporates principles of holistic care. In the area of cultural competence, essential elements include understanding of and respect for the person's specific culture; understanding that racial and ethnic minorities have important and multiple subdivisions or functional units; acknowledging the issues of gender and sexual orientation within the context of cultural competence; and respecting the customs, including modes of communication, of the person's culture. In the area of substance abuse, the following elements are essential for primary care providers: understanding the complex medical picture presented by a person who suffers from both HIV and addiction; understanding the complicated psychosocial, ethical, and legal issues related to care of addicted persons; and being aware of personal attitudes about addiction that may impair providers' ability to give care objectively and nonjudgmentally (e.g., in the administration of pain medication; Gross and Larkin, 1996).

Cost of HIV/AIDS

Medical care for patients with HIV/AIDS is extremely expensive. Pharmaceutical companies claim that the high prices they charge for AIDS drugs reflect their extensive investment in research and development of drugs. Medicaid currently covers more than 240,000 people with HIV (Kaiser Family Foundation, 2016a). In fiscal year (FY) 2016, combined federal and state Medicaid spending on persons with HIV totaled

$9.4 billion, making it the largest source of public financing for HIV/AIDS care in the United States. Of this amount, the federal share was $5.9 billion in FY 2012, or 30% of federal HIV care spending (Kaiser Family Foundation, 2016a). Lack of insurance and underinsurance represent formidable financial barriers to HIV/AIDS care.

The U.S. government also invests substantial amounts of money in research and development through research supported at the NIH and CDC. Government programs spend money in several areas for HIV (**FIGURE 11-12**). Of these expenditures, 73% is devoted to antiretroviral medications, 13% to inpatient care, 9% to outpatient care, and 5% to other HIV-related medications and laboratory costs. For patients who initiate highly active antiretroviral therapy

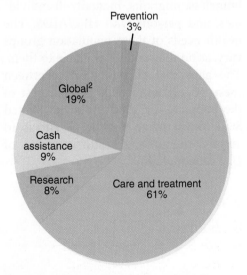

FIGURE 11-12 Federal spending for HIV/AIDS by category,[1] FY 2016.

[1] Categories may include funding across multiple agencies/programs.
[2] The "global" category includes international HIV research at NIH.

Modified from Kaiser Family Foundation. 2016b. *U.S. federal funding for HIV/AIDS: Trends over time.* Available at: http://kff.org/global-health-policy/fact-sheet/u-s-federal-funding-for-hivaids-trends-over-time/. Accessed March 2017.

(HAART) when their CD4 cell count is 200/L, projected life expectancy is 22.5 years, discounted lifetime cost is $354,100 and undiscounted cost is $567,000 (Schackman et al., 2006). Indirect costs attributable to HIV/AIDS include lost productivity, largely because of worker morbidity and mortality. However, other factors affect cost projections associated with the HIV/AIDS epidemic, including the level of employment of HIV-positive people; regional differences in the cost of care, which is often associated with the lack of subacute care in many parts of the country; and the rate at which HIV spreads.

Containment of escalating medical costs, including the coordination of medical care, is the objective of two HIV-specific efforts: the Medicaid waiver program and the Ryan White Comprehensive AIDS Resources Emergency (CARE) Act. Through the **Medicaid waiver program**, states may design packages of services to specific populations, such as the elderly, the disabled, and persons who test HIV positive. At this time, it is unknown whether the program is cost-effective.

The passage of the Ryan White CARE Act in 1990 provided federal funds to develop treatment and care options for persons with HIV/AIDS (Summer, 1991). Title II of this legislation is administered by states and has been used to establish HIV clinics and related services in areas lacking the resources needed to offer this specialty care. Some public health systems have used Ryan White CARE Act money to provide HIV/AIDS services in rural communities in which poor or medically underserved persons lack access to adequate care. Federal spending attributable to the Ryan White CARE Act totaled an estimated $2.4 billion in 2016 (Kaiser Family Foundation, 2016b).

AIDS and the U.S. Health Care System

The course of AIDS is characterized by a gradual decline in the patient's physical, cognitive, and emotional function and well-being. Such a comprehensive decline requires a continuum of care, including emergency care, primary care, housing and supervised living, mental health and social support, nonmedical services, and hospice care. This continuum can encompass elements such as outreach and case finding, preventive services, outpatient and inpatient care, and coordination of private and public insurance benefits.

As HIV disease progresses, many persons become disabled and rely on public entitlement or private disability programs for income and health care benefits. These programs include Social Security Disability Income and Supplemental Security Income, administered by the Social Security Administration.

Medicare and Medicaid become primary payers for health care because of the onset of disability and depletion of personal funds. Approximately 70,000 previously uninsured people with HIV/AIDS were expected to gain coverage under the ACA. Most of them would have gained insurance through Medicaid expansion (Kaiser Family Foundation, 2014b).

▶ Summary

This chapter examines the major characteristics of certain U.S. population groups that face challenges and barriers in accessing health care services—namely, racial/ethnic minorities, children and women, persons living in rural areas, the homeless, migrants, mentally ill individuals, and persons with HIV/AIDS. The health needs of these population groups vary, as do the services available to them. The gaps that currently exist between these population groups and the rest of the population indicate that the United States must make significant efforts to address the unique health concerns of U.S. subpopulations.

▶ Test Your Understanding

Terminology

acquired
   immunodeficiency
   syndrome (AIDS)
chronic
dependency

developmental vulnerability
disability
homophobia
human immunodeficiency
   virus (HIV)

Medicaid waiver program
mental health system
opportunistic infection (OI)
psychiatrists
psychologists

Review Questions

1. How can the framework of vulnerability be used to study vulnerable populations in the United States?
2. What are the racial/ethnic minority categories in the United States?
3. What health challenges do white Americans face, compared with those faced by minorities?
4. Who are the AA/PIs?
5. What is the Indian Health Service?
6. What are the health concerns of children?
7. Which childhood characteristics have important implications for health system design?
8. Which health services are currently available for children?
9. What are the health concerns of women?
10. What are the roles of the Office on Women's Health?
11. What are the challenges faced in rural health?
12. Which measures have been taken to improve access to care in rural areas of the United States?
13. What are the characteristics and health concerns of the homeless population?
14. How are mental health services provided in the United States?
15. Who are the major mental health professionals?
16. How does AIDS affect different population groups in the United States?
17. Which services and policies currently combat AIDS in the United States?
18. What is the impact of the ACA on vulnerable populations?

▶ References

Aday, L. A. 1993. *At risk in America: The health and health care needs of vulnerable populations in the United States.* San Francisco, CA: Jossey-Bass Publishers.

Association of American Medical Colleges (AAMC). 2017. *The state of women in academic medicine: The pipeline and pathways to leadership, 2013-2014.* Available at: https://www.aamc.org/members/gwims/statistics/#bench.

Bircher, H. 2009. Prenatal care disparities and the migrant farm worker community. *MCN American Journal of Maternal-Child Nursing* 34, no. 5: 303-307.

Breakey, W. R., et al. 1989. Health and mental health problems of homeless men and women in Baltimore. *Journal of the American Medical Association* 262 no. 10: 1352-1357.

Burks, L. J. 1992. Community health representatives: The vital link in Native American health care. *IHS Primary Care Provider* 16, no. 12: 186-190.

Centers for Disease Control and Prevention (CDC). 1995. *Facts about women and HIV/AIDS.* Atlanta, GA: CDC.

Centers for Disease Control and Prevention (CDC). 1999a. *CDC fact sheet: Recent HIV/AIDS treatment advances and the implications for prevention.* Available at: http://www.cdc.gov/nchstp/hiv_aids/pubs/facts.htm. Accessed December 2010.

Centers for Disease Control and Prevention (CDC). 1999b. *CDC fact sheet: The deadly intersection between TB and HIV.* Available at: http://www.cdc.gov/nchstp/hiv_aids/pubs/facts.htm. Accessed December 2010.

Centers for Disease Control and Prevention (CDC). 2010a. Vital signs: Health insurance coverage and health care utilization, United States, 2006–2009 and January–March 2010. *Morbidity and Mortality Weekly Report* 59: 1-7.

Centers for Disease Control and Prevention (CDC). 2010b. *Chronic disease and health promotion.* Available at: http://www.cdc.gov /chronicdisease/pdf/2009-Power-of-Prevention .pdf. Accessed January 2011.

Centers for Disease Control and Prevention (CDC). 2011. *HIV surveillance report: Diagnoses of HIV infection and AIDS in the United States and dependent areas, 2011.* Vol. 23. Atlanta, GA: U.S. Department of Health and Human Services.

Centers for Disease Control and Prevention (CDC). 2012a. Deaths: Leading causes for 2009. *National Vital Statistics Reports* 61, no. 7.

Centers for Disease Control and Prevention (CDC). 2012b. Youth Risk Behavior Surveillance— United States, 2011. *Morbidity and Mortality Weekly Report* 61: SS-4.

Centers for Disease Control and Prevention (CDC). 2012c. *HIV surveillance by race /ethnicity.* Available at: http://www.cdc.gov/hiv /pdf/statistics_surveillance_raceEthnicity.pdf. Accessed September 2013.

Centers for Disease Control and Prevention (CDC). 2012d. *HIV among pregnant women, infants, and children in the United States.* Available at: http://img.thebody.com/cdc/2013/hiv_wic _us.pdf. Accessed May 2017.

Centers for Disease Control and Prevention (CDC). 2013a. *HIV among women.* Available at: http://action.naacp.org/page/-/Health%20 Documents/HIV_among_Women_Fact_Sheet .pdf. Accessed May 2017.

Centers for Disease Control and Prevention (CDC). 2013b. HIV infection among heterosexuals at increased risk—United States, 2010. *Morbidity and Mortality Weekly Report* 62 no. 10: 183–188.

Centers for Disease Control and Prevention (CDC). 2013c. Social determinants of health among adults with diagnosed HIV infection in 18 areas, 2005–2009. *HIV Surveillance Supplemental Report* 18, no. 4.

Centers for Disease Control and Prevention (CDC). 2014a. *Behavioral Risk Factor Surveillance System, 2014.* Available at: http://www .americashealthrankings.org/explore/2015 -annual-report/measure/PhysicalHealth/state /ALL. Accessed March 2017.

Centers for Disease Control and Prevention (CDC). 2014b. *Web-based injury statistics query and reporting system (WISQARS).* Available at: http://

www.cdc.gov/ncipc/wisqars. Accessed March 2017.

Centers for Disease Control and Prevention (CDC). 2015a. *Current cigarette smoking among adults in the United States.* Available at: https://www .cdc.gov/tobacco/data_statistics/fact_sheets /adult_data/cig_smoking/. Accessed March 2017.

Centers for Disease Control and Prevention (CDC). 2015b. *Deaths: Leading causes for 2014.* Available at: https://www.cdc.gov/nchs/data/nvsr/nvsr65 /nvsr65_05.pdf. Accessed March 2017.

Centers for Disease Control and Prevention (CDC). 2015c. *At a glance 2015: National Center for Chronic Disease Prevention and Health Promotion.* Available at: https://www.cdc.gov /chronicdisease/resources/publications/aag /pdf/2015/nccdphp-aag.pdf. Accessed March 2017.

Centers for Disease Control and Prevention (CDC). 2015d. *53 million adults in the US live with a disability.* Available at: https://www.cdc.gov /media/releases/2015/p0730-us-disability.html. Accessed March 2017.

Centers for Disease Control and Prevention (CDC). 2016a. *HIV in the United States: At a glance.* Available at: https://www.cdc.gov/hiv/statistics /overview/ataglance.html. Accessed March 2017.

Centers for Disease Control and Prevention (CDC). 2016b. *National Vital Statistics System.* Available at: http://www.cdc.gov/nchs/nvss.htm. Accessed March 2017.

Centers for Disease Control and Prevention (CDC). 2016c. *Chronic disease overview.* Available at: https://www.cdc.gov/chronicdisease/overview/. Accessed March 2017.

Centers for Disease Control and Prevention (CDC). 2016d. *Smoking prevalence and cessation before and during pregnancy: Data from the birth certificate, 2014.* National Vital Statistics Reports 65. Available at: https://www.cdc.gov /nchs/data/nvsr/nvsr65/nvsr65_01.pdf. Accessed July 2017.

Centers for Disease Control and Prevention (CDC). 2016e. *Pregnancy Mortality Surveillance System.* Available at: https://www.cdc.gov /reproductivehealth/maternalinfanthealth /pmss.html. Accessed July 2017.

Centers for Disease Control and Prevention (CDC). 2017. *HIV among women.* Available at: https:// www.cdc.gov/hiv/group/gender/women /#refe. Accessed March 2017.

Congressional Budget Office. 2012. Updated estimates for the insurance coverage provisions of the Affordable Care Act. Washington, DC: Government Printing Office.

Cooper, E. R., et al. 2000. Combination antiretroviral strategies for the treatment of pregnant HIV-1–infected women and prevention of perinatal HIV-1 transmission. *Journal of Acquired Immune Deficiency Syndromes* 29, no. 5: 484–494.

Federal Interagency Forum on Child and Family Statistics. 2016. *America's children in brief: Key national indicators of well-being.* Available at: https://www.childstats.gov/pdf/ac2016/ac_16.pdf. Accessed March 2017.

Finkelstein, E. A., et al. 2009. Annual medical spending attributable to obesity: Payer- and service-specific estimates. *Health Affairs* 28, no. 5: w822–w831.

Gross, E. J., and M. H. Larkin. 1996. The child with HIV in day care and school. *Nursing Clinics of North America* 31, no. 1: 231–241.

Guttmacher Institute. 2013. *Insurance coverage of contraceptives.* Available at: http://www.guttmacher.org/statecenter/spibs/spib_ICC.pdf. Accessed September 2013.

Health Care for the Homeless. 2012. *Client demographics.* Available at: http://www.hchmd.org/demographics.shtml. Accessed September 2013.

Health Resources and Services Administration (HRSA). 2017. *Shortage Areas.* Available at: https://datawarehouse.hrsa.gov/topics/shortageAreas.aspx. Accessed May 2017.

Health Resources and Services Administration (HRSA). 2015. *2015 health center data.* Available at: https://bphc.hrsa.gov/uds/datacenter.aspx. Accessed March 2017.

Health Resources and Services Administration (HRSA), Bureau of Health Professions. 2007. *Shortage designation.* Available at: https://bhw.hrsa.gov/shortage-designation. Accessed December 2008.

Health Resources and Services Administration (HRSA), Bureau of Health Professions. 2013. *National Health Service Corps.* Available at: http://nhsc.hrsa.gov/corpsexperience/aboutus/index.html. Accessed September 2013.

Health Resources and Services Administration (HRSA), National Health Service Corps (NHSC). 2017. *About the NHSC.* Available at: https://nhsc.hrsa.gov/corpsexperience/aboutus/. Accessed May 2017.

Health Resources and Services Administration (HRSA), Office of Rural Health Policy. 2015. *About FORHP.* Available at: https://www.hrsa.gov/ruralhealth/aboutus/index.html. Accessed May 2017.

Hung, M. C., et al. 2016. Racial/ethnicity disparities in invasive breast cancer among younger and older women: An analysis using multiple measures of population health. *Cancer Epidemiology* 45: 112–118.

Indian Health Service (IHS). 1999a. *Fact sheet: Comprehensive health care program for American Indians and Alaskan Natives.* Washington, DC: Public Health Service.

Indian Health Service (IHS). 1999b. *A quick look.* Washington, DC: Public Health Service.

Indian Health Service (IHS). 2010a. *Indian health disparities: IHS fact sheet.* Washington, DC: Public Health Service.

Indian Health Service (IHS). 2010b. *IHS year 2010 profile: IHS fact sheet.* Washington, DC: Public Health Service.

Indian Health Service (IHS). 2013. *Agency overview.* Available at: http://www.ihs.gov/aboutihs/overview/. Accessed September 2013.

Indian Health Service (IHS). 2014. *Trends in Indian health: 2014 edition.* Available at: https://www.ihs.gov/dps/includes/themes/newihstheme/display_objects/documents/Trends2014Book508.pdf. Assessed March 2017.

Institute for Children, Poverty and Homelessness. 2011. *Profiles of risk: Education.* Research Brief No. 2. Available at: https://www.onefamilyinc.org/Blog/wp-content/uploads/2011/10/icph_familiesatrisk_no-2.pdf. Accessed May 2017.

Jasinski, J. L. 2005. *The experience of violence in the lives of homeless women: A research report.* Available at: https://www.ncjrs.gov/pdffiles1/nij/grants/211976.pdf. Accessed January 2014.

Kaiser Family Foundation. 2013. *Health reform: Implications for women's access to coverage and care.* Available at: http://kaiserfamilyfoundation.files.wordpress.com/2012/03/7987-03-health-reform-implications-for-women_s-access-to-coverage-and-care.pdf. Accessed September 2013.

Kaiser Family Foundation. 2014a. *The Affordable Care Act's impact on Medicaid eligibility, enrollment, and benefits for people with disabilities.* Available at: http://kff.org/health-reform/issue-brief/the -affordable-care-acts-impact-on-medicaid -eligibility-enrollment-and-benefits-for -people-with-disabilities/. Accessed March 2017.

Kaiser Family Foundation. 2014b. *Assessing the impact of the Affordable Care Act on health insurance coverage of people with HIV.* http:// kff.org/hivaids/issue-brief/assessing-the -impact-of-the-affordable-care-act-on-health -insurance-coverage-of-people-with-hiv/. Accessed May 2017.

Kaiser Family Foundation. 2015. *Number of Medicare certified rural health clinics.* Available at: http://kff .org/other/state-indicator/total-rural-health -clinics/?currentTimeframe=0&sortModel=%7B %22colId%22:%22Location%22,%22sort%22: %22asc%22%7D. Accessed March 2017.

Kaiser Family Foundation. 2016a. *Medicaid and HIV.* Available at: http://kff.org/hivaids/fact -sheet/medicaid-and-hiv/. Accessed March 2017.

Kaiser Family Foundation. 2016b. *U.S. federal funding for HIV/AIDS: Trends over time.* Available at: http://kff.org/global-health-policy /fact-sheet/u-s-federal-funding-for-hivaids -trends-over-time/. Accessed March 2017.

Kaiser Family Foundation. 2016c. *Women's health insurance coverage.* Available at: http://kff.org /womens-health-policy/fact-sheet/womens -health-insurance-coverage-fact-sheet. Accessed March 2017.

Kaiser Family Foundation. 2016d. *Key Facts about the Uninsured Population.* Available at: http://kff .org/uninsured/fact-sheet/key-facts-about-the -uninsured-population/#footnote-198942-19. Accessed May 2017.

Kaiser Family Foundation. 2017. *Mental health care health profession shortage areas (HPSAs).* Available at: http://kff.org/other/state-indicator /mental-health-care-health-professional -shortage-areas-hpsas/?currentTimeframe=0&s ortModel=%7B%22colId%22:%22Location%22, %22sort%22:%22asc%22%7D. Accessed March 2017.

Kerker, B. D., et al. 2011. A population-based assessment of the health of homeless families in New York City, 2001–2003. *American Journal of Public Health* 101, no. 3: 546–553.

Kessler R. C, et al. 1997. Childhood adversity and adult psychiatric disorder in the US National Comorbidity Survey. *Psychological Medicine* 27, no.5: 1101–1119.

Kraus, L. E., et al. 1996. *Chartbook on disability in the United States, 1996. An InfoUse Report.* Washington, DC: U.S. National Institute on Disability and Rehabilitation Research.

Lam, N., and K. Liu. 1994. Spread of AIDS in rural America, 1982–1990. *Journal of Acquired Immune Deficiency Syndrome* 7, no. 5: 485–490.

Larson, A., and Plascencia, L. 1993. *Migrant enumeration study.* Washington, DC: Office of Minority Health.

Larson, S. L., & Fleishman, J. A. 2003. Rural-urban differences in usual source of care and ambulatory service use: Analyses of national data using Urban Influence Codes. *Medical Care*, III65–III74.

Lloyd-Jones, D., et al. 2009. American Heart Association Statistics Committee and Stroke Statistics Subcommittee. Heart disease and stroke statistics—2009 update: A report from the American Heart Association Statistics Committee and Stroke Statistics Subcommittee. *Circulation* 119: e21–181.

Merson, M. H. 1996. Returning home: Reflections on the USA's response to the HIV/AIDS epidemic. *Lancet* 347, no. 9016: 1673–1676.

Migrant Health Promotion. 2013. *Farmworkers in the United States.* Available at: http://www .migranthealth.org/index.php?option=com _content&view=article&id=38&Itemid=30. Accessed September 2013.

Misra, D., ed. 2001. *Women's health data book: A profile of women's health in the United States,* 3rd ed. Washington, DC: Jacobs Institute of Women's Health and Henry J. Kaiser Family Foundation.

National Alliance to End Homelessness. 2012. *The state of homelessness in America 2012.* Homelessness Research Institute. Available at: http://www.endhomelessness.org/page/-/files /file_FINAL_The_State_of_Homelessness_in _America_2012. Accessed May 2017.

National Center for Farmworker Health. 2011. *HIV /AIDS farmworker factsheet.* Available at: http:// www.ncfh.org/uploads/3/8/6/8/38685499 /fs-hiv_aids.pdf. Accessed March 2017.

National Center for Farmworker Health. 2012. *Facts about Farmworkers.* Available at: http:// www.ncfh.org/uploads/3/8/6/8/38685499

/fs-facts_about_farmworkers.pdf. Accessed May 2017.

National Center for Farmworker Health. 2015. *Tuberculosis.* Available at: http://www.ncfh.org/uploads/3/8/6/8/38685499/fs-what_is_tb.pdf. Accessed March 2017.

National Center for Health Statistics (NCHS). 1996. *Health, United States, 1995.* Hyattsville, MD: U.S. Department of Health and Human Services.

National Center for Health Statistics (NCHS). 2010. *Health, United States, 2009.* Hyattsville, MD: U.S. Department of Health and Human Services.

National Center for Health Statistics (NCHS). 2011. *Health, United States, 2010.* Hyattsville, MD: U.S. Department of Health and Human Services.

National Center for Health Statistics (NCHS). 2013. *Health, United States, 2012.* Hyattsville, MD: U.S. Department of Health and Human Services.

National Center for Health Statistics (NCHS). 2014a. *National Health Interview Survey.* Available at: https://www.cdc.gov/nchs/nhis/. Accessed March 2017.

National Center for Health Statistics (NCHS). 2014b. *National Health and Nutrition Examination Survey 2013-2014.* Available at: https://wwwn.cdc.gov/nchs/nhanes/search/nhanes13_14.aspx. Accessed March 2017.

National Center for Health Statistics (NCHS). 2016a. *Early release of selected estimates based on data from the National Health Interview Survey, January–June 2016.* Available at: https://www.cdc.gov/nchs/data/nhis/earlyrelease/earlyrelease201611_01.pdf. Accessed May 2017.

National Center for Health Statistics (NCHS). 2016b. *Health, United States, 2015.* Hyattsville, MD: U.S. Department of Health and Human Services.

National Conference of State Legislatures. 2013. *Improving rural health: State policy options.* Available at: http://www.ncsl.org/documents/health/RuralHealth_PolicyOptions_1113.pdf. Accessed March 2017.

National Institute of Mental Health (NIMH). 2015. *Any mental illness (AMI) among U.S. adults.* Available at: https://www.nimh.nih.gov/health/statistics/prevalence/any-mental-illness-ami-among-us-adults.shtml. Accessed March 2017.

National Institutes of Health (NIH). 2002. *News release: NHLBI stops trial of estrogen plus progestin due to increased breast cancer risk, lack of overall benefit.* Available at: http://www.nhlbi.nih.gov/new/press/02-07-09.htm. Accessed December 2006.

National Institutes of Health (NIH). 2012. *Guidelines for the use of antiretroviral agents in HIV-1-infected adults and adolescents.* Department of Health and Human Services. Available at: http://aidsinfo.nih.gov/contentfiles/lvguidelines/AdultandAdolescentGL.pdf. Accessed September 2013.

National Law Center on Homelessness and Poverty. 2015. *Homelessness in America: Overview of data and causes.* Available at: https://www.nlchp.org/documents/Homeless_Stats_Fact_Sheet. Accessed May 2017.

National Rural Health Association. 2016. *Rural health care.* Available at: https://www.ruralhealthweb.org/about-nrha/about-rural-health-care. Accessed March 2017.

National Women's Law Center. 2015. *National snapshot: Poverty among women & families, 2015.* Available at: https://nwlc.org/wp-content/uploads/2016/09/Poverty-Snapshot-Factsheet-2016.pdf. Accessed May 2017.

Newcomer, R., et al. 2005. Living quarters and unmet need for personal care assistance among adults with disabilities. *Journals of Gerontology Series B: Psychological Sciences and Social Sciences* 9, no. 4: S205–S213.

O'Neill, J. E., and D. M. O'Neill. 2009. Who are the uninsured? An analysis of America's uninsured population, their characteristics and their health. New York, NY: Employment Policies Institute.

Ostir, G. V., et al. 1999. Disability in older adults 1: Prevalence, causes, and consequences. *Behavioral Medicine* 24, no. 4: 147–156.

Patton, L., and D. Puskin. 1990. *Ensuring access to health care services in rural areas: A half century of federal policy.* Washington, DC: Essential Health Care Services Conference Center at Georgetown University Conference Center.

Population Reference Bureau. 2006. *Elderly white men afflicted by high suicide rates.* Available at: http://www.prb.org/Publications/Articles/2006/ElderlyWhiteMenAfflictedbyHighSuicideRates.aspx. Accessed May 2017.

Reeves, W. C., et al. 2011. *Mental illness surveillance among adults in the United States.*

Available at: https://www.cdc.gov/mmwr/preview/mmwrhtml/su6003a1.htm. Accessed March 2017.

Regier, D. A., et al. 1988. One month prevalence of mental disorders in the United States: Based on five epidemiologic catchment area sites. *Archives of General Psychiatry* 45, no. 11: 977–986.

Rust, G. S. (1990). Health status of migrant farmworkers: A literature review and commentary. *American Journal of Public Health* 80, no. 10: 1213–1217.

Salganicoff, A., et al. 2005. *Women and health care: A national profile.* Menlo Park, CA: Henry J. Kaiser Family Foundation.

Schackman, B. R., et al. 2006. The lifetime cost of current human immunodeficiency virus care in the United States. *Medical Care* 44, no. 11: 990–997.

Schutt, R. K., and S. M. Goldfinger. 1996. Housing preferences and perceptions of health and functioning among homeless mentally ill persons. *Psychiatric Services* 47, no. 4: 381–386.

Sechzer, J. A., et al. 1996. *Women and mental health.* New York, NY: Academy of Sciences.

Shi, L., and G. Stevens. 2010. *Vulnerable populations in the United States.* 2nd ed. San Francisco, CA: Jossey-Bass Publishers.

Shortell, S. M., et al. 1996. *Remaking health care in America.* San Francisco, CA: Jossey-Bass Publishers.

Solis, J. M., et al. 1990. Acculturation, access to care, and use of preventive services by Hispanics: Findings from HHANES 1982–84. *American Journal of Public Health* 80 (suppl): 11–19.

Substance Abuse and Mental Health Services Administration (SAMHSA). 2012a. *Mental health, United States, 2010.* HHS Publication No. (SMA) 12-4681. Rockville, MD: Author.

Substance Abuse and Mental Health Services Administration (SAMHSA). 2012b. *Results from the 2011 National Survey on Drug Use and Health: Mental health findings.* NSDUH Series H-45, HHS Publication No. (SMA) 12-4725. Rockville, MD: Author.

Substance Abuse and Mental Health Services Administration (SAMHSA). 2013. *Behavioral health, United States, 2012.* Available at: http://archive.samhsa.gov/data/2012Behavioral HealthUS/2012-BHUS.pdf.

Substance Abuse and Mental Health Services Administration (SAMHSA). 2014a. National Mental Health Services Survey (N-MHSS): 2010. Data on Mental Health Treatment Facilities. BHSIS Series S-69, HHS Publication No. (SMA) 14-4837. Rockville, MD: Author. Available at: https://www.samhsa.gov/data/sites/default/files/NMHSS2010_Web/NMHSS2010_Web/NMHSS2010_Web.pdf. Accessed May 2017.

Substance Abuse and Mental Health Services Administration (SAMHSA). 2014b. *Projections of national expenditures for treatment of mental and substance use disorders, 2010–2020.* HHS Publication No. SMA-14-4883. Rockville, MD: Author.

Substance Abuse and Mental Health Services Administration (SAMHSA). 2015. *1.5 million young adults do not receive needed mental health services.* Rockville, MD: Author. Available at: https://www.samhsa.gov/data/sites/default/files/report_1975/Spotlight-1975.html. Accessed May 2017.

Summer, L. 1991. *Limited access: Health care for the rural poor.* Washington, DC: Center on Budget and Policy Priorities.

UN Women. 2015. *Facts and figures: HIV and AIDS.* Available at: http://www.unwomen.org/en/what-we-do/hiv-and-aids/facts-and-figures. Accessed March 2017.

U.S. Bureau of Labor Statistics. 2016. *Labor force characteristics by race and ethnicity, 2016.* Washington, DC: Government Printing Office.

U.S. Census Bureau. 2009. *The 2010 census questionnaire: Informational copy.* Available at: https://www.census.gov/history/pdf/2010 questionnaire.pdf. Accessed May 2017.

U.S. Census Bureau. 2010a. *The Two or More Races Population: 2010.* Available at: http://www.census.gov/prod/cen2010/briefs/c2010br-13.pdf. Accessed May 2017.

U.S. Census Bureau. 2010b. *Current population survey, 2010 annual social and economic supplement.* Washington, DC: Government Printing Office.

U.S. Census Bureau. 2010c. *2007–2009 American Community Survey, 3-year estimates.* Washington, DC: Government Printing Office.

U.S. Census Bureau. 2011a. *Overview of race and Hispanic origin: 2010.* Washington, DC: Government Printing Office.

U.S. Census Bureau. 2011b. *The Hispanic population: 2010. 2010 Census Briefs*. Washington, DC: Government Printing Office.

U.S. Census Bureau. 2011c. *Income, poverty, and health insurance coverage in the United States: 2010*. Washington, DC: Government Printing Office.

U.S. Census Bureau. 2011d. *The American Indian and Alaska Native population: 2010. 2010 Census Briefs*. Washington, DC: Government Printing Office.

U.S. Census Bureau. 2011e. *American Community Survey, American FactFinder, Table B18135*. Available at: http://factfinder2.census.gov. Accessed September 2013.

U.S. Census Bureau. 2012a. *Statistical abstract of the United States: 2012*. Washington, DC: Government Printing Office.

U.S. Census Bureau. 2012b. Americans with disabilities: 2010. Household economic studies. *Current Population Reports*. Available at: http://www.census.gov/prod/2012pubs/p70-131.pdf. Accessed September 2013.

U.S. Census Bureau. 2013. *The Hispanic population in the United States: 2013*. Available at: https://www.census.gov/data/tables/2013/demo/hispanic-origin/2013-cps.html. Accessed May 2017.

U.S. Census Bureau. 2014. *Health Insurance Coverage in the United States: 2013*. Washington, DC: Government Printing Office.

U.S. Census Bureau. 2015. *2015 census: Profile of general population and housing characteristics*. Washington, DC: Government Printing Office.

U.S. Census Bureau. 2016. *QuickFacts United States*. Available at: https://www.census.gov/quickfacts/table/PST045216/00. Accessed March 2017.

U.S. Conference of Mayors. 2011. *Hunger and Homelessness Survey*. Available at: http://www.ncdsv.org/images/USCM_Hunger-homelessness-Survey-in-America's-Cities_12%202011.pdf. Accessed May 2017.

U.S. Department of Housing and Urban Development (HUD). 2012. *The 2011 Annual Homeless Assessment Report to Congress*. Available at: https://www.onecpd.info/resources/documents/2011AHAR_FinalReport.pdf. Accessed September 2013.

U.S. Department of Housing and Urban Development (HUD). 2016. *2016 Annual Homeless Assessment Report (AHAR) to Congress.* Available at: https://www.hudexchange.info/resources/documents/2016-AHAR-Part-1.pdf. Accessed March 2017.

U.S. Department of Labor. 2011. *Changing characteristics of U.S. farm workers: 21 years of findings from the National Agricultural Workers Survey*. Available at: http://migrationfiles.ucdavis.edu/uploads/cf/files/2011-may/carroll-changing-characteristics.pdf. Accessed September 2013.

U.S. Department of Labor. 2016. *Findings from the National Agricultural Workers Survey (NAWS) 2013-2014*. Available at: https://www.doleta.gov/agworker/pdf/NAWS_Research_Report_12_Final_508_Compliant.pdf. Accessed March 2017.

U.S. Department of Veteran Affairs. 2012. *Homeless incidence and risk factors for becoming homeless in veterans*. Available at: https://www.va.gov/oig/pubs/VAOIG-11-03428-173.pdf. Accessed March 2017.

U.S. Public Health Service. 2000. *Report of the Surgeon General's Conference on Children's Mental Health: A national action agenda*. Washington, DC: Department of Health and Human Services.

Villarejo, D., et al. 2000. *Suffering in silence: A report on the health of California's agricultural workers*. Davis, CA: California Institute for Rural Studies.

Ward, B. W., and J. S. Schiller. 2013. *Prevalence of multiple chronic conditions among US adults: Estimates from the National Health Interview Survey, 2010*. Available at: http://www.cdc.gov/pcd/issues/2013/12_0203.htm. Accessed September 2013.

Witters, D., and S. Agrawal. 2011. *Unhealthy U.S. workers' absenteeism costs $153 billion*. Available at: http://www.gallup.com/poll/150026/unhealthy-workers-absenteeism-costs-153-billion.aspx. Accessed January 2014.

World Health Organization. 2004. *Antiretroviral drugs for treating pregnant women and preventing HIV infection in infants: Guidelines on care, treatment and support for women living with HIV/AIDS and their children in resource-constrained settings*. Available at: http://www.who.int/hiv/pub/mtct/en/arvdrugsguidelines.pdf. Accessed May 2017.

Yu, S. M., et al. 2004. Health status and health services utilization among US Chinese, Asian

Indian, Filipino, and other Asian/Pacific Islander children. *Pediatrics* 113, no. 1 part 1: 101–107.

Ziller, E. C. 2014. *Access to medical care in rural America*. New York, NY: Springer Publishing.

Ziller, E. C., et al. 2015. *Rural adults delay, forego, and strategize to afford their pre-ACA health care*. Available at: https://muskie.usm. maine.edu/Publications/rural/healthcare-affordability-pre-ACA.pdf. Accessed March 2017.

Zuckerman, S., et al. 2004. Health service access, use, and insurance coverage among American Indians/Alaska Natives and whites: What role does the Indian Health Service play? *American Journal of Public Health* 94, no. 1: 53-59.

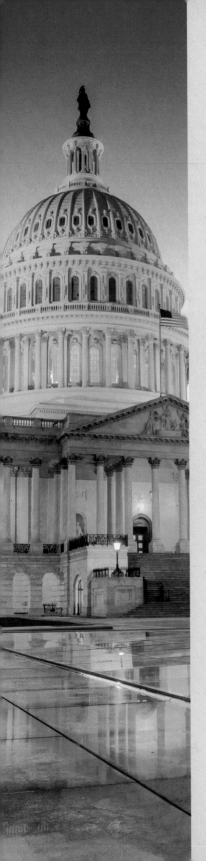

PART IV

System Outcomes

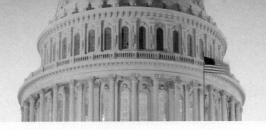

CHAPTER 12

Cost, Access, and Quality

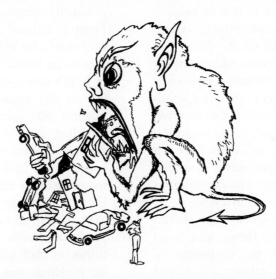

The health care sector of the economy is like a monster with a voracious appetite that needs to be controlled.

▶ Introduction

Cost, access, and quality are three major cornerstones of health care delivery. For many years, employers and third-party payers in the United States have been preoccupied with controlling the growth of health care expenditures. Cost and access go hand in hand; expansion of access will increase health care expenditures. Their intertwined nature is a major reason that attempts to implement universal coverage in the United States have failed in the past and why it remains difficult to achieve this goal even in the post–Affordable Care Act (ACA) era. Although cost and access remain the primary concerns within the U.S. health care delivery system, quality of health care has joined them at center stage in recent years. Cost, access, and quality are interrelated in complex ways.

From a macro perspective, costs of health care are commonly viewed in terms of national health expenditures (NHE). A widely used measure of NHE is the proportion of its gross domestic product (GDP) that a country spends on the delivery of health care services. From a micro perspective, health care expenditures refer to costs incurred by employers to purchase health insurance and out-of-pocket costs incurred by individuals when they receive health care services. Improving access to health care and ensuring equal access to quality health care are contingent on expenditures at both the macro and micro levels.

Sustainable high-quality care should also be cost-effective. Hence, cost is an important factor in the evaluation of quality. In addition, quality is achieved by having up-to-date capabilities, using evidence-based processes, and measuring outcomes. Quality goals are accomplished when the system capabilities and practices employed in the delivery of health care achieve desirable outcomes for individuals and populations.

This chapter discusses the major reasons for the dramatic rise in health care expenditures. Costs are compared with those in other countries, and the impact of cost-containment measures is examined. Dimensions of access are presented. Finally, quality of care and its measurement are discussed.

▶ Cost of Health Care

The term "cost" can carry different meanings in the delivery of health care, depending on whose perspective is considered:

- When consumers and financiers speak of the "cost" of health care, they usually mean the "price" of health care. This could refer to the physician's bill, the price of a prescription, or the cost of health insurance premiums.
- From a national perspective, health care costs refer to how much a nation spends on health care—that is, NHE or health care spending. Since expenditures (E) equal price (P) times quantity (Q), growth in health care spending can be accounted for by growth in prices charged by the providers of health services and by increases in the utilization of services.
- From the perspective of providers, the notion of cost refers to the cost of producing health care services. Such things as staff salaries, capital costs for buildings and equipment, rental of space, and purchase of supplies are included in the cost of production.

Trends in National Health Expenditures

The *Health Services Financing* chapter provided an overview of national and personal health expenditures, their composition, and the proportional share between the private and public sectors. Health care spending spiraled upward at double-digit rates during the 1970s, right after the Medicare and Medicaid programs created a massive growth in access in 1965. By 1970, government expenditures for health care services and supplies had grown by 140%, from $7.9 billion to $18.9 billion (U.S. Department of Health and Human Services [DHHS], 1996). During much of the 1980s, average annual growth in national health spending continued in the double digits, but the rate of increase slowed considerably (**FIGURE 12-1**). In

the 1990s, medical inflation was finally brought under control to a single-digit rate of growth, mainly due to control exerted over payment and utilization through managed care. The rate of growth has again started to accelerate, but at a relatively slow pace (**TABLE 12-1**). In 2010, the United States spent $2.6 trillion on health and health care, which amounts to $8,402 per person (Kaiser Family Foundation, 2012).

Trends in NHE are commonly evaluated in three ways. The first method compares medical inflation to general inflation in the economy, which is measured by annual changes in the consumer price index (CPI). Except for a brief period between 1978 and 1981, when the U.S. economy was experiencing hyperinflation, the rates of change in medical inflation have remained consistently above the rates

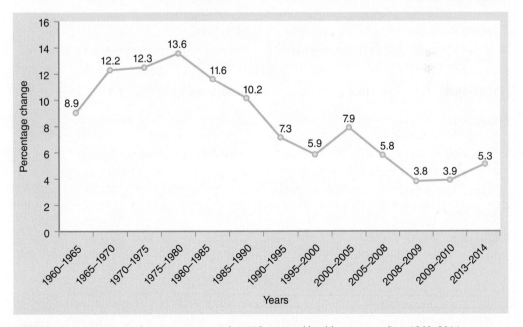

FIGURE 12-1 Average annual percentage growth in U.S. national health care spending, 1960–2014.

Data from Centers for Medicare & Medicaid Services (CMS). 2014. *National health expenditure data.* Available at:https://www.cms.gov/Research-Statistics-Data-and-Systems/Statistics-Trends-and-Reports/NationalHealthExpendData/NationalHealthAccountsHistorical.htm. Accessed February 2017.

TABLE 12-1 Average Annual Percentage Increase in U.S. National Health Care Spending, 1975–2014

Periods	Increase (%)	Periods	Increase (%)
1975–1980	**13.6**	**1990–1995**	**7.3**
1975–1976	14.7	1990–1991	9.2
1976–1977	13.7	1991–1992	9.5
1977–1978	11.9	1992–1993	6.9
1978–1979	12.9	1993–1994	5.1
1979–1980	14.8	1994–1995	4.9
1980–1985	**11.6**	**1995–2000**	**5.9**
1980–1981	16.1	1995–1996	4.6
1981–1982	12.5	1996–1997	4.7
1982–1983	10.0	1997–1998	5.4
1983–1984	9.7	1998–1999	5.7
1984–1985	9.9	1999–2000	6.9
1985–1990	**10.2**	**2000–2005**	**7.9**
1985–1986	7.6	2000–2001	8.7
1986–1987	8.5	2001–2002	9.3
1987–1988	11.9	2002–2003	8.2
1988–1989	11.2	2003–2004	5.9
1989–1990	12.1	2004–2005	6.5

2005–2010	5.0	2010–2014	4.0
2005–2006	6.7	2010–2011	3.9
2006–2007	6.1	2011–2012	3.9
2007–2008	4.7	2012–2013	2.9
2008–2009	3.8	2013–2014	5.3
2009–2010	3.9		

Data from *Health, United States, 1995*, p. 243; *Health, United States, 1996–97*, p. 249; *Health, United States, 1999*, p. 284; *Health, United States, 2000*, p. 322; *Health, United States, 2002*, p. 288; *Health, United States, 2005*, p. 363; *Health, United States, 2006*, p. 377; *Health, United States, 2008*, p. 415; *Health, United States, 2009*, p. 396; *Health, United States, 2011*, p. 374; *Health, United States, 2012*, p. 323; *Health, United States, 2013*, p. 327; *Health, United States, 2015*, p. 293; Levit, K., et al. 2003. Trends in U.S. health care spending, 2001. *Health Affairs* 22, no. 1: 154–164.

of change in the CPI (**FIGURE 12-2**). The second method compares changes in NHE to those in the GDP. With only isolated exceptions, health care spending growth rates have consistently surpassed growth rates in the general economy (**FIGURE 12-3**). When spending on health care grows at a faster rate than GDP, it means that health care consumes a larger share of the total economic output. Put another way, a growing share of total economic resources is devoted to the delivery of health care.

The method is based on international comparisons. Compared to other nations, the United States devotes a larger share of its economic resources to health care (**TABLE 12-2**). In addition, U.S. growth in health care spending has outpaced the growth in health care spending in other countries (**FIGURE 12-4**). Numerous

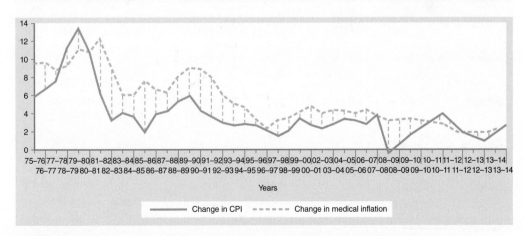

FIGURE 12-2 Annual percentage change in CPI and medical inflation, 1975–2014.

Data from Bureau of Labor Statistics. 2017a. Consumer price index 1975–2014. Available at: https://www.bls.gov/cpi/. Accessed April 2017; Bureau of Labor Statistics. 2017b. Medical care inflation 1975–2014. Available at: https://data.bls.gov/timeseries/CUUR0000SAM?output_view=pct_12mths. Accessed April 2017; *Health, United States, 1995*, p. 241; *Health, United States, 1996–97*, p. 251; *Health, United States, 2002*, p. 289; *Health, United States, 2006*, p. 375; *Health, United States, 2008*, p. 413; *Health, United States, 2009*, p. 394; *Health, United States, 2010*, p. 367; *Health, United States, 2011*, p. 371; *Health, United States, 2012*, p. 321.

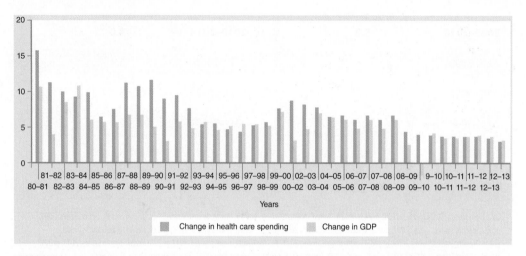

FIGURE 12-3 Annual percentage change in U.S. national health care expenditures and GDP, 1980–2013.

Data from *Health, United States, 1996–97*, p. 249; *Health, United States, 2002*, p. 288; *Health, United States, 2006*, p. 374; *Health, United States, 2008*, p. 412; *Health, United States, 2009*, p. 393; *Health, United States, 2010*, p. 366; *Health, United States, 2011*, p. 370; *Health, United States, 2012*, p. 320, *Health, United States, 2013*, p. 327, *Health, United States, 2015*, p. 293.

TABLE 12-2 Total U.S. Health Care Expenditures as a Proportion of GDP and per Capita Health Care Expenditures (Selected Years, Selected OECD Countries; per Capita Expenditures in U.S. Dollars)

	1990	1995	2000	2005	2009	2014
Australia	7.8%	8.2%	9.0%	8.8%	—	9.0%
	$1,307	$1,745	$2,220	$2,999	—	$4,207
Austria	7.0%	8.0%	7.6%	10.3%	11.0%	10.3%
	$1,338	$1,870	$2,184	$3,507	$4,289	$4,896
Belgium	7.4%	8.4%	8.7%	10.6%	10.9%	10.4%
	$1,345	$1,820	$2,279	$3,385	$3,946	$4,522
Canada	9.0%	9.2%	8.9%	9.9%	11.4%	7.7%
	$1,737	$2,051	$2,503	$3,460	$4,363	$4,496
Denmark	8.5%	8.2%	8.4%	9.5%	11.5%	10.6%
	$1,567	$1,848	$2,382	$3,179	$4,348	$4,857
Finland	7.8%	7.5%	6.7%	8.3%	9.2%	9.5%
	$1,422	$1,433	$1,718	$2,523	$3,226	$3,871
France	8.6%	9.5%	9.3%	11.1%	11.8%	11.1%
	$1,568	$2,033	$2,456	$3,306	$3,978	$4,367

Germany	8.5% $1,748	10.6% $2,276	10.6% $2,761	10.7% $3,251	11.6% $4,218	11.0% $5,119
Italy	7.9% $1,391	7.3% $1,535	8.1% $2,049	8.9% $2,496	9.5% $3,137	9.1% $3,207
Japan	5.9% $1,115	6.8% $1,538	7.6% $1,971	8.2% $2,474	— —	11.4% $4,152
Netherlands	8.0% $1,438	8.4% $1,826	8.3% $2,259	9.5%[1] $3,156[1]	12.0% $4,914	10.9% $5,277
Sweden	8.4% $1,579	8.1% $1,738	8.4% $2,273	9.2% $3,012	10.0% $3,722	11.2% $5,065
United Kingdom	6.0% $986	7.0% $1,374	7.3% $1,833	8.2% $2,580	9.8% $3,487	9.9% $3,971
United States	11.9% $2,738	13.3% $3,654	13.1% $4,539	15.2% $6,347	17.4% $7,960	16.6% $9,024

[1] Data from 2004.

Data from National Center for Health Statistics (NCHS). 2010. *Health, United States, 2009.* Hyattsville, MD: U.S. Department of Health and Human Services. p. 392; National Center for Health Statistics (NCHS). 2012. *Health, United States, 2011.* Hyattsville, MD: U.S. Department of Health and Human Services. p. 369; Organization for Economic Cooperation and Development (OECD). 2016. *Health spending.* Available at: https://data.oecd.org/healthres/health-spending.htm. Accessed April 2017.

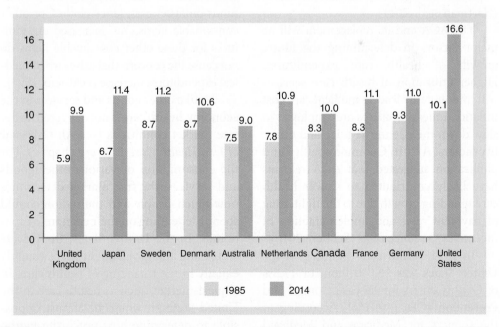

FIGURE 12-4 U.S. health care spending as a percentage of GDP for selected OECD countries, 1985 and 2014.

Data from National Center for Health Statistics (NCHS). 2002. *Health, United States, 2002.* Hyattsville, MD: U.S. Department of Health and Human Services. p. 287; National Center for Health Statistics (NCHS). 2016b. *Health, United States, 2015.* Hyattsville, MD: U.S. Department of Health and Human Services. p. 293; Organization for Economic Cooperation and Development (OECD). 2016. *Health spending.* Available at: https://data.oecd.org/healthres/health-spending.htm. Accessed April 2017.

reasons have been given for the growth of health care expenditures, and several initiatives have been employed over the years to prevent out-of-control spending. These topics are discussed later in this chapter.

The rate of growth in health spending decreased to its lowest level in 4 decades (5.7% average annual growth) between 1993 and 2000 as managed care proliferated, but the good news ended in 2002—a year that recorded the fastest annual growth in NHE (9.3%) since 1992. However, the rate of growth has been slowing down each year (see Table 12-1). In 2009, the rate of growth decreased to 3.9%, a decline largely attributable to the most severe recession the United States had experienced since 1933. As a result of the recession, personal health care expenditures paid mostly by private sources increased just 2.8%, the lowest rate since the 1990s, when managed care implemented tight cost control measures (Hartman et al., 2011).

The ACA and its replacement will be major factors in determining the future growth of health care expenditures. Higher utilization of health care services will undoubtedly lead to medical care cost inflation unless measures are employed to slow down the rise in the price and quantity factors. A 2016 Commonwealth Fund publication suggested that ACA reforms have likely contributed to slower health care spending growth due to the tightening of payment rates and implementation of incentives to reduce costs (Schoen, 2016).

In 2014, health care spending in the United States was $3.0 trillion, or 17.5% of GDP (Centers for Disease Control and Prevention [CDC], 2016a). According to the Centers for Medicare and Medicaid Services (CMS), Office of the Actuary, if present trends continue, health care spending will amount to 19.9% of GDP by 2025.

In 2007, the Congressional Budget Office estimated that health care would consume 37% of GDP by 2050 and 49% by 2082. These forecasts portend that the health care sector will remain one of the fastest-growing components of the U.S. economy.

Should Health Care Costs Be Contained?

Americans view growth in expenditures in other sectors of the economy, such as manufacturing, much more favorably than they do expenditures on medical care. Increased medical expenditures create new health care jobs, do not pollute the air, save rather than destroy lives, and alleviate pain and suffering. Why shouldn't society be pleased that more resources are flowing into a sector that cares for the aged and the sick? It would seem to be a more appropriate use of a society's resources than spending those same funds on faster cars, fancy clothes, or other consumable items. Yet, increased expenditures for these other consumable items do not cause the concern that arises when medical expenditures increase (Feldstein, 1994).

Unlike other goods and services in the economy, health care is not delivered under free market conditions (see *An Overview of U.S. Health Care Delivery* chapter). For the consumption of various other goods and services, the free market determines how much people and the nation should spend, depending on their economic capabilities. In the United States, the private sector and the government share roughly equally in the financing of health care. In a quasi-market, such as health care in the United States, it would be almost impossible to determine how much the nation should spend. Hence, in the United States, we depend on three main sources to assess whether we spend too much:

- The first source, international comparisons (see Table 12-2), is actually not an unbiased tool. In countries other than the United States, the government decides how much should be spent on health care, with various rationing measures—such as supply-side controls, comparatively little spending on developing new technology, and price controls (for pharmaceuticals, for example)—then being used to maintain certain levels of predetermined spending.

- The second source is the rise in health insurance premiums in the private sector. This factor triggered private employers to abandon traditional fee-for-service insurance plans, especially during the 1980s, and to seek employee coverage through health maintenance organization (HMO) plans.

- The third source is government spending on health care for beneficiaries who receive health care through various public insurance programs. Concerns about the short- and long-term sustainability of the Medicare trust funds were discussed in the *Health Services Financing* chapter.

Experts generally agree that the United States spends too much on health care and, therefore, call for expenditures to be controlled. The main reasons are as follows:

- Rising health care costs consume greater portions of the total economic output. Because economic resources are limited, rising health care costs mean that Americans have to forgo other goods and services when more is spent on health care.

- Limited economic resources should be directed to their highest-value uses. In a free market, consumers make purchasing decisions based on their perception of value, knowing that an expenditure on one good means forgoing other goods and services (Feldstein, 1994). In health care delivery, comprehensive health insurance creates moral hazard and provider-induced demand (discussed in *An Overview of U.S. Health Care Delivery* chapter), both of which fuel inefficiencies in the consumption of resources.

- U.S. businesses argue that rising insurance premium costs must be passed on to consumers in the form of higher prices, which may interfere with the ability of businesses to stay globally competitive. For example, health insurance premiums have consistently increased faster than inflation in the general economy or workers' wages in recent years. Between 2006 and 2016, the cumulative growth in health insurance premiums was 58%, whereas cumulative inflation was 19% and cumulative wage growth was 33% (Bureau of Labor Statistics, 2017c, 2017d; Kaiser Family Foundation, 2016).

- Rising premium costs limit the ability of many employers—especially small businesses—to offer health benefits. Even when those benefits are offered, employers may limit the ability of some employees to contribute toward the purchase of employer-sponsored insurance coverage (Kaiser Family Foundation, Health Research and Education Trust, 2010).

- Rising health care costs take a toll on average- and low-income Americans. The 2016 Commonwealth Fund International Health Policy Survey pointed out that affordability of health care was one of the biggest economic problems for many Americans (Commonwealth Fund, 2016). One-third of Americans went without recommended care, did not see a doctor when sick, or failed to fill a prescription because of costs, compared to 7% of survey respondents in the United Kingdom and Germany, and 8% in the Netherlands and Sweden.

- The government has only limited ability to raise people's taxes, given that most American taxpayers believe that they already pay more than their fair share of taxes. Paradoxically, half of Americans, many of whom use tax-financed health care, pay no federal income taxes (*USA Today*, 2010).

▶ Reasons for Cost Escalation

Numerous factors contribute to rising health care expenditures, and they interact in complex ways. Hence, one cannot point to just one or two main causes of this cost escalation. General inflation in the economy is a more visible cause of health care spending because it affects the cost of producing health care services through such factors as higher wages and cost of supplies. Some of the other factors mentioned in this section were also discussed in earlier chapters. They are included here, along with additional pertinent details, to provide a comprehensive picture of the reasons underlying medical cost inflation:

- Third-party payment
- Imperfect market
- Growth of technology
- Increase in the elderly population
- Medical model of health care delivery
- Multipayer system and administrative costs
- Defensive medicine
- Waste and abuse
- Practice variations

Third-Party Payment

Health care is among the few services for which a third party—not the consumer—pays for most services used. Whether payment is made by the government or by a private insurance company, individual out-of-pocket expenses are far lower than the actual cost of the service (Altman and Wallack, 1996). Hence, patients are generally insensitive to the cost of care. Introduction of prospective payment methods and capitation has, to a large extent, minimized provider-induced demand. However, the backlash against managed care (see the *Managed Care and Integrated Organizations* chapter) from consumers and providers alike has, in a sense, kept the door open to the overuse of high-cost technologies and other services. Also, fee-for-service reimbursement and its discounted fee variation are still widely used in the outpatient sector of health care delivery. Hence, provider-induced demand has not been expunged from the system.

Imperfect Market

Prices charged by providers for health care services are likely to be much closer to the cost of producing the services in a highly regulated or highly competitive market (Altman and Wallack, 1996). Because the U.S. health care delivery system follows neither the highly regulated single-payer model nor a free market model, utilization remains largely unchecked; prices charged for health care services remain higher than the true economic costs of production (Altman and Wallack, 1996). A quasi-market results in increased health care expenditures because both the quantity and price factors remain unchecked.

Growth of Technology

The United States has been characterized as following an early start/fast growth pattern in the adoption and diffusion of intensive procedures (TECH Research Network, 2001). Factors that drive technology innovation, diffusion, and utilization and their impact on cost escalation are discussed in the *Medical Technology* chapter. The use of advanced imaging scanning during visits to physician offices and outpatient departments more than tripled from 1996 to 2007 (National Center for Health Statistics [NCHS], 2010). Medicare Part B spending for imaging services under the physician fee schedule more than doubled between 2000 and 2006, from $6.9 billion to $14.1 billion (U.S. Government Accountability Office,

2008). However, following cuts to imaging reimbursements, this growth slowed (American Association of Physicists in Medicine, 2011).

New technology is expensive to develop, and costs incurred in research and development (R&D) are included in total health care expenditures. One reason why Canada and European nations, compared to the United States, have incurred lower health care costs is that they have proportionally invested far less in health care R&D.

Increase in the Elderly Population

Since the early part of the 20th century, life expectancy in the United States has consistently increased (**FIGURE 12-5**). Life expectancy at birth has been extended

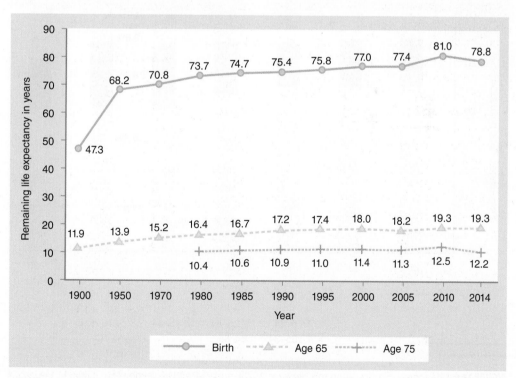

FIGURE 12-5 Life expectancy of Americans at birth, age 65, and age 75, 1900–2014 (selected years).

Data from National Center for Health Statistics (NCHS). 2002. *Health, United States, 2002.* Hyattsville, MD: U.S. Department of Health and Human Services. p. 116; National Center for Health Statistics (NCHS). 2010. *Health, United States, 2009.* Hyattsville, MD: U.S. Department of Health and Human Services. p. 187; National Center for Health Statistics (NCHS). 2016b. *Health, United States, 2015.* Hyattsville, MD: U.S. Department of Health and Human Services. p. 95.

by more than 30 years, from 47.3 years in 1900 to 78.8 years in 2014 (NCHS, 2016b). Consequently, the United States—and other industrialized nations—is experiencing an aging boom. Growth in the U.S. elderly population has outpaced growth in the nonelderly population since 1900. **FIGURE 12-6** shows changes in the demographic makeup of the U.S. population from 1970 to 2014. Most remarkable is the growth in the 85-and-older group, whereas the youngest age group is shrinking (in a relative sense). Growth of the elderly population is projected to continue through the middle of the 21st century. Between 2000 and 2030, the proportion of the U.S. population 65 years and older is

expected to increase from 12.4% to 20%; that is, 1 in 5 Americans will be elderly in 2030. The number in the 85-and-older category is projected to more than double.

Elderly people consume more health care than younger people. In 2012, the average personal health care spending for people 65 and older was $18,988 per person, compared to $3,552 per child and $6,632 per working-age adult (CMS, 2016a). In other words, health care costs for the elderly are 2.6 times more than those for the nonelderly. Given this fact, health care expenditures are sure to rise as the U.S. population continues to age unless drastic steps are taken to curtail spending. Total Medicare expenditures are

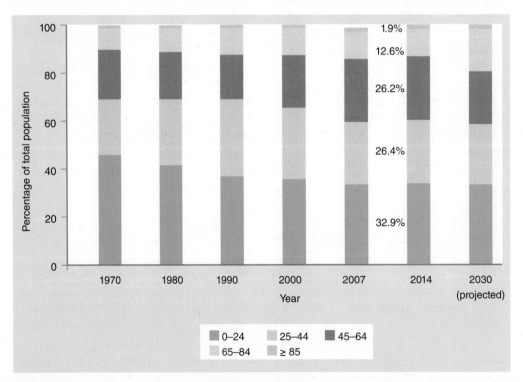

FIGURE 12-6 Change in U.S. population mix between 1970 and 2014, and projections for 2030.

Data from National Center for Health Statistics (NCHS). 2013. *Health, United States, 2012*. Hyattsville, MD: U.S. Department of Health and Human Services. p. 45; U.S. Census Bureau. 2000. *Projections of the total resident population by 5-year age groups, and sex with special age categories: middle series, 2025 to 2045*. Available at: https://www.census.gov/population/projections/files/natproj/summary/np-t3-f.pdf. Accessed April 2017.

projected to increase from 2.7% of GDP in 2005 to 9% of GDP in 2050 (Van de Water and Lavery, 2006).

Medical Model of Health Care Delivery

As discussed in the *Beliefs, Values, and Health* chapter, the medical model emphasizes medical interventions after a person has become sick. It does not put equal emphasis on prevention and lifestyle behavior changes to promote better health. Although health promotion and disease prevention are not the answer to every health problem, these principles have not been accorded their rightful place in the U.S. health care delivery system. Consequently, more costly health care resources must be deployed to treat health problems that could have been prevented. For example, smoking-related illnesses are estimated to cost the United States $75.5 billion annually for direct medical care and an additional $167 billion in lost productivity (CDC, 2005). Evidence suggests that smoking cessation programs have the potential to achieve significant cost savings without imposing an undue cost burden on insurers and employers (Levy, 2006). Although the prevalence of cigarette smoking has been slowly declining, 16.7% of U.S. adult males and 13.6% of U.S. adult women still smoked in 2015 (NCHS, 2016a).

Overweight and obesity rates have shown alarming increases in the United States and in many other developed nations in recent decades. An estimated 70.7% of Americans age 20 and older are overweight, of whom 37.9% are obese (CDC, 2016b). Overweight and obesity substantially elevate a person's risk of developing heart disease, diabetes, some types of cancers, musculoskeletal disorders, and gallbladder problems. Of the total medical spending in the United States, 10% ($147 billion) can be attributed to overweight and obesity, rivaling the spending attributed to smoking (Finkelstein et al., 2009). Both Medicare and Medicaid expend a disproportionate share of their funds to treat overweight- and obesity-related health problems. On average, obese Medicare beneficiaries incur $600 per beneficiary per year in extra costs compared to normal-weight beneficiaries (Finkelstein et al., 2009).

Multipayer System and Administrative Costs

Administrative costs are associated with the management of the financing, insurance, delivery, and payment functions. They include management of the enrollment process, setting up contracts with providers, claims processing, utilization monitoring, denials and appeals of claims, and marketing and promotional expenses.

The enrollment process in private, employer-financed health plans and in publicly financed Medicaid and Medicare programs includes determination of eligibility, enrollment, and disenrollment. Each activity has associated costs. Private insurers also incur marketing costs to promote and sell their plans.

Providers have to deal with numerous plans in which the extent of benefits and reimbursement is not standardized. It is difficult and costly to remain current with the numerous and changing rules and regulations.

Denials of payment result in rebilling and follow-up. Denials of services result in appeals and incur costs for the insurer to review the appeals and for the provider to furnish justifications for the delivery of services. Utilization review and authorization of care incur additional costs for both payers and providers.

According to the CMS (2015), the administrative costs, taxes, profits, and other nonbenefit expenses of private health plans average about 12% of premiums. The ACA requires health plans to standardize electronic data exchange to reduce administrative costs, although it does not provide any specific guidelines on how information must be transferred (Blanchfield et al., 2010). Nevertheless, the ACA addresses only a minute portion of the total administrative costs; hence, its likely effects in reducing these costs will be negligible.

Defensive Medicine

The U.S. health care delivery system is characterized by litigation risks for providers (see *An Overview of U.S. Health Care Delivery* chapter). Fear of legal liability is one of the main reasons for carrying out unnecessary cesarean sections, for example, because it makes it easier to defend a potential birth injury case. Unrestrained malpractice awards by the courts and increased malpractice insurance premiums for physicians significantly add to the cost of health care.

Fraud and Abuse

Fraud and (system) abuse are another type of waste in health care (these concepts were introduced in the *Health Services Financing* chapter). **Fraud**, defined as a knowing disregard of the truth, has been identified as a major problem in the

Medicare and Medicaid programs. Fraud occurs when billing claims or cost reports are intentionally falsified. It may also occur when more services are provided than are medically necessary or when services not provided are billed. **Upcoding** is another fraudulent practice in which a higher-priced service is billed when a lower-priced service is actually delivered. These practices are illegal under the False Claims Act.

Under the anti-kickback statute (Medicare and Medicaid Patient Protection Act of 1987), it is illegal to provide any remuneration to any individual or entity in exchange for a referral for services to be paid by the Medicare or Medicaid program. Knowingly providing such financial inducements amounts to a federal crime, which is punishable by imprisonment. The Stark Laws prohibit physician self-referral for laboratory or other designated health services (see the *Medical Technology* chapter).

Practice Variations

The work of John Wennberg and others brought to the fore a disturbing aspect of physician behavior, which accounts for wide variations in treatment patterns for similar patients. Numerous studies in the United States and abroad have documented notable differences in utilization rates for hospital admissions and surgical procedures among different communities, as well as for the same specialties (Feldstein, 1993). These practice variations are referred to as **small area variations (SAV)** because the differences in practice patterns have been associated with only geographic areas of the country.

For example, in earlier studies, variations in the rate of tonsillectomies in New England counties could not be explained by differences in the demographics or other characteristics of the populations studied (Wennberg and Gittelsohn, 1973). Similarly, the overall inpatient hospital utilization by an aged population in East Boston, Massachusetts, was higher than that by an equivalent population in New Haven, Connecticut (Wennberg et al., 1987). More recent investigations of regional differences in Medicare spending demonstrated that higher rates of inpatient-based care and specialist services were associated with higher costs but not with improved quality of care, health outcomes, access to services, or satisfaction with care (Fisher et al., 2003a, 2003b). This variation, which can be as great as two-fold, cannot be explained by age, gender, race, pricing variations, or health status (Baucus and Fowler, 2002).

A 2016 study found that 40% to 50% of all geographic variations in utilization can be attributed to demand-side factors, including health and preferences, while the remainder may be due to place-specific supply factors (Finkelstein et al., 2016). Such geographic variations signal gross inefficiencies in the U.S. health care delivery system because they increase costs without yielding appreciably better outcomes. They are also unfair because workers and Medicare beneficiaries in low-cost, more-efficient regions subsidize the care of those in high-cost regions (Wennberg, 2002).

SAVs cannot be explained by demand inducement. For example, no incentives exist for physicians to induce demand in Canada or Britain, yet variations similar to those in the United States also exist in those countries. SAVs indicate that patients in some parts of the country are receiving too much treatment, whereas others may be receiving too little. Medical opinions often differ on the appropriateness of clinical interventions because physicians use different criteria for hospital admissions and surgical interventions (Gittelsohn and Powe, 1995).

▶ Cost Containment: Regulatory Approaches

Many attempts to control health care spending have been undertaken in the United States. However, most of these attempts have been met with only limited success, mainly because system-wide cost controls are almost impossible to implement in a quasi-market system. Cost-containment measures in the United States have been piecemeal, affecting only certain targeted sectors of the health care delivery system at a time. For instance, when prices have been regulated, utilization has been left untouched; similarly, when capital expenditures have required preapprovals, operating costs of production have been exempted.

Single-payer systems in other industrialized countries have created national regulatory mechanisms to keep their health care spending in line with their GDPs. Many of these countries enforce **top-down control** over total expenditures. In such a system, the country's government establishes budgets for entire sectors of the health care delivery system. Funds are distributed to providers in accordance with these global budgets, so total spending remains within established budget limits. The downside to this approach is that, under fixed budgets, providers are not as responsive to patient needs and the system provides little incentive to be efficient in the delivery of services. Once budget allocations are used up, providers are forced to cut back services, particularly for illnesses that are not life threatening and that do not represent an emergency.

This top-down approach stands in sharp contrast to the "bottom-up" approach used in the United States, where each provider and managed care organization (MCO) establishes its own fees or premiums (Altman and Wallack, 1996). Competition, created by employers shopping for the best premium rates and by MCOs contracting with providers who agree to favorable fee arrangements, determines what the total expenditures will be. To some extent, the United States also uses regulatory cost control, although it is not as comprehensive as the scheme used in countries with national health care programs.

Cost-control efforts in the United States are characterized by a combination of government regulation and market-based competition. A fragmented approach to cost control allows providers to shift costs (see the *Health Services Financing* chapter), mainly from low payers to higher payers or from one delivery sector to another. For example, when regulatory controls are employed to squeeze costs out of the inpatient sector, providers experience reduced revenues from inpatient services. To make up for the lost revenues, they may increase utilization of outpatient services, if that sector is free of controls. In another scenario, when the government implements cost-control measures, providers may start charging higher prices to private payers. This practice is very common in the nursing home industry, in which reimbursement is restricted under Medicaid rate-setting criteria. In this case, nursing home administrators make a conscious attempt to make up for lost revenues by admitting more private-pay residents and by establishing higher private-pay charges.

Regulatory approaches to cost containment, in the United States and elsewhere, typically control health care supply, prices, and utilization (**EXHIBIT 12-1**). Supply-side controls (health planning) enable policymakers to limit the number of hospital beds and diffusion of costly technology, but regulatory limits on the health care system's capacity inevitably create monopolies on the supply side. To ensure that these artificially created monopolies do not exploit their economic power, health planning is always coupled with stiff price and budgetary controls (Reinhardt, 1994).

Health Planning

Health planning refers to a government undertaking steps to align and distribute health care resources so that—at least in the eyes of government officials—the system will achieve the desired health outcomes for all people. The planning function becomes critical in a centrally controlled national health care program to ensure that the basic health care needs of the population are met and that expenditures are maintained at predetermined levels.

The central planning function does not fit well in a system in which more than

EXHIBIT 12-1 Regulation-Based and Competition-Based Cost-Containment Strategies

	Regulation-Based Cost-Containment Strategies
Supply-side controls	Restrictions on capital expenditures (new construction, renovations, and technology diffusion)
	Example: Certificate of need
	Restrictions on supply of physicians
	Example: Entry barriers for foreign medical graduates
Price controls	Artificially determined prices
	Examples: Reimbursement formulas
	Prospective payment systems
	Diagnosis-related groups
	Resource utilization groups
	Global budgets
Utilization controls	Peer review organizations
	Competition-Based Cost-Containment Strategies
Demand-side incentives	Cost sharing
	Sharing of premium costs
	Deductibles and copayments
Supply-side regulation	Antitrust regulation
Payer-driven competition	Competition among insurers
	Competition among providers
Utilization controls	Managed care

half of health care financing is in private hands and there is no central administrative agency to monitor the system. Instead, the types of health care services, their geographic distribution, access to these services, and the prices charged by providers develop independently of any preformulated plans. Levels of expenditures cannot be predetermined, and such a system is not conducive to achieving broad social objectives. Nevertheless, the United States has tried some forms of health planning on voluntary or mandated bases, although these efforts have met with only limited success.

Health Planning Experiments in the United States

Some of the early efforts to control health care costs in the United States took the form of voluntary health planning, with the goal of minimizing duplication of services. In the 1930s and 1940s, community-wide voluntary organizations, called hospital councils, were established by hospitals in some of the largest cities. Hospitals agreed to share or consolidate services, or they traded the closing of a service in one hospital for the expansion of another service (Williams, 1995). Voluntary planning worked only on a limited basis and only in instances where participating hospitals could gain an advantage through cooperative planning. Consequently, voluntary planning contributed little to increasing the overall efficiency of the health system (Gottlieb, 1974).

The federal government got involved in health planning after the passage of Medicare and Medicaid in the 1960s. Soon after these programs were established, Congress, upon recognizing the increasing dollars the federal government was putting into health care, concluded that it had the right to control escalating costs (Williams, 1995). The comprehensive health planning legislation of the mid-1960s mandated the establishment of local and state health planning agencies. These agencies assessed local health care needs and advocated better coordination and distribution of resources. However, the agencies had little or no actual regulatory power and were largely ineffective (Williams, 1995). When these agencies were evaluated, planned and unplanned areas were found to have the same amount of duplication of facilities and services and their rates of increase in hospital costs were the same (May, 1974).

Certificate-of-Need Statutes

Statutes of **certificate of need (CON)** were state-enacted legislation whose primary purpose was to control capital expenditures by health facilities. The CON process required prior approval from a state government agency for the construction of new facilities, expansion of existing facilities, or acquisition of expensive new technology. Approvals were based on the demonstration of a community need for additional services. Although the CON legislation was justified based on the promise of better planning of resources and greater control over increasing expenditures, its adoption proved easier in states that had greater competition among hospitals (Wendling and Werner, 1980). Essentially, this pattern indicated that hospitals supported CON legislation when it was to their own benefit—that these hospitals did not want additional capital spending on new construction and equipment by their competitors. CON laws did not seem to lower hospital expenditures on a per patient-day basis.

CON statutes also represented a conservative approach to containing rising hospital costs, because they did not address reimbursement and provided no incentives to change utilization behavior in patients or physicians (Feldstein, 1993). In the case of nursing homes, however, CON regulations have been used to contain Medicaid costs. In the face of a growing demand for nursing home beds, CON regulations have restricted the supply of nursing home beds that otherwise would have been utilized. More recently, the Home and Community Based Services (HCBS) waiver program—also referred to as 1915(c) waivers (see the *Long-Term Care* chapter)—has been used to curtail nursing home utilization and costs.

As of 2016, most states have some type of CON program (National Conference of State Legislatures, 2016).

Price Controls

Perhaps the most important effort to control the costs of inpatient hospital care was the conversion of hospital Medicare reimbursement from cost-plus to a prospective payment system (PPS) based on diagnosis-related groups (DRGs) authorized under the Social Security Amendments of 1983 (see the *Health Services Financing* chapter). The DRG-based reimbursement significantly reduced growth in inpatient hospital spending but had little effect on total per capita Medicare cost inflation, because costs were merely shifted from the inpatient to the outpatient sector (**FIGURE 12-7**).

Medicare has implemented other price-control measures through various reimbursement methods that apply to physicians, home health care, and various inpatient service providers. These programs seem to have been successful. For example, before the implementation of the resource-based relative value scale (RBRVS) for physician payments, per capita Medicare spending for physician services had increased at an average annual rate of 11.7% between 1980 and 1990. After the introduction of RBRVS, per capita Medicare spending for physician services increased by only 5% annually between 1995 and 2005, based on data from CMS.

A 2016 MACPAC brief noted that state Medicaid programs can use relative value units and conversion factors established by Medicare, or apply their own conversion factors and update them when appropriate. States have also sought to control their Medicaid expenditures by employing complex formulas that produce arbitrary reimbursement rates and payment ceilings.

Recent proposals have aimed to align Medicare payments with quality of care. In 2003, as part of the Medicare Prescription Drug, Improvement, and Modernization Act, the U.S. Congress asked the Institute of Medicine (IOM) to assess the potential for implementing pay-for-performance (P4P) methods in the Medicare program (IOM, 2004). IOM found mixed evidence regarding the effectiveness of P4P payments, and

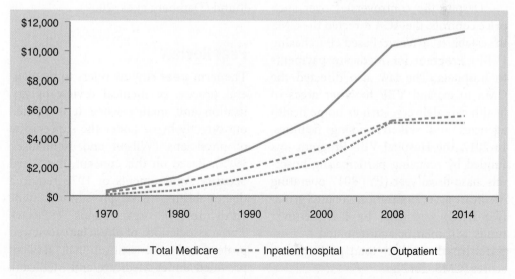

FIGURE 12-7 Increase in U.S. per capita Medicare spending, 1970–2014 (selected years).

Data from National Center for Health Statistics (NCHS). 2016b. *Health, United States, 2015.* Hyattsville, MD: U.S. Department of Health and Human Services. p. 327.

it noted that unintended adverse consequences of P4P could include decreased access to care, increased disparities in care, and impediments to innovation. On the one hand, IOM concluded that careful monitoring of P4P could minimize these adverse consequences. On the other hand, it argued that if Medicare payment structures were left unchanged, they would pose a barrier to improved quality of care.

Research to date does not show that P4P would significantly improve outcomes or control costs (Eijkenaar et al., 2013; Kruse et al., 2012; Ryan, 2009; Shih et al., 2014). In longer term, gains from improvements made in the first few years of implementation tend to fade (Jha et al., 2012; Werner et al., 2011). Also, little evidence supports the contention that hospitals would respond to P4P incentives (Nicholas et al., 2011). To the contrary, if P4P were to result in revenue losses for providers or cost increases for payers, it would have negative repercussions (Kruse et al., 2012).

Despite the controversies over such price controls, the ACA directed the CMS to establish a Value-Based Purchasing (VBP) Program for Medicare payments to hospitals. The law also directed the CMS to expand VBP to other areas of health care delivery, such as home health agencies and skilled nursing facilities. In 2017, the Hospital VBP Program was funded by reducing participating hospitals' base fiscal year (FY) 2017 operating Medicare severity diagnosis-related group (MS-DRG) payments by 2%. Leftover funds will then be redistributed to hospitals based on their total performance scores (CMS, 2017).

The Medicare program is not alone in considering P4P strategies. As of 2012,

19 states had instituted P4P in their Medicaid programs (Hu, 2016). While these programs are in the early stages of development, CMS is offering technical assistance to states for implementing and evaluating P4P. One of the largest efforts is the MassHealth P4P program, implemented in 2008 by the Massachusetts Medicaid Program. Similar to the case for P4P in Medicare, evaluation of this program has so far found only a limited effect on quality improvement (Ryan, 2009). The California Integrated Healthcare Association's (IHA's) statewide P4P program, which has been in operation since 2003, is so far the largest and longest-running private-sector P4P experiment in the United States (James, 2012). However, despite the investment by health care organizations, especially in information technology (IT) adoption and data collection, no "breakthrough quality improvements" have been achieved and no evidence of "any savings or moderation in cost trends" has been found (Damberg et al., 2009).

Peer Review

The term **peer review** refers to the general process of medical review of utilization and quality when it is carried out directly by or under the supervision of physicians (Wilson and Neuhauser, 1985). Based on this concept, the Social Security Amendments of 1972 required the establishment of professional standards review organizations (PSROs). These associations of physicians reviewed professional and institutional services provided under Medicare and Medicaid. The stated purpose of these peer reviews was monitoring and control of both cost and quality. When Congress evaluated the performance of PSROs for their cost-control effectiveness, however, the findings showed that the program had not produced any net savings.

Because of their questionable effectiveness, the PSROs were replaced in 1984 by a new system of peer review organizations (PROs), now called **quality improvement organizations (QIOs)**. QIOs are private organizations composed of practicing physicians and other health care professionals in each state who are paid by the CMS under contract to review the care provided to Medicare beneficiaries. To control utilization, QIOs determine whether care is reasonable, necessary, and provided in the most appropriate setting.

▶ Cost Containment: Competitive Approaches

Competition refers to rivalry among sellers for customers (Dranove, 1993). In health care delivery, it means that providers of health care services try to attract patients who can choose among several different providers. Although competition more commonly refers to price competition, it may also be based on technical quality, amenities, access, or other factors (Dranove, 1993). Because competition is an essential element for the operation of free markets, competitive approaches are also referred to as market-oriented approaches. Competitive strategies fall into four broad categories: demand-side incentives, supply-side regulation, payer-driven price competition, and utilization controls (Exhibit 12-1).

Demand-Side Incentives

The underlying notion of cost sharing is that if consumers pay out of pocket a larger share of the cost of health care services they use, they will consume services more judiciously. In essence, cost sharing encourages consumers to ration their own health care. For example, cost sharing leads people to forgo professional services for minor ailments, but not for serious problems (Wong et al., 2001).

Cost sharing—which is now a common feature of almost all health plans—became popular after the Rand Health Insurance Experiment empirically demonstrated the effects of cost sharing. The most comprehensive study of its type, this experiment ran from 1974 through 1981. It enrolled more than 7,000 people into 1 of 14 different health plans, which included a free plan carrying no deductible or copayments and three other plans with varying degrees of cost sharing. The researchers found that cost sharing resulted in lower costs compared to the free plan. Coinsurance rates of 25% resulted in a 19% decline in expenditures because out-of-pocket costs reduced health care utilization. Increased coinsurance rates resulted in further declines in utilization and expenditures. Another important finding of the Rand Experiment was that lower utilization due to cost sharing did not affect most measures of health status. People enrolled in the free plan did better in three areas—vision, blood pressure, and dental health—but the average appraised mortality risk for people on the free plan was close to the risk for those with cost sharing (Feldstein, 1993).

Supply-Side Regulation

U.S. antitrust laws prohibit business practices that stifle competition among providers. These practices include price fixing, price discrimination, exclusive contracting arrangements, and mergers that the Department of Justice deems anticompetitive. The purpose of antitrust policy is to ensure competitiveness and in turn the efficiency of economic markets. In a competitive environment, MCOs, hospitals, and other health care organizations have to be cost-efficient to survive.

Payer-Driven Price Competition

Generally speaking, consumers drive competition. However, health care markets are imperfect because patients are not typical consumers in the marketplace—insured patients lack the incentive to be good shoppers. Patients also face information barriers that prevent them from being efficient shoppers. Despite the information boom, it is extremely difficult for individual patients or their surrogates to obtain needed information on cost and quality.

Payer-driven competition in the form of managed care has overcome the drawbacks of patient-driven competition (Dranove, 1993). Payer-driven competition occurs at two different points. First, employers shop for the best value, in terms of the cost of premiums and the benefits package (competition among insurers). Second, MCOs shop for the best value from providers of health services (competition among providers).

Utilization Controls

Managed care also helps overcome some of the other inefficiencies of an imperfect health care market. The utilization controls established by managed care (discussed in the *Managed Care and Integrated Organizations* chapter) have cut through some of the unnecessary or inappropriate services provided to consumers. Managed care is designed to intervene in the decisions made by care providers to ensure that they give only appropriate and necessary services and that they provide these services efficiently. MCOs base this intervention on information that is not generally available to consumers. In this way, MCOs act on the consumer's behalf (Dranove, 1993).

▶ Cost Containment Under Health Reform

To keep the costs from spiraling upward in an unsustainable manner, some cost-control measures are essential. The main cost-control measures under the ACA pertain to Medicare payment cuts to providers. Also, it was believed that competition among health plans through the exchanges may control the cost of health insurance premiums. Yet, various mandates imposed on health plans actually increased premium costs. It is not clear whether expansion of the prescription drug benefit under Medicare Part D, by phasing out the coverage gap, is cost neutral. Another major impact on costs comes from the various new taxes imposed under the ACA. The House version of the American Health Care Act, passed in May 2017, however, proposes to repeal most of these taxes. To assess the ACA's future impact on health care costs is difficult, as it is unclear how the government will report health care expenditures. For example, will the government subsidies paid to millions of

Americans to purchase health insurance be fully captured as health care costs? What about the costs associated with the expansion of the Internal Revenue Service necessary to collect the various taxes and penalties specified by the ACA?

Some advocates of the ACA have asserted that this act would control rising health care costs (Kaiser Family Foundation, 2013; Zuckerman and Holahan, 2012). According to the Commonwealth Fund, ACA reforms have contributed to the slowdown in health care spending growth by tightening provider payment rates and providing incentives to reduce costs. Under the ACA, Medicare alone is projected to spend $1 trillion less by 2020 (Schoen, 2016).

▶ Access to Care

Access refers to the ability of a person to obtain health care services when needed. More broadly, access to care is the ability to obtain needed, affordable, convenient, acceptable, and effective personal health services in a timely manner. It may also refer to whether an individual has a usual source of care (such as a primary care physician), indicate the ability to use health care services (based on availability, convenience, referral, or some other criterion), or reflect the acceptability of particular services (according to an individual's preferences and values). Access has several key implications for health and health care delivery:

- Access to medical care is one of the key determinants of health, along with environment, lifestyle, and heredity factors.
- Access is a significant benchmark in assessing the effectiveness of the medical care delivery system. For example,

access can be used to evaluate national trends against specific goals, such as those proposed in *Healthy People 2010* and *2020*.
- Measures of access reflect whether the delivery of health care is equitable.
- Access is linked to quality of care and the efficient use of needed services.

Framework of Access

The conceptualization of access to care can be traced to Andersen (1968) and was later refined by Aday and Andersen (1975) and Aday and colleagues (1980). Andersen (1968) believed that, in addition to need, predisposing and enabling conditions prompt some people to use more medical services than others. Predisposing conditions include an individual's sociodemographic characteristics, such as age, sex, education, marital status, family size, race and ethnicity, and religious preference. These factors indicate a person's propensity to use medical care. For example, holding everything else constant, elderly people are more likely to use medical care than young people. Enabling conditions include income, socioeconomic status, price of medical services, financing of medical services, and occupation. These factors focus on the individual's means, which support that person's ability to use medical care. For example, holding everything else constant, individuals with high incomes are more likely to use medical care than individuals with low incomes, particularly in countries that do not provide national health insurance.

The distinction between predisposing and enabling conditions can be applied to assess the equity of a health care system (Aday et al., 1993). To the extent that significant differences in medical care utilization can be explained by need and certain predisposing characteristics (e.g., age, gender), the delivery of medical care is considered equitable. When enabling characteristics create significant differences in medical care utilization, the delivery of medical care is considered inequitable.

This access to care model has been expanded to include characteristics of health policy and the health care delivery system (Aday et al., 1980). Examples of health policy include major health care financing initiatives (Medicare, Medicaid, and the Children's Health Insurance Program [CHIP]) and organization of health services delivery (Medicaid managed care, community health centers). Characteristics of the health care delivery system include availability (volume and distribution of services) and organization (mechanisms of entry into and movement within the system). Both health policy and the health care delivery system are aggregate components, in contrast to the individual components of predisposing, enabling, and need characteristics. The expanded access to care model recognizes the importance of systemic and structural barriers to access and is useful in comparing access to care among countries with different health policies and health care delivery systems.

Because of managed care's dominance in U.S. health care delivery, the revised version of the access framework was updated by Docteur and colleagues (**FIGURE 12-8**). According to this model, access to care is a two-stage process in a managed care environment. In the first stage, individuals select among the health plans available to them, with those choices being constrained by structural, financial, and personal characteristics. In the second stage, individuals seek medical care, while being constrained by both plan-specific and nonplan factors. The access to care framework accounts for people enrolling and staying with the plan or disenrolling, and it links actual utilization with clinical and policy outcomes. Although comprehensive models are useful in conceptualizing access to care, they are difficult to test because of the range of variables and the differing levels of analysis they require.

Dimensions of Access

Penchansky and Thomas (1981) described access to care as consisting of five dimensions: availability, accessibility, accommodation, affordability, and acceptability. *Availability* refers to the fit between service capacity and individuals' requirements. Availability-related issues include whether primary and preventive services are available to patients; whether enabling services, such as transportation, language, and social services, are made available by the provider; whether the health plan has sufficient specialists to care for patients' needs; and whether access to primary care services is provided 24 hours a day, 7 days a week.

Accessibility refers to the fit between the locations of providers and patients. It is likely that individuals with different enabling conditions (e.g., transportation) may have different perceptions of accessibility. Accessibility-related issues include convenience (Can the provider be reached by public or private transportation?), design (Is the provider site designed for convenient use by disabled or elderly patients?), and payment options (Will the

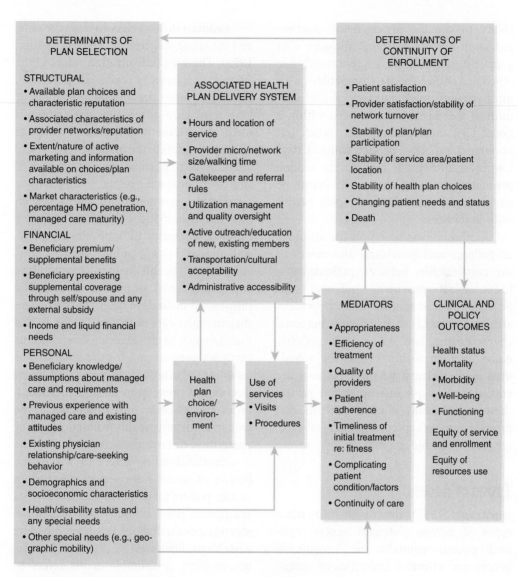

FIGURE 12-8 Framework for access in the managed care context.

Reproduced from Docteur, E. R., et al. 1996. Shifting the paradigm: monitoring access in Medicare managed care. *Health Care Financing Review* 17, no. 4: 5–21.

provider accept patients regardless of payment source [e.g., Medicare, Medicaid]?).

Affordability refers to individuals' ability to pay. Even individuals with insurance often have to consider deductibles and copayments prior to utilization. Affordability-related questions include:

Are insurance premiums too high? Are deductibles and copayments reasonable for the services covered under the plan? Is the cost of prescription drugs affordable?

Accommodation refers to the fit between how resources are organized to provide services and the individual's ability to use the arrangement. Accommodation-related questions include: Can a patient schedule an appointment? Are scheduled office hours compatible with most patients' work and way of life? Can most of the urgent cases be seen within 1 hour? Can most patients with acute, but nonurgent, problems be seen within 1 day? Can most appropriate requests for routine appointments, such as preventive exams, be met within 1 week? Does the plan permit walk-in services?

Acceptability is based on the attitudes of patients and providers, and refers to the compatibility between patients, attitudes about providers' personal and practice characteristics and providers' attitudes toward their clients' personal characteristics and values. Acceptability issues include waiting time for scheduled appointments; whether patients are encouraged to ask questions and review their records; and whether patients and providers are accepted regardless of race, religion, or ethnic origin.

Types of Access

Andersen (1997) described four main types of access: potential access, realized access, equitable or inequitable access, and effective and efficient access. *Potential access* refers to both health care system characteristics and enabling characteristics. Examples of health care system characteristics include capacity (e.g., physician–population ratio), organization (e.g., managed care penetration), and financing mechanisms (e.g., health insurance coverage). Enabling characteristics include personal (e.g., income) and community resources (e.g., public transportation).

Realized access refers to the type, site, and purpose of health services (Aday, 1993). The type of utilization refers to the category of services rendered: physician, dentist, or other practitioners; hospital or long-term care admission; prescriptions; medical equipment; and so on. The site of utilization refers to the place where services are received (e.g., inpatient setting, such as short-stay hospital, mental institution, or nursing home; or ambulatory setting, such as hospital outpatient department, emergency department (ED), physician's office, staff-model HMO, public health clinic, community health center, freestanding emergency center, or patient's home). The purpose of utilization refers to the reason that medical care was sought: for health maintenance in the absence of symptoms (primary prevention), for the diagnosis or treatment of illness to return to well-being (secondary prevention or illness related), or for rehabilitation or maintenance in the case of a chronic health problem (tertiary prevention or custodial care).

Equitable access refers to the distribution of health care services according to the patient's self-perceived need (e.g., symptoms, pain, physical and functional status) or evaluated need as determined by a health professional (e.g., medical history, test results). *Inequitable access* refers to services distributed according to enabling characteristics (e.g., income, insurance status).

Effective and efficient access links realized access to health outcomes (IOM, 1993). For example, does adequate prenatal care lead to successful birth outcomes as measured by birth weight? Is immunization related to reduction of vaccine-preventable childhood diseases, such as diphtheria, measles, mumps, pertussis, polio, rubella, and tetanus? Are preventive services related to the early detection and diagnosis of treatable diseases? The concepts of effectiveness and efficiency link access to quality of care.

Measurement of Access

Using the conceptual models, access can be measured at three different levels: individual, health plan, and delivery system. Access indicators at the individual level include: (1) measures of medical services utilization relative to enabling and predisposing factors, while controlling for need for care (Aday and Andersen, 1975), and (2) the patient's assessment of the interaction with the provider. Examples include differences in physician visits by race/ethnicity, gender, age, income, and insurance. Patients' perceived level of access is closely related to patient satisfaction with care and is part of the access to care framework (Aday et al., 1984).

At the health plan level, there are three types of indicators:

- Plan characteristics that affect enrollment, such as cost of premium, deductibles, copayments, coverage for preventive care, authorization of new and expensive procedures, physician referral incentives, and out-of-plan use
- Plan practices that affect access, such as travel time to a usual source of care and waiting time to see a physician (accessibility); whether an appointment is necessary, hours of operation, language, and other enabling services (accommodation); the content of provider–patient encounters, including tests ordered and done, and referral to specialists (contact)

- Plan quality as measured by the Healthcare Effectiveness Data and Information Set (HEDIS; see the *Managed Care and Integrated Organizations* chapter) and patient satisfaction surveys

Indicators of access at the level of the health care delivery system comprise ecological measures that affect populations rather than individuals. System indicators help researchers study access in an environmental context—that is, how context affects the access of persons and groups. Examples of system access indicators include health policies or programs related to access, physician–population ratio, hospital beds per 1,000 population, percentage of population with insurance coverage, median household income, state per capita spending on welfare and preventive care, and percentage of population without access to primary care physicians.

Population-based surveys supported by federal statistical agencies are the major sources of data for conducting access-to-care analyses. Large national surveys, such as the National Health Interview Survey, the Medical Expenditure Panel Survey (MEPS), and the Community Tracking Survey, are the leading data sources used to monitor access trends and other issues of interest. Other well-known national surveys include the Current Population Survey, the National Hospital Discharge Survey, the Ambulatory Medical Care Survey, the National Nursing Home Survey, and the National Home and Hospice Care Survey. In addition, the federal government periodically collects data on special topics, such as human immunodeficiency virus (HIV)/acquired immunodeficiency syndrome (AIDS); mental health; health care utilization by veterans, military staff, and their dependents; patient satisfaction; and community health centers.

States, professional associations, and research institutions also regularly collect data on health care topics of interest to them. Examples of state-based initiatives include state health services utilization data (all-payer hospital discharge data systems), state managed care data (managed care encounter data), and state Medicaid enrollee satisfaction data (Medicaid enrollee satisfaction surveys). Examples of association-based initiatives include data on physicians (the American Medical Association's Physician Masterfile and the Periodic Survey of Physicians, which was first conducted in 1969 and is still performed today) and hospitals (the American Hospital Association's Annual Survey of Hospitals, which was first conducted in 1946 and continues to be performed today). Examples of research institution-based initiatives include collecting data on the health care delivery system (Center for Evaluative Clinical Sciences: Dartmouth Atlas of Health Care in the United States), women's health (Kaiser Family Foundation: Women's Health Survey), minority health (Commonwealth Fund: Minority Health Survey), family health (Urban Institute: National Survey of America's Families), health insurance (Commonwealth Fund: Biennial Health Insurance Survey), and access to care (Robert Wood Johnson Foundation [RWJF]: National Access Surveys).

Current Status of Access

In the United States, barriers to access still exist at both the individual and the system levels. Many of these barriers are experienced by vulnerable population groups (discussed in the *Health Services for Special Populations* chapter). Access is best predicted by race, income, and occupation. These three factors are interrelated. People belonging to minority groups tend to be poor, not well educated, and more likely to work in jobs that pose greater health risks.

TABLE 12-3 and **TABLE 12-4** summarize physician contacts by categories of age, sex, race, income, and geographic location. **TABLE 12-5** summarizes dental visits. However, these results are not adjusted for health need, so they are not true indicators of access. Rather, they provide utilization measures as a proxy for access.

▶ The Affordable Care Act and Access to Care

Overall insurance coverage and access to health care have increased under the ACA. For example, the proportion of the U.S. population without a regular source of care decreased from 29.8% in 2013 to 26% in 2014 (Karpman et al., 2015). By March 2015, 73.9% of nonelderly adults reported having a usual source of care, an increase of 3.4% from September 2013 (Shartzer et al., 2016). This change was even more pronounced among low-income adults targeted by the Medicaid expansion: The proportion with a usual source of care increased by 5.2 percentage points in this population (Shartzer et al., 2016). There was also a significant decline in the proportion of adults who reported difficulty finding a doctor or other provider in the same time period (Karpman et al., 2015). Fewer people are reporting problems with medical bills and financial barriers to obtaining care (Collins et al., 2015). The ACA is also associated with significantly improved trends in self-reported coverage

TABLE 12-3 Visits to Office-Based Physicians, 2012

Characteristic	Number of Visits (Millions)	Percentage Distribution	Visits per 100 Persons/Year
All visits	928.6	100.0	292
Age			
Younger than 18 years	171.0	18.4	232
18–44 years	234.6	25.3	211
45–64 years	275.3	29.6	335
65–74 years	126.4	13.6	532
85 years and older	121.2	13.1	670

Data from National Center for Health Statistics (NCHS). 2016b. *Health, United States, 2015*. Hyattsville, MD: U.S. Department of Health and Human Services. p. 265.

TABLE 12-4 Number of Health Care Visits According to Selected Patient Characteristics, 2014

Characteristic	None	1–3 Visits	4–9 Visits	≥ 10 Visits
Total	15.3%	50.4%	22.8%	11.5%
Sex				
Male	19.7%	51%	20.1%	9.3%
Female	11.1%	49.9%	25.4%	13.6%
Race				
White	15.2%	49.6%	23.3%	11.9%
Black	14.8%	52.1%	22.8%	10.3%
Income as a Percentage of the Federal Poverty Level				
Below 100%	18.9%	42.5%	22.9%	15.7%

(continues)

TABLE 12-4 Number of Health Care Visits According to Selected Patient Characteristics, 2014 (*continued*)

Characteristic	None	1–3 Visits	4–9 Visits	≥ 10 Visits
100–200%	19.2%	45.9%	22.3%	12.6%
More than 200%	26.9%	99.1%	45.6%	21%
Geographic Region				
Northeast	13.3%	51.6%	23.1%	12.0%
Midwest	13.6%	50.9%	23.3%	12.2%
South	16%	49.7%	23.1%	11.2%
West	17.2%	50.5%	21.4%	110.8%
Location of Residence				
Within metropolitan statistical area	15.3%	51%	22.5%	11.3%
Outside metropolitan statistical area	15.3%	47.2%	24.6%	12.9%

Data from National Center for Health Statistics (NCHS). 2016b. *Health, United States, 2015*. Hyattsville, MD: U.S. Department of Health and Human Services. p. 235.

TABLE 12-5 Dental Visits in the Past Year Among Persons 18–64 Years of Age, 2014

Characteristic	Percentage of Population
All persons	66.6
Income as a Percentage of the Federal Poverty Level	
Below 100%	52.5
100–199%	54.4
200–399%	65.8

400% or more	80.4
Race and Hispanic Origin	
White, non-Hispanic	69.7
Black, non-Hispanic	60.6
Hispanic	59.7
Sex	
Male	64.1
Female	68.9

Data from National Center for Health Statistics. 2016b. *Health, United States, 2015*. Hyattsville, MD: U.S. Department of Health and Human Services. p. 270.

and access to primary care and medications. Compared to pre-ACA trends, the proportions of Americans reporting that they lack a personal physician, lack easy access to medicine, and are unable to afford care have all decreased significantly (Sommers et al., 2015).

Despite the welcome progress made, there are still gaps in access to and affordability of health care, particularly for low-income adults. Moreover, the newly insured face challenges such as changing their care-seeking patterns and behaviors, and some may run into provider capacity issues. More than 25% of nonelderly adults report having no source of usual care; among those who have reported access problems, more than one-third could not find a doctor that would see them, and almost 70% delayed care because they could not get an appointment. These adults were more likely to be younger, male, Hispanic, and low income compared to those persons who had a usual source of care (Shartzer et al., 2016).

The ACA also improved access to certain services for people who already had health insurance coverage. In 2011, 71 million Americans in private insurance plans received expanded coverage of preventive services, such as cancer screenings, flu shots, and cholesterol checks, without cost sharing (Skopec and Sommers, 2013). Under the ACA, preventive services covered without cost sharing have expanded to include more services for women, such as well-women visits, contraception, and breastfeeding comprehensive support and counseling.

▶ Quality of Care

One reason the pursuit of quality in health care has trailed behind the emphasis on cost and access is the difficulty of defining and measuring quality. Since the 1990s, health care cost inflation slowed after several years of rapidly rising when cost intuitive concerns that cost control may negatively impact quality. In spite of the progress made, there is still a long road ahead in deciding what constitutes good quality in medical care, how to ensure it for patients, and how to reward providers and health plans whose outcomes indicate successes in quality improvement. One challenge in achieving this goal is that patients, providers, and payers all define quality differently, which translates into different expectations of the health care delivery system and, in turn, differing evaluations of its quality (McGlynn, 1997).

The IOM has defined **quality** as "the degree to which health services for individuals and populations increase the likelihood of desired health outcomes and are consistent with current professional knowledge" (McGlynn, 1997). This definition has several implications:

- Quality performance occurs on a continuum, theoretically ranging from unacceptable to excellent.
- The focus is on services provided by the health care delivery system, as opposed to individual behaviors.
- Quality may be evaluated from the perspective of individuals and populations or communities.
- The emphasis is on desired health outcomes, and scientific research must identify the services that improve health outcomes.

For example, Blum's model of health and wellness (discussed in the *Beliefs, Values, and Health* chapter) clearly points to a more significant role for numerous factors—other than medical care—in determining health and well-being of individuals and populations. Therefore, more health care expenditures will not necessarily produce better health, and high-quality

care must also be cost-effective. The observation that most medical care is delivered at the flat of the curve (see the *Medical Technology* chapter) clearly points to a greater need to incorporate the cost of care into the assessment of quality.

▶ Dimensions of Quality

Quality needs to be viewed from both micro and macro perspectives. The micro view focuses on services at the point of delivery and their subsequent effects. It is associated with the performance of individual caregivers and health care organizations. The macro view looks at quality from the standpoint of populations. It reflects the performance of the entire health care delivery system by evaluating indicators such as life expectancy, mortality rates, incidence and prevalence of certain health conditions, and so on.

Micro View

The micro dimension of health care quality encompasses the clinical aspects of care delivery, the interpersonal aspects of care delivery, and quality of life.

Clinical Aspects

Clinical aspects of care deal with technical quality, such as the facilities where care is delivered, the qualifications and skills of caregivers, the processes and interventions used, the cost-efficiency of care, and the results or effects on patients' health.

One example of lack of clinical quality is medical errors. According to IOM (2000), 44,000 to 98,000 patients die in U.S. hospitals each year because of medical errors. A 2016 study suggested that medical errors are the third leading cause of death in the United States, behind heart disease and cancer (Makary and Daniel, 2016). The Agency for Healthcare Research and Quality (AHRQ, 2000) has identified four types of medical errors:

- Medication errors, or adverse drug events (ADEs), are errors in prescribing and administering medicines to patients.
- Surgical errors are errors in performing surgical operations.
- Diagnostic inaccuracies may lead to incorrect treatment or unnecessary testing.
- Systemic factors, such as organization of health care delivery and distribution of resources, may contribute to preventable adverse events.

Interpersonal Aspects

When quality is viewed from the patient's perspective, interpersonal aspects of care become essential. Patients lack technical expertise, so they often judge the quality of technical care indirectly based on their perceptions of the practitioner's interest, concern, and demeanor during clinical encounters (Donabedian, 1985). Interpersonal relations and satisfaction become even more important when placed within the holistic context of health care delivery. Positive interactions between patients and practitioners are major contributors to treatment success through greater patient compliance and return for care (Svarstad, 1986). Expressions of love, hope, and compassion can enhance the healing effects of medical treatments.

Interpersonal aspects of quality are also important from the standpoint of organizational management. Consumers— that is, patients and their surrogates—gain lasting impressions of organizational quality from the way they are treated by an organization's employees. Such employee-customer interactions include not just the direct caregivers but a variety of other employees associated with the health care organization, such as receptionists, cafeteria workers, housekeeping employees, and billing clerks.

To measure interpersonal aspects of quality, patient satisfaction surveys have been widely used by various types of health care organizations. Ratings by consumers provide the most appropriate method for evaluating interpersonal quality (McGlynn and Brook, 1996). Satisfaction surveys have been used to give physicians feedback on important dimensions of interpersonal communication and service quality.

Quality of Life

The concept of quality of life has drawn greater attention in recent years because patients with chronic and debilitating diseases are now living longer but in a declining state of health. Chronic problems often impose serious limitations on patients' functional status (physical, social, and mental functioning), access to community resources and opportunities, and sense of well-being (Lehman, 1995).

In a composite sense, during or subsequent to disease, a person's own perception of health, ability to function, role limitations stemming from physical or emotional problems, and personal happiness are referred to as **health-related quality of life (HRQL)**. General HRQL refers to the essential or common components of overall well-being that are more broadly applicable to almost everyone. Disease-specific HRQL focuses entirely on impairments that are caused by a specific disorder and the effects and side effects of treatments for that disorder. For example, arthritis quality of life is concerned with joint pain and mobility and the side effects of anti-inflammatory agents; depression quality of life deals with the symptoms of depression, such as suicidal thoughts, and medication side effects, such as blurred vision, dry mouth, constipation, and impotence (Bergner, 1989); and cancer-specific HRQL may include anxiety about cancer recurrence (Ganz and Litwin, 1996) and pain management.

Institution-related quality of life is another important attribute of quality in addition to the clinical and interpersonal aspects. It refers to a patient's quality of life while confined in an institution as an inpatient. Factors contributing to institutional quality of life can be classified into three main groups: environmental comfort, self-governance, and human factors. Cleanliness, safety, noise levels, odors, lighting, air circulation, environmental temperature, and furnishings are some of the key comfort factors that are particularly relevant to the physical aspects of institutional living. Self-governance means autonomy to make decisions, freedom to air grievances without fear of reprisal, and reasonable accommodation of personal likes and dislikes. Human factors are associated with caregiver attitudes and practices; they include privacy and confidentiality, treatment from staff in a manner that maintains respect and dignity, and freedom from physical and/or emotional abuse.

▶ Quality Assessment and Assurance

The terms "quality assessment" and "quality assurance" are often encountered in literature on health care quality, but are not always well defined or differentiated. **Quality assessment** refers to the measurement of quality against an established standard. It includes the process of defining how quality is to be determined, identification of specific variables or indicators to be measured, collection of appropriate data to make the measurement possible, statistical analysis, and interpretation of the results of the assessment (Williams and Brook, 1978). **Quality assurance** is synonymous with quality improvement. It is the process of institutionalizing quality through ongoing assessment and using the results of assessment for continuous quality improvement (CQI) (Williams and Torrens, 1993). Quality assurance goes a step beyond quality assessment. It is a system-wide or organization-wide commitment to engage in the improvement of quality on an ongoing basis.

Although the two activities of quality assessment and quality assurance are related, quality assurance cannot occur without quality assessment. Quality assessment becomes an integral part of the process of quality assurance. Conversely, it is possible to conduct quality assessment without engaging in quality assurance.

In the past, quality assurance focused on observing deviations from established standards by using inspection techniques, and was used in conjunction with punitive actions for noncompliance. The nursing home industry presents a typical case. Standards of patient care in nursing homes and the system for evaluating performance were developed mainly in conjunction with the certification of facilities for Medicare and Medicaid. Federal regulations developed by CMS are viewed as minimum standards or baseline criteria for defining quality of resident care in certified facilities. Compliance with the standards is monitored through periodic inspections of the facilities, and serious noncompliance is punishable by monetary fines and threats of expulsion from Medicare and Medicaid.

Quality assurance is based on the principles of **total quality management (TQM)**, also referred to as CQI. The philosophy of TQM was developed and used in other industries before it was adapted for health care delivery. The adoption of TQM by many hospitals and health systems has streamlined administration, reduced lengths of stay, improved clinical outcomes, and produced higher levels of patient satisfaction (HCIA Inc. and Deloitte & Touche, 1997).

The Donabedian Model

In his well-known model to help define and measure quality in health care organizations, Donabedian (1985) proposed three domains in which health care quality could be examined: structure, process, and outcomes. These three domains are both closely linked and hierarchical (**FIGURE 12-9**). Structure is the foundation of the quality of health care. Good processes require a good structure; in other words, deficiencies in structure have a negative effect on the processes of health care delivery. Structure and process together influence quality outcomes. Structure primarily influences process and has only a

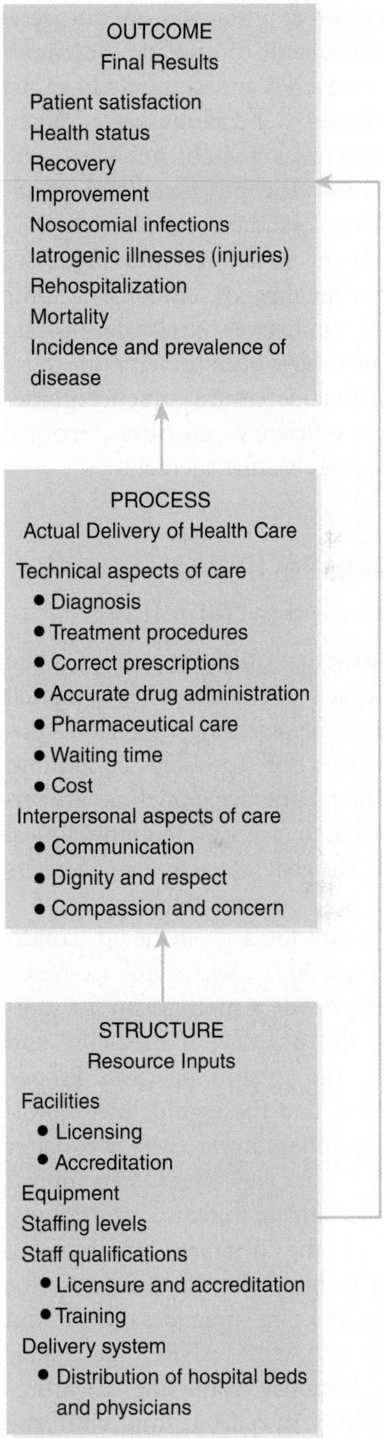

OUTCOME
Final Results

Patient satisfaction
Health status
Recovery
Improvement
Nosocomial infections
Iatrogenic illnesses (injuries)
Rehospitalization
Mortality
Incidence and prevalence of disease

PROCESS
Actual Delivery of Health Care

Technical aspects of care
- Diagnosis
- Treatment procedures
- Correct prescriptions
- Accurate drug administration
- Pharmaceutical care
- Waiting time
- Cost

Interpersonal aspects of care
- Communication
- Dignity and respect
- Compassion and concern

STRUCTURE
Resource Inputs

Facilities
- Licensing
- Accreditation

Equipment
Staffing levels
Staff qualifications
- Licensure and accreditation
- Training

Delivery system
- Distribution of hospital beds and physicians

FIGURE 12-9 The Donabedian model.

secondary direct influence on outcome. For improvement of quality, outcomes must be measured and compared against pre-established benchmarks. When desired outcomes are not achieved, one must examine the processes and structures to identify and correct deficiencies.

Quality of structures and processes determines quality of outcomes. Some significant initiatives toward process improvement have been undertaken; these initiatives include clinical practice guidelines, cost-efficiency measures, critical pathways, and risk management.

Processes That Improve Quality
Clinical Practice Guidelines

Clinical practice guidelines (also called medical practice guidelines) are explicit descriptions representing preferred clinical processes for specified conditions. Hence, clinical practice guidelines are scientifically based protocols to guide clinical decisions. The goal is to assist practitioners in adopting a "best practice" approach in delivering care for a given health condition (Ramsey, 2002). Such evidence-based guidelines provide a mechanism for standardizing the practice of medicine and improving the quality of care. Proponents believe that these guidelines simultaneously promote lower costs and better outcomes. Critics view them as an administrative mechanism to reduce utilization.

One of the primary mandates of AHRQ is to build the scientific base for which health care practices work and which do not work. AHRQ has established a National Guideline Clearinghouse (NGC) in partnership with the American Medical Association (AMA) and America's Health Insurance Plans.

The NGC is a comprehensive database of evidence-based clinical practice guidelines and related documents. It facilitates access to information produced by different organizations by making it all available at one site. This Internet-based resource enables health care professionals to compare clinical recommendations. Guidelines have been catalogued in the areas of diseases; chemicals and drugs; analytical, diagnostic, and therapeutic techniques and equipment; and behavioral disciplines and activities.

Cost-Efficiency

Also referred to as cost-effectiveness, **cost-efficiency** is an important concept in quality assessment. A service is cost-efficient when the benefit received is greater than the cost incurred to provide the service. Medical care delivered at the flat of the curve is not cost-effective (see the *Medical Technology* chapter).

Overutilization (overuse) occurs when the costs or risks of a treatment outweigh its benefits, but additional care is still delivered. When health care is overused, its value is diluted because resources are wasted. Hence, inefficiency can also be regarded as unethical because it deprives someone else of the potential benefits of health care. **Underutilization** (underuse) occurs when the benefits of an intervention outweigh its risks or costs, yet it is not used (Chassin, 1991). Potential adverse health outcomes related to underutilization include hospitalizations that could be avoided by providing better medical access and timely care, low birth weight due to lack of prenatal care, infant mortality due to lack of early pediatric care, and low cancer survival rates due to lack of early detection and treatment.

The principles of cost-efficiency indicate that health care costs can be reduced without lowering quality of care. Conversely, quality can be improved without increasing costs. A trade-off does not have to occur between cost and quality. Introduction of PPS by Medicare is an example. The resulting discharge of patients "quicker and sicker" triggered by PPS initially raised some alarm concerning decreased quality, but it was found that processes of care in hospitals actually improved and mortality rates were unchanged or lower (Rogers et al., 1990). Other potential negative health outcomes that can be avoided by curtailing overuse include life-threatening drug interactions, nosocomial infections, and iatrogenic illnesses.

Critical Pathways

Critical pathways are outcome-based and patient-centered case management tools that are interdisciplinary in nature, facilitating coordination of care among multiple clinical departments and caregivers. Such a timeline identifies planned medical interventions, along with expected patient outcomes, for a specific diagnosis or class of cases, often defined by a DRG. The outcomes and interventions included in the critical pathway are broadly defined. In addition to technical outcomes, pathways may measure such factors as patient satisfaction, self-reported health status, mental health, and activities of daily living (ADLs). Interventions include treatments, medications, diagnostic tests, diet, activity regimens, consultations, discharge planning, and patient education. A critical pathway serves as a plan of action for all disciplines caring for a patient and incorporates a system for documenting and evaluating variances from the critical path plan.

Critical pathways are unique to the institutions that develop them because they are based on the particular practices of that facility and its caregivers. A pathway also is customized to the patient population being served and the available patient care resources.

Critical pathways are meant to promote interdisciplinary collaboration with in the environment of the hospital and its market. The latter occurs by making patients and families active participants in the process. For these reasons, critical pathways are difficult to replicate from one organization to another. Use of critical pathways reduces costs and improves quality by reducing errors, improving coordination among interdisciplinary players, streamlining case management functions, providing systematic data with which to assess care, and reducing variations in practice patterns (Giffin and Giffin, 1994).

Risk Management

Risk management consists of proactive efforts to prevent adverse events related to clinical care and facilities operations and is especially focused on avoiding medical malpractice (Orlikoff, 1988). In response to the threat of lawsuits, initiatives undertaken by a health care organization to review clinical processes and establish protocols for the specific purpose of reducing malpractice litigation can actually enhance quality. Because malpractice concerns also result in **defensive medicine**, risk management approaches should employ the principles of cost-efficiency along with standardized practice guidelines and critical pathways.

Perhaps not surprisingly, the threat of malpractice litigation also has a downside. Fear of litigation actually leads to a reluctance by hospitals and physicians to disclose preventable harm and actual medical errors. In this respect, it is believed that fear of litigation may actually conceal problems that may compromise patient safety (Lamb et al., 2003).

▶ Public Reporting of Quality

Public reporting on macro levels of quality expanded in the early 2000s. This section summarizes the major public reporting initiatives.

CMS Programs on Quality

CMS started launching quality initiatives in 2001 (CMS, 2013a). Quality programs specific to Medicare include the Home Health Quality Initiative, Hospital VBP Program, Hospice Quality Reporting Program, Inpatient Rehabilitation Facilities Quality Reporting, Long-Term Care Hospitals Quality Reporting, Measures Management System, Nursing Home Quality Initiative, Outcome and Assessment Information Set (OASIS), Physician Compare Initiative, End-Stage Renal Disease (ESRD) Quality Incentive Program, and Post-Acute Care Quality Initiatives (http://www.cms.gov/Medicare/Medicare .html). CMS also has initiatives to improve the quality of care provided to Medicaid and CHIP enrollees related to early periodic screening, diagnosis, and treatment (EPSDT); dental care; obesity; maternal and infant health; home and community-based services; vaccines;

prevention; health disparities; performance measurement; patient safety; external quality review; state quality strategies; and improving care transitions (http:// www.medicaid.gov/Medicaid-CHIP -Program-Information/By-Topics/Quality -of-Care/Quality-of-Care.html).

The following are examples of CMS's efforts to enhance quality:

- CMS developed a large public reporting program known as Hospital Compare, which provides information about the quality of care at more than 4,000 Medicare-certified hospitals across the United States (https://www .medicare.gov/hospitalcompare). Hospital Compare has expanded beyond the 10 process measures available at the beginning of this program and now includes data on structural measures, ED throughput, compliance, and hospital outpatient facilities; hospital 30-day risk standardized mortality and readmission rates for acute myocardial infarction, heart failure, and pneumonia; patient experience and satisfaction; medical imaging usage (Medicare.gov, 2016; Ross et al., 2010); and data on the Hospital VBP Program under the ACA (CMS, 2013b).
- CMS and AHRQ jointly developed the Hospital Consumer Assessment of Healthcare Providers and Systems (CAHPS) survey, which collects uniform measures of patients' perspectives on various aspects of their inpatient care (CMS, 2005). Results are publicly reported on the CMS Hospital Compare website. Health care organizations, public and private purchasers, consumers, and researchers can use the CAHPS results to inform their

purchasing or contracting decisions and to improve the quality of health care services (AHRQ, 2010). CAHPS surveys ask about experiences with health plans, clinicians, and specific facilities, including hospitals and nursing homes (https://www.ahrq.gov /cahps).

- The Physician Quality Reporting System allows physicians and other eligible professions to participate by reporting quality measures to CMS about specific services provided to their Medicare patients with specific conditions (http:// www.cms.gov/PQRS). Physicians can earn incentives by reporting. In 2015, the program began applying negative payment adjustment to individuals and practices who did not adequately report data.

- Quality improvement organizations (QIOs) are contracted by CMS for each state to review medical care and help beneficiaries with concerns about quality of care. QIO contracts are 3 years in length. The core functions of the QIO program are to improve quality of care for beneficiaries, protect the integrity of the Medicare Trust Fund, and protect beneficiaries by addressing individual complaints (CMS, 2013a).The two types of QIOs that work under the direction of CMS in support of the QIO program are beneficiary and family-centered care QIOs, which focus on helping Medicare beneficiaries exercise their right to high-quality health care, and quality innovation network QIOs, which bring beneficiaries, providers, and communities together in initiatives to increase patient safety and health (CMS, 2016b).

- Ambulatory Surgical Center Quality Reporting is a pay-for-reporting, quality-data program, in which ambulatory care centers report quality of care for standardized measures to receive the full annual update to their annual payment rates (CMS, 2013b). Measures included in payment determination are patient burns, patient falls, hospital transfers/admissions, and incidents involving the wrong site, wrong side, wrong patient, wrong procedure, or wrong implant (CMS, 2016c).

AHRQ Quality Indicators

Since 2003, AHRQ has published the annual National Healthcare Quality Report and National Healthcare Disparities Report (AHRQ, 2012, 2013a). In identifying key measures for these reports, the Federal Interagency Workgroup focused on priority areas established in *Healthy People 2010* (AHRQ, 2005). AHRQ has developed a set of quality indicators (QIs) that measure the quality of the process of care in an outpatient or inpatient setting (Farquhar, 2008). Prevention QIs identify hospital admissions that could have been avoided. Inpatient QIs and patient safety indicators both reflect quality of care inside hospitals, with the former focusing on inpatient mortality and the latter on potentially avoidable complications and iatrogenic events. Pediatric quality indicators reflect quality of care received by children inside hospitals and identify potentially avoidable hospitalizations.

Current AHRQ QI modules include Prevention Quality Indicators, Inpatient Quality Indicators, Patient Safety Indicators, and Pediatric Quality Indicators. These measures expand upon Healthcare

Cost and Utilization Project (HCUP) QIs, and several are endorsed by the National Quality Forum (NQF). Specific information on individual quality indicators within each module can be found at http://www.qualityindicators.ahrq.gov/. Select indicators are also used by CMS's Hospital Compare website (https://www .medicare.gov/hospitalcompare/search .html; AHRQ, 2013b; NQF, 2013).

An example of an ongoing AHRQ quality initiative is the AHRQ's Patient Safety Network (PSNet). PSNet is a Web-based resource that features news and resources on patient safety. The site offers updates on literature, news, tools, and meetings, and it provides browsing capability and site customization (https://psnet.ahrq.gov).

States' Public Reporting of Hospital Quality

Many states also provide data on hospital outcomes of care, typically focusing on acquired infections, readmission rates, and mortality rates following hospitalization for the same clinical conditions reported by CMS (acute myocardial infarction, heart failure, and pneumonia). One of the advantages of state-based public reporting programs is that their reporting is not limited to Medicare fee-for-service beneficiaries, but also includes younger adults and older adults insured through private plans and Medicaid-affiliated HMOs.

▶ The Affordable Care Act and Quality of Care

The ACA includes some provisions for improving quality of care, through programs that link payment to quality

outcomes in Medicare, strengthening of the quality infrastructure, and encouraging the development of new patient care models, such as patient-centered medical homes (see the *Outpatient and Primary Care Services* chapter) and accountable care organizations (see the *Managed Care and Integrated Organizations* chapter).

The ACA initiated the National Quality Strategy (NQS) to set national goals to improve the quality of health care. To date, three objectives have been established: (1) to make health care more accessible, safe, and patient centered; (2) to address environmental, social, and behavioral influences on health and health care; and (3) to make care more affordable (RWJF, 2013).

New payment models in the ACA, such as accountable care organizations (ACOs), use a value-based model in which health care organizations are reimbursed based on quality measures. ACOs are intended to promote integration and coordination of care for patients over the spectrum of health care services, such as ambulatory, inpatient, and postacute services. The value-based payment model is designed to ensure that patients receive high-quality care by evaluating organizations on numerous quality measures related to patient safety, care coordination, and patient/caregiver experience while generating financial savings (CMS, 2016d). Organizations are incentivized to provide high-quality care in two ways: (1) by being penalized for failing to report these quality measures and (2) by sharing in the savings generated due to the implementation of these quality measures.

In addition to ACOs, a number of value-based payment models are being explored, including pay-for-performance report cards for physicians, bundled payments for care improvement, numerous state innovation models, and initiatives to transform primary care (CMS, 2015). Most of these value-based models are still in their early phases, and evidence of their effectiveness and impact has not yet been published.

Through efforts to improve the quality of care, the number of patient safety and medical errors has decreased since 2010. Incidents involving patient harm fell by 17% from 2010 to 2013, which translates to approximately 50,000 fewer people dying as a result of preventable errors and infections (AHRQ, 2014). The decline in hospital-acquired conditions is estimated to have prevented more than 87,000 deaths from 2010 to 2014 (AHRQ, 2015). The rate of hospital readmissions among Medicare beneficiaries has also declined, from a mean of 19.1% in 2010 to a mean of 17.8% during 2015, resulting in 565,000 fewer readmissions (Zuckerman et al., 2016).

Moreover, self-reports of timely access to care and primary physicians' being informed about specialty care have significantly improved since ACO contracts came into being. Patients with chronic conditions and high predicted spending have also reported significantly improved ratings of physicians, interactions with physicians, and overall care (McWilliams et al., 2014).

The Patient-Centered Outcomes Research Institute (PCORI) was established through funding provided by the ACA. This institute is responsible for comparative effectiveness research, which studies health outcomes, clinical effectiveness, and the appropriateness of different medical treatments (Frank et al., 2014).

PCORI's main mission is to improve the quality and relevance of evidence available to help patients, caregivers, clinicians, employers, and insurers make informed health decisions. The goal is to improve health care outcomes by providing patients with high-quality evidence they can use to make informed health care decisions.

Evidence of the ACA's overall impact on health outcomes is limited, but its effects may be similar to those of other health care provisions that have provided health insurance to a previously uninsured group. In the past, Medicaid expansions have increased self-reported overall physical and mental health and reduced mortality (Baicker et al., 2013; Sommers et al., 2012). Young adults covered under the ACA have an increased probability of self-reporting excellent physical and mental health (Barbaresco et al., 2015).

Although the ACA has led to a number of innovative performance-based delivery systems intended to improve the quality of care, a fair amount of work still needs to be done to fully understand how to best design and implement value-based payment programs (Damberg et al., 2014). Moreover, it is still too early to draw definite conclusions about the quality effects of the ACA. Although the preliminary data are promising, showing reductions in hospital-acquired conditions and Medicare readmissions, the causes of these trends need further investigation. More evidence and time are needed to fully assess the ACA's impact on quality of care.

▶ Summary

Increasing costs, lack of access, and concerns about quality pose the greatest challenges to health care delivery in the United States. To some extent, these three issues are interrelated. Increasing costs limit the system's ability to expand access. A lack of universal coverage negatively affects the health status of uninsured groups. Despite spending the most resources on health care, the United States continues to rank in the bottom quartile among developed countries on outcome indicators such as life expectancy and infant mortality.

Nations that have national health insurance can control system-wide costs through top-down controls, mainly in the form of global budgets. This approach is not possible in the United States, which has a multipayer system. In the United States, regulatory approaches have been used to try to constrain the supply side, but the major emphasis has been on limiting reimbursement to providers. Several competitive approaches have been used, mainly through the expansion of managed care. A move toward prospective payments and the growth of managed care can be largely credited with the brakes put on rising health care spending during the 1990s.

Access to medical care is one of the key determinants of health status, along with environment, lifestyle, and hereditary factors. Access is also regarded as a significant benchmark in assessing the effectiveness of the medical care delivery system. Access is explained in terms of enabling and predisposing factors, as well as factors related to health policy and health care delivery. It has five dimensions: availability, accessibility, accommodation, affordability, and acceptability. Measures of access can relate to individuals, health care plans, and the health care delivery system.

Quality in health care has been difficult to define and measure, although it has received increasing emphasis in recent years. At the micro level, health care quality encompasses the clinical aspects of care delivery, the interpersonal aspects of care delivery, and quality of life. Indicators of quality at the macro level are commonly associated with life expectancy, mortality, and morbidity. Quality assessment is the measurement of quality against an established standard, whereas quality assurance emphasizes improvement of quality using the principles of continual quality improvement. Donabedian proposed that quality should be assessed along three dimensions: structure, process, and outcomes. These three dimensions are complementary and should be used collectively to monitor quality of care. Reliability and validity are important concepts in the measurement of quality. Since 2000, several federal and state initiatives have been implemented to report on certain macro levels of quality.

▶ Test Your Understanding

Terminology

access	cost-efficiency	health-related quality
administrative costs	critical pathways	of life (HRQL)
certificate of need	defensive medicine	institution-related quality
clinical practice guidelines	fraud	of life
competition	health planning	outcomes

overutilization
peer review
quality
quality assessment
quality assurance

quality improvement
   organization (QIO)
risk management
small area variations (SAV)
top-down control

total quality
   management (TQM)
underutilization
upcoding

Review Questions

1. What is meant by the term "health care costs"? Describe the three meanings of the term "cost."

2. Why should the United States control the rising costs of health care?

3. How do the findings from the Rand Health Insurance Experiment reinforce the relationship between growth in third-party reimbursement and increase in health care costs? Explain.

4. Explain how, under imperfect market conditions, both prices and quantity of health care are higher than they would be in a highly competitive market.

5. What are some of the reasons for increased health care costs that are attributed to the providers of medical care?

6. What are some of the main differences between the broad cost-containment approaches used in the United States and those used in countries with national health insurance?

7. Discuss the effectiveness of CON regulation in controlling health care expenditures.

8. Discuss price controls and their effectiveness in controlling health care expenditures.

9. Discuss the role of quality improvement organizations in cost containment.

10. What are the four competition-based cost-containment strategies?

11. What are the implications of access for health and health care delivery?

12. What is the role of enabling and predisposing factors in access to care?

13. Briefly describe the five dimensions of access.

14. What are the four main types of access described by Andersen?

15. Describe the measurement of access to care at the individual, health plan, and delivery system levels.

16. What are some of the implications of the definition of quality proposed by the Institute of Medicine? In which way is the definition incomplete?

17. Discuss the dimensions of quality from the micro and macro perspectives.

18. Discuss the two types of health-related quality of life.

19. Distinguish between quality assessment and quality assurance.

20. What are the basic principles of total quality management (continual quality improvement)?

21. Give a brief description of the Donabedian model of quality.

22. Discuss the main developments in process improvement that have occurred in recent years.

23. Discuss the implications of the ACA for health care access, cost, and quality.

▶ References

Aday, L. A. 1993. Indicators and predictors of health services utilization. In: *Introduction to health services*. 4th ed. S. J. Williams and P. R. Torrens, eds. Albany, NY: Delmar Publishers. pp. 46–70.

Aday, L. A., and R. Andersen. 1975. *Development of indices of access to medical care*. Ann Arbor, MI: Health Administration Press.

Aday, L. A., et al. 1980. *Health care in the US: Equitable for whom?* Newbury Park, CA: Sage.

Aday, L. A., et al. 1984. *Access to medical care in the US: Who has it, who doesn't?* Research Series No. 32. Chicago, IL: Center for Health Administration Studies, University of Chicago, Pluribus Press.

Aday, L. A., et al. 1993. *Evaluating the medical care system: Effectiveness, efficiency, and equity*. Ann Arbor, MI: Health Administration Press.

Agency for Healthcare Research and Quality (AHRQ). April 2000. *Reducing errors in health care: Translating research into practice*. AHRQ Publication No. 00-PO58. Available at: https://archive.ahrq.gov/qual/errors.htm. Accessed May 2017.

Agency for Healthcare Research and Quality (AHRQ). 2005. *National healthcare quality report: Background on the measures development process*. Available at: https://archive.ahrq.gov/research/findings/nhqrdr/nhqr02/nhqrprelim.html. Accessed May 2017.

Agency for Healthcare Research and Quality (AHRQ). 2010. *Consumer Assessment of Health—care Providers and Systems (CAHPS)*. Available at: http://www.cahps.ahrq.gov. Accessed January 2011.

Agency for Healthcare Research and Quality (AHRQ). 2012. *Annual progress report to Congress: National strategy for quality improvement in health care*. Available at: from http://www.ahrq.gov/workingforquality/nqs/nqs2012annlrpt.pdf. Accessed January 2014.

Agency for Healthcare Research and Quality (AHRQ). 2013a. *National healthcare quality & disparities reports*. Available at: http://www.ahrq.gov/research/findings/nhqrdr/index.html. Accessed September 2013.

Agency for Healthcare Research and Quality (AHRQ). 2013b. *AHRQ quality indicators*. Available at: http://www.qualityindicators.ahrq.gov/. Accessed January 2014.

Agency for Healthcare Research and Quality (AHRQ). 2014. *Interim update on 2013 annual hospital-acquired condition rate and estimates of cost savings and deaths averted from 2010 to 2013*. Available at: https://www.ahrq.gov/sites/default/files/wysiwyg/professionals/quality-patient-safety/pfp/interimhacrate2013.pdf. Accessed February 2017.

Agency for Healthcare Research and Quality (AHRQ). 2015. *Saving lives and saving money: Hospital-acquired conditions update*. Available at https://www.ahrq.gov/professionals/quality-patient-safety/pfp/interimhacrate2014.html. Accessed February 2017.

Altman, S. H., and S. S. Wallack. 1996. Health care spending: Can the United States control it? In: *Strategic choices for a changing health care system*. S. Altman and U. Reinhardt, eds. Chicago, IL: Health Administration Press.

American Association of Physicists in Medicine. 2011. *MedPAC verifies drop in imaging spending, utilization*. Available at: http://www.aapm.org/pubs/enews/documents/MedPACverifies.pdf. Accessed February 2017.

Andersen, R. 1968. *A behavioral model of families' use of health services*. Research Series No. 25. Chicago, IL: Center for Health Administration Studies, University of Chicago.

Andersen, R. 1997. *Too big, too small, too flat, too tall: Search for "just right" measures of access in the age of managed care*. Chicago, IL: Paper presented at the Association for Health Services Research Annual Meeting.

Baicker, K., et al. 2013. The Oregon experiment: Effects of Medicaid on clinical outcomes. *New England Journal of Medicine* 368, no. 18: 1713–1722.

Barbaresco, S., et al. 2015. Impacts of the Affordable Care Act dependent coverage provision on health-related outcomes of young adults. *Journal of Health Economics* 40: 54–68.

Baucus, M., and E. J. Fowler. 2002. Geographic variation in Medicare spending and the real focus of Medicare reform. *Health Affairs* (Suppl Web Exclusives): W115–W117.

Bergner, M. 1989. Quality of life, health status, and clinical research. *Medical Care* 27, no. 3 (Suppl): S148–S156.

Blanchfield, B. B., et al. 2010. Saving billions of dollars and physicians' time by streamlining billing practices. *Health Affairs*, 29, no. 6: 1248–1254.

Bureau of Labor Statistics. 2017a. *Consumer price index 1975–2014.* Available at: https://www.bls.gov/cpi/. Accessed April 2017.

Bureau of Labor Statistics. 2017b. *Medical care inflation 1975–2014.* Available at: https://data.bls.gov/timeseries/CUUR0000SAM?output_view=pct_12mths. Accessed April 2017.

Bureau of Labor Statistics. 2017c. *CPI inflation calculator.* Available at: https://www.bls.gov/data/inflation_calculator.htm. Accessed February 2017.

Bureau of Labor Statistics. 2017d. *Employment, hours, and earnings from the Current Employment Statistics survey.* Available at: https:// www.bls.gov/ces/. Accessed May 2017.

Centers for Disease Control and Prevention (CDC). 2005. Annual smoking-attributable mortality, years of potential life lost, and productivity losses—United States, 1997–2001. *Morbidity and Mortality Weekly Report* 54, no. 25: 625–628.

Centers for Disease Control and Prevention (CDC). 2016a. *Health expenditures.* Available at: https://www.cdc.gov/nchs/fastats/health-expenditures.htm. Accessed February 2017.

Centers for Disease Control and Prevention (CDC). 2016b. *Obesity and overweight.* Available at: https://www.cdc.gov/nchs/fastats/obesity-overweight.htm. Accessed February 2017.

Centers for Medicare and Medicaid Services (CMS). 2005. *Costs and benefits of HCAHPS.* Available at: http://www.cms.gov/HospitalQualityInits/downloads/HCAHPSCostsBenefits200512.pdf. Accessed January 2011.

Centers for Medicare and Medicaid Services (CMS). 2013a. *Quality improvement organizations.* Available at: https://www.cms.gov/medicare/quality-initiatives-patient-assessment-instruments/qualityimprovementorgs/index.html. Accessed January 2014.

Centers for Medicare and Medicaid Services (CMS). 2013b. *ASC quality reporting.* Available at: https://www.cms.gov/Medicare/Quality-Initiatives-Patient-Assessment-Instruments/ASC-Quality-Reporting/. Accessed January 2014.

Centers for Medicare & Medicaid Services (CMS). 2014. *National health expenditure data.* Available at: https://www.cms.gov/Research-Statistics-Data-and-Systems/Statistics-Trends-and-Reports/NationalHealthExpendData/NationalHealthAccountsHistorical.htm. Accessed February 2017.

Centers for Medicare and Medicaid Services (CMS). 2015. *Better care, smarter spending, healthier people: Improving our health care delivery system.* Available at: https://www.cms.gov/Newsroom/MediaReleaseDatabase/Fact-sheets/2015-Fact-sheets-items/2015-01-26.html. Accessed February 2017.

Centers for Medicare and Medicaid Services (CMS). 2016a. *NHE fact sheet.* Available at: https://www.cms.gov/research-statistics-data-and-systems/statistics-trends-and-reports/nationalhealthexpenddata/nhe-fact-sheet.html. Accessed February 2017.

Centers for Medicare and Medicaid Services (CMS). 2016b. *Quality improvement organizations.* Available at: https://www.cms.gov/Medicare/Quality-Initiatives-Patient-Assessment-Instruments/QualityImprovementOrgs/index.html?redirect=/QualityImprovementOrgs/. Accessed February 2017.

Centers for Medicare and Medicaid Services (CMS). 2016c. *ASC quality reporting.* Available at: https://www.cms.gov/Medicare/Quality-Initiatives-Patient-Assessment-Instruments/ASC-Quality-Reporting/. Accessed February 2017.

Centers for Medicare and Medicaid Services (CMS). 2016d. *Improving quality of care for Medicare patients: Accountable care organizations.* Medicare Learning Network. Available at: https://www.cms.gov/medicare/medicare-fee-for-service-payment/sharedsavingsprogram/downloads/aco_quality_factsheet_icn907407.pdf. Accessed February 2017.

Centers for Medicare and Medicaid Services (CMS). 2017. *Hospital value-based purchasing.* Available at: https://www.cms.gov/Medicare/Quality-Initiatives-Patient-Assessment-Instruments/hospital-value-based-purchasing/index.html?redirect=/hospital-value-based-purchasing/. Accessed February 2017.

Chassin, M. R. 1991. Quality of care: Time to act. *Journal of the American Medical Association* 266, no. 24: 3472–3473.

Collins, S. R., et al. 2015. The rise in health care coverage and affordability since health reform took effect. New York, NY: Commonwealth Fund.

Commonwealth Fund. 2016. *2016 Commonwealth Fund International Health Policy Survey of Adults.* Available at: http://www.commonwealthfund .org/interactives-and-data/surveys /international-health-policy-surveys/2016/2016 -international-survey. Accessed February 2017.

Congressional Budget Office. November 2007. *The long-term outlook for health care spending.* Available at: http://www.cbo.gov/ftpdocs/87xx /doc8758/11-13-LT-Health.pdf. Accessed January 2011.

Damberg, C. L., et al. 2009. Taking stock of pay-for-performance: A candid assessment from the front lines. *Health Affairs* 28, no. 2: 517–525.

Damberg, C. L., et al. 2014. *Measuring success in health care value-based purchasing programs: Summary and recommendations.* Available at: http://www.rand.org/pubs/research_reports /RR306z1.html. Accessed February 2017.

Docteur, E. R., et al. 1996. Shifting the paradigm: monitoring access in Medicare managed care. *Health Care Financing Review* 17, no. 4: 5–21.

Donabedian, A. 1985. *Explorations in quality assessment and monitoring: The methods and findings of quality assessment and monitoring.* Vol. 3. Ann Arbor, MI: Health Administration Press.

Dranove, D. 1993. The case for competitive reform in health care. In: *Competitive approaches to health care reform.* R. J. Arnould et al., eds. Washington, DC: Urban Institute Press. pp. 67–82.

Eijkenaar, F., et al. 2013. Effects of pay for performance in health care: A systematic review of systematic reviews. *Health Policy* 110, no. 2: 115–130.

Farquhar, M. 2008. Chapter 45. AHRQ quality indicators. In *Patient safety and quality: An evidence-based handbook for nurses.* R. G. Hughes, ed. Rockville, MD: Agency for Healthcare Research and Quality). Available at: https://www .ncbi.nlm.nih.gov/books/NBK2664/. Accessed February 2014.

Feldstein, P. J. 1993. *Health care economics.* 4th ed. Albany, NY: Delmar Publishers.

Feldstein, P. 1994. *Health policy issues: An economic perspective on health reform.* Ann Arbor, MI: AUPHA Press/Health Administration Press.

Finkelstein, A., et al. 2016. Sources of geographic variation in health care: Evidence from patient migration. *Quarterly Journal of Economics*, 131, no. 4: 1681–1726.

Finkelstein, E. A., et al. 2009. Annual medical spending attributable to obesity: Payer- and service-specific estimates. *Health Affairs* 28, no. 5: W822–W831.

Fisher, E. S., et al. 2003a. The implications of regional variations in Medicare spending. Part 1: The content, quality, and accessibility of care. *Annals of Internal Medicine* 138, no. 4: 273–287.

Fisher, E. S., et al. 2003b. The implications of regional variations in Medicare spending. Part 2: Health outcomes and satisfaction with care. *Annals of Internal Medicine* 138, no. 4: 288–298.

Frank, L., et al. 2014. The PCORI perspective on patient-centered outcomes research. *Journal of the American Medical Association* 312, no. 15: 1513–1514.

Ganz, P. A., and M. S. Litwin. 1996. Measuring outcomes and health-related quality of life. In: *Changing the US health care system: Key issues in health services, policy, and management.* R.M. Andersen et al., eds. San Francisco, CA: Jossey-Bass Publishers.

Giffin, M., and R. B. Giffin. 1994. Market memo: Critical pathways produce tangible results. *Health Care Strategic Management* 12, no. 7: 1–6.

Gittelsohn, A., and N. R. Powe. 1995. Small area variation in health care delivery in Maryland. *Health Services Research* 30, no. 2: 295–317.

Gottlieb, S. R. 1974. A brief history of health planning in the United States. In: *Regulating health facilities construction.* C. C. Havighurst, ed. Washington, DC: American Enterprise Institute for Public Policy Research.

Hartman, M., et al. 2011. Health spending growth at a historic low in 2008. *Health Affairs* 29, no. 1: 147–155.

HCIA Inc., and Deloitte & Touche. 1997. *The comparative performance of US hospitals: The sourcebook.* Baltimore, MD: HCIA Inc.

Hu, T., et al. (2016). Medicaid pay for performance programs and childhood immunization status. *American Journal of Preventive Medicine* 50, no. 5: S51–S57.

Institute of Medicine (IOM). 1993. *Access to health care in America*. M. Millman, ed. Washington, DC: National Academy Press.

Institute of Medicine (IOM). 2000. *To err is human: Building a safer health system*. L. T. Kohn et al., eds. Washington, DC: National Academy Press.

Institute of Medicine (IOM). 2004. *Rewarding provider performance: Aligning incentives in Medicare*. Washington, DC: National Academies Press.

James, J. October 11, 2012. Health Policy Briefs: Pay-for-performance. *Health Affairs*. Available at: http://www.healthaffairs.org/health policybriefs/brief.php?brief_id=78. Accessed September 2013.

Jha, A. K., et al. 2012. The long-term effect of premier pay for performance on patient outcomes. *New England Journal of Medicine* 366: 1606–1615.

Kaiser Family Foundation. May 2012. *How much does the U.S. spend on health and how has it changed?* Available at: http://kff.org/report -section/health-care-costs-a-primer-2012 -report/. Accessed February 2017.

Kaiser Family Foundation. 2013. *Health costs*. Available at: http://www.kaiseredu.org/issue -modules/us-health-care-costs/background -brief.aspx. Accessed January 2014.

Kaiser Family Foundation. 2016. *2016 Employer health benefits survey*. Available at: http://kff .org/report-section/ehbs-2016-summary-of -findings/. Accessed February 2017.

Kaiser Family Foundation, Health Research and Education Trust. 2010. *Employer health benefits 2010 annual survey*. Available at: http://kaiserfamilyfoundation.files.wordpress .com/2013/04/8085.pdf. Accessed May 2017.

Karpman, M., et al. 2015. QuickTake: Access to health care providers improved between September 2013 and September 2014. Health Reform Monitoring Survey 2015. Available at: http://hrms.urban.org/quicktakes/Access -to-Health-Care-Providers-Improved.html. Accessed February 2017.

Kruse, G. B., et al. 2012. The impact of hospital pay-for-performance on hospital and Medicare costs. *Health Services Research* 47, no. 6: 2118–2136.

Lamb, R. M., et al. 2003. Hospital disclosure practices: Results of a national survey. *Health Affairs* 22, no. 2: 73–83.

Lehman, A. F. 1995. Measuring quality of life in a reformed health system. *Health Affairs* 14, no. 3: 90–101.

Levit, K., et al. 2003. Trends in U.S. health care spending, 2001. *Health Affairs* 22, no. 1: 154–164.

Levy, D. E. 2006. Employer-sponsored insurance coverage of smoking cessation treatments. *American Journal of Managed Care* 12, no. 9: 553–562.

MACPAC. 2016. *Issue brief: Medicaid physician payment policy*. Available at: https://www .macpac.gov/wp-content/uploads/2016/04 /Medicaid-Physician-Payment-Policy.pdf. Accessed February 2017.

Makary, M. A., & M. Daniel. 2016. Medical error: The third leading cause of death in the US. *BMJ* 353: i2139.

May, J. 1974. The planning and licensing agencies. In: *Regulating health facilities constructions*. C. C. Havighurst, ed. Washington, DC: American Enterprise Institute for Public Policy Research.

McGlynn, E. A. 1997. Six challenges in measuring the quality of health care. *Health Affairs* 16, no. 3: 7–21.

McGlynn, E. A., and R. H. Brook. 1996. Ensuring quality of care. In: *Changing the US health care system: Key issues in health services, policy, and management*. R. M. Andersen et al., eds. San Francisco, CA: Jossey-Bass Publishers.

McWilliams, J. M., et al. 2014. Changes in patients' experiences in Medicare accountable care organizations. *New England Journal of Medicine* 371, no. 18: 1715–1724.

Medicare.gov. 2016. *Hospital Compare: Measures and current data collection periods*. Available at: https://www.medicare.gov/hospitalcompare /Data/Data-Updated.html#. Accessed February 2017.

National Center for Health Statistics (NCHS). 1996. *Health, United States, 1995*. Hyattsville, MD: U.S. Department of Health and Human Services.

National Center for Health Statistics (NCHS). 1997. *Health, United States, 1996–97*. Hyattsville, MD: U.S. Department of Health and Human Services.

National Center for Health Statistics (NCHS). 1999. *Health, United States, 1999*. Hyattsville,

MD: U.S. Department of Health and Human Services.

National Center for Health Statistics (NCHS). 2000. *Health, United States, 2000*. Hyattsville, MD: U.S. Department of Health and Human Services.

National Center for Health Statistics (NCHS). 2002. *Health, United States, 2002*. Hyattsville, MD: U.S. Department of Health and Human Services.

National Center for Health Statistics (NCHS). 2005. *Health, United States, 2005*. Hyattsville, MD: U.S. Department of Health and Human Services.

National Center for Health Statistics (NCHS). 2006. *Health, United States, 2006*. Hyattsville, MD: U.S. Department of Health and Human Services.

National Center for Health Statistics (NCHS). 2009. *Health, United States, 2008*. Hyattsville, MD: U.S. Department of Health and Human Services.

National Center for Health Statistics (NCHS). 2010. *Health, United States, 2009*. Hyattsville, MD: U.S. Department of Health and Human Services.

National Center for Health Statistics (NCHS). 2011. *Health, United States, 2010*. Hyattsville, MD: U.S. Department of Health and Human Services.

National Center for Health Statistics (NCHS). 2012. *Health, United States, 2011*. Hyattsville, MD: U.S. Department of Health and Human Services.

National Center for Health Statistics (NCHS). 2013. *Health, United States, 2012*. Hyattsville, MD: U.S. Department of Health and Human Services.

National Center for Health Statistics (NCHS). 2014. *Health, United States, 2013*. Hyattsville, MD: U.S. Department of Health and Human Services.

National Center for Health Statistics (NCHS). 2016a. *Early release of selected estimates based on data from the 2015 National Health Interview Survey*. Available at: https://www.cdc.gov/nchs /data/nhis/earlyrelease/earlyrelease201605.pdf. Accessed February 2017.

National Center for Health Statistics (NCHS). 2016b. *Health, United States, 2015*. Hyattsville,

MD: U.S. Department of Health and Human Services.

National Conference of State Legislatures. 2016. CON: Certificate of need state laws. Available at: http://www.ncsl.org/research/health/con -certificate-of-need-state-laws.aspx. Accessed February 2017.

National Quality Forum (NQF). 2013. *Endorsed individual and composite measures*. Available at: https://www.qualityindicators.ahrq.gov /Downloads/Modules/V45/Module_NQF _Endorsement_V4.5.pdf. Accessed May 2017.

Nicholas L. H., et al. 2011. Do hospitals alter patient care effort allocations under pay-for-performance? *Health Services Research* 46, no. 1: 61–81.

Organization for Economic Cooperation and Development (OECD). 2016. *Health spending*. Available at: https://data.oecd.org/healthres /health-spending.htm. Accessed April 2017.

Orlikoff, J. E. 1988. *Malpractice prevention and liability control for hospitals*. 2nd ed. Chicago, IL: American Hospital Publishing.

Penchansky, R., and J. W. Thomas. 1981. The concept of access: Definition and relationship to consumer satisfaction. *Medical Care* 19: 127–140.

Ramsey, S. D. 2002. Economic analyses and clinical practice guidelines: Why not a match made in heaven? *Journal of General Internal Medicine* 17, no. 3: 235–237.

Reinhardt, U. E. 1994. Providing access to health care and controlling costs: The universal dilemma. In: *The nation's health*. 4th ed. P. R. Lee and C. L. Estes, eds. Boston, MA: Jones and Bartlett Publishers. pp. 263–278.

Robert Wood Johnson Foundation (RWJF). 2013. *What is the national quality strategy?* Available at: http://www.rwjf.org/en/research-publications /find-rwjf-research/2012/01/what-is-the-national -quality-strategy-.html. Accessed January 2014.

Rogers, W. H., et al. 1990. Quality of care before and after implementation of the DRG-based prospective payment system: A summary of effects. *Journal of the American Medical Association* 264, no. 15: 1989–1994.

Ross, J. S., et al. 2010. State-sponsored public reporting of hospital quality: Results are hard to find and lack uniformity. *Health Affairs* 29, no. 12: 2317–2322.

Ryan, A. M. 2009. Effects of the Premier Hospital Quality Incentive demonstration on Medicare patient mortality and cost. *Health Services Research* 44, no. 3: 821–842.

Schoen, C. February 2016. *The Affordable Care Act and the U.S. economy: A five-year perspective.* Commonwealth Fund. Available at: http://www.commonwealthfund.org/publications/fund-reports/2016/feb/aca-economy-five-year-perspective. Accessed February 2017.

Shartzer, A., et al. 2016. Access to care and affordability have improved following Affordable Care Act implementation; problems Remain. *Health Affairs (Millwood)* 35, no. 1: 161–168.

Shih, T., et al. 2014. Does pay-for-performance improve surgical outcomes? An evaluation of phase 2 of the Premier Hospital Quality Incentive Demonstration. *Annals of Surgery* 259, no. 4: 677.

Skopec, L., and B. D. Sommers. 2013. *Seventy-one million additional Americans are receiving preventive services coverage without cost-sharing under the Affordable Care Act.* Available at: https://aspe.hhs.gov/basic-report/seventy-one-million-additional-americans-are-receiving-preventive-services-coverage-without-cost-sharing-under-affordable-care-act. Accessed May 2017.

Sommers, B. D., et al. 2012. Mortality and access to care among adults after state Medicaid expansions. *New England Journal of Medicine* 367, no. 11: 1025–1034.

Sommers, B. D., et al. 2015. Changes in self-reported insurance coverage, access to care, and health under the affordable care act. *Journal of the American Medical Association* 314, no. 4: 366–374.

Svarstad, B. L. 1986. Patient–practitioner relationships and compliance with prescribed medical regimens. In: *Applications of social sciences to clinical medicine and health policy.* L. H. Aiken and D. Mechanic, eds. New Brunswick, NJ: Rutgers University Press.

TECH Research Network. 2001. Technology change around the world: Evidence from heart attack care. *Health Affairs* 20, no. 3: 25–42.

U.S. Census Bureau. 2000. *Projections of the total resident population by 5-year age groups, and sex with special age categories: middle series, 2025 to 2045.* Available at: https://www.census.gov/population/projections/files/natproj/summary/np-t3-f.pdf. Accessed April 2017.

U.S. Department of Health and Human Services (DHHS). 1996. *Health, United States, 1995.* Hyattsville, MD: National Center for Health Statistics.

U.S. Government Accountability Office. 2008. *Medicare Part B imaging services: Rapid spending growth and shift to physician offices indicate need for CMS to consider additional management practices.* Available at: http://www.gao.gov/products/GAO-08-452. Accessed January 2011.

USA Today. 2010. *Our view on financing government: When 47% don't pay income tax, it's not healthy for USA.* Available at: https://usatoday30.usatoday.com/news/opinion/editorials/2010-04-16-editorial16_ST_N.htm. Accessed May 2017.

Van de Water, P. N., and J. Lavery. 2006. Medicare finances: Findings of the 2006 trustees report. *Medicare Brief* 13: 1–8.

Wendling, W., and J. Werner. 1980. Nonprofit firms and the economic theory of regulation. *Quarterly Review of Economics and Business* 20, no. 3: 6–18.

Wennberg, J. E. 2002. Unwarranted variations in healthcare delivery: Implications for academic medical centres. *British Medical Journal* 325, no. 7370: 961–964.

Wennberg, J. E., and A. Gittelsohn. 1973. Small area variations in health care delivery. *Science* 183: 1102–1108.

Wennberg, J. E., et al. 1987. Are hospital services rationed in New Haven or over-utilized in Boston? *Lancet* 1, no. 8543: 1185–1189.

Werner, R. M., et al. 2011. The effect of pay-for-performance in hospitals: Lessons for quality improvement. *Health Affairs* 30, no. 4: 690–698.

Williams, K. N., and R. H. Brook. 1978. Quality measurement and assurance. *Health Medical Care Services Review* 1: 3–15.

Williams, S. J. 1995. *Essentials of health services.* Albany, NY: Delmar Publishers.

Williams, S. J., and P. R. Torrens. 1993. Influencing, regulating, and monitoring the health care system. In: *Introduction to health services.* 4th ed. S. J. Williams and P. R. Torrens, eds. Albany, NY: Delmar Publishers. pp. 377–396.

Wilson, F. A., and D. Neuhauser. 1985. *Health services in the United States*. 2nd ed. Cambridge, MA: Ballinger Publishing.

Wong, M. D., et al. 2001. Effects of cost sharing on care seeking and health status: Results from the Medical Outcomes Study. *American Journal of Public Health* 91, no. 11: 1889–1894.

Zuckerman, R. B., et al. 2016. Readmissions, observation, and the hospital readmissions reduction program. *New England Journal of Medicine* 374, no. 16: 1543–1551.

Zuckerman, S., and J. Holahan. 2012. *Despite criticism, the Affordable Care Act does much to contain health care costs*. Available at: http://www.urban.org/UploadedPDF/412665-Despite-Criticism-The-Affordable-Care-Act-Does-Much-to-Contain-Health-Care-Cost.pdf. Accessed January 2014.

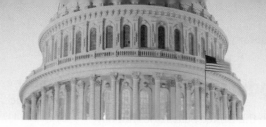

CHAPTER 13

Health Policy

LEARNING OBJECTIVES

- Discuss the definition, scope, and role of health policy in the United States.
- Recognize the principal features of U.S. health policy.
- Describe the process by which legislative health policy is developed.
- Identify critical health policy issues in the United States.
- Discuss the passage, implementation, and repeal of the Affordable Care Act from a political perspective.

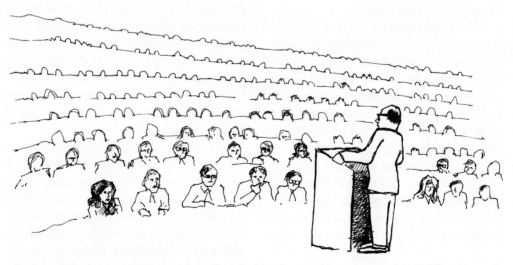

"Ladies and gentlemen, to come up with a uniform health policy, we will now break up into 31 different groups."

▶ Introduction

Even though the United States does not have a centrally controlled system of health care delivery, it does have a history of federal, state, and local government involvement in health care and health policy. Government involvement in social welfare programs can be traced back to almshouses and pesthouses, the two well-known government-run institutions of the 19th century (see *The Evolution of Health Services in the United States* chapter). Perhaps the most visible policy efforts, which continue to have implications today, are the social programs created under the Social Security legislation during Franklin Roosevelt's presidency in the 1940s. Amendments to the Social Security Act later created the massive public health insurance programs, Medicare and Medicaid in 1965, the Children's Health Insurance Program (CHIP) in 1997, and the recently enacted Affordable Care Act (ACA).

The government's success in bringing about social change through health policy has given it a solid footing to engage in further expansion of tax-financed health care. Hence, the government continues to find new opportunities to mold health care delivery through health policy. This chapter defines what health policy is and explores the principal features of health policy in the United States. It describes how legislative policy is developed and provides a policy context for many past developments in health care delivery, including the ACA.

▶ What Is Health Policy?

Public policies are authoritative decisions made in the legislative, executive, or judicial branch of government intended to direct or influence the actions, behaviors, or decisions of others (Longest, 2010; Shi, 2014). When public policies pertain to or influence the pursuit of health, they become health policies. **Health policy** can be defined as "the aggregate of principles, stated or unstated, that . . . characterize the distribution of resources, services, and political influences that impact on the health of the population" (Shi, 2014).

Public policies are supposed to serve the interests of the public; however, the term "public" has been interpreted differently in the political landscape. At the most general level, the term "public" refers to all Americans. "Public" can also refer to voters or likely voters in political elections. Finally, this term can refer to only those who are politically active—that is, those Americans who communicate directly with their representatives by writing or calling them, who contribute money to politicians or political groups, who attend protests or other forums on behalf of a particular interest or candidate, or who, in other ways, make their voices and policy preferences heard. People who are older, have more years of education, and have strong party identification are more likely to be politically active.

Legislators and policymakers tend to be responsive to the views or wishes of these active Americans, particularly when they are constituents from within their legislative districts. In contrast, politicians tend to strongly lean toward supporting policies that agree with their own ideologies or advance their own political agendas. Because most policymakers are also politicians, policy making and politics are often closely intertwined. The danger is that policy making often becomes highly politicized and is held hostage to the ideologies of the political party that happens to be in power at a given time. The party in power also exerts considerable peer pressure on its own members to support policies along party lines. For most politicians, their primary concern may be getting elected or reelected. Hence, certain policies are driven by a strong desire to keep campaign promises or to please some powerful constituent group.

This kind of policy-for-politics approach does not ask for or consider the cost-benefit trade-offs of a proposed policy. Policies driven by political considerations are likely to be near-sighted. In addition, party-line politics keep the American public deeply divided on major issues, as witnessed during the 2016 presidential election.

Uses of Policy

Regulatory Tools

Health policies may be used as **regulatory tools** (Longest, 2010). They call on government to prescribe and control the behavior of a particular target group by monitoring the group and imposing sanctions if it fails to comply. Examples of regulatory policies are abundant in the health care system. Federally funded quality improvement organizations (QIOs; formerly called peer review organizations), for instance, develop and enforce standards concerning appropriate care under the Medicare program (see the *Cost, Access, and Quality* chapter). State insurance departments across the country regulate insurance companies and managed care organizations in an effort to protect customers from default on coverage in case of financial failure of the insurer, excessive premiums, and mendacious practices. Since the passage of the ACA, the U.S. Department

of Health and Human Services (DHHS) has been charged with the responsibility of implementing many of its provisions, whereas the U.S. Department of the Treasury, through the Internal Revenue Service (IRS), has been charged with the responsibility of regulating the individual and employer mandates and collecting the many taxes imposed by the ACA.

Some health policies are "self-regulatory." For example, physicians set standards of medical practice, hospitals accredit one another as meeting the standards that the Joint Commission has set, and schools of public health decide which courses should be part of their graduate programs in public health. Similarly, managed care organizations (MCOs) voluntarily collect and report on quality measures, using Healthcare Effectiveness Data and Information Set (HEDIS) data (see the *Managed Care and Integrated Organizations* chapter), to the National Committee for Quality Assurance, which is a voluntary, nongovernmental agency.

Allocative Tools

Health policies may also be used as **allocative tools** (Longest, 2010). They involve the direct provision of income, services, or goods to certain groups of individuals or institutions. Allocative tools in the health care arena may be either distributive or redistributive.

Distributive policies spread benefits throughout society. Typical distributive policies include funding of medical research through the National Institutes of Health (NIH), the development of medical personnel (e.g., medical education through the National Health Service Corps), the construction of facilities (e.g., hospitals under the Hill-Burton Act program during the 1950s and 1960s), and the initiation of new institutions (e.g., health maintenance organizations [HMOs] under the Health Maintenance Organization Act of 1973).

Redistributive policies are designed to benefit only certain groups of people by taking money from one group and using it for the benefit of another. This system often creates visible beneficiaries and payers. For this reason, health policy is often most visible and politically charged when it performs redistributive functions. Redistributive policies include Medicaid, which takes tax revenue from the more affluent and spends it on the poor in the form of free health insurance. Other redistributive policies include CHIP, welfare, and public housing programs.

Redistributive policies, in particular, are believed to be essential for addressing the fundamental causes of health disparities. Expansion of health insurance for the uninsured—a key goal of the ACA—is also based on a redistributive approach.

Different Forms of Health Policies

Health policies often emerge as a by-product of social policies enacted by the government. For example, the Social Security Act of 1935 was passed mainly as a retirement income security measure for the elderly, but it also contained the Old Age Assistance program that enabled the elderly to pay for services in homes for the aged and boarding homes. After World War II, policies that excluded fringe benefits from income or Social Security taxes and a 1948 Supreme Court ruling that employee benefits, including health insurance, could be legitimately included in the collective bargaining process (see *The Evolution of Health Services in the United States* chapter) had the effect of promoting employment-based private health insurance. Consequently, employer-based health benefits grew rapidly in the mid-20th century.

The extraordinary growth of medical technology in the United States can also be traced to health policies that directly support biomedical research and encourage private investments in such research. NIH had a budget of approximately $10 million when the agency was established in the early 1930s. Following exponential growth in its funding, the proposed fiscal year 2017 budget for NIH is $33.1 billion (NIH, 2016). Encouraged by policies, such as patent laws, that permit firms to recoup their investments in research and development, private industry is the largest financier of biomedical research and development in the United States.

Health policies affect groups or classes of individuals, such as physicians, the poor, the elderly, and children. They can also affect various types of organizations, such as medical schools, HMOs, hospitals, nursing homes, manufacturers of medical technology, and employers. Examples include licensing of physicians and nurses by states; federal certification of health care institutions, which enables them to receive public funds to care for patients covered by the Medicare and Medicaid programs; court decisions that may prevent the merger of two hospitals on the grounds of violating federal antitrust laws; and local ordinances banning smoking in public places.

Statutes or laws, such as the statutory language contained in the 1983 Amendments to the Social Security Act that authorized the prospective payment system (PPS) for reimbursing hospitals for Medicare beneficiaries, are also considered policies.

Another example is the certificate-of-need (CON) programs, through which many states seek to regulate capital expansion in their health care systems (see the *Medical Technology* and *Cost, Access, and Quality* chapters). While CON programs have changed significantly over the past 30 years, as of 2016, 34 states maintained some type of CON program, while 14 states had discontinued their CON programs, and 3 states had some variations of the program. States that maintain CON programs often target expansion of outpatient and long-term care facilities, which make up a growing segment of the health care market (National Conference of State Legislatures, 2016).

The scope of health policy is limited by the political and economic system of a country. In the United States, where pro-individual and pro-market sentiments dominate, public policies have been incremental and noncomprehensive. Even the massive ACA is regarded as a major incremental reform. National policies and programs are typically based on the notion that local communities are in the best position to identify the most desirable strategies to address their unique needs. The type of change that can be enacted at the community level is clearly limited, however, because communities are bounded by policies and regulations formulated at the national and state levels.

▶ Principal Features of U.S. Health Policy

Several features characterize U.S. health policy, including the position of the government as subsidiary to the private sector; fragmented, incremental, and piecemeal reform; pluralistic politics associated with demanders and suppliers of policy; a decentralized role for the states; and the impact of presidential leadership. These features often act or interact to influence the development and evolution of health policies.

Government as Subsidiary to the Private Sector

In much of the developed world, national health care programs are built on a consensus that health care is a right of citizenship and that government should play a leading role in the delivery of health care. In the United States, health care has not been seen as a right of citizenship or as a primary responsibility of government. Instead, the private sector has played a dominant role. Traditionally, Americans have been opposed to any major government interventions in health care financing and delivery, except for helping the underprivileged. Over the past few years, an argument has been made that health care should also be a right in the United States, and this view finally prevailed and became the basis for the ACA. Because not all Americans espouse liberal views, however, the ACA has deeply divided the nation, and its repeal has been promised by the Trump administration.

Americans' general mistrust of government dates back to the founding of the United States. The Declaration of Independence defined the new nation by making a great protest over government intrusion on personal liberty. It outlined the individual's right to life, liberty, and the pursuit of happiness. The Constitution further limited the powers of government. The fundamental beliefs and values that most Americans still subscribe to (see the *Beliefs, Values, and Health* chapter) evolved from these earlier founding documents.

Generally speaking, the government's role in U.S. health care has grown incrementally, mainly to address perceived problems and negative health consequences for the underprivileged. Also, the most credible argument for policy intervention in the nation's domestic activities begins with the identification of situations in which markets fail or do not function efficiently. In an ironic twist, even though health care in the United States functions under imperfect market conditions (see the *Overview of U.S. Health Care Delivery* chapter), problems and issues in health care are often blamed on "the market," which prompts politicians to further regulate health care through policy interventions. For example, cost escalations in the health care delivery system were assumed to reflect on the inability of private parties to control health care costs, which paved the way for various prospective payment methods.

Unfortunately, certain policy interventions have also fueled the growth of health care expenditures, at least indirectly. The legislation passed in many states to rein in managed care's initiatives to contain escalating health care costs is a prime example. Yet, for lack of other cost-control alternatives, several states passed laws to enroll all of their Medicaid beneficiaries in managed care programs. Conversely, voluntary enrollment by Medicare enrollees in the federal Medicare Advantage (Part C) program has been less successful (see the *Managed Care and Integrated Organizations* chapter).

Government spending for health care has been largely confined to filling the gaps in areas where the private sector has been unwilling or unable to address certain issues. For example, court decisions such as *Duggan v. Bowen* and *Olmstead v. L.C.* were largely responsible for promoting large-scale transfers of people with mental illness and disabilities from institutions to community-based settings across the United States. Other policy interventions include various public health measures, such as environmental protection, communicable disease control, and preparedness for disasters and bioterrorism.

Fragmented Policies

Fragmentation of the government's power in the United States follows the design of the Founding Fathers, who developed a structure of "checks and balances" to limit government's power. Federal, state, and local governments pursue their own policies, with little coordination of purpose or programs occurring. The subsidiary role of the government and the attendant mixture of private and public approaches to the delivery of health care have also resulted in a complex and fragmented pattern of health care financing in which (1) the employed are predominantly covered by voluntary insurance provided through contributions that they and their employers make; (2) the elderly are insured through a combination of private–public financing of Medicare; (3) the poor are covered by Medicaid through a combination of federal and state tax revenues; and (4) special population groups—for example, veterans, American Indians, members of the armed forces, Congress, and employees of the executive branch—have coverage provided directly by the federal government.

Incremental and Piecemeal Policies

Incremental and piecemeal health policies in the United States have been the result of compromises made to accommodate a variety of competing interests. An example is the broadening of the Medicaid program since its introduction in 1965. In 1984, the first steps were taken to mandate coverage of pregnant women and children in two-parent families who met income requirements and to mandate coverage for all children 5 years or younger who met the Medicaid's financial requirements. In 1986, states were given the option of covering pregnant women and children up to 5 years of age in families with incomes below 100% of the federal poverty level (FPL). In 1988, that option was increased to cover families at 185% of the FPL. In 1997, under CHIP, states were allowed to use Medicaid to extend coverage to uninsured children who otherwise did not qualify for the existing Medicaid program. The Medicaid experience illustrates how a program is reformed and/or expanded through successive legislative action achieved through compromises between the two opposite political parties.

The Medicare program was also expanded incrementally. At first, it covered only the elderly under Parts A and B in 1965. Since then, Medicare has been expanded to include benefits for speech, physical, and chiropractic therapy in 1972. In the 1980s, the Medicare program added the payments option to HMOs. Over the years, Congress expanded Medicare eligibility to younger people with permanent disabilities who receive Social Security Disability Insurance payments and those who have end-stage renal disease (ESRD).

In 1982, the program also added hospice benefits, and in 2001, Medicare was further expanded to cover younger people with amyotrophic lateral sclerosis.

Interest Groups as Demanders of Policy

Health policy outcomes in the United States are heavily influenced by the demands of interest groups and the compromises struck to satisfy those demands. **EXHIBIT 13-1** summarizes the major concerns of the dominant interest groups. The powerful interest groups involved in health care politics have historically resisted any major changes in the existing health care system (Alford, 1975). Each group fights hard to protect its own best interests; however, the result for any single group is less than optimal. Well-organized interest groups are the most effective "demanders" of policies. By combining and concentrating their members' resources, organized interest groups can dramatically change the ratio between the costs and benefits of participation in the political process for policy change. These interest groups represent a variety of individuals and entities, such as physicians in the American Medical Association (AMA); senior citizens allied with AARP (formerly called the American Association of Retired Persons); institutional providers, such as hospitals belonging to the American Hospital Association (AHA); nursing homes belonging to the American Health Care Association; and the companies making up the Pharmaceutical Research and Manufacturers of America (PhRMA).

Physicians have often found it hard to lobby for their interests with a single voice because they include so many specialty groups. For example, the American Academy of Pediatrics is involved in advocacy for children's health issues. Other specialty groups include Physicians for a National Health Program, the American Society of Anesthesiologists, and the Society of Thoracic Surgeons. These groups can come together on issues that threaten the interests of the entire group. For example,

the various physician groups coalesced in 1992, when Medicare decided to change the reimbursement system from fee for service to a resource-based relative value scale (RBRVS). Notably, the physicians did not prevail in this case.

The policy agendas of interest groups reflect the interests of their members. For example, the AARP advocates programs to expand health care financing for the elderly. It became a major advocate for prescription drug coverage for Medicare beneficiaries by supporting the Medicare Prescription Drug Improvement and Modernization Act of 2003. In a surprising move, the AARP enthusiastically supported the ACA even though the law had proposed Medicare cuts, which were opposed by the elderly. It has been suggested that payment cuts to Medicare Advantage (MA) plans could trigger a withdrawal of participating insurers from MA, which would financially benefit the AARP, as it is the largest sponsor of Medigap plans (Roy, 2012). For once, this organization seems to have abandoned its primary mission to champion the interests of its elderly members.

Other examples of interest groups include labor unions, which have become the staunchest supporters of national health insurance. The primary concerns of educational and research institutions and accrediting bodies are embedded in policies that would generate higher funding to support their educational and research activities.

Pharmaceutical and medical technology organizations are concerned with detecting changes in health policy and influencing the formulation of policies concerning approval and monitoring of drugs and devices. Three main factors drive health policy concerns about medical technology:

- Medical technology is an important contributor to rising health costs.
- Medical technology often provides health benefits.
- The utilization of medical technology provides economic benefits by creating jobs in health care and other sectors of the economy.

These factors are likely to remain important determinants of U.S. policies on medical technology. Another factor driving U.S. technology policy is policymakers' desire to develop cost-saving technology and expand access to it. The government is spending large amounts of money on outcomes studies and comparative effectiveness studies to identify the value of alternative technologies that promise better care at lower costs.

Business also is a major interest group, although it is generally split into two factions along the lines of large and small employers. U.S. employers' health policy concerns are shaped mostly by the degree to which they provide health insurance benefits to their employees, their employees' dependents, and their retirees. Many small business owners adamantly oppose health policies requiring them to cover employees, because they believe they cannot afford to provide this benefit. Employees also pay attention to health policies that affect worker health or the labor–management relations experienced by employers. For example, employers must comply with federal and state regulations on employee health and well-being and on the prevention of job-related illnesses and injuries. Employers are often inspected by regulatory agencies to ensure that they adhere to workplace health and safety policies.

Other relatively newer members of the health policy community represent consumer interests. For example, the Tea Party movement representing conservative Americans actively demonstrated in Washington, D.C., and around the United States during the legislative battle to pass the ACA, although they ultimately lost this fight. Consumer representation on the liberal side during the ACA debate was noticeably silent, perhaps for two main reasons: (1) It was believed that a liberal majority in Congress and a liberal president were already taking action on their behalf, and (2) the Tea Party movement was often marginalized in the news media (based largely on false reports).

Pluralistic Suppliers of Policy

In the United States, each branch and level of government can influence health policy. For example, both the executive and legislative branches at the federal, state, and local levels can establish health policies, and the judicial branch can uphold, strike down, or modify existing laws affecting health and health care at federal, state, or local levels. Perhaps the biggest factor is shifts in control of the presidency and the Congress, which can either create or close down opportunities for reform (Oliver et al., 2004). Fundamental ideologies, leaning toward the left or the right, come to the fore when advocates of these ideologies seek to take policy action as control passes from one political party to the other. The dominant political party often ends up sweeping its agenda through as long as there is little resistance from powerful interest groups and the American people. For either meaningful support or resistance to occur toward a proposed policy, transparency and truthful information must be made available by the policymakers, and it must be faithfully carried to the public by the news media.

All three branches of government—legislative, executive, and judicial—are suppliers of policy. Of these, the legislative branch is the most active in policy making, a point that is particularly evident with policies that take the form of statutes or laws. Legislators play central roles in providing policies demanded by their various constituencies.

Members of the executive branch also act as suppliers of policies. Presidents, governors, and other high-level public officials propose policies in the form of proposed legislation and push legislators to enact their preferred policies. Executives and administrators in charge of departments and agencies of government make policies in the form of rules and regulations used to implement statutes and programs. In this manner, they interpret congressional interest, thereby becoming intermediary suppliers of policies.

The judicial branch of government is a policy supplier as well. Whenever a court interprets an ambiguous statute, establishes judicial precedents, or interprets the Constitution, it makes policy. These activities are not conceptually different from legislators enacting statutes or members of the executive branch establishing rules and regulations for the implementation of the statutes. All three activities concur with the definition of policy, in that they are authoritative decisions made within government to influence or direct the actions, behaviors, and decisions of others.

Decentralized Role of the States

In the United States, under the theory of federalism, political power is shared between the federal government and the governments in each state. Hence, individual states play a significant role in the development and implementation of health policies. An example is the state governments' dominant role in regulating managed care in the delivery of health care. Other examples of states' roles include financial support for the care and treatment of the poor and chronically disabled, oversight of health care practitioners and facilities through state licensure and regulation, training of health personnel (states pay most of the costs to train health care professionals), and authorization of health services available through local governments. **EXHIBIT 13-2** lists the arguments often cited in favor of decentralizing health programs at the state level.

Many of the incremental policy actions related to health care have originated in state governments. One such action by states was to create "insurance risk pools," a type of program that helped people acquire private insurance otherwise unavailable to them because of the medical risks they posed to insurance companies. These special programs were financed by a combination of individual premiums and taxes on insurance carriers. The ACA does away with the need for state-based risk pools under the assumption that insurers cannot legally deny insurance to anyone with a preexisting medical condition, no matter how severe the condition.

Other state-initiated programs have been created to address the needs of vulnerable populations. For example, New Jersey developed a program to ensure access to care for all pregnant women. Florida set up a program called Healthy Kids Corporation, which linked health insurance to schools. Washington developed a special program

EXHIBIT 13-2 Arguments for Enhancing States' Role in Health Policy Making

- Americans distrust centralized government in general and lack faith in the federal government as an administrator in particular.
- The federal government has grown too large, intrusive, and paternalistic.
- The federal government is too impersonal, distant, and unresponsive.
- State and local governments are closer to the people and more familiar with local needs; therefore, they are more accessible and accountable to the public and better able to develop responsive programs than federal agencies.
- National standards reduce flexibility and seriously constrain the ability of states to experiment and innovate.
- States are equipped to take on such functions (i.e., they have more full-time legislators, professional staffs, and bureaucrats).
- States are more likely to implement and enforce programs of their own making.
- States have served as important laboratories for testing different structures, approaches, and programs and for providing insight into the political and technical barriers encountered in enactment and implementation.
- States respond to crises more quickly.
- It is easier to change a state law than a federal one.
- States are more willing to take risks.

for the working poor that used HMOs and preferred provider organizations (PPOs) to provide care within the state's counties. Maine established MaineCare, a program that offered HMO-based coverage at moderate prices to small businesses with 15 or fewer employees. Minnesota created the Children's Health Plan, a program designed to provide benefits to children up to 9 years of age who lived in families with incomes below 185% of the FPL but who did not qualify for Medicaid.

Two states in particular took bold policy initiatives to expand health insurance coverage. In 1989, Oregon embarked on a controversial experiment that expanded Medicaid coverage to more than 100,000 additional people, by reducing the Medicaid benefit package (Bodenheimer, 1997). In 2006, Massachusetts passed a universal health insurance program based on employer and employee mandates (see *The Evolution of Health Services in the United States* chapter).

There are disadvantages to the dichotomous federal–state approach to policy making. For one thing, the divergence between states and the federal government makes it difficult to coordinate a national strategy in many areas. For example, it is difficult to plan a national disease-control program if some states do not participate or if states do not collect and report data in a uniform manner.

States may also interpret federal incentives in ways that jeopardize the policy's original intent. For example, many states took advantage of federal matching grants for Medicaid by including a number of formerly state-funded services under an "expanded" Medicaid program. This allowed states to obtain increased federal funding, while providing exactly the same level of services they had provided prior to the "expansion." This phenomenon, called Medicaid maximization, although pursued by only a few states, had an impact outside of those states and may have contributed to rising national health care costs in the early 1990s (Coughlin et al., 1999). Subsequent to the 2012 U.S. Supreme Court decision, states have a choice to expand or not expand their Medicaid programs, as was originally mandated by the ACA, and not risk losing federal matching funds. Under the ACA, states are promised that their additional expenses incurred as a result of Medicaid expansion will be paid by the federal government.

Impact of Presidential Leadership

To pass national policy initiatives, a strong presidential role is almost always necessary. Lyndon Johnson's role in the passage of the Medicare and Medicaid legislation, George W. Bush's role in adding prescription drug coverage to Medicare, and Barack Obama's role in the enactment of the ACA are key examples. Presidents have important opportunities to influence congressional outcomes through their efforts to bring about compromises, to engage in political maneuvering, or to take advantage of economic and political situations, particularly when policies concern their own preferred agendas.

Even under the most auspicious political circumstances, however, presidents are often hampered from getting their agendas fully adopted by Congress. For example, while running for a Senate seat in Congress, candidate Barack Obama made it clear that he was a proponent of a single-payer health care system. This position was opposed by hospitals, insurance companies, and the pharmaceutical industry. Only after President Obama's administration reached compromises with this powerful industry block did the ACA become a reality.

Sometimes presidents' political agendas result, years later, in unintended and undesirable consequences. In 1946,

President Harry Truman took advantage of reports that the United States had severe capacity deficits in the hospital sector and that many Americans across the country were unable to access acute care services, which was the stepping stone to the Hill-Burton Act, a law passed by Congress in 1946 that gave grants and loans to hospitals, nursing homes, and other health facilities for construction and modernization. In 1965, President Lyndon Johnson dreamed of a "great society" to push his Medicare and Medicaid agenda through Congress. Both the Truman- and Johnson-advocated programs were passed through political compromises. Over time, however, overbuilding of hospitals and unrestrained use of Medicare and Medicaid funding sent health care costs into an uncontrolled upward spiral. Paradoxically, just when the nation achieved its goal of 4.5 community hospital beds per 1,000 population in 1980, as envisioned under the Hill-Burton Act program (see the *Inpatient Facilities and Services* chapter), the government concluded that the Medicare and Medicaid programs were no longer sustainable due to the rapid rise in health care costs. Subsequently, President Ronald Reagan authorized the PPS method of payment to reduce hospital utilization, which started a downward trend in inpatient stays and created a glut of unoccupied hospital beds in many parts of the United States.

Rising health care costs shortly after Medicare and Medicaid were implemented also presented an economic opportunity for President Richard Nixon to pass the Health Maintenance Organization Act in 1973. In addition, Nixon succeeded in getting the CON legislation enacted under the National Health Planning and Resources

Development Act of 1974. This act represented another effort to restrain rapidly rising health care costs, as it required approvals for purchases of new health care technology and new hospital construction.

In the 1990s, even though President Bill Clinton's comprehensive health care reform efforts failed, his incremental initiatives did succeed in the creation of CHIP and enactment of the Health Insurance Portability and Accountability Act (HIPAA) of 1996. Clinton's first term in office was marked by a relatively high level of public interest in health care reform (see *The Evolution of Health Services in the United States* chapter), but his administration did not act on it quickly enough. Also, the ever-changing details of his proposal, when made public, proved too complex for most people to grasp. Moreover, Americans did not want their taxes increased to pay for health care reform.

Politics of the Affordable Care Act

Prior to Barack Obama's victory in the 2008 presidential election, there was much excitement among his supporters about the prospect of the first black U.S. president, especially one whose campaign mantra was "hope and change." Anyone asking pointed questions about Obama's vision of hope and change ran the risk of the queries becoming distorted into a racial issue by the U.S. media. Hence, amid the excitement of the election, pertinent issues often went unaddressed. On health care, Obama simply stated that everyone would have health insurance. Perhaps by design, not even a general model of the proposed plan was ever made public. Nonetheless, Obama had overwhelming support from the members of his own party.

The enactment of the ACA became reality following a unique set of political circumstances that is perhaps unparalleled in the history of U.S. policy making. At the time, both houses of Congress had solid Democratic majorities and strong Democratic leadership—Nancy Pelosi in the House of Representatives and Harry Reid in the Senate. The United States was then in the middle of the worst economic downturn since the Great Depression, with an unemployment rate that exceeded 10%. Obama and his Democratic colleagues blamed former President George W. Bush for the nation's various malaises. In addition, they portrayed the insurance industry as the villain responsible for rising health care costs.

Whereas the Clinton plan had been presented in full to the public in 1993, details of the ACA legislation were largely kept secret from the public. Democrats made little effort to make passage of the ACA a bipartisan process. Ultimately, Republicans, who were in the minority in both houses of Congress, made few contributions to the debate on health care reform. In the end, the ACA passed without a single Republican vote.

Oberlander (2010) has identified other factors that contributed to the passage of the ACA. Instead of employing different reform strategies, members of the House of Representatives introduced a single health reform bill that combined three bills from three House committees, demonstrating greater agreement among Democrats. The final legislation also allowed certain exemptions from individual and employer mandates.

Oberlander (2010) also credits weak opposition to the bill from health industry stakeholders as playing a key role. Instead of waging a war against the industry,

Obama and congressional Democrats were willing to compromise. By promising millions of newly insured people who would use health care, they received pledges from stakeholders, including PhRMA and the AHA, to support health care reform. Even the insurance industry and the AMA endorsed the legislation, although their support faded over time.

Another key factor behind the ACA's success was the speed with which the reform was pushed through the legislative process. A notable drawback was that the general public was confused about the legislation and was not supportive (Patel and McDonough, 2010). In the end, however, that did not seem to have mattered. The public now has remained deeply divided on the legislation. Tracking polls showed that 42% hold unfavorable views of the ACA versus 49% holding favorable views in May 2017 (Kaiser Family Foundation, 2017d).

▶ The Development of Legislative Health Policy

The making of U.S. health policy is a complex process that involves the private and public sectors, including multiple levels of government. It reflects several unique aspects of the U.S. system of government and the U.S. populace:

- The relationship of the government to the private sector
- The distribution of authority and responsibility within a federal system of government
- The relationship between policy formulation and implementation

- A pluralistic ideology as the basis of politics
- Incrementalism as the strategy for reform

▶ The Policy Cycle

The formation and implementation of health policy occurs in a policy cycle comprising five components: (1) issue raising, (2) policy design, (3) public support building, (4) legislative decision making and policy support building, and (5) legislative decision making and policy implementation. These activities are likely to be shared by Congress and interest groups in varying degrees.

Issue raising is clearly essential in the policy formation cycle. The enactment of a new policy is preceded by a variety of actions that first create a widespread sense that a problem exists and needs to be addressed. The president may form policy concepts from a variety of sources, including campaign information; recommendations from advisers, cabinet members, and agency chiefs; personal interests; expert opinions; and public opinion polls.

The second component of policy making is the design of specific policy proposals. Presidents have substantial resources to develop new policy proposals. They may call on segments of the executive branch of government, such as the Centers for Medicare and Medicaid Services and policy staffs within the DHHS. An alternative—and one that was preferred by both Presidents John Kennedy and Lyndon Johnson—is to use outside task forces.

In building public support, presidents can choose from a variety of strategies, including major addresses to the nation and efforts to mobilize their administration to make public appeals and organized attempts to increase support among interest groups. To facilitate legislative decision making and policy support building, presidents, key staff, and department officials interact closely with Congress. Presidents generally meet with legislative leaders several mornings each month to shape the coming legislative agenda and identify possible problems as bills move through various committees.

Legislative Committees and Subcommittees

The legislative branch creates health policies and allocates the resources necessary to implement them. Congress has three important powers that make it extremely influential in the health policy process.

First, the Constitution grants Congress the power to "make all laws which shall be necessary and proper for carrying into execution." The doctrine of implied powers states that Congress may use any reasonable means not directly prohibited by the Constitution to carry out the will of the people. This mandate gives it great power to enact laws influencing all manner of health policy.

Second, Congress possesses the power to tax, which allows it to influence and regulate the health behavior of individuals, organizations, and states. Taxes on cigarettes, for example, are intended to reduce individual cigarette consumption, whereas tax relief for employer benefits is designed to promote increased insurance coverage for working people.

Third, Congress possesses the power to spend. This ability to allocate resources not only allows for direct expenditures on the public's health through federal programs, such as Medicare and the NIH, but also gives

Congress the ability to induce state conformance with federal policy objectives. Congress may prescribe the terms under which it dispenses funds to the states, such as mandating the basic required elements of the federal-/state-funded Medicaid program.

At least 14 committees and subcommittees in the House of Representatives, 24 committees and subcommittees in the Senate, and more than 60 other such legislative panels directly influence legislation (Falcone and Hartwig, 1991; Morone et al., 2008). The conglomeration of reform proposals that emerge from these committees face a daunting political challenge—separate consideration and passage in each chamber, negotiations in a joint conference committee to reconcile the bills passed by the two houses, and then return to each chamber for approval. In the Senate, 41 of the 100 members can thwart the whole process at any point. In some circumstances, the nuclear option can be applied, which is a parliamentary procedure that allows the Senate to override a rule or precedent by a simple majority of 51 votes.

Five committees—three in the House and two in the Senate—control most of the legislative activity in Congress (Longest, 2010). They are discussed in the following subsections.

House Committees

The Constitution provides that all bills involving taxation must originate in the House of Representatives. The organization of the House gives this authority to the Ways and Means Committee. Hence, the Ways and Means Committee is the most influential by virtue of its power to tax. This committee was the launching pad for much of the health financing legislation passed in the 1960s and early 1970s under the chairmanship of Representative Wilbur Mills (Democrat-Arkansas). Ways and Means has sole jurisdiction over Medicare Part A, Social Security, unemployment compensation, public welfare, and health care reform. It also shares jurisdiction over Medicare Part B with the House Energy and Commerce Committee. The latter committee has jurisdiction over Medicaid, Medicare Part B, matters of public health, mental health, health personnel, HMOs, foods and drugs, air pollution, consumer products safety, health planning, biomedical research, and health protection.

The Committee on Appropriations is responsible for funding substantive legislative provisions. Its subcommittee on Labor, Health and Human Services, Education, and Related Agencies is responsible for health appropriations. Essentially, this committee holds the power of the purse. The committee and the subcommittee are responsible for allocating and distributing federal funds for individual health programs, except for Medicare and Social Security, which are funded through their respective trust funds.

Senate Committees

The Committee on Labor and Human Resources has jurisdiction over most health bills, including the Public Health Service Act; the Food, Drug, and Cosmetic Act; HMOs; health personnel; and mental health legislation (e.g., Community Mental Health Centers Act). This committee formerly included a subcommittee on Health and Scientific Research, which was used by its then chairman, Senator Edward Kennedy (Democrat-Massachusetts), as a forum for debating whether the United States should have a national health care

program. When the full committee came under Republican control in the 1980s, the subcommittee was abolished.

The Committee on Finance and its Subcommittee on Health, similar to the Ways and Means Committee in the House, have jurisdiction over taxes and revenues, including matters related to Social Security, Medicare, Medicaid, and Maternal and Child Health (Title V of the Social Security Act). It is responsible for many of the Medicare and Medicaid amendments, such as QIOs, PPS, and amendments controlling hospital and nursing home costs.

The Legislative Process

When a bill is introduced in the House of Representatives, the House leader (the Speaker of the House of Representatives) assigns it to an appropriate committee. The committee chair forwards the bill to an appropriate subcommittee. The subcommittee forwards proposed legislation to agencies that will be affected by the legislation, holds hearings ("markup") and testimonies, and may add amendments. The subcommittee and committee may recommend, not recommend, or recommend tabling the bill. Diverse interest groups, individuals, experts in the field, and business, labor, and professional associations often exert influence on the bill through campaign contributions and intense lobbying. The full House then hears the bill and may add amendments. The bill can be approved with or without amendments. The approved bill is then sent to the Senate.

In the Senate, the bill is sent to an appropriate committee and then forwarded to an appropriate subcommittee. The subcommittee may send the bill to agencies that will be affected. It also holds hearings and testimonies from all interested parties (e.g., private citizens, business, labor, agencies, and experts). The subcommittee votes on and forwards the proposed legislation with appropriate recommendations. Amendments may or may not be added. The full Senate hears the bill and may add amendments. If the bill and House amendments are accepted, the bill goes to the president. If the Senate adds amendments that have not been voted on by the House, the bill must go back to the House floor for a vote.

If the amendments are minor and noncontroversial, the House may vote to pass the bill. If the amendments are significant and controversial, the House may call for a conference committee to review the amendments. The conference committee consists of members from equivalent committees of the House and Senate. If the recommendations of the conference committee are not accepted, another conference committee is called.

After the bill has passed both the House and the Senate in identical form, it is forwarded to the president for signature. If the president signs the legislation, it becomes law. If the president does not sign the legislation, at the end of 21 days, it becomes law unless the president vetoes the legislation. If less than 21 days are left in the congressional session, presidential inaction results in a veto—a so-called "pocket veto." The veto can be overturned by a two-thirds majority of the Congress; otherwise, the bill is dead.

▶ Policy Implementation

Once legislation has been signed into law, it is not a fait accompli. The new law is forwarded to the appropriate agency of the executive branch, where multiple levels of federal bureaucracy must interpret and implement the legislation. Rules and regulations must be written, detailing what the entities affected by the legislation must do to comply with it. During this process, politicians, interest groups, or program beneficiaries may influence the legislation's ultimate design. Sometimes, the result can differ significantly from its sponsors' intent. The process of policy making is complex enough; its implementation can be quite daunting as well.

The agency publishes proposed regulations in the *Federal Register* and holds hearings on how the law is to be implemented. A bureaucracy, only loosely controlled by either the president or Congress, writes (publishes, gathers comments about, and rewrites) regulations. Then the program goes on to the 50 states for enabling legislation, if appropriate. There, organized interests hire local lawyers and lobbyists, and a completely new political cycle begins. Finally, all parties may adjourn to the courts, where long rounds of litigation may shape the final outcome.

Implementation of the ACA

Since the signing of the ACA into law on March 23, 2010, several provisions have gone into effect, including 26 provisions in 2010, 18 provisions in 2011, and 10 provisions in 2012 (Kaiser Family Foundation, 2017e). As of August 2013, an additional 11 provisions had gone into effect with 2013 deadlines, 15 provisions with 2014 deadlines, and 3 provisions with 2015 and later deadlines (Kaiser Family Foundation, 2017e).

State take-up of the ACA provisions has varied. For example, only 31 states and the District of Columbia had signed Medicaid expansion legislation into effect as of January 2017 (Kaiser Family Foundation, 2017a). Twelve states had decided to create state-based health insurance exchanges as of January 2017, with another 5 opting for a state-based marketplace through the federal platform, and 6 selecting state-partnership marketplaces (Kaiser Family Foundation, 2017b); the remaining 28 states' health insurance exchanges were created by the federal government.

▶ Critical Policy Issues

Most past health policy initiatives have focused on access to care, cost of care, and quality of care. Some Americans contend that they have the right (access) to the best care (quality) at the least expense (cost) despite their level of income or social class. Legislative efforts, by comparison, have been specific to issues related to access (expanding insurance coverage, outreach programs in rural areas), cost containment (PPS, RBRVS), and quality (creating the Agency for Healthcare Research and Quality [AHRQ] and calling for clinical practice guidelines; see the *Cost, Access, and Quality* chapter).

With the publication of the *Healthy People 2010* and *2020* initiatives, elimination of health disparities across sociodemographic subpopulations has emerged as a bold policy objective. Since health disparities are caused primarily by nonmedical factors (see the *Beliefs, Values, and Health* chapter), the advancement of this goal signals a new policy direction that integrates health policy with broader social policies. Although it is highly unlikely that this goal will be fulfilled in the near future, the promotion of this policy objective reflects a significant government commitment. In the remainder of this section, the three areas of greatest health policy concerns are highlighted.

Access to Care

The underlying support for government policies to enhance access to care is the social justice principle that access to health care is a right that should be guaranteed to all American citizens. There are two variations on this argument: (1) All citizens have a right to the same level of care and (2) all citizens have a right to some minimum level of care. Which position the United States should espouse has never been openly debated in policy circles. In the past, efforts to ensure access to comprehensive services were aimed primarily at the most needy and underserved populations, as was the case with Medicaid. Medicare, in contrast, does not incorporate the same level of access, as its coverage is limited by high deductibles and copayments and exclusion of certain services (see the *Health Services Financing* chapter).

Providers

Policy issues include ensuring a sufficient number and desirable geographic distribution of various types of providers. The debate over the supply of physicians is an important public policy issue because policy decisions influence the number of persons entering the medical profession; that number, in turn, has implications for policies related to access and cost. The number of new entrants into the profession is influenced by programs of government assistance for individual students and by government grants made directly to educational institutions. An increased supply of physicians—particularly specialists—may result in increased health care expenditures because of increased demand for care induced by those physicians. An increased supply of physicians, particularly primary care physicians, is necessary to provide basic health care to the newly insured under any expansion of health insurance coverage. For example, the ACA will likely remain ineffective in achieving its access goals if the supply of primary care physicians does not increase.

One goal on which both Republicans and Democrats seem to agree is preserving community health centers as a safety net for the underprivileged. Consequently, federal support for these centers has been boosted. Funding for community health centers was doubled over a 5-year period under the George W. Bush administration, and this program received $2 billion in the American Recovery and Reinvestment Act of 2009. In addition, the ACA established the Community Health Center Fund, which provided $11 billion in funding over a 5-year period for the expansion of health centers across the United States (Health Resources and Services Administration, 2013).

Integrated Access

Access to care continues to be a problem in many communities, partly because health policies enacted since 1983 have focused on narrowly defined elements of the delivery system. The United States has not had a unified strategy of reforming the overall system based on a policy of integrated services. Despite an increased reliance on accountable care organizations proposed in the ACA, and other provisions such as integration of long-term care services, it is too early to forecast whether the ACA will make significant headway in making integrated access a reality. For example, long-term care services need to be integrated not just within their own orbit of services, but also with the larger health care delivery system.

Access and the Elderly

Three main concerns dominate the debate about Medicare policy: (1) Spending should be restrained to keep the program viable, (2) the program is not adequately focused on the management of chronic conditions, and (3) the program does not cover long-term nursing home care. These concerns originate from the assumption that the elderly need public assistance to finance their health care. The ACA's proposed Community Living Assistance Services and Supports (CLASS) provision was repealed in 2012 due to concerns about its stability and feasibility (Colello and Mulvey, 2013). While the CLASS provision will not be implemented, the requirements it established were taken into consideration by the Commission on Long-Term Care, which made recommendations for Congress in 2013 on the development and implementation of a long-term care system (American Taxpayer Relief Act of 2012, P.L. 112-240; Colello and Mulvey, 2013; Commission on Long-Term Care, 2016).

Access and Minorities

As pointed out in the *Health Services for Special Populations* chapter, minorities are more likely than whites to face problems with accessing health care services. However, with the exception of Native Americans, no minority population within the United States has programs specifically designed to serve its needs. Resolving the problems confronting minority groups would require policies designed to target the special needs of minorities, to encourage professional education programs sensitive to their special needs, and to develop programs to expand the delivery of services to areas populated by minorities.

The Office of Minority Health was reauthorized by the ACA in 2010 to "improve the health of racial and ethnic minority populations through the development of health policies and programs that will eliminate health disparities" (DHHS, 2016). In 2011, two strategic plans were launched to reduce disparities: the HHS Action Plan to Reduce Racial and Ethnic Health Disparities and the National Stakeholder Strategy for Achieving Health Equity. In 2013, the National Standards for Culturally and Linguistically Appropriate Service in Health and Health Care (National CLAS Standards) were updated in an attempt to further improve health equity (DHHS, 2016).

Access in Rural Areas

Delivery of health care services in rural communities has always raised the question of how to bring advanced medical care to residents of sparsely settled areas. In the area of acute and long-term care, policies have been crafted in the form of the swing bed program and critical access hospitals (see the *Inpatient Facilities and Services* chapter).

In the medical care arena, financing high-tech equipment for a few people is not cost-efficient, and finding physicians who want to live in rural areas can be difficult. The use of telemedicine, especially as a means to increase access for patients with chronic diseases in rural areas, is expected to increase in coming years. A recent report projected that the number of consumers using telecommunication applications in the home will grow to 78.5 million by 2020 (Tractica, 2015). As health systems face increasing pressure to deliver high-quality care within strict financial constraints, telemedicine may prove a valuable way to use health care resources more cost-effectively. For example, it is estimated that chronic

diabetes care costs could be reduced by an average of 9% per year with the effective use of telemedicine as opposed to expensive office visits and hospitalizations (Wilson and Maeder, 2015). Furthermore, the uptake of telemedicine will most likely improve with the increasing availability of reliable wireless communication and user interface devices; these devices may allow telemedicine to be more easily used at the point of care.

A recent review of the literature concluded that there are two major drivers of telemedicine development (Wilson and Maeder, 2015). The first driver is high-volume demand for a particular service in which it is difficult to physically connect a patient and the expert needed to deal with the patient's needs. The second driver arises within high-criticality applications, in which the clinical expertise to deliver a service is needed urgently. The use of telemedicine is expanding beyond just providing care to rural areas and is increasingly used to provide cost-effective care to an increasing number of patients.

The *Health Services for Special Populations* chapter discussed various policy attempts that intend to alleviate shortages of health care professionals in rural areas. They include federal designation of health professional shortage areas (HPSA) and funding for the National Health Service Corps. The latter funding covers only a limited period of time per physician, however, so it does not help alleviate the health care workface shortages over a longer term. The ACA contains provisions to boost the health care workforce and funding for the National Health Service Corps.

Access and Low Income

In the United States, low-income mothers and their children are more likely to be uninsured than other groups. Many of these families also live in medically underserved areas, such as inner cities. Pregnant women in low-income families are far less likely to receive prenatal care than women in higher income categories. CHIP requires periodic reauthorization, which can hamper continuity of services to those enrolled. The Medicare Access and CHIP Reauthorization Act of 2015 (MACRA) extended the authorization of CHIP through September 30, 2017 (Congress.gov, 2015).

Access and Persons with HIV/AIDS

People with human immunodeficiency virus (HIV)/acquired immunodeficiency syndrome (AIDS) can face significant barriers in obtaining insurance coverage, and their illness can lead to catastrophic health care expenditures. The ACA makes it illegal to deny insurance coverage to people with HIV/AIDS. However, because of the many legal requirements that place increased burdens on health insurers, premiums for many insureds are expected to skyrocket. If this happens, people with HIV/AIDS and other individuals with serious preexisting conditions could well end up on Medicaid rolls.

In 2003, President George W. Bush pledged $15 billion over 5 years to combat HIV/AIDS in developing countries, with a particular focus on Africa. In 2010, the White House released the National HIV/AIDS Strategy, which outlined goals for reducing infection rates, increasing access to care, and reducing the disparities experienced in receiving care (White House, 2010). To support the achievement of these goals, federal funding for domestic and global HIV/AIDS programs and policies has increased, with a proposed $34 billion in funding requested for fiscal year 2017 (Kaiser Family Foundation, 2016).

Cost of Care

No other aspect of health care policy has received more attention during the past 30-plus years than efforts to contain health care costs. As pointed out elsewhere in this text, the government's main weapon of cost control has been payment cuts to providers. PPS has achieved success in curtailing inpatient costs, but outpatient costs have continued to climb. Direct control over utilization has not been tried by public payers (the Medicaid program in the state of Oregon is an exception), but it became widely unpopular when HMOs tried it. Whether public policy can be used to impose explicit rationing of health care services in the United States remains to be seen. The fragmented multipayer system does not lend itself to a centralized policy of cost containment.

As an example, prescription drug spending has been rising rapidly over the last few years, significantly driving up overall health care costs. Overall spending on prescription drugs increased more than 12% in 2014 and 2015, the largest increase in more than 10 years; by comparison, the U.S. drug prescription market grew at an average annual pace of only 2% from 2003 to 2013 (Aitken et al., 2016). The recent increase in drug expenditures has been driven by both brand-name entries into the market and price increases for generic drugs. More than 3,500 generic drugs at least doubled in price from 2008 to 2015, with increases up to 1,000% for some drugs (Jaret, 2015). Manufacturers cited research and development costs to justify these high pharmaceutical prices (Pharmaceutical Research and Manufacturers of America, 2016). In conjunction with this trend, several new high-value drugs obtained marketing approval from the Food and Drug Administration (FDA) and their launch into the U.S. market further drove up the overall cost of prescription drugs (PwC Health Research Institute, 2016).

The increasing drug prices have drawn considerable public attention, such as the outcry over Mylan's increase of the price for its EpiPen from $100 to $600 in 2016. Nevertheless, no government action has been taken to prevent pharmacy companies from hiking prices in the future. Thus, the prices of prescription drugs may well continue to rise in the upcoming years.

Quality of Care

Along with access and cost, quality of care is the third main concern of health care policy. In March 2001, the Institute of Medicine issued a comprehensive report, *Crossing the Quality Chasm*. Building on the extensive evidence collected by the IOM committee, the report identified six areas for quality improvement (Berwick, 2002):

- Safety: Patients should be as safe in health care facilities as they are in their homes.
- Effectiveness: The health care system should avoid overuse of ineffective care and underuse of effective care.
- Patient centeredness: Respect for the patient's choices, culture, social context, and special needs must be incorporated into the delivery of services.
- Timeliness: Waiting times and delays should be continually reduced for both patients and caregivers.
- Efficiency: Health care should engage in a never-ending pursuit to reduce total costs by curtailing waste, such as waste of supplies, equipment, space, capital, and the innovative human spirit.
- Equity: The system should seek to close racial and ethnic gaps in health status.

Research on Quality

Funding to evaluate new treatment methods and diagnostic tools has increased dramatically; so has funding for research to measure the outcomes of medical interventions and appropriateness of medical procedures. The mission of AHRQ (one of the 12 agencies within the DHHS) is to improve the quality, safety, efficiency, and effectiveness of health care for all Americans. AHRQ fulfills this mission by developing and working with the health care system to implement information that does the following:

- Reduces the risk of harm from health care services by using evidence-based research and technology to promote the delivery of the best possible care
- Transforms the practice of health care to achieve wider access to effective services and reduce unnecessary health care costs
- Improves health care outcomes by encouraging providers, consumers, and patients to use evidence-based information to make informed treatment decisions

Ultimately, AHRQ achieves its goals by translating research into improved health care practice and policy. Health care providers, patients, policymakers, payers, administrators, and others use AHRQ research findings to improve health care quality, accessibility, and outcomes of care (AHRQ, 2013).

Comparative effectiveness research (CER) is a relatively recent undertaking by the AHRQ. The Effective Health Care Program (EHCP) funds researchers, research centers, and academic organizations in working with AHRQ to produce effectiveness and comparative effectiveness

research. This program was created as a result of the Medicare Prescription Drug, Improvement, and Modernization Act (MMA) of 2003. EHCP reviews and synthesizes published and unpublished evidence, generates new evidence and tools, and translates research findings into more helpful formats. The program produces research reviews, original research reports, and research summaries (AHRQ, 2017).

Malpractice Reform

The federal government began its actions to relieve the malpractice crisis and devote greater attention to policing the quality of medical care with the Health Care Quality Act of 1986. This legislation mandated the creation of a national database within the DHHS to provide data on legal actions against health care providers. The database helps people recruiting physicians in one state discover actions against those physicians in other states. To date, though, comprehensive tort reform has failed to materialize despite much talk from politicians about its desirability.

Recent literature has both reported an association between medical malpractice expenditures and health care spending (Bilimoria et al., 2016; Popescu, 2015), and suggested that there is little evidence showing that reforms are an effective method for dealing with medical malpractice (Born and Karl, 2016). Some states have limited damage awards in malpractice cases, but no uniform national policy has emerged. One main reason for the inertia in this area is opposition from trial lawyers and consumer groups, who contend that limiting lawsuit awards hurts victims of egregious medical mistakes and reduces incentives to protect patient safety.

Role of Research in Policy Development

The research community can influence health policy making through documentation, analysis, and prescription (Longest, 2010). The first role of research in policy making is documentation—that is, the gathering, cataloging, and correlating of facts that depict the state of the world that policymakers face. This process may help define a given public policy problem or raise its political profile.

A second way in which research informs and influences policy making is through analysis of what does and does not work. Examples include program evaluation and outcomes research. Often taking the form of demonstration projects intended to provide a basis for determining the feasibility, efficacy, or practicality of a possible policy intervention, and analysis can help define solutions to health policy problems.

The third way in which research influences policy making is through prescription. Research demonstrating that a course of action being contemplated by policymakers may (or may not) lead to undesirable or unexpected consequences and can contribute significantly to policy making.

Future Considerations in Health Policy

Domestic Health Policy

With the enactment and promised repeal of the ACA, the landscape of health policy in the United States is again on the verge of undergoing significant change. While the health policy reforms after the ACA will impact access to health services, increased attention must also be given to ensuring high-quality, personalized, and

effective care for each and every patient. This consideration is especially important in the area of primary and preventive health policy, which can be used as a tool to both improve health outcomes and ensure long-term cost containment. Currently, initiatives are under way to expand and evaluate primary care delivery models, such as patient-centered medical homes, that aim to provide consistent, continuous, and high-quality care.

International Health Policy

Like domestic health policy efforts, international health initiatives have faced challenges in recent years as a result of continuing attempts to reduce government spending. In turn, government spending on global health initiatives has remained largely stable. For example, the Global Health Initiative (2014)—the umbrella for the global health programs launched by President Obama between 2009 and 2014—dedicated more than $50 billion to achieve health goals, including $13 billion to maternal health and child survival and $39 billion to HIV/AIDS funding.

Within the current budget constraints, initiatives must attempt to address immediate health concerns and build the capacity of the United States and other countries to address evolving health issues, which in turn requires a greater emphasis on innovation in global health policy. Global public health policies often vacillate with a changing political climate. In January 2017, for example, President Donald Trump reinstated the Mexico City Policy, which bans foreign nongovernmental organizations from performing or actively promoting abortion if they want to receive U.S. global health funding. This policy was first enacted under the Reagan administration in 1984, and as of 2017, had been in place for 17 of the past 32 years (Kaiser Family Foundation, 2017c.)

▶ Summary

The U.S. health care delivery system is the product of many health policies, which over the years have brought about incremental changes. Health policies are developed to serve the public interests; however, public interests are diverse. On the one hand, interest group politics often have a remarkable influence on policy making. On the other hand, a complex process and divided opinions may leave the public out of even major policy decisions. Although the public wants the government to control health care costs, it also believes that the federal government already controls too much of Americans' daily lives. Presidential leadership and party politics played a major role in the passage of the ACA, but several critical policy issues pertaining to access, cost, and quality remain unresolved. Among future challenges, cost containment will be the most daunting. The political feasibility of adopting a public policy to impose explicit rationing in the United States is unknown as of now.

▶ Test Your Understanding

Terminology

allocative tools	health policy	redistributive policies
distributive policies	public policies	regulatory tools

Review Questions

1. What is health policy? How can health policies be used as regulatory or allocative tools?

2. What are the principal features of U.S. health policy? Why do these features characterize U.S. health policy?

3. Identify health care interest groups and their concerns.

4. Why do you think the Clinton health reform failed but the Obama health reform succeeded?

5. What is the process of legislative health policy in the United States? How is this process related to the principal features of U.S. health policy?

6. Describe the critical policy issues related to access to care, cost of care, and quality of care.

▶ References

Agency for Healthcare Research and Quality (AHRQ). 2013. *AHRQ annual highlights, 2012.* Available at: http://www.ahrq.gov/news /newsroom/highlights/highlt12.html. Accessed August 2013.

Agency for Healthcare Research and Quality. Effective Health Care Program. 2017. *What is the Effective Health Care Program?* Available at: https://effectivehealthcare.ahrq.gov/index.cfm /what-is-the-effective-health-care-program1/. Accessed February 2017.

Aitken, M., et al. 2016. Has the era of slow growth for prescription drug spending ended? *Health Affairs* 35, no. 9: 1595–1603.

Alford, R. R. 1975. *Health care politics: Ideology and interest group barriers to reform.* Chicago, IL: University of Chicago Press.

American Taxpayer Relief Act of 2012 (ATRA). Pub. L. 112-240, Sec 643.

Berwick, D. M. 2002. A user's manual for the IOM's "Quality Chasm" report. *Health Affairs* 21, no. 3: 80–90.

Bilimoria, K. Y., et al. 2016. Association between state medical malpractice environment and surgical quality and cost in the United States. *Annals of Surgery* 263, no. 6: 1126–1132.

Bodenheimer, T. 1997. The Oregon health plan: Lessons for the nation. *New England Journal of Medicine* 337, no. 9: 651–655.

Born, P. H., and J. B. Karl. 2016. The effect of tort reform on medical malpractice insurance market trends. *Journal of Empirical Legal Studies* 13, no. 4: 718–755.

Colello, K. J., and J. Mulvey. 2013. *Community Living Assistance Services and Supports (CLASS): Overview and summary of provisions.* CRS Report R40847. Washington, DC: Congressional Research Service.

Commission on Long-Term Care. 2016. *Home.* Available at: http://www.ltccommission.org/. Accessed February 2017.

Congress.gov. 2015. *H.R.2: Medicare Access and CHIP Reauthorization Act of 2015.* Available at: https://www.congress.gov/bill/114th-congress /house-bill/2. Accessed February 2017.

Coughlin, T., et al. 1999. A conflict of strategies: Medicaid managed care and Medicaid maximization. *Health Services Research* 34, no. 1: 281–293.

Falcone, D., and L. C. Hartwig. 1991. Congressional process and health policy: Reform and retrenchment. In: *Health policies and policy.* 2nd ed. T. Litman and L. Robins, eds. New York, NY: John Wiley & Sons. pp. 126–144.

Global Health Initiative. 2014. *U.S. global health programs.* Available at: https://www.ghi.gov /about/index.html#.WJy0mm8rLIU. Accessed February 2017.

Health Resources and Services Administration. 2013. *The Affordable Care Act and health centers.* Available at: http://bphc.hrsa.gov/about /healthcenterfactsheet.pdf. Accessed August 2013.

Jaret, P. 2015. *Prices spike for some generic drugs: Costs for brand names also increasing.* Available at: http://www.aarp.org/health/drugs-supplements /info-2015/prices-spike-for-generic-drugs. html. Accessed January 2017.

Kaiser Family Foundation. 2016. *U.S. federal funding for HIV/AIDS: Trends over time.* Available at: http://kff.org/global-health-policy/fact-sheet /u-s-federal-funding-for-hivaids-trends-over -time/#footnote-190024-2. Accessed February 2017.

Kaiser Family Foundation. 2017a. *Status of state action on the Medicaid expansion decision, as of January 1, 2017.* Available at: http://kff.org /health-reform/state-indicator/state-activity -around-expanding-medicaid-under-the -affordable-care-act. Accessed February 2017.

Kaiser Family Foundation. 2017b. *State Health Insurance Marketplace Types, 2017, as of January 2017.* Available at: http://kff.org/health -reform/state-indicator/state-health-insurance -marketplace-types. Accessed February 2017.

Kaiser Family Foundation. 2017c. *The Mexico City Policy: An explainer.* Available at: http://kff.org /global-health-policy/press-release/the-mexico -city-policy-an-explainer/. Accessed February 2017.

Kaiser Family Foundation. 2017d. *Kaiser Health Tracking Poll: The Public's Views on the ACA.* Available at: http://www.kff.org/interactive /kaiser-health-tracking-poll-the-publics -views-on-the-aca/#?response=Favorable --Unfavorable&aRange=twoYear. Accessed June 2017.

Kaiser Family Foundation. 2017e. *Summary of the Affordable Care Act.* Available at: http://www .kff.org/health-reform/fact-sheet/summary-of -the-affordable-care-act/. Accessed June 2017.

Longest, B. B. 2010. *Health policymaking in the United States.* 5th ed. Ann Arbor, MI: Health Administration Press.

Lowry, R. October 29, 2013. Obama's false insurance promise. *New York Post.* Available at: http://nypost.com/2013/10/29/obamas-false -insurance-promise. Accessed October 2013.

Morone J. A., et al. 2008. *Health policies and policy.* 4th ed. New York, NY: Delmar.

National Conference of State Legislatures. 2016. *CON: Certificate of need state laws.* Available at: http:// www.ncsl.org/research/health/con-certificate-of -need-state-laws.aspx. Accessed May 2017.

National Institutes of Health (NIH). 2016. *NIH FY 2017 budget roll-out.* Available at: https:// www.nih.gov/sites/default/files/about-nih /nih-director/testimonies/fy17-budget-rollout -slides-20160209.pdf. Accessed February 2017.

Oberlander, J. 2010. Long time coming: Why health reform finally passed. *Health Affairs* 29, no. 6: 1112–1116.

Oliver, T. R., et al. 2004. A political history of Medicare and prescription drug coverage. *Milbank Quarterly* 82, no. 2: 283–354.

Patel, K., and J. McDonough. 2010. From Massachusetts to 1600 Pennsylvania Avenue: Aboard the health reform express. *Health Affairs* 29, no. 6: 1106–1111.

Pharmaceutical Research and Manufacturers of America. 2016. *Prescription medicines: Costs in context.* Available at: http://phrma-docs .phrma.org/sites/default/files/pdf/prescription -medicines-costs-in-context-extended.pdf. Accessed January 2017.

Popescu, G. H. 2015. Increased medical malpractice expenditures as a main determinant of growth in health care spending. *American Journal of Medical Research* 2, no. 1: 80.

PwC Health Research Institute. 2016. *Medical cost trend: Behind the Numbers 2016.* Washington, DC: PwC.

Roy, A. 2012. *How the AARP made $2.8 billion by supporting Obamacare's cuts to Medicare.* Available at: http://www.forbes.com/sites/aroy /2012/09/22/the-aarps-2-8-billion-reasons -for-supporting-obamacares-cuts-to-medicare. Accessed October 2013.

Shi, L. 2014. *Introduction to health policy.* Chicago, IL: Health Administration Press, AUPHA.

Tractica. 2015. *Home health technologies.* Available at: https://www.tractica.com/research/home -health-technologies/. Accessed June 2017.

U.S. Department of Health and Human Services (DHHS). 2016. *HHS finalizes streamlined Medicare payment system that rewards clinicians for quality patient care.* Available at: https:// wayback.archive-it.org/3926/20170127192642 /https://www.hhs.gov/about/news/2016/10/14 /hhs-finalizes-streamlined-medicare-payment -system-rewards-clinicians-quality-patient -care.html. Accessed May 2017.

White House. 2010. *National HIV/AIDS strategy for the United States.* Available at: http://aids.gov /federal-resources/national-hiv-aids-strategy /nhas.pdf. Accessed August 2013.

Wilson, L. S. and A. J. Maeder. 2015. Recent directions in telemedicine: Review of trends in research and practice. *Healthcare Informatics Research* 21, no. 4: 213–222.

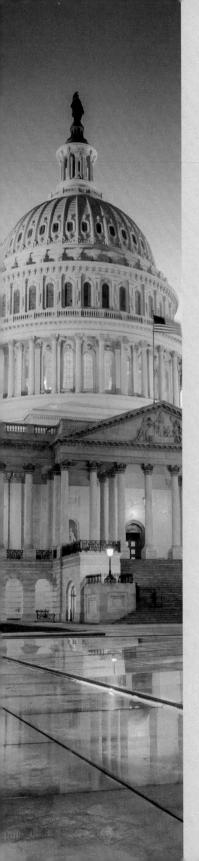

PART V

System Outlook

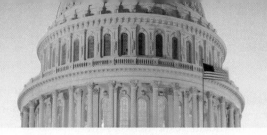

CHAPTER 14

The Future of Health Services Delivery

LEARNING OBJECTIVES

- Identify the major forces of future change that affect health care delivery.
- Assess health care reform in transition in the United States.
- Discuss the evolving health care delivery infrastructure and the progress in population health.
- Describe the special skills needed by future nurses, physicians, and other health care workers.
- Evaluate the future of long-term care.
- Describe the role of international cooperation in dealing with global threats.
- Provide an overview of new frontiers in clinical technology.
- Survey the future of evidence-based health care based on comparative effectiveness research and patient-oriented outcomes research.

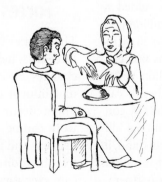

"Will the U.S. have a single-payer system?"

▶ Introduction

The outlook for health care delivery in the United States is predicated on major current developments and the course that these developments might take in the foreseeable future. Any attempts to project the future of health care inevitably provoke more questions than answers, however, the future often turns out differently than people anticipate (Kenen, 2011). Indeed, prognostication is an art that is fraught with assumptions that may not materialize and other developments may yet be unforeseen (Vitalari, 2016).

In spite of the employer and individual mandates contained in the Affordable Care Act (ACA), employer-based health insurance has eroded in case of both small and large employers. The main beneficiaries of the ACA were those who obtained coverage under Medicaid (11 million people in 2016; Congressional Budget Office [CBO], 2016), those who were able to obtain private insurance coverage through the government-sponsored exchanges thanks to federal subsidies that lowered their cost of premiums (12 million people enrolled in 2016, of whom 10 million received subsidies; CBO, 2016), and adults younger than age 26 who were added to their parents' health plans (4.5 million people; Furman and Fiedler, 2015). In 2016, the number of uninsured Americans was estimated at approximately 27 million (CBO, 2016). On the supply side, the health care industry has reacted to these trends by consolidating and forming organizational alliances in which hospitals, physicians, and, in many instances, managed care organizations (MCOs) have integrated as major partners.

When we look at health care delivery as an institution in and of itself, several external factors can be identified that exert powerful influences in causing this institution to change and conform. Certain forces, such as demographic trends and political dynamics, can be expected to follow a foreseeable course, so that some predictions can be made on this basis. For other external factors, even short-term predictions are difficult. For instance, it is impossible to predict the future course of the U.S. economy and family incomes, both of which will affect what individual Americans and the nation may or may not be able to afford.

Future change also relies on historical precedents. Certain fundamental features of U.S. health care delivery, such as a largely private infrastructure and the society's fundamental values, have, in the past, prompted resistance to any proposals for a sweeping transformation of health care. Yet, certain historical precedents have also been used as a springboard for current change, and they will no doubt influence future change as well.

This chapter puts the future of health care in the larger national and global context. It also assesses the likely future course of health care reform, clinical technology, and new models of delivering health care.

▶ Forces of Future Change

The framework presented here includes forces that help us understand why certain changes have occurred in the past, and that inform the direction of change that might occur in the future. This framework can be used for viewing health care delivery and policy from a macro perspective. In addition, it can be used by health care executives to craft strategies for their organizations that are aligned with the changes occurring in the broader health care environment.

The eight forces included in the framework are (1) social and demographic, (2) political, (3) economic, (4) technological, (5) informational, (6) ecological, (7) global, and (8) anthro-cultural. These forces often interact in complex ways, and these interactions are generally difficult to interpret. Keen observation of these forces, however, can create opportunities for change.

How those opportunities are either realized or forgone determines the nature of change. With the passage of time, some forces become more dominant than others. The directions of change that these forces may portend have implications for cost and, therefore, affordability of health care; access to health care services; and power balancing within the health care system among the powerful players. Hence, the U.S. health care system will continue to evolve, but no one truly knows its ultimate destiny.

For several decades, the U.S. health care delivery system has not been driven by free-market forces. Over the years, the government has become a major player that controls a growing segment of health care financing, and it has increasingly wielded control over the private sector through its legal and regulatory powers. Yet, the government needs the private health care sector to serve its millions of beneficiaries in public health insurance programs. At least for the foreseeable future, tension and power balancing between the private and public sectors will continue and, for better or for worse, we will see ongoing changes in the way Americans receive health care.

Currently, health care expenditures account for almost one-fifth of the U.S. economy. The ongoing ability to deliver health care is, therefore, closely tied to the nation's economic health, regardless of whether health care is delivered through private or public insurance programs.

Social and Demographic Forces

From a demographic standpoint, the United States is getting bigger, older, and more ethnically diverse. Shifts in the demographic composition of the population, cultural factors, and lifestyles affect not only the need for health care, but also the means by which those needs will be met. Demographic trends will also continue to affect the United States' ability to afford health care services.

The elderly, vulnerable populations, and people with certain high-cost health conditions all present varied needs. These groups also have the highest costs, so they are essentially drivers of change in the health care system. Vulnerable populations in the United States receive health care mainly through Medicaid and Medicare. Between 2004 and 2014, the proportion of Medicaid adult beneficiaries with complex activity limitation[1] increased from 28.9% to 39.7% (National Center for Health Statistics [NCHS], 2016, p. 320). Limitation of activities has also increased among the Medicare population (NCHS, 2016, p. 330). One study found that the annual average health care spending per person among the high-needs population—defined as adults with three or more chronic conditions and a functional limitation—is four times higher than the spending per person for the general adult U.S. population, and three times higher than the spending per person for adults

---

[1] Limitations in core areas of functioning that include physical, cognitive, emotional, and social domains.

with chronic conditions but no functional limitation. The high-needs population is predominantly covered under Medicare and Medicaid (Hayes et al., 2016).

These expanding government programs are currently on an unsustainable financial path: Spending growth in these programs is expected to exceed growth of the overall economy. The Congressional Budget Office (2017) has projected that the U.S. gross domestic product (GDP) will grow by 2.1% in 2017, but the rate of growth in outlays is expected to be 4.1% for Medicare (net of premiums paid by the beneficiaries) and 5.5% for Medicaid. Subsequently, the net spending for both Medicaid and Medicare is expected to rise at an average annual rate of 7% (CBO, 2017), which is substantially higher than general inflation and the rate of national economic growth. Moreover, while the elderly population continues to grow, growth in the size of the working age population is moderating. Hence, a larger number of beneficiaries must be supported by fewer taxpayers.

For many years, the trustees of the Medicare trust funds have projected the number of years until the trust funds become insolvent. In the past, those dates have come and gone, while the trust funds remained solvent. While it is impossible to forecast future economic conditions, in 2016 the Hospital Insurance trust fund was projected to be insolvent by 2028 (Davis, 2016). The fate of this trust fund will ultimately depend on the ability of taxpayers to support the program through mandatory tax deductions. The same applies to the Supplementary Medical Insurance (SMI) trust fund and Medicaid. For SMI, which mainly covers payments to physicians (Part B) and cost of prescription drugs (Part D), premiums have been increased for the beneficiaries to buffer the growth in spending. Both Medicare and Medicaid face future challenges that remain unresolved as yet. Whether benefit cuts may have to be applied to Medicare and Medicaid in the future is anyone's guess.

An equally challenging factor is how population shifts affect the composition of the health care workforce, because health care delivery is a labor-intensive enterprise. In a free society, people choose their professions and where they work. Hence, social and demographic factors play a significant role in determining the number of health care professionals and their geographic distribution. Future immigration may be one factor that affects the supply of health care professionals.

The U.S. society's cultural mix, which also reflects the rate and nature of immigration, will continue to slowly transform health care delivery in this country. For example, language and other cultural barriers affect both patients and caregivers. Language training and posting of signs in different languages are just small pieces of this more complex cultural puzzle. Social and cultural factors affect exposure and vulnerability to disease, risk-taking behaviors, health promotion and disease prevention, and health care–seeking behavior. For example, emergency department (ED) use is disproportionately higher among blacks compared to whites (NCHS, 2016). A large population of illegal immigrants, estimated to number approximately 11.3 million (Krogstad et al., 2017) and not covered by any health insurance program, also taps into the nation's health care resources through ED use and charity care. Historically, the

United States has failed to craft and pursue a well-thought-out immigration policy. Hence, the effects of immigration on the economy and on health care remain unclear. Social and cultural factors also play a role in shaping perceptions of and responses to health problems.

To a large extent, population growth and aging are uncontrollable factors. Even individual responsibility for one's own health is largely beyond the control of employers and the government, except when they offer incentives to persuade people to engage in healthy behaviors to prevent disease and disability. Personal lifestyles will significantly impact the future of wellness, prevention, health promotion, and the burden associated with financing and delivery of health care.

Economic Forces

Economic growth, employment, household incomes, and the national debt are major forces that will determine the availability of health care services, their cost, and their affordability. Household incomes, especially for middle-class families, largely determine the affordability of health care, and household incomes depend on the nation's economic health and quality of employment. In a survey reported by the Federal Reserve Board (2016), almost one-third of American adults stated that they were "struggling to get by" or "just getting by" financially. A little more than one-fifth of employed adults indicated that they were either working multiple jobs, doing informal work for pay in addition to their main job, or both.

Jobs requiring above-average education, training, and experience have been growing faster than those requiring below-average preparation. Yet, the earnings of American workers have increased only modestly (16% in 25 years), and both employer-based health care and retirement benefits have decreased (Pew Research Center, 2016).

In a survey conducted by the Pew Research Center (2016), a large proportion of Americans expressed concern that outsourcing of jobs to other countries has been particularly damaging to the U.S. workforce. It appears that outsourcing of jobs affects mostly well-educated people, because households with higher incomes and people with higher levels of education have been more discouraged about workplace trends than those with lower incomes and less education.

Americans have also expressed mixed views about how well colleges and universities are preparing students for today's job market. For example, only 16% of Americans think that a 4-year degree prepares students "very well" for good-paying jobs, 29% think that it prepares students "not too well" or "not at all well," and approximately half think it prepares students "somewhat well" (Pew Research Center, 2016). Clearly, institutions of higher education have an immense responsibility to furnish job-related skills for the future. Better-paying jobs can be brought to the United States, as President Donald Trump has promised, but the workforce may not be adequately prepared for them. To address future challenges in health care delivery, such conditions need to change dramatically.

The federal debt is projected to grow from $20.3 trillion in 2017 to $30.0 trillion in 2027 (CBO, 2017). There are opinions, but no plausible solutions to address this issue. Some experts even claim that the national debt does not need to be paid off. Economists often disagree on key issues because of the different assumptions they make, yet a simple argument can be made in this case: Debts must be paid off in private life; otherwise, a default occurs that often has unpleasant consequences. The same must be true for national debt: If a default occurs, there will be unpleasant consequences for many Americans. Any default would negatively affect the economy, households, and entitlement programs such as Medicaid, Medicare, and Social Security. Hence, there are obvious concerns that the public debt must be reduced. Solutions for debt reduction are the reverse of what creates debt—a combination of spending cuts, tax increases, and economic growth. Spending cuts and tax hikes are both unpalatable and highly unpopular politically. Even if U.S. economic growth can be stimulated so that it reaches 4% or 5% per year (in 2016, the GDP grew at a measly 1.6%; Trading Economics, 2017), it will still fall short of the projected rate of growth for public health care programs.

The Trump presidency had just begun at the time this manuscript was completed. From the little that is known, it appears that the economic outlook for the United States—and its implications for health care—may hinge on several factors in the context of the Trump agenda:

- Success in bringing jobs to the United States from non-U.S. locations. A manufacturing recovery within the United States would add to both household incomes and tax revenues.
- Development of domestically produced energy. The United States has some of the largest oil and gas reserves in the world. Hence, energy self-sufficiency would provide a tremendous boost to the U.S. economy, increased wages, and lower energy prices for consumers.
- The effects of "repealing and replacing" the ACA. If more part-time jobs can be converted into full-time positions, thereby boosting household incomes, and if health care can be made more affordable, millions of Americans will reap the benefits.
- A "border tax" on goods produced overseas by U.S. corporations and brought into the country for sale. Such a tax could cause consumer prices to rise. It could have a negative effect on consumers, unless the other factors discussed here could more than offset this factor.
- Tax cuts, increased defense spending, and spending on the infrastructure. These expenditures could improve employment, but would cause the national debt to rise.
- Less regulation. Scaling back stifling regulations could jump-start businesses and hiring of workers.

At this point, it is unclear how the combined effects of these initiatives might eventually play out.

Political Forces

Public policy is closely intertwined with almost all aspects of health care delivery. Policies that affect education at home, as well as immigration policies, can determine not only the number but also the qualifications of the future health care workforce. Controls over the nation's total economic spending and tax policies also lie in the hands of politicians. Will they have the resolve, for example, to cut runaway government spending?

The history of health care in the United States and in other countries is replete with examples of major changes brought about through political will, depending on which party has the legislative majority. Party politics along ideological lines can hold up major initiatives from moving forward. Politics, however, serve a nation best when it is subservient to the people's needs and wants. Americans have remained divided over major policy issues, however, and health care is one such issue. Politicians, therefore, must try to assess the needs and wants of their main constituents.

Trump's presidential victory in 2016 also coincided with Republican majorities in both the House of Representatives and the Senate, for the first time since 2003–2007 under President George W. Bush. Hence, it is possible that much of Trump's agenda could pass through Congress. The three branches of government—executive, legislative, and judicial—are independent entities, however, and serious disagreements can arise among them. That is especially the case when the Congress and the courts in the United States are divided along ideological lines. Given this reality, regardless of Trump's previous successes as a businessman, he will face a quite different playing field in the political arena.

Technological Forces

It is widely believed that technological innovation in medical sciences will continue to revolutionize health care. Americans strongly favor ongoing innovation, availability, and use of new technology. One recent example of this preference is the passage into law of the 21st Century Cures Act of 2016, which is aimed at advancing medical innovation and quick access to new treatments. The high cost of research and development and the subsequent costs associated with unrestrained use of technology do raise questions about how long this pattern can go on, given that growth in health care spending will continue to surpass GDP growth. Technologies that promote a greater degree of self-reliance or achieve cost-efficiencies will almost certainly receive much attention in the future. Nevertheless, the overall effect of technology is to increase costs unless it is accompanied by utilization control measures.

Informational Forces

Information technology (IT) has numerous applications in health care delivery. IT has also become an indispensable tool for managing today's health care organizations. Realization of IT's full potential is still evolving and will continue well into the future. The use of smart cards in health care, for example, can combat forgery and identity theft, thereby curtailing fraud and abuse (Horowitz, 2012). Americans have often viewed smart cards with suspicion and distrust, mainly because of fears that their personal health information could be compromised. Smart cards are already in wide use in European health systems, and it is only a matter of time before their use becomes more common in the United States. That use could well begin with Medicare and Medicaid beneficiaries.

Ecological Forces

New diseases, natural disasters, and bioterrorism have major implications for public health, and potentially even global consequences. Communicable diseases—such as new strains of influenza—and disease related to environmental agents—such as vector-borne diseases (e.g., West Nile virus and chikungunya virus)—can trigger mass hysteria, particularly in large population centers, especially when the disease remains mysterious and treatments are not readily available. For example, some cases of the deadly Ebola virus infection created widespread concern, especially among health care workers, in the United States in 2014. The mosquito-borne Zika virus has caused concerns among the general U.S. population. **Zoonoses** are diseases or infections that are naturally transmittable from vertebrate animals to humans. Growth of populations around the globe will intensify interactions at the human–animal–ecosystems interface, raising the probability of engendering diseases that are as yet unknown.

When a significant number of people are affected or threatened by disease, research and technological innovation go into high gear. Technologies, such as remote sensing and geographic information systems (GIS), will find ongoing applications in public health and safety in such circumstances.

Natural disasters not only disrupt people's daily lives, but also create conditions that pose serious health risks through contamination of food and water. Health problems and psychological distress often follow. The roles of the Centers for Disease Control and Prevention (CDC) and other partnering agencies will continue to evolve as new challenges emerge. On the down side, the growing need to combat new ecological threats will divert resources from the provision of routine health care to patients.

Global Forces

The economies of the world have become progressively more interdependent. Globalization has become an extremely complex phenomenon, because the various forces discussed here interact as this process continues to evolve (Huynen et al., 2005). For example, Rennen and Martens (2003) define contemporary globalization in terms of an intensification of cross-national cultural, economic, political, social, and technological interactions. Hence, health and health care in various countries will continue to be affected in diverse ways through multiple pathways.

To give a simple example of how globalization affects health care, consider the "brain drains" of physicians, therapists, and nurses from developing countries to relieve shortages in developed countries. This sort of immigration generally occurs for personal economic reasons, but social, cultural, and technological factors may hinder the full utilization of these health care professionals' talents and learning. Economically backward countries have experienced "brain gains" as the number of health professionals from developed countries on medical missions to provide care in poorer countries has grown globally (Martiniuk et al., 2012). Medical missionaries do charity work out of a sense of deeply rooted personal ethics and compassion, but cross-cultural factors have at least some diluting effects on their optimal performance.

There are indications that the trend toward globalization in health care will intensify. Increasingly, generic drugs are being manufactured in Asian countries for export to Europe, Canada, and the United States. This trend has made drugs more affordable in the United States, but ensuring the drugs' safety and securing adequate supplies to meet demand on a consistent basis pose major challenges for the Food and Drug Administration (FDA).

Medical tourism is likely to increase as more people opt for consumer-driven health plans, which give greater control to consumers on how to spend their own savings on health care. Given the high cost of health care services in the United States and Europe, providers in other countries will continue to offer a wider array of lower-cost but almost identical high-quality health services, with these services often coming with greater amenities (Reeves, 2011).

Finally, cross-border telemedicine used in conjunction with medical tourism is becoming a rapidly developing trend (George and Henthorne, 2009). Several U.S. hospitals have established affiliations with hospitals in foreign countries. In future, foreign hospitals and clinics are likely to provide services within the United States.

Anthro-Cultural Forces

In the health care context, the term *anthro-cultural* refers to a society's beliefs, values, ethos, traditions, and experiences. In the United States, the beliefs and values have traditionally been those espoused primarily by middle-class Americans. These beliefs and values have historically acted as a strong deterrent against attempts to initiate radical changes in the financing and delivery of health care. In a society that is becoming more culturally diverse, however, Americans are now evenly split on the question of whether providing health insurance to all Americans is a government responsibility: In 2015, 47% of Americans stated that it was the responsibility of the federal government to

make sure all Americans had health care coverage (Gallup, 2016a). Such a belief reflects a gradual shift away from traditional American views. In terms of their experiences, while 65% of Americans are satisfied with the health care services they receive, in 2016, there was a 2% drop in the satisfaction rating since the ACA was implemented in 2014. The drop was noted among people covered under various types of health insurance (Gallup, 2016b).

▶ The Future of Health Care Reform

The prospects of a single-payer system have been pushed back for several reasons. The ACA is likely to be rolled back, though some of its features will be retained. Universal coverage in the United States is possible, but under certain conditions of austerity.

No Single-Payer System

With the anticipated demise of the ACA (at the time of this writing), the prospect of U.S. health care being transformed into a **single-payer system**—that is, a national health care program in which the financing and insurance functions are taken over by the federal government—may have been averted. During the congressional deliberations among the Democrats that led to the ACA in 2010, it appeared that some legislators wanted to create a single-payer system, dubbed the "public option" (McHugh, 2013). Because of a lack of support for this proposal within the ACA from some Democrats, and to build the consensus that became essential to pass the ACA, the single-payer option was eventually dropped (Halpin and Harbage, 2010).

Although Trump had praised a single-payer system as something that was working well in countries such as Canada and Scotland (Camp, 2016), any proposals from the White House to move in that direction will undoubtedly draw strong opposition from the Republicans in Congress, at the risk of fracturing the party. Yet, 58% of U.S. adults seem to favor the idea of replacing the ACA with a federally funded health care system that provides insurance for all Americans (Gallup, 2016c).

There are six main contentious issues in establishing a single-payer plan in the United States.

- Such a plan would shift a major segment of the costs from the private sector to the public sector, meaning the taxpayers. Hence, taxes would have to be increased—a notion that Americans have historically rejected.
- A single-payer system would require overt rationing[2] to curtail runaway costs, something that has been unpopular with the majority of Americans. In other developed nations, **universal access**—that is, basic health care for all—has been a part of the cultural ethos, combined with the realization that some form of rationing and higher taxes would be the cost that came with it. These nations have been able to achieve universal access thanks to a robust primary care system that is lacking in the United States.
- A single-payer system would cause major disruptions in well-ingrained programs, such as Medicare and Medicaid. The elderly, in particular, would be skeptical of any attempts by the government to take away Medicare, a plan in which they invested throughout their working lives.
- The government would assume the functions of insurance and financing. In turn, a single-payer system would increase the size of government bureaucracy, which would become necessary to manage expenditures amounting to one-fifth of the nation's economy. Hence, a single-payer system would suffer from government inefficiency.
- Government control over insurance and financing would cause major disruptions within the health care industry. These changes would undoubtedly inspire opposition from insurers and health care providers.
- From a historical and cultural standpoint, under the U.S. Constitution, delivery of health care to all citizens is not the primary function of government.

Proponents of a single-payer system will likely continue to push their agenda forward. For example, Gaffney and colleagues (2016) would like to see the ACA transformed into a single-payer system. According to these authors:

> Despite the ACA, many serious problems remain in American health care. Uninsurance and underinsurance endure, bureaucracy is growing, costs are likely to rise, and caring relationships take second place to the financial

---

[2] Certain forms of covert rationing exist in the United States. For example, self-rationing exists in health plans that have high deductibles, and consumers decide whether and when to obtain certain types of services. Overt rationing is deliberately imposed by the government who is the payer for health care services in single-payer systems.

prerogatives of health insurers and providers. A single-payer NHP [national health program] offers a salutary alternative.

A single-payer system is not necessarily a cure for the issues of cost, access, and quality in the current health care system. Years of experience with Medicare and Medicaid bear that statement out. Medicaid and its accompanying government bureaucracy remain unpopular with physicians. Furthermore, middle-class Americans do not appear to have the appetite for an overhaul of the U.S. health care system through government fiat, as the polls concerning the ACA suggest. In a 2016 Gallup poll, 55% of Americans expressed their preference for a privately run health care system, whereas only 41% preferred a government-run system. Discontent with the ACA—which had become a campaign issue—among middle-class voters may well have been a significant factor that resulted in the defeat of Hillary Clinton (Trump's opponent) in the 2016 presidential election. After the economy, health care and the ACA were top concerns in voters' minds during this election (Gallup, 2016a). Hence, a single-payer system in the United States does not appear to be a possibility for the foreseeable future.

Reforming the Reform

Health care reform is no longer a dead issue because of the campaign promises made by Trump to "repeal and replace Obamacare." The ACA is a complex piece of legislation, and its total repeal and replacement will be a daunting task. If handled haphazardly, any new reform initiatives could risk destabilizing some key areas of health care. Hence, the promised reforms would very likely retain some of the provisions of the existing law. In essence, the ACA could be transformed, albeit in some major ways, in lieu of being scrapped entirely. The most unpopular parts of the ACA, such as the individual and business mandates and penalties, are also the most likely parts to be repealed.

Future health care reform will have to address two broad issues: cost of health insurance for businesses and individuals, and cost of health care services (discussed in the next section). In essence, overall costs need to be reduced to a level that will allow most people to afford health insurance, and enable them to access health care services when necessary. Unfortunately, these issues have persisted under the ACA.

Trump has proposed that insurance companies should be allowed to sell health plans across the states. That prospect, it is argued, would stimulate competition, provide more options to people, and bring down prices. Critics have countered that selling health plans on a national scale would be difficult to implement because of varying state regulations and the overwhelming task of having to establish provider networks (Sanger-Katz, 2015). If interstate marketing of health plans is to become feasible, it must be done in a way that reduces the high administrative costs associated with the ACA. For example, new administrative costs attributable to the ACA were estimated to total $273.6 billion, which translated into $1,375 for each newly insured person, or 22.5% of the total federal government expenditures for the ACA program (Himmelstein and Woolhandler, 2015).

Federal subsidies, in one form or another, to assist low-income people to buy health insurance are likely to be retained in any new reform proposals. In the past, Republican lawmakers have proposed tax credits and vouchers to help such individuals purchase health insurance. More importantly, people who have benefited from federal subsidies are not likely to give them up.

Consumer-directed high-deductible health plans (HDHPs), coupled with a tax-free spending account, may play a significant role in any future health care reform, because these plans are especially appealing to young healthy people. HDHPs provide an incentive to curtail unnecessary care that other types of health insurance plans actually encourage through the phenomena of moral hazard and provider-induced demand. A multiyear study demonstrated that HDHPs do indeed curtail health care spending, with long-lasting effects. Moreover, at least over a 3-year period, this study found no evidence that decreased spending resulted in complications from foregone care (Haviland et al., 2016).

Defined contribution programs, similar to those found in employer-based retirement plans, could also be a part of health care reform. Under such a program, the benefit to the employee is a fixed amount paid by the employer. The employee can then decide on the type of health insurance plan that would be most appropriate for him or her as an individual and for the employee's family.

A critical issue with individual enrollments in the ACA plans offered through the exchanges was that fewer young and healthy people enrolled than had been expected. Only 28% of those people who enrolled in the exchange plans were members of the 18–34 age group, a percentage well below the 40% needed to make the plans actuarially stable (Herman, 2016). This pattern constitutes a phenomenon called adverse selection. In it, people who really need to use health care—for instance, people with preexisting medical conditions—enroll in larger numbers than those who are healthy. The result of such adverse selection with the ACA was that premiums had to be raised to unaffordable levels, and some large insurers simply left the exchanges because of financial losses sustained. Prior to the ACA, many states had managed their own **high-risk pools** to enable people with preexisting conditions to purchase health insurance at more affordable rates than was possible otherwise. To reduce premium costs, high-risk pools would be reestablished under new reform proposals.

Medicaid has historically and legally been within each state's domain to implement and modify. Each state's administrative right with regard to Medicaid was upheld by the 2012 U.S. Supreme Court decision in the first major challenge to the constitutionality of the ACA. It remains to be seen what the states that have expanded Medicaid under the ACA will do in the future, mainly because loss of federal funds would be at stake. The ACA provided federal funding to cover the cost of Medicaid expansion at 100% through 2016, then rolled this rate back gradually to 90% in 2020.

According to Trump's campaign promises, reform of the Veterans Health Administration (VHA) will be part of the broader health care reform. Trump has promised that veterans can obtain timely physical and mental health services by seeking care either at VHA facilities or from private providers.

Other changes could include tort reform to mitigate the effects of malpractice lawsuits against physicians and hospitals. Meaningful tort reform could lower the cost of health care, as the costs of malpractice lawsuits are eventually passed on to consumers in the form of higher insurance premiums. The CBO

(2013) has estimated that reducing the size of very large malpractice claims could save $57 billion over 10 years in the public programs alone, thereby reducing federal deficit spending (which ultimately increases the national debt).

The regulatory burden that ails the U.S. health care system must also be trimmed. Ever-increasing government regulations stifle economic growth, and result in inefficiencies and loss of productivity.

Going forward, reform initiatives to dismantle some of the contentious areas of the ACA will not be simple to achieve. Experts have already lined up with their predictive speculations, with many claiming that harm will inevitably ensue from any changes. Battles between ideologues are likely to intensify in the future. In any event, the U.S. government does need to address the nagging issues that the ACA either failed to solve or helped to create.

Universal Coverage and Access

There is no question that the United States needs some type of universal coverage, but the nation also needs to strengthen the health delivery infrastructure. As Lamm and Blank (2005) cogently stated, universal coverage is feasible but, to financially sustain such a system, Americans will have to "give up a cherished dream: the dream of total, universal care for any ailment freely available on demand." Hence, a change in mindset will be necessary. As Paulus and colleagues (2008) have proposed, the underpinnings for a change in philosophy should be to seek value in health care. Such a change necessitates asking the questions: What do we propose to get in return for what we pay? How much should we pay for what we should reasonably expect to get?

The ACA's push for IT adoption by health care organizations and promotion of care coordination of defined populations through accountable care organizations (ACOs) and patient-centered medical home models were perhaps steps in the right direction in achieving value-based health care. The ACA also promoted some innovative payment methods—for example, shared savings in the payment arrangements with ACOs. The effects of these delivery and payment models need close examination to determine which models have been successful in delivering the best value. Future health care reform should build on the best-value approaches.

▶ The Health Care Delivery Infrastructure of the Future

The health care delivery infrastructure will continue to evolve as some innovative models demonstrate success in providing better value for the money and improved patient outcomes. ACOs and patient-centered medical homes are still in their infancy. Newer models are likely to emerge and be adopted if they prove adept at delivering value. To serve a variety of needs, several different models of care will find a footing in the U.S. health care delivery system. Yet, having different models of care by no means suggests a dismantling of the traditional infrastructure consisting of hospitals of different types, small and large clinics, and other existing settings for care. By taking advantage of certain incentives in the payment systems, providers could align themselves into formal and informal structures that promote the desirable goals of providing better care at reduced cost.

Certain organizational and patient-related challenges will have to be overcome to achieve these goals. Adoption of new models of care often requires organizational changes and staff realignments, which pose leadership challenges. Providers participating in these alliances will need assurances that reimbursement will be adequate to cover their services. Patient skepticism will need to be addressed because patients will not choose an ACO or a medical home, for instance, but rather will be assigned to one by the payer. Hence, practical implications must be considered when implementing any new model. Moving from concept to practice is not always an easy transition.

Care coordination, ease of navigating the system by patients, preventive care, and management of chronic conditions will continue to be the focus as the health care delivery infrastructure continues to evolve. Patient activation and patient-centered care will remain the driving forces from the standpoint of individual patients. In addition, community-oriented primary care and population health will receive increased attention. Ongoing adoption of IT, use of cost-saving technology, and evidence-based care will undergird the system to eliminate waste, improve efficiencies, and produce better patient outcomes. IT systems, for instance, will be essential for the information exchange that is necessary for care coordination across several providers. Payers will hold health care organizations accountable for achieving the desired goals in the areas just mentioned. Collectively, these factors suggest that health care reform is not likely to be a static, one-time achievement.

Physicians and nurses must be trained to practice in a wellness-oriented model of care delivery. To some extent, the delivery system will evolve to replace periodic encounters between patients and providers with an ongoing relationship that includes remote monitoring of health status and virtual consultations (Adler et al., 2009). By some estimates, the number of virtual video consultations between primary care providers and patients will double by 2020, with 25% annual growth in such encounters being anticipated. Large insurance companies, such as United Health, are strong proponents of this model (Japsen, 2015). In contrast, in the public sector, there is currently limited reimbursement for such services. That situation is likely to change, however, if virtual consultations can be shown to produce good value, such as reductions in ED visits given the same or better outcomes.

Health care and insurance senior executives have provided some insights into how care delivery might evolve over the next few years (Phillips, 2015). Cost control will be a major driving force going forward. Patients are likely to see fewer disruptions in their lives caused by frequent office visits, as much more care will be delivered where the patients are. For example, home care will be used extensively to manage higher-risk populations. Sensors, early warning systems, and remote monitoring will enable this shift. Many patients in need of acute care for non-life-threatening conditions, such as wounds and fractures, will go to freestanding emergent and urgent care clinics; the number of these clinics has been increasing. Nonphysician practitioners will deliver most health care, leaving physicians to work with the sickest 5% to 10% of patients. Similarly, nurse extender clinical aides will take over some functions currently performed by nurses. Use of mobile communication devices will provide the needed support.

Clinical decision support systems and evidence-based treatment protocols will become indispensable. Value-based payment models will become the norm.

conditions can increase the risk of developing chronic conditions, reduce a person's ability to manage those conditions, and lead to avoidable health care utilization.

Toward Population Health

In the past, the community-oriented primary care (COPC) model and ACOs have demonstrated shortcomings in achieving population health improvements. The COPC model has been known for its distinctive integration of public health and medicine. ACOs drew much attention after the passage of the ACA, and their role in delivering integrated care will continue. Unfortunately, these organizations have not been able to successfully structure community linkages to improve population health (Tipirneni et al., 2015). Perhaps the reason for this lack of success is that most ACOs are sponsored by physician groups, hospitals, and insurers (Muhlestein, 2013), rather than by community organizations.

Accountable Care Communities

To achieve population health improvement, an emerging model—called accountable health communities (AHCs)—has been sponsored by the Centers for Medicare and Medicaid Services (CMS). These organizations seek to address population health from a community perspective by integrating health care, public health, and social services. In some cases, AHCs may be able to join hands with ACOs to form community coalitions to address broad social determinants of health (Tipirneni et al., 2015) by combining health-sector efforts with efforts to mitigate social forces that negatively impact patient care and health outcomes (Chaiyachati et al., 2016). For example, inadequate nutrition and unhealthy living

The Vermont Blueprint

In 2006, Vermont launched the Vermont Blueprint for Health—a program designed to meet the medical and social needs of people in the state's communities. Medical homes are the foundation of this program. In addition, practice facilitators are employed to help with continuous quality improvement. The medical homes are integrated with community health teams that expand medical care to include care coordination, counseling, substance abuse treatment support, and health coaching, among other services (State of Vermont, 2017). The aim is to improve overall population health through enhanced access to and coordination of medical and nonmedical services. The model has managed to deliver high-quality care while reducing expenditures from lower hospitalization rates and outpatient facility use (Jones et al., 2016).

Patient Activation

Patient activation refers to a patient's skills, confidence, ability, and motivation to become actively engaged in his or her own health care. It differs from compliance, in which the emphasis is on getting patients to follow medical advice given by providers (Hibbard and Greene, 2013). Activation often coincides with actual changes in behavior, such as changing one's diet, engaging in physical activity, and having regular checkups.

Activation goes a step beyond **patient-centered care**, in which patients are allowed to make choices that best fit their individual circumstances (Institute of Medicine [IOM], 2001). With this type of care, health professionals take the time to understand patients' individual needs, preferences, and values, and invite patients' participation in their care. In turn, activated patients are more actively engaged and take a greater degree of responsibility for their own health compared to patient-centered care.

A growing body of research points to patient activation as a promising new approach to improving health outcomes and lowering health care costs. The approach requires communication to engage patients and instill in them the knowledge and confidence needed to maintain behaviors that promote better health (Tufts University School of Medicine, 2014). Innovative delivery systems are measuring activation in an attempt to improve and individualize patient care and to strengthen patients' roles in improving health outcomes (Hibbard and Greene, 2013).

Activation can be improved over time through information, education, support, and encouragement. The challenge is that activation levels differ considerably across socioeconomic and health status characteristics. For example, among all groups covered by health insurance, people enrolled in Medicaid are the least activated (Hibbard and Cunningham, 2008).

Future Workforce Challenges

An adequate and well-trained workforce is a critical component of the health care delivery infrastructure. Workforce-related issues and challenges will continue to require attention, especially in light of the emerging models of care discussed in the previous sections. This section highlights future needs and recommendations for change.

The Nursing Profession

In 2010, the Institute of Medicine released its report titled *The Future of Nursing: Leading Change, Advancing Health*, which offered recommendations for nursing in the new health care landscape. This section briefly outlines the main recommendations from that report, and offers an update to drive future change. The content here is attributed to the IOM (2016). As the following points emphasize, the nursing profession will face ongoing challenges that also have implications for health care organizations, educational institutions, and policymakers.

Nurses should practice to the full extent of their education and training. In 2015, only 21 states had passed laws to give nurse practitioners (NPs) full practice and prescriptive authority, an increase of 8 states since 2010. As they have sought to expand their scope of practice, advanced practice nurses (APNs) have encountered barriers imposed by physician organizations. The new models of care will require that all health professionals practice to the full extent of their education and training so as to deliver greater efficiency and quality of services, and they will improve satisfaction among professionals. It is, therefore, recommended that health care professionals find common ground to remove scope-of-practice restrictions, increase interprofessional collaboration, and work with policymakers to bring about necessary changes in health policy.

Nurses should obtain higher levels of education and training to adequately address the needs of a patient population with complex needs. Nurse competencies should include leadership, health policy, system improvement, research in evidence-based practices, teamwork and collaboration, and competency in specific content areas, including community health, public health, and geriatrics. Nurses are also being called upon to fill expanding roles and to master technological tools and information management systems, while collaborating with and coordinating care across teams of health professionals. Baccalaureate programs that confer the BSN degree have substantially increased their enrollments since 2010. Upon entering the profession, however, nurses experience a high turnover rate. There is a great need to enhance transition-to-practice residencies, which have been found to improve skills in organization, management, and communication, and to lead to higher retention. In addition, there is a great need to prepare nurses at the doctoral level to undertake teaching and research, and to serve as leaders in clinical practice and advocacy for health policy change. Finally, there is a great need for nurses' continuing education to keep pace with the needs of an increasingly complex, team-based health care system.

Achieving cultural diversity in the nursing workforce remains a challenge, particularly in regard to blacks and Hispanics. Likewise, men make up less than 10% of the registered nurse (RN) workforce. It is believed that a more diverse workforce will be better suited to delivering more culturally relevant care.

Collaboration will require all members of a team to work together to their full potential on behalf of patients. Nurses are needed in leadership positions to contribute their unique perspective and expertise in the areas of care delivery, quality, and safety. In 2014, for example, nurses accounted for only 5% of hospital board membership, whereas physicians represented 20%. In addition, members of the nursing profession need to communicate effectively with key stakeholders and the media about the ongoing needs related to health care.

Effective workforce planning and policy making require better data and improved information systems. Data collection and analysis should drive the systematic assessment and projection of workforce requirements by role, skill mix, region, and demographics to inform changes in nursing practice and education.

Primary Care Physicians

The current shortage of PCPs, and its exacerbation in the future, is just one aspect of the health care workforce challenges that must be addressed. Caudill and colleagues (2011) have argued that the PCPs trained today will not have the requisite skills to fulfill their contemplated responsibilities because of a variety of factors. Future health care demands—mainly because of a growing number of people with complex chronic conditions—will require PCPs to function as "comprehensivists." These comprehensivists will need to be experts in multiple areas:

- Anticipating, preventing, and managing the progression and/or complications of common complex conditions
- Managing complex pharmacology
- Understanding end-of-life issues and medical ethics
- Coordinating care
- Leading health care teams

The practice environments for these physicians will need to contain the elements and systems to support comprehensive care, such as advanced information systems. Comprehensivists will also need to be able to direct and coordinate a health care team that includes expertise in patient education, mental health and behavioral modification, physical and occupational therapy, pharmacy, and home health. Care delivery will have to be consistent with evidence-based medicine, while incorporating the patient's values (Caudill et al., 2011).

To train future PCPs, physicians' education must be more efficient, integrated, and longitudinal. Time must be created for medical students to learn essential elements of patient safety and quality, teamwork in the health care environment, health maintenance, and continuity of care, without sacrificing fundamental knowledge. A "pay for educational performance and outcomes" model, with organizational bundling of educational costs, may need to be piloted in a similar way to the piloting of new care delivery models (Caudill et al., 2011).

Leaders in the academic field have also identified a lack of focus on population health in their family medicine residency programs. Resident/faculty time demands are cited as barriers to curricular success (Vickery et al., 2015).

Training in Geriatrics

Growth of the elderly population in the United States is attributed to increases in life expectancy and aging of the baby boomer generation. By 2030, more than one-fifth of the U.S. population is projected to be 65 years or older, compared with 13% in 2010 (Ortman et al., 2014).

According to the IOM (2008), the U.S. health care workforce is not prepared to deliver the best care to older patients. Geriatric care has not attracted health care

professionals in sufficient numbers. Geriatricians will be needed in large numbers because of their clinical expertise and their role in educating and training the rest of the health care workforce in geriatric principles. In 2007, slightly more than 7,000 physicians in the United States were certified in geriatric medicine; by 2030, that number will have increased by less than 10%. Yet, to adequately care for the growing elderly population, 36,000 geriatricians will be needed.

While this goal may never be met, the IOM has put forth several recommendations that would alleviate the problem to some extent. They include residency training, improved recruitment and retention, financial incentives to attract geriatric specialists in various health professions, enhancement of reimbursement for practitioners, federal programs such as loan forgiveness and scholarships for specialization in geriatrics, better pay and benefits for direct care workers in geriatric settings, and support for technological innovation to enhance the capacity of caregivers to deliver services to older adults (IOM, 2008).

▶ The Future of Long-Term Care

In the future, significant demographic and economic trends will make long-term care (LTC) less affordable for most people in the United States, and increase the already high level of dependency on Medicaid. Several factors make it extremely difficult for individuals to plan for future LTC—namely, unpredictability of the future need for LTC (many elders will not need it), escalating costs of these services, erosion of people's ability to save for retirement to pay for out-of-pocket costs, and unaffordability of LTC insurance because of high premiums. Hence, there have been calls to make LTC a national priority (Kwak and Polivka, 2014). Medicaid cannot continue to cover the increasing costs of LTC for too long without the program eventually collapsing. Proposals for direct cuts to this benefit are likely to fall victim to partisan politics. Any meaningful reform will have to look at the entire welfare system—for example, by formulating programs to take people who can work off the welfare rolls.

Long-term care has undergone some structural changes in the past years, as more people in need of LTC have been receiving services at home and in other community-based settings. Consequently, the demand for nursing homes has declined. This trend has become firmly entrenched in the U.S. culture based on people's own preferences about where they would like to receive LTC services. Yet, the need for nursing home care will not disappear. Both institutional skilled nursing care and assisted living care will continue to have a place in the LTC spectrum of services. Three main current trends will support the need for institutional care:

- The number of informal caregivers, such as family and friends, has been declining relative to the growth of the elderly population.
- Victims of serious accidents, dementia, and serious illnesses will need institutional care.
- Current policy, under the ACA, penalizes hospitals with excessive readmissions within 30 days.

Hence, postacute services will continue to have a place in LTC.

From a social standpoint, the culture change movement that has led to the creation of enriched living environments in LTC facilities will continue. Culture change emphasizes provision of living environments that enhance overall quality of life, offer sensory stimulation to overcome boredom and lethargy, and empower patients to make individual decisions based on their preferences.

The LTC sector is not impervious to the workforce issues discussed previously. Indeed, LTC may be affected more adversely by these issues than other areas of health care because of employee preferences to work in hospitals and clinics rather than LTC settings. Based on current trends, the occupations anticipated to grow the most in the LTC sector include social workers, community and social services coordinators, and home health and personal care aides (Spetz et al., 2015).

New technology, however, will either replace some human functions or improve worker efficiency and productivity. For example, LTC requires frequent monitoring of patients—a function that can be partially replaced by sensor technology. Sensor technology can also measure blood pressure and heart rate. IT advances will facilitate transfers of patients between facilities, such as hospitals and nursing homes. This will free up some social work and nursing time. Robotic exoskeleton technology will be used to assist patients with mobility and body mechanics to compensate for disability. Similar technology will be used to prevent the worker injuries that are often sustained when moving and transferring a patient, as from bed to the toilet.

▶ Global Threats and International Cooperation

The world faces many challenges. At least for the foreseeable future, the nations of the world will continue to face shortages of resources to meet their populations' demands, and these shortages will continue to affect people disproportionately. Thus, rationed health care has inevitably, but unintentionally, become a reality in most countries.

Disease and disability will continue to pose major challenges globally. Natural disasters occur without warning, causing large-scale devastation followed by disease and disability. Examples include the Haiti earthquake in January 2010; the earthquake and tsunami that killed thousands in Japan in March 2011; and industrial accidents, such as the oil rig explosion in the Gulf of Mexico in April 2010. Large-scale bioterrorism has not yet occurred, but global unrest amid the rise of extremism makes it a real possibility in the future. Such prospects necessitate ongoing preparations, rapid deployment of resources, and sufficient capacity of the health care infrastructure to deal with mass casualties. When major disasters strike, the need for resources is often far greater than the available supply. Hence, responses to disasters will require international assistance, cooperation, and joint efforts.

Increased air travel has enabled infectious diseases to spread quickly around the globe, as evidenced by the spread of severe acute respiratory syndrome (SARS) from China to Canada in 2003 and the spread of the polio virus from India to northern Minnesota in 2005 (Milstein et al., 2006). SARS, in fact, eventually spread to more than 20 countries. These examples highlight the importance of early identification of infectious threats and subsequent rapid response to prevent further spread, which is often difficult without international cooperation (Johns et al., 2011). For example, ending an outbreak of Ebola virus disease (EVD) required 3 years of unprecedented international cooperation (Mackey, 2016).

Given the scope of such efforts, protecting global health has become the subject of international law. The International Health Regulations (IHR), for example, constitute an international legal instrument that is binding on 194 countries. IHR's aim is to facilitate international efforts to prevent and respond to acute public health risks that have the potential to cross borders and threaten people worldwide. Detecting and tracking significant public health threats that may emerge in countries that cannot or might not report such events to the global health community will remain an ongoing challenge. For example, the reemergence of EVD—an old but powerful infectious disease—has put increased pressure on the World Health Organization (WHO) to reform its role in global health issues. At the same time, there is increased awareness that the responsibility for meeting complex global health challenges can no longer be borne by WHO alone (Mackey, 2016).

Wars and terrorism in the Middle East and Africa have created failed states, displacing millions of people from their homes and communities, and magnifying health emergencies. In 2015, the world refugee population totaled a staggering 65.3 million people (UN Refugee Agency, 2015). Resources have been stretched as aid workers have sought to deal with these people's physical and emotional distress and need for medical services. Trends suggest that this situation will get worse before it gets better.

Emerging antibiotic resistance among infectious agents is another public health and security threat. Almost all of the antibiotic-resistant pathogens that exist naturally can be bioengineered through forced mutation or cloning. In addition, existing pathogens can be genetically manipulated to make them resistant to available antibiotics. Efforts to strengthen global health security include disease surveillance for outbreaks of international importance and urgency, exchange of technical information on new pathogens, early warning and control of serious animal disease outbreaks, prevention of drug-resistant infections, and development of new antimicrobial drugs.

Despite international treaties, such as the 1972 Biological and Toxin Weapons Convention (BWC), which prohibits the development, possession, acquisition, stockpiling, and transfer of biological and toxin agents, compliance with and enforcement of such bans have remained ongoing concerns. Some countries are believed to have active biological warfare programs. Cooperation on the part of individual nations often amounts to nothing more than voluntary adherence to international law, even as some countries openly defy international conventions with impunity.

Adequate delivery of health care to millions around the world depends on an adequate and well-trained workforce. WHO (2016) has estimated that the supply of various categories of health care workers will increase significantly between 2013 and 2030, but anticipates that a need-based shortage of 14 million workers will persist worldwide, mostly in Africa and Eastern Mediterranean nations. The problem in many countries is compounded by unequal distributions of workers, lack of training, and "brain drains." Also, in spite of the pivotal role that community health workers play in scaling up essential services, this workforce category does not receive adequate support in most nations (Chatterjee, 2011).

▶ New Frontiers in Clinical Technology

Despite its association with cost escalation, technological progress will continue. Increased efforts in technology assessment will go hand in hand with new innovations. To what extent clinical decisions will be influenced by the cost-effectiveness of technology, however, remains an open question. As cost-effectiveness research continues to advance, its results will likely find their way into health policy.

Medicine is advancing on several fronts. The future looks bright owing to the promise of better cures, higher quality of care, and improved quality of life. Understanding of the human genome has paved the way for a number of new approaches to prevent and treat disease. Future innovation and progress, however, will not come automatically. Much will depend on future regulations, insurance coverage, and reimbursement from payers.

Genetic medicine has opened a pathway for understanding the association of genes with specific disease traits. One application of genetic medicine is **gene therapy**, which involves the use of genes to prevent or treat a wide array of diseases such as hypertension, diabetes, and cancer. Currently at an experimental stage, gene therapy may eventually allow doctors to insert a functioning gene into a patient's targeted cells to correct an inborn defect or provide the cell with a new function. This technique is expected to replace treatment with medications or surgery in some areas. The future challenge is to develop methods that deliver just enough genetic material to only the right cells. Cancer treatment is receiving much attention as a prime candidate for gene therapy since current techniques (surgery, radiation, and chemotherapy) are effective in only half of all cases and can greatly reduce a patient's quality of life.

Personalized and precision medicine will drive developments in the pharmacotherapeutic arena. Personal characteristics of individual patients can vary so much that not all medications work for everyone. Hence, a one-size-fits-all approach can be both wasteful and ineffective. In **personalized medicine**, specific gene variations among patients will be matched with responses to selected medications to increase effectiveness and reduce unwanted side effects. Going a step further, **precision medicine** will take into account not only variability in genes, but also the environment and lifestyle factors.

Rational drug design will replace the trial-and-error method of discovering new drugs, which is very expensive. Rational design will utilize multidisciplinary advances in various sciences to address specific targets such as a microorganism that causes disease or a defective human body molecule that activates a disease. The objective is to shorten the drug discovery process, thereby reducing the cost of finding new drugs.

Targeted drug delivery has the potential to provide more effective treatment by using nanoparticles as drug delivery vehicles. For example, cellular uptake of nanoparticles may efficiently translocate drug molecules into cancer tumors without damaging healthy tissues (Ding and Ma, 2013). Nanotechnology also has the potential to deliver antiviral formulations to specific targeted sites and viral reservoirs in the body (Lembo and Cavalli, 2010).

Imaging technologies have accounted for some of the most dramatic advances in health care mainly because of the exponential growth in the performance of silicon devices (Busse, 2006). Current research focuses on four areas:

- Finding new energy sources and focusing energy beams so as to avoid damage to adjacent tissue and to minimize residual damage
- Use of microelectronics in digital detectors and advances in the contrast media for finer detection of abnormalities
- Faster and more accurate analysis of images using three-dimensional (3D) technology
- Improvements in display technology to produce higher-resolution displays

For example, EchoPixel's 3D technology can take hundreds of two-dimensional magnetic resonance imaging (MRI) and computed tomography (CT) scans and produce 3D images that enable physicians to not only view but also interact with patient tissues and organs. In trying to decipher two-dimensional images, important information may be overlooked.

Advances in *minimally invasive surgery* include image-guided brain surgery, minimal-access cardiac procedures, and endovascular placement of grafts for abdominal aneurysms. Robotic surgery is in its early stages, but it will be used in many different procedures in the future. "Liquid biopsies" involving blood tests are an emerging technology that will replace some of the traditional biopsies to diagnose cancer.

Vaccines have traditionally been used prophylactically to prevent specific infectious diseases, such as diphtheria, smallpox, and whooping cough. However, the therapeutic use of vaccines in the treatment of noninfectious diseases, such as cancer, has opened new fronts in medicine. At the same time, development of new vaccines for emerging infectious diseases remains on the research agenda. Making vaccines safer for wide-scale preventive use against bioterrorism in which such agents as smallpox and anthrax may be used will also be an ongoing pursuit.

Immunotherapy is a promising field in the treatment of cancers. New technologies can genetically modify a patient's own immune system to recognize and kill cancer cells.

Blood substitutes will likely be available one day for large-scale use. Even though the safety of blood used in transfusions has been greatly enhanced, substitutes for real blood are necessary when supplies fall short, particularly in war and in natural disasters.

Xenotransplantation, in which animal tissues are used for transplants in humans, is a growing research area. It holds promise as a means to overcome the critical shortages of available donor organs. Organs from genetically engineered animals may one day be available for transplantation (Schneider and Seebach, 2013). 3D bioprinting is also an emerging science that may one day enable the production of human organs for transplant. In the operating room, surgeons can use this technology to create tailor-made implants.

Regenerative medicine is the first truly interdisciplinary field that utilizes and brings together nearly every field in science. This new field holds the realistic promise of regenerating damaged tissues and organs in vivo (in the living body) through reparative techniques that stimulate previously irreparable organs into healing themselves. Regenerative medicine also enables scientists to grow tissues and organs in vitro (in the laboratory) and safely implant them when the body is unable to be prompted into healing itself. This revolutionary technology has the potential to develop therapies for previously untreatable diseases and conditions.

▶ The Future of Evidence-Based Health Care

Evaluating the effectiveness of care is the primary goal of evidence-based medicine (EBM). In EBM, the onus is on showing, with a sufficiently high degree of certainty, that a new practice of care is superior to the usual practice (Fischer and Ghelardi, 2016). Evidence-based practice guidelines are intended to represent "best practices" and "proven therapies."

Research has demonstrated that providers who charge more for their services do not necessarily deliver better outcomes. Incorporation of EBM into medical practice would increase the value of health care services. Quality of care can actually be improved while reducing costs—thereby increasing the value of medical care—by reducing misuse and overuse (Slawson and Shaughnessy, 2001). Halm and colleagues (2007), for example, reported a remarkable reduction in the proportion of patients undergoing carotid endarterectomy (a surgical procedure that removes the inner lining of the carotid artery if it has become thickened or damaged by plaque) for inappropriate reasons. EBM has also attracted a great deal of international interest and activity (Kredo et al., 2016). However, EBM's full potential has not yet been realized, and work in this area is ongoing.

Comparative effectiveness research (CER) is a novel concept in which a chosen intervention is guided by scientific evidence of how well it would work, compared to other available treatments. Hence, CER will play a critical role in deciding which therapies are better practices than others. In 2009, the Institute of Medicine defined CER as follows:

> The generation and synthesis of evidence that compares the benefits and harms of alternative methods to prevent, diagnose, treat, and monitor a clinical condition or to improve the delivery of care. The purpose of comparative effectiveness research is to assist consumers, clinicians, purchasers, and policy makers to make informed decisions that will improve health care at both the individual and population levels.

One important element of CER is ensuring that appropriate outcomes are measured in research, so that findings can be compared and contrasted across different studies, and useful evidence can be provided to both clinical and policy decision makers (Gorst et al., 2016). A key concern has been which outcomes should be measured. Hence, it is critical to have a standard collection of outcomes that researchers can agree upon. Ongoing work is needed to determine such core outcome sets (COS), which would then be measured and reported in clinical research.

While efforts to promote health services research are commendable, EBM has remained underutilized in practice, and the adoption of research-based evidence into routine clinical practice has been slow. Thus, a significant gap exists between knowledge and practice. Implementation of EBM is complex, and the whole discipline of implementation research has been evolving. Any change in provider behavior is unlikely to occur on the basis of receiving information alone, and even training may not produce the desired results by modifying provider practices (Leathers et al., 2016). Hence, any research efforts will need to be accompanied by appropriate strategies that would motivate providers to make use of research findings. Some critical areas that will require close attention include robustness of research studies, sound interpretation of results, relevance to clinical practice, formulation of clear and specific clinical practice guidelines, performance measures, clinical decision support tools, and properly aligned financial incentives (Timbie at al., 2012). Because compliance is influenced by multiple factors, a comprehensive strategy to changing providers' practices must be adopted.

Implementation Strategies for Evidence-Based Care

Future strategies to improve guidelines and protocols and their adherence should include the following measures:

- Health care leaders must continue to emphasize the adoption of evidence-based guidelines in their organizations. The primary impetus for EBM adoption must come from governance and senior management, with adequate commitment and support for implementing EBM.

- Systems consultation is a relatively new strategy. It includes translation of a clinical practice guideline into a checklist-based implementation plan; use of physician peer coaches, called systems consultants, to train physicians and assist with guideline implementation; and a focus on reducing variation in practices among practitioners (Quanbeck et al., 2016).
- Ongoing development of computer-based models incorporating EBM will facilitate multidisciplinary caregiving based on best practices by various practitioners, including physicians and nurses. EBM should be incorporated into clinical decision support systems (Stijn et al., 2016). Clinical guidelines should be updated as new evidence becomes available.
- A mechanism for auditing and providing feedback to staff has been shown to improve compliance with EBM (Munn et al., 2015).
- Future practice guidelines must incorporate economic analysis to promote the delivery of cost-effective health care.
- Financial incentives, including provider reimbursement, must be restructured. Reimbursement methods should focus on paying for best achievable outcomes and the most effective care over the course of treatment, instead of paying for units of service (Gauthier et al., 2006).

Strategies for Comparative Effectiveness and Patient-Centered Research

When conducting CER, there are seven key steps:

1. Identify new and emerging clinical interventions.
2. Review and synthesize current medical research.
3. Identify gaps between existing medical research and the needs of clinical practice.
4. Promote and generate new scientific evidence and analytic tools.
5. Train and develop clinical researchers.
6. Translate and disseminate research findings to diverse stakeholders.
7. Reach out to stakeholders via a citizens forum (Agency for Healthcare Research and Quality, 2011).

Etheredge (2010) has suggested that our collective knowledge about comparative effectiveness will grow more quickly if we can draw on the voluminous information that already exists in clinical trial databases and in other research data sets, rather than relying solely on new CER studies. Problems of noncomparability notwithstanding, if existing information can be extracted in a meaningful way, CER could then be used to fill research gaps.

Future priorities for CER include the capacity to conduct experimental and quasi-experimental comparative studies; evaluation of broad, system-level strategies, such as benefit designs and payment reforms; focus on population subgroups, including vulnerable groups, most likely to benefit from a given intervention; dissemination of research results; and the actual use of evidence in the delivery of care (Benner et al., 2010). At present, much remains unknown about the extent to which important stakeholders, such as physicians and patients, will be involved in patient-centered research.

Americans support research that would provide information on treatment options. In contrast, public support for research is contingent upon how medical evidence will be used in practice. The public remains opposed to the use of research for allocation of resources or for mandating certain treatment decisions (Gerber et al., 2010). Public attitudes may well become the biggest obstacle to cost-efficient delivery of health care in the future and to any attempts by the government to mandate certain types of care or to ration services.

▶ Summary

Health care delivery in the United States and abroad will undoubtedly continue to change. The framework of future change presented in this chapter can help inform the nature and direction of change. Regardless of the shape the health care delivery system might take under current and future reform efforts, major challenges related to cost, access, and quality will not simply go away.

The U.S. demographic landscape continues to change, and various models and concepts of health care delivery remain at an experimental stage. The future delivery system will likely incorporate several models of care to address the needs of a diverse population at both the individual and population levels. However, an infrastructure that fails to ensure primary care delivery presents a major obstacle to achieving this goal. The financing and delivery of long-term care will put further strains on the U.S. health care system. Nevertheless, technology will play a major role in shaping the future system of health care.

International threats will continue to be an unwelcome aspect of globalization. Rapid responses in dealing with infectious diseases that can quickly spread around the world, natural disasters, and human-made threats of terrorism will increasingly require global assistance, cooperation, and joint efforts. Both now and in the future, many developing and underdeveloped countries will face critical shortages of trained health care workers.

New frontiers in clinical technology will continue to unfold. Medical treatments in the next 10 to 15 years are likely to be very different from the ones in vogue now, although proven traditional methods will not be wholly abandoned.

Standardized protocols for practitioners will continue to be informed by scientific evidence, including results from comparative effectiveness research and patient-oriented research. Their adoption into clinical practice will not be automatic, but rather will require strategies that include financial incentives.

▶ Test Your Understanding

Terminology

comparative effectiveness research (CER)	patient activation	single-payer system
gene therapy	patient-centered care	universal access
genetic medicine	personalized	xenotransplantation
high-risk pools	medicine	zoonoses
	precision medicine	

Review Questions

1. Explain the eight main forces that will determine future change in health care.
2. Discuss the main elements of the evolving health care delivery infrastructure in the United States.
3. What is patient activation? What are the main challenges in activation?
4. What recommendations have been made to transform the nursing profession?
5. What type of training is needed for primary care physicians to become "comprehensivists"?
6. What are some of the main reasons behind the deficits in geriatric training?
7. What are the main challenges faced by long-term care in the future?
8. Give an overview of what new technology might achieve in the delivery of health care.
9. What role does international cooperation play in globalization?
10. What can be done to achieve greater adoption of evidence-based medicine in the delivery of health care?

References

Adler, R., et al. 2009. *Healthcare 2020*. Palo Alto, CA: Institute for the Future.

Agency for Healthcare Research and Quality (AHRQ). 2011. *What is comparative effectiveness research?* Available at: http://www.effectivehealthcare.ahrq .gov/index.cfm/what-is-comparative -effectiveness-research1/. Accessed January 2011.

Benner, J. S., et al. 2010. An evaluation of recent federal spending on comparative effectiveness research: Priorities, gaps, and next steps. *Health Affairs* 29, no. 10: 1768–1776.

Busse, F. 2006. Diagnostic imaging. In: *Advances in healthcare technology: Shaping the future of medical care*. G. Spekowius and T. Wendler, eds. Dordrecht, Netherlands: Springer. pp. 15–34.

Camp, F. 2016. 5 times Donald Trump praised socialized healthcare. *Independent Journal Review*. Available at: http://ijr.com/2016/02/537107-5 -times-donald-trump-praised-socialized -healthcare. Accessed February 2017.

Caudill, T., et al. 2011. Health care reform and primary care: Training physicians for tomorrow's challenges. *Academic Medicine* 86, no. 2: 158–160.

Chaiyachati, K. H., et al. 2016. Health systems tackling social determinants of health: Promises, pitfalls, and opportunities of current policies. *American Journal of Managed Care* 22, no. 11: e393–e394.

Chatterjee, P. 2011. Progress patchy on health-worker crisis. *Lancet* 377, no. 9764: 456.

Congressional Budget Office (CBO). 2013. *Limit medical malpractice torts*. Available at: https:// www.cbo.gov/budget-options/2013/44892. Accessed February 2017.

Congressional Budget Office (CBO). 2016. *Federal subsidies for health insurance coverage for people under age 65: 2016 to 2026*. Available at: https://www.cbo.gov/sites/default/files/114th -congress-2015-2016/reports/51385 -HealthInsuranceBaseline_OneCol.pdf. Accessed January 2017.

Congressional Budget Office (CBO). 2017. *The budget and economic outlook: 2017 to 2027*. Available at: https://www.cbo.gov/sites/default /files/115th-congress-2017-2018/reports/52370 -outlook.pdf. Accessed January 2017.

Davis, P. A. 2016. *Medicare: Insolvency projections*. Congressional Research Service. Available at: https://fas.org/sgp/crs/misc/RS20946.pdf. Accessed January 2017.

Ding, H. M., and Y. Q. Ma. 2013. Controlling cellular uptake of nanoparticles with pH-sensitive polymers. *Scientific Reports* 3: 2804.

Etheredge, L. M. 2010. Creating a high-performance system for comparative effectiveness research. *Health Affairs* 29, no. 10: 1761–1767.

Federal Reserve Board. 2016. *Report on the economic well-being of U.S. households in 2015*. Available at: https://www.federalreserve.gov/2015-report -economic-well-being-us-households-201605 .pdf. Accessed February 2017.

Fischer, A. J., and G. Ghelardi. 2016. The precautionary principle, evidence-based medicine, and decision theory in public health evaluation. *Frontiers in Public Health* 4: 107.

Furman, J., and M. Fiedler. 2015. *4.5 million young adults have gained coverage since 2010, improving access to care and benefitting our economy*. Available at: https://obamawhitehouse.archives .gov/blog/2015/01/29/45-million-young-adults -have-gained-coverage-2010-improving-access -care-and-benefitt. Accessed January 2017.

Gaffney, A., et al. 2016. Moving forward from the Affordable Care Act to a single-payer system. *American Journal of Public Health* 106, no. 6: 987–988.

Gallup. 2016a. *Gallup review: Healthcare and the election*. Available at: http://www.gallup.com /opinion/polling-matters/196814/gallup-review -healthcare-election.aspx. Accessed February 2017.

Gallup. 2016b. *Americans' satisfaction with healthcare system edges down*. Available at: http://www .gallup.com/poll/195605/americans-satisfaction -healthcare-system-edges-down.aspx?g _source=satisfaction+with+healthcare&g _medium=search&g_campaign=tiles. Accessed May 2017.

Gallup. 2016c. *Majority in U.S. support idea of fed-funded healthcare system*. Available at: http://www.gallup.com/poll/191504/majority -support-idea-fed-funded-healthcare-system .aspx. Accessed May 2017.

Gauthier, A., et al. 2006. *Toward a high performance health system for the United States*. New York, NY: Commonwealth Fund.

George, B. P., and T. L. Henthorne. 2009. The incorporation of telemedicine with medical tourism: A study of consequences. *Journal of Hospitality Marketing and Management* 18, no. 5: 512–522.

Gerber, A. S., et al. 2010. The public wants information, not board mandates, from comparative effectiveness research. *Health Affairs* 29, no. 10: 1872–1881.

Gorst, S. L., et al. 2016. Choosing important health outcomes for comparative effectiveness research: An updated review and identification of gaps. *PLoS One* 11, no. 12: 1–14.

Halm, E. A., et al. 2007. Has evidence changed prac-tice? Appropriateness of carotid endarterectomy after the clinical trials. *Neurology* 68, no. 3: 187–194.

Halpin, H. A., and P. Harbage. 2010. The origins and demise of the public option. *Health Affairs* 29, no. 6: 1117–1124.

Haviland, A. M., et al. 2016. Do "consumer-directed" health plans bend the cost curve over time? *Journal of Health Economics* 46: 33–51.

Hayes, S. L., et al. 2016. *High-need, high-cost patients: Who are they and how do they use health care? A population-based comparison of demographics, health care use, and expenditures*. Issue Brief (August, Pub. 1897, Vol. 26). Washington, DC: Commonwealth Fund.

Herman, B. 2016. What, me buy insurance? *Modern Healthcare* 46, no. 20: 20–22.

Hibbard, J. H., and P. J. Cunningham. 2008. *How engaged are consumers in their health and health care, and why does it matter?* Research Brief No. 8. Washington, DC: Center for Studying Health System Change.

Hibbard, J. H., and J. Greene. 2013. What the evidence shows about patient activation: Better health outcomes and care experiences; fewer data on costs. *Health Affairs* 32, no. 2: 207–214.

Himmelstein, D., and S. Woolhandler. 2015. The post-launch problem: The Affordable Care Act's persistently high administrative costs. *Health Affairs Blog*. Available at: http://healthaffairs .org/blog/2015/05/27/the-post-launch -problem-the-affordable-care-acts-persistently -high-administrative-costs. Accessed February 2017.

Horowitz, B. T. March 28, 2012. Smart card use surging in health care, government. *eWeek*, p. 7.

Huynen, M. M. T. E., et al. 2005. The health impacts of globalisation: A conceptual framework. *Globalization and Health* 1: 1–12.

Institute of Medicine (IOM). 2001. *Crossing the quality chasm: A new health system for the 21st century*. Washington, DC: National Academies Press.

Institute of Medicine (IOM). 2008. *Retooling for an aging America: Building the health care workforce*. Washington, DC: National Academies Press.

Institute of Medicine (IOM). 2009. *Initial national priorities for comparative effectiveness research*. Washington, DC: National Academies Press.

Institute of Medicine (IOM). 2010. *The future of nursing: Leading change, advancing health*. Washington, DC: National Academy of Sciences.

Institute of Medicine (IOM). 2016. *Assessing progress on the Institute of Medicine report: The Future of Nursing*. Washington, DC: National Academies Press.

Japsen, B. 2015. *Doctors' virtual consults with patients to double by 2020*. Available at: http://www .forbes.com/sites/brucejapsen/2015/08/09 /as-telehealth-booms-doctor-video-consults -to-double-by-2020/#7cf82a25d66d. Accessed February 2017.

Johns, M. C., et al. 2011. A growing global network's role in outbreak response: AFHSC-GEIS 2008–2009. *BMC Public Health* 11 (Suppl 2): S3.

Jones, C., et al. 2016. Vermont's community-oriented all-payer medical home model reduces expenditures and utilization while delivering high-quality care. *Population Health Management* 19, no. 3: 196–205.

Kenen, J. 2011. Dx on the preexisting condition insurance plan. *Health Affairs* 30, no. 3: 379–382.

Kredo, T., et al. 2016. Guide to clinical practice guidelines: The current state of play. *International Journal for Quality in Health Care* 28, no. 1: 122–128.

Krogstad, J. M., et al. 2017. *5 facts about illegal immigration in the U.S. Pew Research Center*. Available at: http://www.pewresearch.org /fact-tank/2017/04/27/5-facts-about-illegal -immigration-in-the-u-s/. Accessed February 2017.

Kwak, J., and L. J. Polivka. 2014. The future of long-term care and the aging network. *Generations* 38, no. 2: 67–73.

Lamm, R. D., and R. H. Blank. July–August 2005. The challenge of an aging society. *The Futurist*, pp. 23–27.

Leathers, S. J., et al. 2016. The effect of a change agent on use of evidence-based mental health practices. *Administration and Policy in Mental Health* 43, no. 5: 768–782.

Lembo, D., and R. Cavalli. 2010. Nanoparticulate delivery systems for antiviral drugs. *Antiviral Chemistry & Chemotherapy* 21, no. 2: 53–70.

Mackey, T. K. 2016. The Ebola outbreak: Catalyzing a "shift" in global health governance? *BMC Infectious Diseases* 16, no. 1: 699.

Martiniuk, A. L. C., et al. 2012. Brain gains: A literature review of medical missions to low and middle-income countries. *BMC Health Services Research* 12, no. 1: 134–141.

McHugh, K. August 10, 2013. Reid says Obamacare will lead to a single-payer healthcare system. *The Daily Caller*. Available at: http://dailycaller .com/2013/08/10/absolutely-yes-reid-says -obamacare-will-lead-to-a-single-payer -healthcare-system. Accessed January 2017.

Milstein, J. B., et al. 2006. The impact of globalization on vaccine development and availability. *Health Affairs* 25, no. 4: 1061–1069.

Muhlestein, D. 2013. Continued growth of public and private accountable care organizations. *Health Affairs Blog*. Available at: http:// healthaffairs.org/blog/2013/02/19/continued -growth-of-public-and-private-accountable -care-organizations. Accessed February 2017.

Munn, Z., et al. 2015. The implementation of best practice in medication administration across a health network: A multisite evidence-based audit and feedback project. *JBI Database of Systematic Reviews and Implementation Reports* 13, no. 8: 338–352.

National Center for Health Statistics (NCHS). 2016. *Health, United States, 2015*. Hyattsville, MD: U.S. Department of Health and Human Services.

Ortman, J. M., et al. 2014. *An aging nation: The older population in the United States*. Washington, DC: U.S. Census Bureau.

Paulus, R. A., et al. 2008. Continuous innovation in health care: Implications of the Geisinger experience. *Health Affairs* 27, no. 5: 1235–1245.

Pew Research Center. 2016. *The state of American jobs*. Available at: http://assets.pewresearch .org/wp-content/uploads/sites/3/2016/10 /ST_2016.10.06_Future-of-Work_FINAL4.pdf. Accessed February 2017.

Phillips, L. 2015. *What will health care look like in 5–15 years?* Available at: http://www .hfma.org/Leadership/E-Bulletins/2015/April /What_Will_Health_Care_Look_Like_in _5-15_Years_/. Accessed February 2017.

Quanbeck, A., et al. 2016. Systems consultation: Protocol for a novel implementation strategy designed to promote evidence-based practice in primary care. *Health Research Policy & Systems* 14: 1–10.

Reeves, T. C. 2011. Globalizing health services: a policy imperative? *International Journal of Business and Management* 6, no. 12: 44–57.

Rennen, W., and P. Martens. 2003. The globalisation timeline. *Integrated Assessment* 4: 137–144.

Sanger-Katz, M. 2015. The problem with G.O.P. plans to sell health insurance across state lines. *New York Times*. Available at: https://www .nytimes.com/2015/09/01/upshot/the-problem -with-gop-plans-to-sell-health-insurance-across -state-lines.html?_r=0. Accessed February 2017.

Schneider, M. K. J., and J. D. Seebach. 2013. Xenotransplantation literature update, July– August 2013. *Xenotransplantation* 20, no. 5: 308–310.

Slawson, D. C., and A. F. Shaughnessy. 2001. Using "medical poetry" to remove the inequities in health care delivery. *Journal of Family Medicine* 50, no. 1: 51–65.

Spetz, J., et al. 2015. Future demand for long-term care workers will be influenced by demographic and utilization changes. *Health Affairs* 34, no. 6: 936–945.

State of Vermont. 2017. *Vermont Blueprint for Health*. Department of Vermont Health Access. Available at: http://blueprintforhealth.vermont .gov. Accessed February 2017.

Stijn, V. V., et al. 2016. Tailoring implementation strategies for evidence-based recommendations using computerized clinical decision support systems: Protocol for the development of the GUIDES tool. *Implementation Science* 11: 1–8.

Timbie, J. W., et al. 2012. Five reasons that many comparative effectiveness studies fail to change patient care and clinical practice. *Health Affairs* 31, no. 10: 2168–2175.

Tipirneni, R., et al. 2015. Accountable communities for health: Moving from providing accountable care to creating health. *Annals of Family Medicine* 13, no. 4: 367–369.

Trading Economics. 2017. *United States GDP growth rate: 1947–2017*. Available at: http:// www.tradingeconomics.com/united-states /gdp-growth. Accessed February 2017.

Tufts University School of Medicine. 2014. *New tool for health communicators: The patient activation model*. Available at: http://sites.tufts.edu /healthcomm/2014/04/27/new-tool-for-health -communicators-the-patient-activation-model. Accessed February 2017.

UN Refugee Agency. 2015. *Fact sheet: Global forced displacement*. Available at: http:// w w w . u n h c r . o r g / e n - u s / p u b l i c a t i o n s /brochures/579b31e54/fact-sheet-global -forced-displacement.html?query=fact%20 sheets. Accessed February 2017.

Vickery, K. D., et al. 2015. Preparing the next generation of family physicians to improve population health: A CERA study. *Family Medicine* 47, no. 10: 782–788.

Vitalari, N. P. 2016. Prospects for the future of the U.S. healthcare industry: A speculative analysis. *American Journal of Medical Research* 3, no. 2: 7–52.

World Health Organization (WHO). 2016. *Global strategy on human resources for health: Workforce 2030*. Available at: http://www.who.int/hrh /resources/global_strategy_workforce2030 _14_print.pdf?ua=1. Accessed February 2017.

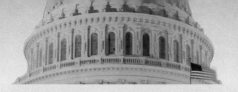

Glossary

A

Academic medical center The organization of one or more hospitals around a medical school. Apart from the training of physicians, research activities and clinical investigations become an important undertaking in these institutions.

Access The ability of persons needing health services to obtain appropriate care in a timely manner. Can you get medical care when you need it? If so, you have access to medical care. Access is not the same as health insurance coverage, although insurance coverage facilitates access to health care services.

Accountability The responsibility of clinicians and patients, respectively, for the provision and receipt of efficient and quality health care services.

Accountable care organization (ACO) An integrated group of providers who are willing and able to take responsibility for improving the overall health status, care efficiency, and satisfaction with care for a defined population.

Accreditation A private mechanism designed to assure that accredited health care facilities meet certain basic standards.

Acquired immunodeficiency syndrome (AIDS) The occurrence of immune deficiency caused by the human immunodeficiency virus (HIV).

Acquisition Purchase of one organization by another.

Activities of daily living (ADLs) The most commonly used measure of disability, which includes whether an individual needs assistance to perform basic activities, such as eating, bathing, dressing, toileting, and getting into or out of a bed or chair. *See* **functional status** and **instrumental activities of daily living (IADLs)**.

Actuary A person professionally trained in the technical aspects of insurance and related fields, particularly in the mathematics of insurance, such as the calculation of premiums, reserves, and other values.

Acupuncture Use of long, thin needles passed through the skin to specific reflex points to treat chronic pain or to produce regional anesthesia.

Acute condition Short-term, intense medical care for an illness or injury, usually requiring hospitalization. *See* **subacute care**.

Adjusted community rating Also called modified community rating; a method of determining health insurance premiums that takes into account demographic factors such as age, gender, geography, and family composition, while ignoring other risk factors.

Administrative costs Costs that are incidental to the delivery of health services. They are not only associated with the billing and collection of claims for services delivered, but also include numerous other costs, such as time and effort incurred by employers for the selection of insurance carriers, costs incurred by insurance and managed care organizations to market their products, and time and effort involved in the negotiation of rates.

Administrative information systems Systems designed to assist in carrying out financial and administrative support activities such as payroll, patient accounting, materials management, and office automation.

Adult day care (ADC) A community-based, long-term care service that provides a wide range of health, social, and recreational services to elderly adults who require supervision and care while members of the family or other informal caregivers are away at work.

Adult foster care (AFC) Long-term care services provided in small, family-operated homes, located in residential communities, which provide room, board, and varying levels of supervision, oversight, and personal care to nonrelated adults.

Advance directives A patient's wishes regarding continuation or withdrawal of treatment when the patient lacks decision-making capacity.

Advanced practice nurse (APN) A general name for nurses who have education and clinical experience beyond that required of a registered nurse (RN). APNs include four areas of specialization in nursing: clinical nurse specialists (CNSs), certified registered nurse anesthetists (CRNAs), nurse practitioners (NPs), and certified nurse-midwives (CNMs).

Adverse selection A phenomenon in which individuals who are likely to use more health care services than other persons due to their poor health enroll in health insurance plans in greater numbers, compared to people who are healthy. *See* **favorable risk selection**.

Affective disorders A group of disorders characterized by severe mood changes, often accompanied by a manic or depressive syndrome.

Affordable Care Act (ACA) The Patient Protection and Affordable Care Act of 2010, as amended by the Health Care and Education Reconciliation Act of 2010; nicknamed Obamacare.

Agency for Healthcare Research and Quality (AHRQ) A federal agency within the U.S. Department of Health and Human Services whose mission is to improve the quality, safety, efficiency, and effectiveness of health care through research activities.

Agent One of the factors of the epidemiology triangle, which must be present for an infectious disease to occur; in other words, an infectious disease cannot occur without an agent.

Aging-in-place Older people's preference and expectation to stay in one place for as long as possible, and to delay or avoid transfer to an institution where the acuity level of patients is higher.

Alliance A joint agreement between two organizations to share their resources without having joint ownership of assets.

Allied health A broad category that includes services and professionals in many health-related technical areas. Allied health professionals include technicians, assistants, therapists, and technologists.

Allied health professional Someone who has received a certificate; associate's, bachelor's, or master's degree; doctoral-level preparation; or post-baccalaureate training in a science related to health care and has responsibility for the delivery of health or related services.

Allocative tools Use of health policy in which there is a direct provision of income, services, or goods to groups of individuals who usually reap benefits from receiving them.

Allopathic medicine A philosophy of medicine that views medical treatment as active intervention to counteract the effects of disease through medical and surgical procedures that produce effects opposite those of the disease. *See* **homeopathy** and **osteopathic medicine**.

Almshouse A poorhouse; an unspecialized institution existing during the 18th and mid-19th centuries that mainly served general welfare functions, essentially providing shelter to the homeless, the insane, the elderly, orphans, and the sick who had no family to care for them.

Alternative medicine Also called alternative and complementary medicine; nontraditional remedies, such as acupuncture, homeopathy, naturopathy, biofeedback, yoga exercises, chiropractic, and herbal therapy.

Alzheimer's disease A progressive degenerative disease of the brain that leads to loss of memory, confusion, irritability, severe loss of functioning, and ultimately death. The disease is named after German neurologist, Alois Alzheimer (1864–1915).

Ambulatory Having the ability to move about at will.

Ambulatory care Also referred to as outpatient services. It includes (1) services rendered to patients who come to physicians' offices, outpatient departments of hospitals, and health centers to receive care; (2) outpatient services intended to serve the surrounding community (community medicine); and (3) certain services that are transported to the patient.

Ancillary services Hospital or other inpatient services other than room and board and professional medical services, such as physician and nursing care. Examples include radiology, pharmacy, laboratory, bandages and other supplies, and physical therapy.

Anesthesiology Administration of drugs for the prevention or relief of pain during surgery.

Anorexia nervosa A mental disturbance characterized by self-imposed starvation because the patient may claim to feel fat even when emaciated.

Antiretroviral A drug that stops or suppresses the activity of a retrovirus, such as human immunodeficiency virus (HIV).

Antitrust Federal and state laws that make certain anticompetitive practices illegal, including price fixing, price discrimination, exclusive contracting arrangements, and mergers among competitors.

Assisted living facility (ALF) A residential setting that provides personal care services, 24-hour supervision, scheduled and unscheduled assistance, social activities, and some health care services.

Asynchronous technology Use of store-and-forward technology that allows the user to review the information at a later time.

Audiology Identification and evaluation of hearing disorders and correction of hearing loss through rehabilitation and prostheses.

Average daily census Average number of hospital beds occupied daily over a given period of time; it provides an estimate of the number of inpatients receiving care each day at a hospital.

Average length of stay (ALOS) The average number of days each patient stays in the hospital. For individual or specific categories of patients, this measure indicates severity of illness and resource use.

B

Baby boom A sudden, large increase in the birth rate, especially that of the United States after World War II from 1946 through 1964. This generation, known as baby boomers, includes approximately 77 million adults.

Balance bill The practice in which the provider bills the patient for the leftover sum after insurance has only partially paid the charge initially billed.

Beneficiary Anyone covered under a particular health insurance plan.

Benefit period The period of illness beginning with hospitalization and ending when the beneficiary has not been an inpatient in a hospital or a skilled nursing facility for 60 consecutive days.

Benefits Services covered by an insurance plan.

Biofeedback A training program that uses relaxation and visualization to develop the ability to control one's involuntary nervous system as an aid to reducing stress, lowering blood pressure, and alleviating headaches.

Biologics Biological products such as vaccines, blood and blood components, allergenics, somatic cells, gene therapy, tissues, and recombinant therapeutic proteins.

Bioterrorism The use of chemical, biological, and nuclear agents to cause harm to relatively large civilian populations.

Board of trustees The governing body of a hospital; it is legally responsible for hospital operations, and is charged with defining the mission and long-term direction of the hospital.

Brokerage model A model of long-term care case management in which patients' needs are independently assessed by a freestanding case manager, who then arranges services through other providers.

Bulimia A mental disturbance that leads to bouts of overeating followed by induced vomiting.

C

Capitation A reimbursement mechanism under which the provider is paid a set monthly fee per enrollee (sometimes referred to as per member per month [PMPM] rate) regardless of whether the enrollee sees the provider and how often the enrollee sees the provider.

Cardiology Medical science pertaining to the study of the heart and its diseases.

Cardiopulmonary resuscitation (CPR) Medical procedure used to restart a patient's heart and breathing when the patient has suffered a heart failure.

Carriers Private claims processors for Medicare Part B services.

Carve-out The assignment through contractual arrangements of specialized services to an outside organization because these services are not included in the contracts that the managed care organization (MCO) has with its providers or the MCO does not provide the services.

Cases Individuals who acquire a certain disease or condition.

Case management An organized approach to evaluating and coordinating care, particularly for patients who have complex, potentially costly problems that require a variety of services from multiple providers over an extended period.

Case mix An aggregate of the severity of conditions requiring medical intervention. Case-mix categories are mutually exclusive and differentiate patients according to the extent of resource use.

Catastrophic care Medical care needed when a patient suffers a major injury or life-threatening illness that requires expensive long-term treatment.

Categorical programs Public health care programs designed to benefit only a certain category of people.

Centers for Disease Control and Prevention (CDC) The federal public health agency of the United States.

Centers for Medicare and Medicaid Services (CMS) The federal agency that administers the Medicare and Medicaid programs.

Certificate of need (CON) Control exercised by a government planning agency over expansion of medical facilities—for example, determination of whether a new facility should be opened in a certain location, whether an existing facility should be expanded, or whether a hospital should be allowed to purchase major equipment.

Certification A status conferred by the U.S. Department of Health and Human Services, which entitles a hospital to participate in Medicare and Medicaid. A necessary condition is for the hospital to comply with the conditions of participation.

Certified nurse-midwives (CNMs) Registered nurses with additional training from a nurse-midwifery program in areas such as maternal and fetal procedures, maternity and child nursing, and patient assessment. CNMs deliver babies, provide family planning education, and manage gynecologic and obstetric care. They can substitute for obstetricians/gynecologists in prenatal and postnatal care. *See* **nonphysician practitioner**.

Charge The amount a provider bills for rendering a service. *See* **cost**.

Chief of service A physician who is in charge of a specific medical specialty in a hospital, such as cardiology.

Chief of staff Also known as the medical director; a physician who supervises the medical staff in a hospital.

Children's Health Insurance Program (CHIP) A joint federal–state program established as Title XXI of the Social Security Act under the 1997 Balanced Budget Act. CHIP provides health insurance for children from low-income families who do not qualify for Medicaid.

Chiropractic A system of medicine based on manipulation of the spine, physiotherapy, and dietary counseling to treat neurologic, muscular, and vascular problems. Chiropractic care is based on the belief that the body is a self-healing organism.

Chiropractors Licensed practitioners who have completed the doctor of chiropractic (DC) degree. Requirements for licensure include completion of an accredited program that awards a DC degree and an examination by the state chiropractic board.

Chronic Refers to diseases or health conditions that last for significant amount of time (3 months or more) and often with no complete cure or recovery.

Chronic condition Also referred to as chronic disease. A medical condition that persists over time (3 months or longer). Chronic diseases may lead to a permanent medical condition that is nonreversible and/or leaves residual disability.

Churning A phenomenon in which people gain and lose health insurance periodically.

Claim A demand for payment of covered medical expenses sent to an insurance company.

Clinical information systems Systems that provide for organized processing, storage, and retrieval of information to support patient care processes.

Clinical practice guidelines Also known as medical practice guidelines; standardized guidelines in the form of scientifically established protocols, representing preferred processes in medical practice.

Clinical trial A research study, generally based on random assignments, designed to study the effectiveness of a new drug, device, or treatment.

Closed-panel Also called closed network, in network, or closed access; a health plan that pays for services only when they are provided by physicians and hospitals within the plan's network.

Cognitive impairment A mental disorder in which a person has difficulty remembering, learning new things, concentrating, or making decisions that affect the individual's everyday life.

Coinsurance A set proportion of the medical costs that the insured must pay out of pocket when health care services are received. *See* **copayment**.

Community health assessment A method used for conducting broad assessments of populations at a local or state level.

Community health center (CHC) Local, nonprofit, community-owned organization of health care providers serving low-income and medically underserved communities.

Community hospital A nonfederal (i.e., Veterans Affairs and military hospitals are excluded), short-term, general or specialized hospital whose services are available to the public.

Community-oriented primary care (COPC) The combination of the elements of good primary care delivery with a population-based approach to identifying and addressing community health problems.

Community rating A system in which all members of a community are charged the same insurance rate.

Comorbidity The presence of more than one health problem in an individual.

Comparative effectiveness research (CER) A concept in which a chosen medical intervention is guided by scientific evidence on how well it would work compared to other available treatments.

Competition Rivalry among sellers for the purpose of attracting customers.

Concurrent utilization review A process that determines, on a daily basis, the length of stay necessary in a hospital. It also monitors the use of ancillary services and ensures that the medical treatment provided is appropriate and necessary.

Conditions of participation Standards developed by the U.S. Department of Health and Human Services that a facility must comply with to participate in the Medicare and Medicaid programs.

Consumer-directed health plans High-deductible health plans that include a savings option to pay for routine health care expenses.

Continuing care retirement community (CCRC) An organization that integrates and coordinates the independent living and institutional components of the long-term care continuum. As a convenience factor, different levels of services are all located on one campus. CCRCs also guarantee delivery of higher-level services as future needs arise.

Continuous quality improvement (CQI) *See* **total quality management**.

Continuum A range or spectrum of health care services, spanning basic to complex services.

Copayment A flat amount the insured person must pay each time health services are received. *See* **coinsurance**.

Cost What it costs the provider to produce a service. *See* **charge**.

Cost-benefit analysis Evaluation of benefits in relation to costs when both are expressed in dollar terms.

Cost-effectiveness analysis Analysis that goes a step beyond the determination of efficacy (i.e., the benefit derived from the use of technology) by evaluating the additional (marginal) benefits to be derived in relation to the additional (marginal) costs to be incurred.

Cost-efficiency Also known as cost-effectiveness; a state in which the benefit received from a service is greater than the cost incurred to provide that service. *See* **efficiency**.

Cost-plus reimbursement A payment scheme in which reimbursement to a provider is based on cost plus a factor to cover the value of capital.

Cost sharing Sharing of the cost of health insurance premiums by those enrolled and/or payment of certain medical costs out of pocket, such as copayments and deductibles.

Cost-shifting Also known as cross-subsidization; in general, shifting of costs from one entity to another as a way of making up losses in one area by charging more in other areas. For example, when care is provided to the uninsured, the provider compensates for the costs for those services by charging more to the insured.

Cost-utility analysis Analysis that includes the use of quality-adjusted life years.

Credentials committee A committee that reviews the qualifications of clinicians so as to decide whether those clinicians should have admitting privileges.

Critical access hospital (CAH) Medicare designation for small rural hospitals with 25 or fewer beds that provide emergency medical services in addition to short-term hospitalization for patients with noncomplex health care needs. CAHs receive cost-plus reimbursement.

Critical pathways Outcome-based, patient-centered, interdisciplinary case management tools designed to facilitate coordination of care among multiple clinical departments and caregivers. A critical pathway identifies planned medical interventions in a given case, along with expected outcomes.

Cross-subsidization Also known as cost shifting; in general, shifting of costs from one entity to another as a way of making up losses in one area by charging more in other areas. For example, when care is provided to the uninsured, the provider compensates for the costs for those services by charging more to the insured.

Crude rates Measures referring to the total population; they are not specific to any age groups or disease categories.

Cultural authority The general acceptance of professional judgment as valid. Physicians' cultural authority is reflected in the reliance placed on their evaluation of signs and symptoms, diagnosis of disease, and suggested prognosis.

Current Procedural Terminology (CPT) An accepted standard for coding physician services.

Custodial care Nonmedical care provided to support and maintain the patient's condition, generally requiring no active medical or nursing treatments.

D

Days of care Cumulative number of patient days over a given period of time.

Decision support systems Computer-based information and analytical tools to support managerial decision making in health care organizations.

Deductible The portion of health care costs that the insured must first pay (generally up to an annual limit) before insurance payments kick in. Insurance payments may be further subject to copayment.

Deemed status A designation used when a hospital, by virtue of its accreditation by the Joint Commission or the American Osteopathic Association, does not require separate certification from the Department of Health and Human Services to participate in the Medicare and Medicaid programs.

Defensive medicine Excessive medical tests and procedures performed as a protection against malpractice lawsuits, and otherwise regarded as unnecessary.

Demand The quantity of health care purchased by consumers based solely on the price of those services.

Demand-side rationing Barriers to obtaining health care faced by individuals who do not have sufficient income to pay for services or purchase health insurance.

Dementia A general term for progressive and irreversible decline in cognition, thinking, and memory. Alzheimer's disease is one disorder that leads to severe dementia.

Denial of claim Refusal by a payer to reimburse a provider for services rendered.

Dental assistants Health care professionals who usually work for dentists in the preparation, examination, and treatment of patients.

Dental hygienists Health care professionals who work under the supervision of dentists and provide preventive dental care, including cleaning teeth and educating patients on proper dental care.

Dentists Professionals who diagnose and treat dental problems related to the teeth, gums, and tissues of the mouth.

Department of Health and Human Services (DHHS) The principal U.S. federal agency responsible for protecting the health of all Americans and providing essential human services.

Dependency (1) A person's reliance on another for assistance with common daily functions, such as bathing and grooming. *See* **activities of daily living**. (2) Children's reliance on adults, such as parents or school officials, to recognize and respond to their health needs.

Dermatology Medical science pertaining to the study of the skin and its diseases.

Developmental disability (DD) A physical incapacity that generally accompanies intellectual disability (mental retardation) and often arises at birth or in early childhood.

Developmental vulnerability Rapid and cumulative physical and emotional changes that characterize childhood and the potential impact that illness, injury, or untoward family and social circumstances can have on a child's life-course trajectory.

Diagnosis-related group (DRG) A diagnostic category associated with a fixed payment to an acute care hospital under the prospective payment system.

Disability Physical or mental handicap—partial or total—resulting from sickness or injury.

Discharge A patient who has received inpatient services. The total number of discharges indicate access to hospital inpatient services as well as the extent of utilization.

Discharge planning Part of the overall treatment plan that is designed to facilitate discharge from an inpatient setting. It includes, for example, an estimate of how long the patient will be in the hospital, what the expected outcome is likely to be, whether any special requirements will be needed at discharge, and what needs to be facilitated to ensure postacute continuity of care.

Disease management Used primarily by health plans, a population-oriented strategy involving patient education, training in self-management, ongoing monitoring of the disease process, and follow-up aimed at people with chronic conditions, such as diabetes, asthma, depression, and coronary artery disease.

Disparities Differences in the quality of health care or the health outcomes of different groups of people (e.g., racial/ethnic, socioeconomic, gender) that are not due to access-related factors or clinical needs, preferences, and appropriateness of interventions.

Distinct part A section of a nursing home that is distinctly certified from the rest of the facility; it generally refers to a skilled nursing facility.

Distributive policies Policies intended to spread benefits throughout society. Examples are funding of medical research through the National Institutes of Health, the training of medical personnel through the National Health Services Corps, the construction of health facilities under the Hill-Burton Act program, and the initiation of new institutions (e.g., health maintenance organizations).

Diversification Addition of new services that the organization has not offered before.

Do-not-resuscitate order Advance directive telling medical professionals not to perform cardiopulmonary resuscitation. Through these orders, patients can make their wishes known regarding aggressive efforts at resuscitation.

Doctoral nursing degrees These include the Doctor of Nursing Practice (DNP), Doctor of Nursing Science (DNS), and Doctor of Philosophy in Nursing (PhD).

Dual certification Having both skilled nursing facility (SNF) and nursing facility (NF) certifications. Dual certification allows a facility to admit both Medicaid and Medicare patients.

Durable medical equipment (DME) Supplies and equipment not immediately consumed, such as ostomy supplies, wheelchairs, and oxygen tanks.

Durable power of attorney A written document that provides a legal means for a patient to delegate authority to another to act on the patient's behalf, even after the patient has been incapacitated.

E

Effectiveness Also known as efficacy; the health benefits of a medical intervention.

Efficacy *See* **effectiveness**.

Efficiency Provision of higher-quality and more-appropriate services at a lower cost, generally measured in terms of benefits relative to costs. *See* **cost-efficiency**.

E-health Health care information and services offered over the Internet by professionals and nonprofessionals alike.

Electronic health records (EHRs) Information technology applications that enable the processing of any electronically stored information pertaining to individual patients for the purpose of delivering health care services.

Eligibility The process of determining whether a patient qualifies for benefits, based on such factors as age, income, and veteran status.

Emergency department Hospital facilities for the delivery of unscheduled outpatient services to patients whose conditions require immediate care. Emergency departments must be staffed 24 hours a day.

Emergent conditions Acute conditions that require immediate medical attention.

Emigration Migration out of a defined geographic area.

Employer mandate A legal requirement for U.S. employers to help pay for their employees' health insurance.

Enabling services Services that enable people to receive medical care that otherwise would not be received despite insurance coverage—for example, transportation and translation services.

Enrollee A person enrolled in a health plan, especially a managed care plan.

Entitlement A health care program to which certain people are entitled by right. For example, almost everyone at 65 years of age is entitled to Medicare coverage because of contributions made through taxes.

Environment One of the factors of the epidemiology triangle, which is external to the host; it includes the physical, social, cultural, and economic aspects of the environment.

Environmental health The field that focuses on the environmental determinants of health.

Epidemic An outbreak of an infectious disease that spreads rapidly and affects many individuals within a population. *See* **pandemic**.

Epidemiology The study of the distribution and determinants of health, health-related behavior, disease, disorder, and death in a population group.

E-therapy Any type of professional therapeutic interaction that makes use of the Internet to connect qualified mental health professionals and their clients.

Ethics committees Interdisciplinary committees that are responsible for developing guidelines and standards for ethical decision making in the provision of health care and for resolving issues related to medical ethics.

Etiology Study of the causes of disease or dysfunction.

Evidence-based care Delivery of health care that incorporates the use of best practices that have been evaluated for effectiveness and safety through clinical research. Best practices are often found in clinical practice guidelines.

Exclusive provider plan A health plan that is very similar to those offered by preferred provider organizations, except that insureds are restricted to in-network providers.

Executive committee A committee within the governing body that has monitoring responsibility and authority over the hospital. Usually it receives reports from other committees, monitors policy implementation, and makes recommendations. The medical staff also have a separate executive committee that establishes policy and has oversight regarding medical matters.

Experience rating Setting of insurance rates based on a group's actual health care expenses in a prior period, which allows healthier groups to pay less. *See* **community rating**.

F

Family medicine A branch of medical practice based on a core of knowledge that enables the medical professional to function as the primary provider of health care and to perform the roles of patient management, problem solving, counseling, and coordination of care.

Favorable risk selection A phenomenon in which healthy people are disproportionately enrolled into a health plan. *See* **adverse selection**.

Fee for service Payment of separate fees to providers for each separate service, such as examination, administering a test, and hospitalization.

Fee schedule A list of fees charged for various health care services.

Fertility The capacity of a population to reproduce.

Fiscal intermediaries Private-sector insurers, such as Blue Cross/Blue Shield and commercial insurance companies, that process provider claims under contracts from Medicare and Medicaid.

First-dollar insurance Health care coverage with no cost sharing.

Flat of the curve Medical care that produces relatively few or no benefits for the patient because of diminishing marginal returns.

Formulary A list of prescription drugs approved by a health plan.

Fraud Intentional filing of false billing claims or cost reports and provision of services that are not medically necessary.

Free clinic A general ambulatory care center serving primarily the poor and the homeless who may live next to affluent neighborhoods. Free clinics are staffed predominantly by trained volunteers, and care is given for free or at a nominal charge.

Free market A competitive market characterized by the unencumbered operation of the forces of supply and demand and where numerous buyers and sellers freely interact.

Fringe benefits A term loosely denoting life insurance, health insurance, or pension benefits provided in whole or in part by an employer to its employees.

Functional status A person's ability or inability to cope with the activities of daily living.

G

Gatekeeper A primary care physician who functions as the provider of first contact to deliver primary care services and to make referrals for specialty care.

Gatekeeping The use of primary care physicians to coordinate health care services needed by enrollees in a managed care plan.

Gene therapy A therapeutic technique in which a functioning gene is inserted into targeted cells to correct an inborn defect or to provide the cell with a new function.

General hospital A hospital that provides a variety of services, including general medicine, specialized medicine, general surgery, specialized surgery, and obstetrics, to meet the general medical needs of the community it serves. Such a facility provides diagnostic, treatment, and surgical services for patients with a variety of medical conditions.

Generalists Physicians in family practice, general internal medicine, or general pediatrics. *See* **specialists**.

Genetic medicine In the treatment of certain diseases, the association of genes with specific disease traits.

Genometrics The association of genes with specific disease traits.

Geriatrics The branch of medicine dealing with the problems and diseases that accompany aging.

Gerontology Study of the aging process and the special problems associated with aging.

Global budgets Allocation of pre-established total expenditures for a health care system or subsystem.

Global health Efforts to protect the entire global community against threats to people's health and to deliver cost-effective public health and clinical services to the world's population.

Globalization Various forms of cross-border economic activities driven by the global exchange of information, production of goods and services more economically in developing countries, and increased interdependence of mature and emerging world economies.

Gross domestic product (GDP) A measure of all the goods and services produced by a nation in a given year.

Group insurance An insurance policy obtained through an entity, such as an employer, a union, or a professional organization, under the assumption that a substantial number of people in the group will participate in purchasing insurance through that entity.

Group model A health maintenance organization (HMO) model in which the HMO contracts with a multispecialty group practice and separately with one or more hospitals to provide comprehensive services to its members.

Group policy An insurance policy purchased by an organization or association as a benefit to its employees or members. Typical groups are employers, union or trade organizations, and professional associations.

H

Habilitation Services that enable a person to maintain skill or function, and prevent deterioration.

Head Start A federal government–funded program that provides child development services to children in low-income families, including services in education, health care, nutrition, and mental health.

Health care The treatment of illness and the maintenance of health.

Health care reform In the U.S. context, expansion of health insurance to cover the uninsured.

Health determinants Factors that contribute to the general well-being of individuals and population.

Health informatics The application of information science to improve the efficiency, accuracy, and reliability of health care services. Health informatics requires the use of information technology (IT), but goes beyond IT by emphasizing the improvement of health care delivery.

Health information organization (HIO) An independent organization that brings together health care stakeholders within a defined geographic area and governs electronic information exchange among these stakeholders, with the objective of improving the delivery of health care in the community.

Health maintenance organization (HMO) A type of managed care organization that provides comprehensive medical care for a predetermined annual fee per enrollee.

Health plan The contractual arrangement between a managed care organization and an enrollee, including the collective array of covered health services to which the enrollee is entitled.

Health planning Decisions made by governments to limit health care resources, such as hospital beds and diffusion of costly technology.

Health policy public policy that pertains to or influences the pursuit of health.

Health professional shortage area (HPSA) A federal designation indicating an area has shortages of primary medical care, dental, or mental health providers. HPSAs may be urban or rural areas, population groups, or medical or other public facilities.

Health reimbursement arrangement (HRA) An account set up and funded by an employer that can be used by an employee or a retiree to pay for health care expenses.

Health-related quality of life (HRQL) In a composite sense, a person's own perception of health, ability to function, role limitations stemming from physical or emotional problems, and personal happiness during or subsequent to disease experience.

Health Resources and Services Administration (HRSA) A federal agency of the Department of Health and Human Services whose mission is to improve access to health care services for people who are uninsured, isolated, or medically vulnerable.

Health risk appraisal The evaluation of risk factors and their health consequences for individuals.

Health technology assessment (HTA) Any process of examining and reporting the properties of a medical technology used in health care, such as safety, effectiveness, feasibility, and indications for use, cost, and cost-effectiveness, as well as social, economic, and ethical consequences, whether intended or unintended.

Healthcare Effectiveness Data and Information Set (HEDIS) The standard for reporting quality information on managed care plans; developed by National Committee for Quality Assurance, a private nonprofit organization.

Hemiplegia Paralysis of half of the body.

Hemodialysis A mechanical procedure used to cleanse the blood by removing toxic chemicals in patients who have lost the function of one or both kidneys.

High-deductible health plans (HDHPs) Health plans that combine a savings option with a health insurance plan carrying a high deductible.

High-risk pools State-based pools, which existed before 2014, to make health insurance available to people who otherwise would have been uninsurable because of preexisting health conditions.

Holistic health The well-being of every aspect of what makes a person whole and complete.

Holistic medicine A philosophy of health care that emphasizes the well-being of every aspect of a person, including the physical, mental, social, and spiritual aspects of health.

Home health care Services such as nursing, therapy, and health-related homemaker or social services that are brought to patients in their own homes because such patients are generally unable to leave their homes safely to get the care they need.

Homemaker services Nonmedical support services given to a homebound individual—for example, bathing, food preparation, house repairs, and shopping.

Homeopathy A system of medicine based on the theory that "like cures like," meaning large doses of substances that produce symptoms of a disease in healthy people can be administered in small and diluted doses to cure the same illness. The system was founded in the late 18th century by German physician, Samuel Hahnemann (1755–1843). *See* **allopathic medicine**.

Homophobia Prejudice against, fear if, and/or hatred of gays and lesbians.

Horizontal integration A growth strategy in which an organization extends its core product or service. *See* **vertical integration**.

Hospice A cluster of special services for the dying, which blends medical, spiritual, legal, financial, and family-support services. The venue in which services are provided can vary from a specialized facility to a nursing home to the patient's own home.

Hospital A licensed institution with at least six beds, whose primary function is to deliver diagnostic and therapeutic patient services for various medical conditions. A hospital must have an organized physician staff, and it must provide continuous nursing services under the supervision of registered nurses.

Hospitalists Physicians who specialize in the care of hospitalized patients.

Host One of the factors of the epidemiology triangle; an organism, generally a human, who receives the agent and becomes sick.

Human immunodeficiency virus (HIV) A virus that can destroy the immune system and lead to acquired immunodeficiency syndrome (AIDS).

Hypertension High blood pressure.

I

Iatrogenic illnesses Illnesses or injuries caused by the process of medical care.

Immigration Migration to a defined geographic area.

Incidence The number of new cases of a disease in a defined population within a specified period.

Indemnity insurance Also referred to as fee-for-service health insurance; a health insurance plan that allows the insured to obtain health care services anywhere and from any physician or hospital. Indemnity insurance and fee-for-service reimbursement to providers are closely intertwined.

Independent practice association (IPA) A legal entity that physicians in private practice can join so that the organization can represent them in the negotiation of managed care contracts.

Infection control committee A medical committee that is responsible for reviewing policies and procedures for minimizing infections in the hospital.

Information technology (IT) Technology used for the transformation of data into useful information; it focuses on determining data needs, gathering appropriate data, storing and analyzing the data, and reporting the information generated in a user-friendly format.

Informed consent A fundamental patient right to make an informed choice regarding medical treatment based on full disclosure of medical information by the providers.

Inpatient A term used in conjunction with an overnight stay in a health care facility, such as a hospital.

Inpatient day A night spent in the hospital by a person admitted as an inpatient; also called a patient day or a hospital day.

Inpatient services Services delivered on the basis of an overnight stay in a health care institution.

Institution-related quality of life A patient's quality of life while confined in an institution as an inpatient. Examples include comfort factors (e.g., cleanliness, safety, noise levels, environmental temperature) and factors related to emotional well-being (e.g., autonomy to make decisions, freedom to air grievances without fear of reprisal, reasonable accommodation of personal likes and dislikes, privacy and confidentiality, treatment from staff in a manner that maintains respect and dignity, freedom from physical and/or emotional abuse).

Instrumental activities of daily living (IADLs) A person's ability to perform household and social tasks, such as home maintenance, cooking, shopping, and managing money. *See* **activities of daily living (ADLs)**.

Insurance A mechanism for protection against risk.

Insured The individual who is covered for risk by insurance.

Insurer An insurance agency or managed care organization that offers insurance.

Integrated delivery system (IDS) A network of organizations that provides, or arranges to provide, a coordinated continuum of services to a defined population and is willing to be held clinically and fiscally accountable for the outcomes and health status of the population serviced.

Integration Various strategies that health care organizations employ to achieve economies of operation, diversify existing operations by offering new products or services, or gain market share.

Intellectual disability (ID) Below-average intellectual capacity, which can be caused by a disorder such as Down syndrome.

Interest group An organized sector of society, such as a business association, citizen group, labor union, or professional association, whose main purpose is to protect members' interests through active participation in the policy-making process.

Internal medicine General diagnosis and treatment for problems involving one or more internal organs in adults.

Internal Revenue Service The tax collection agency in the United States.

***International Classification of Diseases, Ninth Version, Clinical Modification* (ICD-9-CM)** The official system of assigning codes to diagnoses and procedures.

Investor-owned hospital Also referred to as proprietary hospitals; for-profit hospitals owned by individuals, partnerships, or corporations.

IPA model An organizational arrangement in which a health maintenance organization contracts with an independent practice association for the delivery of physician services.

J

Joint Commission Previously called the Joint Commission on Accreditation of Healthcare Organizations (JCAHO); a private, nonprofit organization that sets standards and accredits hospitals and various other types of health care facilities.

Joint venture Creation of a new organization in which two or more institutions share resources to pursue a common purpose.

L

Licensed practical nurses (LPNs) Also known as licensed vocational nurses (LVNs) in some states; nurses who have completed a state-approved program in practical nursing and a national written examination. LPNs often work under the supervision of registered nurses to provide patient care. *See* **registered nurses**.

Licensure Licensing of a health care facility that an organization must obtain to operate. Licensure is conferred by each state upon compliance with its standards.

Life expectancy Actuarial determination of how long, on average, a person of a given age is likely to live.

Lifetime cap The maximum amount of money a health insurance policy will pay over the lifetime of the insured.

Living will A legal document in which a patient puts into writing what his or her preferences are regarding treatment during terminal illness and the use of life-sustaining technology. Such a directive instructs a physician to withhold or discontinue medical treatment when the patient is terminally ill and unable to make decisions.

Long-term care (LTC) A variety of individualized, well-coordinated services that are designed to promote the maximum possible independence for people with functional limitations. These services are provided over an extended period to meet the patients' physical, mental, social, and spiritual needs, while maximizing quality of life.

Long-term care hospitals (LTCHs) These are a special type of long-stay hospital described in section 1886(d)(1)(B)(iv) of the Social Security Act. LTCHs must meet Medicare's conditions of participation for acute (short-stay) hospitals and must have an average length of stay greater than 25 days. LTCHs serve patients who have complex medical needs and may suffer from multiple chronic problems requiring long-term hospitalization.

Low birth weight A weight of less than 2,500 grams at birth.

M

Magnet hospital A special designation conferred by the American Nurses Credentialing Center, an affiliate of the American Nurses Association, that recognizes high-quality patient care, nursing excellence, and innovations in professional nursing practice in hospitals.

Magnetic resonance imaging (MRI) The use of a uniform magnetic field and radio frequencies to study body tissues and structures.

Maldistribution An imbalance (i.e., surplus in some but shortage in others) of the distribution of health professionals, such as physicians, needed to maintain the health status of a given population at an optimal level. Geographic maldistribution refers to the surplus in some regions (e.g., metropolitan areas) but shortage in other regions (e.g., rural and inner-city areas) of needed health professionals. Specialty maldistribution refers to the surplus in some specialties (e.g., physician specialists) but shortage in others (e.g., primary care).

Mammography The use of breast x-rays to detect unsuspected breast cancer in asymptomatic women.

Managed care A system of health care delivery that (1) seeks to achieve efficiencies by integrating the four functions of health care delivery, (2) employs mechanisms to control (manage) utilization of medical services, and (3) determines the price at which the services are purchased and, consequently, how much the providers get paid.

Management services organization (MSO) An organization that brings management expertise and, in some instances, capital for expansion to physician group practices.

Margin (Total revenues − Total costs)/Total revenues; generally shown as a percentage.

Market justice A distributional principle according to which health care is most equitably distributed through the market forces of supply and demand rather than government interventions. *See* **social justice**.

Meals-on-wheels A program of home-delivered meals for the elderly, which is administered by Area Agencies on Aging under Title VII of the Older Americans Act.

Means test A program in which eligibility depends on income.

Means-tested program A government-run health insurance program in which eligibility depends on people's financial resources.

Medicaid A joint federal–state program of health insurance for the poor.

Medicaid waiver program A program that enables states to design packages of services targeted at specific populations, such as the elderly, the disabled, and those who test positive for human immunodeficiency virus. The waiver is an alternative to some form of institutional care.

Medical home The quality features of primary health care delivery in settings such as a physician office or community health center.

Medical loss ratio (MLR) The percentage of premium revenue spent on medical expenses.

Medical model Delivery of health care that places its primary emphasis on the treatment of disease and relief of symptoms instead of prevention of disease and promotion of optimum health.

Medical practice guidelines *See* **clinical practice guidelines**.

Medical records committee A medical committee that is responsible for certifying complete and clinically accurate documentation of the care given to each patient.

Medical staff committee A committee within the governing body that is charged with medical staff relations in a hospital. For example, it reviews admitting privileges and the performance of the medical staff.

Medical technology Practical application of the scientific body of knowledge for the purpose of improving health and creating efficiencies in the delivery of health care.

Medical tourism Travel abroad to receive elective, non-emergency medical care.

Medically underserved A designation determined by the federal government that indicates a dearth of primary care providers and delivery settings, as well as poor health indicators of the populace. The majority of this population group are Medicaid recipients.

Medically underserved area (MUA) A federal designation for a geographic area that has a shortage of personal health services for its residents.

Medically underserved population (MUP) A federal designation for a group of persons who face economic, cultural, or linguistic barriers to health care.

Medicare A federal program of health insurance for the elderly, certain disabled individuals, and people with end-stage renal disease.

Medicare Advantage Also called Part C of Medicare; an option in which a Medicare beneficiary receives all health care services through a managed care plan.

Medicare Physician Fee Schedule (MPFS) A national price list for physician services established by Medicare.

Medigap Commercial health insurance policies purchased by individuals covered by Medicare to insure the expenses not covered by Medicare.

Mental health system In the United States, combination of two subsystems that provide mental health care services: one primarily for individuals with insurance coverage or money, and one for those without. Patients without insurance coverage or personal financial resources are primarily treated in state and county mental health hospitals, or in community mental health clinics. Patients with insurance coverage or the personal ability to pay receive care from both inpatient and ambulatory mental health care systems.

Mental retardation *See* **intellectual disability**.

Merger Unification of two or more organizations into a single entity through mutual agreement.

Metropolitan statistical area (MSA) According to the U.S. Bureau of Census, a geographic area that includes at least (1) one city with a population of 50,000 or more or (2) an urbanized area of at least 50,000 inhabitants and a total MSA population of at least 100,000 (75,000 in the New England Census Region).

M-health Mobile health; the use of wireless communication devices to support public health and clinical practice.

Migration The geographic movement of populations between defined geographic units, which involves a permanent change of residence.

Minimum data set (MDS) An assessment instrument used for determining the case mix in a skilled nursing facility.

Mixed model An organizational arrangement in which a health maintenance organization cannot be categorized neatly into a single model type because it features some combination of large medical group practices, small medical group practices, and independent practitioners, most of whom have contracts with a number of managed care organizations.

Molecular medicine A branch of medicine that deals with the understanding of the role that genes play in disease processes and treatment of diseases through gene therapy.

Money Follows the Person (MFP) A demonstration program codified in the Deficit Reduction Act of 2005 to provide adequate federal funding to states for the sole purpose of moving qualified people whose care is funded by Medicaid from nursing homes back into community-based settings.

Moral agent A person, such as a health care executive, who has the moral responsibility to ensure that the best interest of patients takes precedence over fiduciary responsibility toward the organization.

Moral hazard Consumer behavior that leads to a higher utilization of health care services because people are covered by insurance.

Morbidity Sickness.

Mortality Death.

Multihospital system (MHS) Operation of two or more hospitals owned, leased, sponsored, or contractually managed by a central organization.

N

Nanomedicine A new area, still in its infancy, which involves the application of nanotechnology for medical use. This cutting-edge advancement within science and engineering is not a single field, but rather an intense collaboration between disciplines to manipulate materials on the atomic and molecular level (one nanometer is one-billionth of a meter).

Natality The birth rate.

National Committee on Quality Assurance (NCQA) A private organization that accredits managed care organizations and establishes standards for reporting quality.

National health expenditures Total amount spent for all health services and supplies and health-related research and construction activities consumed in a country during a calendar year.

National health insurance (NHI) A tax-supported national health care program in which services are financed by the government but are rendered by private providers (Canada is an example of a country that has NHI).

National Health Service Corps (NHSC) Administered by the Health Resources and Services Administration, a program that recruits health professionals to work in medically underserved rural and urban communities. Education loan repayment is a major incentive for providers to join the NHSC.

National health system (NHS) A tax-supported national health care program in which the government finances and also controls the service infrastructure (the United Kingdom is an example of a country that has an NHS).

Naturopathy A system of medicine based on such natural remedies as nutrition, use of herbs, massage, and yoga exercises.

Need Obtaining health care services based on individual judgment (in contrast to demand for health services). The patient makes the primary determination of the need for health care and, under most circumstances, initiates contact with the system. The physician may make a professional judgment and determine need for referral to higher-level services.

Network model An organizational arrangement in which a health maintenance organization contracts with more than one medical group practice.

Neurology The branch of medicine that specializes in the nervous system and its diseases.

New morbidities Dysfunctions, such as drug and alcohol abuse, family and neighborhood violence, emotional disorders, and learning problems, from which older generations do not suffer.

Noncertified A nursing facility that cannot admit Medicaid or Medicare patients.

Nonphysician practitioner (NPP) One of many clinical professionals who practice in areas similar to those in which physicians practice, but who do not have a medical doctor (MD) or doctor of osteopathy (DO) degree. NPPs are sometimes called midlevel practitioners because they receive less advanced training than physicians but more training than registered nurses.

Nonprofit (organization) Also called a not-for-profit organization; a private organization, such as a hospital, that operates under Internal Revenue Code, Section 501(c)(3). These organizations are tax exempt; in exchange for tax exemption, they must provide some defined public good, such as service, education, or community welfare, and not distribute profits to any individuals.

Nonurgent conditions Conditions that do not require the resources of an emergency service, and in which the disorder is nonacute or minor in severity.

Nosocomial infections Infections acquired while receiving health care.

Nurse practitioners (NPs) Individuals who have completed a program of study leading to competence as registered nurses in an expanded role. NP specialties include pediatric, family, adult, psychiatric, and geriatric programs. *See* **nonphysician practitioner**.

Nursing facility (NF) A nursing home (or part of a nursing home) certified to provide services to Medicaid beneficiaries. *See* **skilled nursing facility**.

O

Obamacare *See* **Affordable Care Act**.

Obesity For adults, a body mass index (BMI) of 30 or greater, where BMI is calculated by dividing a person's body weight in kilograms by the square of his or her height in meters. *See* **overweight**.

Obstetrics/gynecology Diagnosis and treatment relating to the sexual and reproductive system of women using surgical and nonsurgical techniques.

Occupancy rate The percentage of a hospital's total inpatient capacity that is actually utilized.

Occupational therapists (OTs) Health care professionals who help people of all ages improve their ability to perform tasks in their daily living and working environments. OTs work with individuals who have conditions that are mentally, physically, developmentally, or emotionally disabling.

Occupational therapy Therapy to help people improve their ability to perform tasks in their daily living and working environments.

Oncology The medical specialty dealing with cancers and tumors.

Open-panel Also known as open access; a health care plan that allows insureds access to providers outside the panel, but some conditions apply, such as higher out-of-pocket costs.

Ophthalmology The branch of medicine specializing in the eye and its diseases.

Opportunistic infection An infection that occurs when the body's natural immune system breaks down.

Optometrists Professionals who possess a doctor of optometry degree and have passed a written and clinical state board examination. An optometrist provides vision care—examination, diagnosis, and correction of vision disorders.

Organization for Economic Cooperation and Development (OECD) A forum of approximately 30 countries, including all Western European nations, the United States, Canada, New Zealand, Australia, Japan, and others, committed to a market economy. Representatives of member nations meet and discuss global economic and social policies.

Organized medicine Concerted activities of physicians, mainly to protect their own interests, through such associations as the American Medical Association.

Orphan drugs Certain new drug therapies for conditions that affect fewer than 200,000 people in the United States.

Orthopedics The branch of medicine dealing with the skeletal system (i.e., bones, joints, muscles, ligaments, and cartilage).

Osteopathic medicine A medical philosophy based on the holistic approach to treatment. It uses the traditional methods of medical practice, which include pharmaceuticals, laboratory tests, x-ray diagnostics, and surgery, and supplements them by advocating treatment that involves correction of the position of the joints or tissues and emphasizes diet and environment as factors that might destroy natural resistance. *See* **allopathic medicine**.

Outcomes The end results of health care delivery; often viewed as the bottom-line measure of the effectiveness of the health care delivery system.

Outliers Unusual cases that call for additional reimbursement under a payment method; these atypical cases require an exceptionally long inpatient stay or incur exceptionally high costs compared to the overall distribution of cases.

Out-of-pocket costs Costs of health care paid by the recipient of care. For an individual covered by health insurance, these costs generally include the deductible, copayments, cost of excluded services, and costs in excess of what the insurer has determined to be "customary, prevailing, and reasonable."

Outpatient services Any health care services that are not provided based on an overnight stay in which room and board costs are incurred. *See* **ambulatory care**.

Overutilization Also known as overuse; utilization of medical services, the cost of which exceeds the benefit to consumers or the risks of which outweigh potential benefits.

Overweight For adults, a body mass index (BMI) of 25 or greater, where BMI is calculated by dividing a person's body weight in kilograms by the square of his or her height in meters. *See* **obesity**.

P

Package pricing Bundling of fees for an entire package of related services.

Palliation Serving to relieve or alleviate, such as pharmacologic pain management and nausea relief.

Pandemic Relating to the spread of disease in a large segment of the population. *See* **epidemic**.

Panel Providers selected to render services to the members of a managed care plan; the plan generally refers to them as "preferred providers."

Paramedic A health care worker other than a physician who works as an emergency medical technician.

Paraprofessionals Personnel, such as certified nursing assistants and therapy aides, who provide basic assistance with activities of daily living and/or assist licensed and professional staff.

Parenteral feeding Total parenteral nutrition (TPN); the infusion of nutrients and water into the veins through a catheter, bypassing the gastrointestinal tract.

Parkinson's disease A chronic disease of the nervous system characterized by tremor and muscular debility. Named after British physician, James Parkinson (1755–1824).

Part A The component of Medicare that provides coverage for hospital care and limited nursing home care.

Part B Federal government–subsidized voluntary insurance for physician services and outpatient services.

Pathology The study of the nature and cause of disease that involves changes in structure and function.

Patient activation A person's ability to manage his or her own health and utilization of health care.

Patient-centered care Delivery of health care that respects and responds to patients' wants, needs, and preferences so that they can make choices about their care that best fit their individual circumstances.

Patient's bill of rights A document that reflects the law concerning the rights a patient has while confined to an institution such as a hospital. Issues addressed in the bill of rights include confidentiality, consent, and the right to make decisions regarding medical care, to be informed about diagnosis and treatment, to refuse treatment, and to formulate advance directives.

Pay for performance A reimbursement plan that links payment to quality and efficiency as an incentive to improve the quality of health care and to reduce costs. *See* **value-based reimbursement**.

Payer The party who actually makes payment for services under the insurance coverage policy. In most cases, the payer is the same as the insurer.

Pediatrics General diagnosis of and treatment for children.

Peer review The general process of medical review of utilization and quality when it is carried out directly or under the supervision of physicians.

Per diem A type of reimbursement mechanism for inpatient care in a health care institution. The reimbursement comprises a flat rate for each day of inpatient stay.

Per member per month (PMPM) A capitated rate. *See* **capitation**.

Personal care Assistance with basic activities of daily living.

Personal emergency response system (PERS) A system that provides at-risk elderly persons with an effective and convenient means to summon help if an emergency occurs. Using a transmitter unit, the individual can activate an alarm that sends a medical alert to a local 24-hour response center.

Personal health expenditures The portion of national health expenditures remaining after expenditures for research and construction, administrative expenses incurred in health insurance programs, and costs of government public health activities are subtracted. These expenditures go toward services and goods related directly to patient care.

Personalized medicine A treatment approach in which gene variations among patients are matched with responses to selected medications to increase effectiveness and reduce unwanted side effects.

Pesthouse A type of facility operated by local governments during the 18th and mid-19th centuries to quarantine people who had contracted a contagious disease such as cholera, smallpox, or typhoid. The primary function of a pesthouse was to protect the community from the spread of contagious disease; medical care was a secondary consideration.

Phantom providers Practitioners who generally function in an adjunct capacity; the patient does not receive direct services from them. They bill for their services separately, and the patients often wonder why they have been billed. Examples include anesthesiologists, radiologists, and pathologists.

Pharmaceutical care A mode of pharmacy practice in which the pharmacist takes an active role on behalf of patients, which includes giving information on drugs and advice on their potential misuse and assisting prescribers in appropriate drug choices. In so doing, the pharmacist assumes direct responsibility, in collaboration with other health care professionals and with patients, to achieve the desired therapeutic outcomes.

Pharmacists Professionals who have graduated from an accredited pharmacy program that awards a bachelor of pharmacy or doctor of pharmacy degree and have successfully completed a state board examination and a supervised internship.

Pharmacology The body of science dealing with drugs, their nature, properties, and effects.

Physical therapists (PTs) Health care professionals who provide care for patients with movement dysfunction.

Physical therapy The evaluation and treatment of physical problems resulting from injury or disease, including problems with joint motion, muscle strength, endurance, and heart and lung function.

Physician assistants (PAs) Health care professionals who work in a dependent relationship with a supervising physician to provide comprehensive medical care to patients. The major services provided by PAs include evaluation, monitoring, diagnostics, therapeutics, counseling, and referral. *See* **nonphysician practitioner**.

Physician extender *See* **nonphysician practitioner**.

Physician–hospital organization (PHO) A legal entity formed between a hospital and a physician group to achieve shared market objectives and other mutual interests.

Plan The form in which health insurance, particularly private health insurance, is obtained. The plan specifies, among other details, information pertaining to costs, covered services, and how to obtain health care when needed.

Planned rationing Also called supply-side rationing; government efforts to limit the availability of health care services, particularly expensive technology.

Play-or-pay A type of employer mandate in which employers must choose to provide health insurance to employees ("play") or pay a penalty.

Podiatrists Health care professionals who treat patients with foot diseases or deformities.

Point-of-service (POS) plan A managed care plan that allows its members to decide at the time they need medical care (at the point of service) whether to go to a provider on the panel or to pay more to receive services out of network.

Population at risk All of the people in the same community or population group who are susceptible to acquiring a disease or a negative health condition.

Practice profiling Use of provider-specific practice patterns and comparing individual practice patterns to some norm.

Preadmission Screening and Resident Review (PASRR) An evaluation required under federal regulations before a patient can be admitted to a Medicaid-certified nursing facility, which determines whether a nursing facility is the best alternative for individuals with serious mental illness or intellectual disability or whether their needs can be adequately met in community-based settings.

Precision medicine A treatment approach that takes into account not only variability in genes, but also the environment and lifestyle factors.

Preexisting conditions Physical and/or mental conditions that existed before the effective date of an insurance policy.

Preferred provider organization (PPO) A type of managed care organization that has a panel of preferred providers who are paid according to a discounted fee schedule. The enrollees have the option to go to out-of-network providers, but incur a higher level of cost sharing for doing so.

Premium The insurer's charge for insurance coverage; the price for an insurance plan.

Premium cost sharing Employers' requirement that their employees pay a portion of the health insurance cost.

Prepaid plan A contractual arrangement under which a provider must provide all needed services to a group of members (or enrollees) in exchange for a fixed monthly fee paid in advance to the provider on a per-member basis (called capitation).

Prevalence The number of cases of a given disease in a given population at a certain point in time.

Primary care Basic and routine health care provided in an office or clinic by a provider (physician, nurse, or other health care professional) who takes responsibility for coordinating all aspects of a patient's health care needs; an approach to health care delivery that is the patient's first contact with the health care delivery system and the first element of a continuing health care process.

Primary care case management (PCCM) A managed care arrangement in which a state contracts directly with primary care providers, who agree to be responsible for the provision and/or coordination of medical services for Medicare recipients under their care.

Primary health care Essential health care that constitutes the first level of contact by a patient with the health delivery system and the first element of a continuing health care process.

Primary prevention In a strict epidemiologic sense, the prevention of disease—for example, health education, immunization, and environmental control measures.

Prior approval A form of utilization review in which an insurance company requires a provider to get permission from the insurance company before providing care (usually surgery).

Private-pay patients Patients not covered by either Medicare or Medicaid.

Program of All-Inclusive Care for the Elderly (PACE) An example of the integrated care model of long-term care case management for clients who have been certified as eligible for nursing home placement. PACE has had a high success rate of keeping clients in the community.

Proprietary hospitals Also referred to as investor-owned hospitals; for-profit hospitals owned by individuals, a partnership, or a corporation.

Prospective payment system (PPS) A payment scheme in which criteria for how much will be paid for a particular service are predetermined.

Prospective reimbursement A method of payment in which certain preestablished criteria are used to determine in advance the amount of reimbursement.

Prospective utilization review A process that determines the appropriateness of utilization before the care is actually delivered.

Provider Any entity that delivers health care services and can either independently bill for those services or is tax supported. Examples of providers include physicians, dentists, optometrists, and therapists in private practices; hospitals; diagnostic and imaging clinics; and suppliers of medical equipment (e.g., wheelchairs, walkers, ostomy supplies, oxygen).

Provider-induced demand Artificial creation of demand by providers that enables them to deliver unneeded services to boost their incomes.

Provider-sponsored organization (PSO) Also known as a provider service organization; a quasi-managed care organization that is a risk-bearing entity sponsored by physicians, by hospitals, or jointly by physicians and hospitals to compete with regular managed care organizations.

Psychiatrists Physicians who receive postgraduate specialty training in mental health after completion of medical school. These professionals treat patients with mental disorders, prescribe drugs, and admit patients to hospitals.

Psychiatry The branch of medicine that specializes in mental disorders.

Psychologists Mental health professionals who must be licensed or certified to practice. These professionals may specialize in such areas as clinical, counseling, developmental, educational, engineering, personnel, experimental, industrial, psychometric, rehabilitation, school, and social psychology.

Public health A wide variety of activities undertaken by state and local governments to ensure conditions that promote optimal health for society as a whole.

Public hospitals Hospitals owned by the federal, state, or local government.

Public policies Authoritative decisions made in the legislative, executive, or judicial branches of government that are intended to direct or influence the actions, behaviors, or decisions of others.

Q

Quad-function model The four key functions necessary for health care delivery: financing, insurance, delivery, and payment.

Quality The degree to which health services for individuals and populations increase the likelihood of desired health outcomes and are consistent with current professional knowledge.

Quality-adjusted life year (QALY) The value of 1 year of high-quality life, used as a measure of health benefit.

Quality assessment The process of defining quality and deciding how quality is to be measured according to established standards.

Quality assurance The process of ongoing quality measurement and use of the results of assessment for ongoing quality improvement. *See* **total quality management**.

Quality improvement committee A medical committee that is responsible for overseeing the program for continuous quality improvement.

Quality improvement organization (QIO) A private organization composed of practicing physicians and other health care professionals in each state that is paid by the Centers for Medicare and Medicaid Services under contract to review the care provided to Medicare beneficiaries.

Quality of life (1) Factors considered important by patients, such as environmental comfort, security, interpersonal relations, personal preferences, and autonomy in making decisions when institutionalized. (2) Overall satisfaction with life during and following a person's encounter with the health care delivery system.

R

R&D Research and development.

Radiology The branch of medicine that involves the use of radioactive substances, such as x-rays, to diagnose, prevent, and treat disease.

Rate The price for a health care service set by a third-party payer.

Rationing Any process of limiting the utilization of health care services; it can be achieved by price, waiting lists, or deliberately limiting access to certain services.

Redistributive policies Policies that take money or power from one group and give it to another. An example is the Medicaid program, which takes tax revenue and spends it on the poor in the form of health insurance.

Registered nurses (RNs) Nurses who have completed an associate's degree (ADN), a diploma program, or a bachelor's degree (BSN) and are licensed to practice.

Regulatory tools Uses of health policy in which the government prescribes and controls the behavior of a particular target group by monitoring the group and posing sanctions if it fails to comply.

Rehabilitation Therapies that restore lost functioning or maintain the current levels of functioning and prevent further decline.

Rehabilitation hospitals Hospitals that specialize in providing restorative services to rehabilitate chronically ill and disabled individuals to a maximum level of functioning.

Reimbursement The amount insurers pay to a provider. The payment may be just a portion of the actual charge.

Reinsurance Stop-loss coverage that self-insured employers purchase to protect themselves against any potential risk of high losses.

Relative value units (RVUs) Measures based on physicians' time, skill, and intensity required to provide a service.

Reliability The extent to which repeated applications of a measure produce the same results.

Residency Graduate medical education in a specialty that takes the form of paid on-the-job training, usually in a hospital.

Resident (1) A patient in a nursing home or some other long-term care facility. (2) A physician in residency.

Resource-based relative value scale (RBRVS) A system instituted by Medicare for determining physicians' fees. Each treatment or encounter by the physician is assigned a "relative value" based on the time, skill, and training required to treat the condition.

Resource utilization groups (RUGs) A classification system designed to differentiate nursing home patients by their levels of resource use.

Respiratory therapy Treatment for various acute and chronic lung conditions, using oxygen, inhaled drugs, and various types of mechanical ventilation.

Respite care A service that provides temporary relief to informal caregivers, such as family members.

Restorative care Short-term therapy to help a person regain or improve physical function.

Retrospective reimbursement A payment scheme in which reimbursement rates are based on costs actually incurred.

Retrospective utilization review A review of utilization after services have been delivered.

Risk The possibility of a substantial financial loss from an event for which the probability of occurrence is relatively small.

Risk adjustment Any adjustment made for people who are likely high users of health care services—for example, adjustment of payments based on the proportion of high-risk patients.

Risk factors Environmental elements, personal habits, or living conditions that increase the likelihood of developing a particular disease or negative health condition in the future.

Risk management Limiting risks against lawsuits or unexpected events.

Risk rating Insurance rating according to which high-risk individuals pay more than the average premium price, and low-risk individuals pay less than the average price.

Rural hospitals Hospitals located in counties that are not part of a metropolitan statistical area.

S

Safety net Programs, generally government financed, that enable people to receive health care services when they lack private resources to pay for them. Without these programs, many people would have to forgo the services. For example, Medicaid becomes a safety net for long-term care services once a patient has exhausted private funds; community health centers are safety net providers for many uninsured and vulnerable populations.

Secondary care Routine hospitalization, routine surgery, and specialized outpatient care, such as consultation with specialists and rehabilitation. Compared to primary care, these services are usually brief and more complex, involving advanced diagnostic and therapeutic procedures.

Secondary prevention Efforts to detect disease in early stages so as to provide a more effective treatment—for example, screening.

Self-insured plan A health plan in which a large company acts as its own insurer by collecting premiums and paying claims. Such businesses most often purchase reinsurance against unusually large claims.

Self-referral The practice in which physicians order services from laboratories or other medical facilities in which they have a direct financial interest, usually without disclosing this conflict of interest to the patient.

Senior centers Local community centers for older adults that provide opportunities to congregate and socialize. Many centers offer subsidized meals, wellness programs, health education, counseling, and referral services.

Short-stay hospital A hospital in which the average length of stay is less than 25 days.

Single-payer system A national health care program in which the financing and insurance functions are taken over by the federal government.

Skilled nursing care Medically oriented care provided mainly by a licensed nurse under the overall direction of a physician.

Skilled nursing facility (SNF) A nursing home (or part of a nursing home) certified to provide services under Medicare. *See* **nursing facility**.

Small area variations (SAVs) Unexplained variations in the treatment patterns for similar patients and medical conditions.

Smart card A credit card-like device with an embedded computer chip and memory to hold personal medical information that can be accessed and updated at a hospital or physician's office.

Social contacts The number of activities a person engages in within a specified period of time. Examples include visits with friends and relatives, and attendance at social events, such as conferences, picnics, or other outings.

Social justice A distribution principle according to which health care is most equitably distributed by a government-run national health care program. *See* **market justice**.

Social resources Social contacts that can be relied upon for support, such as family, relatives, friends, neighbors, and members of a religious congregation; they are indicative of adequacy of social relationships.

Socialized health insurance (SHI) Health care that is financed through government-mandated contributions by employers and employees, and delivered by private providers (Germany, Israel, and Japan are examples of countries with SHI).

Socialized medicine Any large-scale government-sponsored expansion of health insurance or intrusion in the private practice of medicine.

Specialists Physicians who specialize in specific health care problems; examples include anesthesiologists, cardiologists, and oncologists. *See* **generalists**.

Specialty care Care that tends to be limited to illness episodes, the organ system, or the disease process involved. Specialty care, if needed, generally follows primary care.

Specialty hospitals Hospitals that admit only certain types of patients or those with specified illnesses or conditions. Examples include rehabilitation hospitals, tuberculosis hospitals, children's hospitals, cardiac hospitals, and orthopedic hospitals.

Speech therapy Therapy focusing on individuals with communication problems, including using the voice correctly, speaking fluently, and feeding or swallowing.

Spina bifida A deformity of the spine.

Staff model A health maintenance organization (HMO) arrangement in which the HMO employs salaried physicians.

Standards of participation Minimum quality standards established by government regulatory agencies to certify providers for delivery of services to patients covered by Medicare and Medicaid.

Subacute care Clinically complex services that are beyond traditional skilled nursing care.

Subacute condition A condition that requires technically complex services that are beyond traditional skilled nursing care.

Supplemental Food Program for Women, Infants, and Children (WIC) A program created in 1972 as an amendment to the Child Nutrition Act of 1966, with the objective of providing sufficient nutrition for pregnant women, mothers, infants, and children.

Supplemental Security Income (SSI) A federal program of income support for disabled individuals, including those with mental illness and some infectious diseases.

Supply-side rationing Also called planned rationing; government efforts to limit the availability of health care services, particularly expensive technology.

Surge capacity The ability of a health care facility or system to expand its operations to safely treat an abnormally large influx of patients.

Surgicenters Freestanding, ambulatory surgery centers that perform various types of surgical procedures on an outpatient basis.

Swing bed A hospital bed used for acute care or skilled nursing care, depending on fluctuations in demand.

Synchronous technology Technology in which telecommunications occur in real time.

System A set of interrelated and interdependent components that are logically coordinated to achieve a common goal.

T

Teaching hospital A hospital with an approved residency program for physicians.

Technological imperative The use of technology without cost considerations, especially when the benefits to be derived from the use of technology are small compared to the costs.

Technology assessment *See* **health technology assessment**.

Technology diffusion The proliferation of technology once it is developed.

Telehealth Educational, research, and administrative uses of telecommunications technology in health care, as well as clinical applications that involve nurses, psychologists, administrators, and other nonphysicians.

Telematics The combination of information and communications technology to meet user needs.

Telemedicine Use of telecommunications technology that enables physicians to conduct two-way, interactive video consultations or transmit digital images, such as x-rays and magnetic resonance imaging results, to other sites.

Telephone triage Telephone access to a trained nurse for expert opinion and advice, especially during the hours when physicians' offices are closed.

Tertiary care The most complex level of care, which is typically institution based, highly specialized, and highly technological. Examples include burn treatment, transplantation, and coronary artery bypass surgery.

Tertiary prevention Interventions to prevent complications from chronic conditions and avoid further illness, injury, or disability.

Third party An intermediary between patients and providers, which carries out the functions of insurance and payment for health care delivery.

Third-party administrator (TPA) An administrative organization, other than the employee benefit plan or health care provider, that collects premiums, pays claims, and/or provides administrative services.

Third-party payers In a multipayer system, the payers for covered services—for example, insurance companies, managed care organizations, and the government. They are neither the providers nor the recipients of medical services.

Title XVIII Title XVIII (18) of the Social Security Amendment of 1965; the Medicare program.

Title XIX Title XIX (19) of the Social Security Amendment of 1965; the Medicaid program.

Top-down control Use of global budgets in a health care system to control total expenditures in accordance with preestablished limits. *See* **global budgets**.

Total care In the context of long-term care delivery, recognition of any health care need that may arise, with that need then being evaluated and addressed by appropriate clinical professionals.

Total quality management (TQM) Also known as continuous quality improvement (CQI); an environment in which all aspects of health services within an organization are oriented to patient-related objectives and the production of desirable health outcomes. TQM holds the promise of not only improving quality, but also increasing efficiency and productivity by identifying and implementing less costly ways to provide services; it is viewed as an ongoing effort to improve quality.

Trauma center An emergency unit specializing in the treatment of severe injuries.

Triage A system of prioritizing treatment when demand for medical care exceeds supply.

Triple-option plans Health insurance plans that combine the features of indemnity insurance, a health maintenance organization, and a preferred provider organization; the insured has the flexibility to choose which feature to use when using health care services.

U

Uncompensated care Charity care provided to the uninsured who cannot pay for such care.

Underinsurance Medical insurance coverage considered inadequate to cover the costs of a major illness.

Underutilization Withholding of medical care services particularly when potential benefits may exceed the cost or the risks.

Underwriting A systematic technique used by an insurer for evaluating, selecting (or rejecting), classifying, and rating risks.

Uninsured People who lack health insurance coverage.

Universal access The ability of all citizens to obtain health care when needed. It is a misnomer because timely access to certain services may still be a problem because of supply-side rationing.

Universal coverage Health insurance coverage for all citizens.

Upcoding A fraudulent practice in which a higher-priced service is billed when a lower-priced service is actually delivered.

Urban hospitals Hospitals located in counties that are part of a metropolitan statistical area.

Urgent care centers Walk-in clinics that are generally open to see patients after normal business hours in the evenings and weekends, and for which patients do not have to make an appointment.

Urgent conditions Conditions that require medical attention within a few hours; a longer delay presents possible danger to the patient. This kind of disorder is acute but not necessarily severe.

Urology The branch of medicine concerned with the urinary tract in both sexes and the sexual/reproductive system in males.

Utilization The extent to which health care services are actually used.

Utilization review (UR) The process of evaluating the appropriateness of services provided.

Utilization review committee A process by which an insurer reviews decisions made by physicians and other providers on how much care to provide.

V

Value Provision of greater benefits or higher quality at the same or lower price levels (costs).

Value-based reimbursement A payment mechanism that takes into account quality improvement and cost reduction. *See* **pay for performance**.

Venous stasis Stagnation of normal blood flow causing swelling and pain, generally in the legs.

Ventilator A mechanical device for artificial breathing, which forces air into the lungs.

Vertical integration Linking of services that are at different stages in the production process of health care. Examples include a hospital system that acquires a firm that produces medical supplies, and a physician group practice or a hospital that launches hospice, long-term care, or ambulatory care services. *See* **horizontal integration**.

Virtual integration The formation of networks based on contractual arrangements.

Virtual physician visits Online clinical encounters between a patient and a physician.

Voluntary health insurance Private health insurance (in contrast to government-sponsored compulsory health insurance).

Voluntary hospitals Nonprofit hospitals.

Voucher An approach to health insurance reform that relies on individual decisions to purchase health insurance. Tax credits are issued in advance to individuals to offset the costs of purchasing health insurance.

W

Walk-in clinic A freestanding, ambulatory clinic in which patients are seen without appointments on a first-come, first-served basis.

Welfare program A means-tested program for which only people below certain income levels qualify. Medicaid is an example of a welfare program. *See* **entitlement**.

Workers' compensation An employer-paid benefit that compensates workers for medical expenses and wages lost due to work-related injuries or illnesses.

X

Xenotransplantation Also known as xenografting; transplanting of animal tissue into humans.

Y

Yoga exercises Use of physical postures and regulation of breathing to treat certain chronic conditions and to achieve overall health benefits.

Z

Zoonoses Any disease or infection that is naturally transmittable from vertebrate animals to humans.

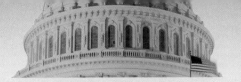

Index

Note: Page numbers followed by *t* or *f* indicate tables or figures, respectively. Page numbers in *italics* indicate exhibits.